KU-256-569

COLLINS FAMILY MEDICAL HANDBOOK

COLLINS FAMILY MEDICAL HANDBOOK

Collins
London and Glasgow

First published 1981

© **Wm. Collins Sons & Co. Ltd.**

ISBN 0 00 434322 0

Collins Family Medical Handbook
is based on and abridged from
Collins Family Health Medical Encyclopedia

Printed in Great Britain by
Wm. Collins Sons & Co. Ltd.

INTRODUCTION

Nobody who reads newspapers or magazines, listens to radio, watches television, or even talks with relatives and neighbours can avoid receiving a lot of information about matters of health and disease; but the information tends to concentrate on the new and the glamorous, is not always accurate, and is inevitably patchy. Thus a scriptwriter preparing a programme on Legionnaires' disease has to assume, because of the short duration of his item, that the audience will understand terms like 'incubation period', 'symptoms like those of pneumonia' and 'erythromycin or tetracycline'. A journalist writing a short article on sickle cell disease lacks space to discuss the normal formation of blood corpuscles, the Mendelian inheritance of abnormal haemoglobin and the possible role of folic acid in treatment, and if he mentions enlargement of the spleen he certainly has to take it for granted that the reader is aware of the position and main functions of that organ. Again, a health educator in a brief radio interview about whooping cough vaccination cannot hope to deal with the spread of the disease, its main complications, the subject of immunity, and the history of the particular vaccine.

Yet many people, without being preoccupied with illness and without having the time or the inclination to study medical or nursing text-books full of terms unfamiliar to them, are keen to acquire a reasonable knowledge of health matters. They are interested in how their minds and bodies work, and in how best to maintain their own and their children's physical and emotional health amid the stresses of modern life. They want to know how to prevent those diseases which are preventable, and to be able to cope when confronted with sudden illness or accident.

This *Handbook* attempts to provide such knowledge. Scientifically accurate but written in simple language, it seeks to include within a limited space important aspects of health improvement, disease prevention, anatomy and physiology, the working of the mind in health and in sickness, causes of physical and mental disease, brief descriptions of many diseases and injuries, treatment – especially first aid treatment – and indications of sources of help.

The *Handbook* can be used in two ways. Firstly, it is a dictionary or a condensed encyclopedia. At the end of the book (for very rapid reference) there is an alphabetically arranged section on first aid, containing such headings as bleeding, choking, fractures, etc. However, it is hoped that the wise reader, if ignorant of first aid, will read through these pages at leisure before any emergency occurs. The rest of the book is completely alphabetical. So if the reader wishes to know the meaning of a term (perhaps one that the doctor has mistakenly assumed that the patient understood), a quick reference to the book will suffice. Again, if a patient suspects that her child has a particular disease, she can check the description in the book and can also see whether the disease is likely to need medical treatment. Yet again, the parent can quickly answer the question in her mind – 'What exactly is the health visitor who visited me, and what is the infant welfare clinic to which she advised me to take the baby?'

Secondly, and perhaps more excitingly, the handbook can be used systematically to gain a reasonable knowledge of matters related to health and disease. Perhaps this use can best be illustrated by a series of examples.

1. To study the body and how it works the reader might start either from SKELETON and BONES, working outwards, or from SKIN, working inwards; and having appreciated some of the main organs (e.g., the HEART), he might proceed to study the various systems of the body – CIRCULATION OF THE BLOOD, RESPIRATORY SYSTEM, DIGESTIVE SYSTEM, REPRODUCTIVE SYSTEM, ENDOCRINE GLANDS, and so on. Inevitably some of these systems would draw his interest to other entries: e.g., reading about the circulation might make him desire to study BLOOD, and reading about the digestive system might turn his mind to DIET and NUTRITION. By systematic study of a couple of dozen relevant entries, often aided by cross-references, he could acquire a good working knowledge of anatomy and physiology.

2. If interested in the functioning of the mind, he might usefully first read three physiological entries – BRAIN, NERVOUS SYSTEM and ENDOCRINE GLANDS. He could then turn to PSYCHOLOGY, MENTAL HEALTH, MENTAL EFFICIENCY, PERSONALITY, the SUBCONSCIOUS and CONFLICT. If becoming interested in the mind's malfunctioning he could read STRESS, PSYCHIATRY, PSYCHOSOMATIC DISEASES and MENTAL DISEASES.

3. If concerned with improvement of health he might start with KEEPING FIT and pass to such entries as EXERCISE and REST; or he might start with HEALTH and HEALTH EDUCATION, and, since nutrition plays an important part in health preservation or health loss, he would inevitably find his attention directed to such entries as NUTRITION, DIET, OBESITY, SLIMMING, and the various constituents of food (e.g., VITAMINS).

4. If seeking information about common diseases and injuries he might begin with CAUSES OF DISEASE, and then pass to such conditions as he cared to study, from ACCIDENTS and ARTERIOSCLEROSIS to YELLOW FEVER and the ZOONOSIS. In diseases with sizable entries he would find that the normal order used is causes, clinical appearances, treatment and methods of prevention.

5. For social factors affecting health he might start with SOCIAL ASPECTS OF HEALTH, and then turn to such topics as BEREAVEMENT, BIRTH CONTROL, ONE PARENT FAMILIES, ALCOHOL and MARITAL DISHARMONY.

6. If he sought to study prevention, he might consult PREVENTABLE DISEASES, and then make a threefold choice: reading about prevention of infections, in such entries as HYGIENE, EPIDEMIOLOGY, IMMUNITY and many individual infections from SMALLPOX to TUBERCULOSIS; steeping himself in NUTRITION and DEFICIENCY DISEASES; or turning to GENETICS and GENETIC GUIDANCE.

7. Again the reader could study children's health through such entries as CHILDBIRTH, INFANCY (PSYCHOLOGY OF), GROWTH IN CHILDHOOD, CHILDHOOD (PSYCHOLOGY OF), and ADOLESCENCE.

8. To give some final examples for the systematic reader, he could find sources of available help under such headings as GENERAL PRACTITIONER, HEALTH VISITOR, DENTIST, and so on; modern drugs under headings like ANTIBIOTICS, SULPHONAMIDES and INTERFERON; and matters of current discussion in such entries as SMOKING, FLUORIDATION, BIRTH CONTROL, ACUPUNCTURE, and DIVORCE.

The handbook assumes no medical or scientific knowledge. It is intended for intelligent people (outside the various health professions), but, since all the health professions are becoming increasingly specialized, it may perhaps occasionally serve as a quick reminder to health workers who have encountered something outside their recent experience.

Inevitably, a book that tries to cover, in condensed but intelligible form, the entire field of health and disease will be criticized by a few professional workers. Some will maintain, seeking to preserve medical mystique, that any book describing diseases and their symptoms will encourage hypochondria and imagined illness. The answers are (a) that virtually everybody has some knowledge of diseases nowadays and that accurate knowledge is better than inaccurate and partial information, (b) that the emphasis throughout the book is on improvement of health and prevention of illness, and (c) that medical and nursing students although devoting long years to the study of diseases seldom become hypochondriacs. A few other health workers, again anxious to preserve professional mystique, will assert that this little book seeks to convert its readers into amateur doctors, unqualified health visitors or untrained nurses. The answers are (a) that it takes over four years of intensive, full-time preparation for a health visitor to qualify, three years for a nurse or physiotherapist to qualify and two years for a social worker to qualify, and clearly no intelligent person could imagine that the study of one small book could establish its reader as an imitation health professional; (b) that the book again and again indicates situations in which expert professional advice is essential; and (c) that a modicum of knowledge both helps the individual to maintain his own health and enables him to follow more easily the advice of the doctor or other health expert when skilled guidance is needed.

The World Health Organization, the supreme authority on all matters of health and disease, defines health as physical, mental and social well-being. It claims as its main objective the attainment by all peoples of the highest possible level of health, and maintains that for the attainment of health there are required firstly the extension to all peoples of the benefits of medical, psychological and related knowledge, and secondly informed opinion and active cooperation on the part of the public. It is in the spirit of that declaration that this book is offered to those who care to read it.

I.A.G.M.

GENERAL EDITOR

Ian A.G. MacQueen, OBE, MA, MD, DPH, FFCM, DSCHE
Formerly Medical Officer of Health, Aberdeen, and
Chairman, Scottish Council for Health Education.

ORIGINAL CONTRIBUTORS

Andrew P. Curran, KSS, BSc. MD, FRCP, FRCP(G), DPH, DIH
Senior Lecturer in Epidemiology & Preventive
Medicine, University of Glasgow

Prof Derek J. Gill, BSc (Soc), PhD,
University of Missouri, Columbia, USA

The late John D. Kershaw, MD, DPH, FFCM
Formerly Medical Officer of Health, Colchester

D. Joan Lamont, SRN, SCM, HV Tutor's Cert, DSCHE
Formerly Head of School of Health Visiting,
Robert Gordon's Institute of Technology, Aberdeen

Robert J. Lumsden, MB, ChB, DPH, MFCM
Formerly Medical Officer of Health, Airdrie

George A. Venters, MB, ChB, PhD, MFCM
Community Medicine Specialist, Lothian Health Board

A

abdomen. The abdomen or belly is the part of the trunk bounded above by the diaphragm, below by the pelvic bones, and at the back by the spine and strong muscles, but protected in front only by the muscles of the abdominal wall. It contains the digestive, renal and genital organs, and can be considered as consisting of two parts, the upper abdomen and the pelvis. The liver (on the right), stomach, and the spleen are situated at the top of the abdomen immediately below the diaphragm, which spreads out like a dome and separates the abdomen from the chest. The large intestine lies at each side with a central connecting loop while the small intestine occupies most of the middle. The kidneys and ureters lie at the back, and the rectum, bladder, and internal genital organs (e.g., uterus and ovaries) are mainly in the pelvis.

The muscles of the abdominal wall play an important part in supporting various organs: over-lax muscles may cause organ displacement with repercussions on the efficiency of the particular organ, e.g., lack of support of the intestines leads to constipation. Hence it is necessary to keep these muscles in good tone by suitable exercise and sometimes massage. There are natural weak spots in the abdominal wall through which the intestines can sometimes protrude to form a HERNIA.

The interior of the abdominal wall is lined with a membrane, the peritoneum, which also passes from the wall to form a suspending and supporting band to cover the contained organs.

Abdominal injuries. The effects of violence to the abdomen depend both on its nature and degree and on whether the muscles are relaxed or contracted. Well developed muscles, if fully contracted, can give considerable protection to the abdominal organs and to the solar plexus. Nevertheless the belly is, with the single exception of the external genital organs, the most unprotected part of the body.

Where violence produces signs of SHOCK these should be treated. Additionally, vomiting, persistent pain, and rigidity of the abdominal wall suggest bruising or rupture of an organ, in which case the victim should be kept warm and moved as little as possible until the arrival of expert help. Where the wall has actually been broken, the patient should be treated for shock, kept warm and at rest with the knees bent over a pillow, and a bandage applied to the wound. In no case should a patient with abdominal injury be given anything by mouth until he has either recovered from signs of shock and from abdominal symptoms, or been seen by a doctor.

Until almost the middle of this century serious abdominal wounds were usually fatal, but the advent of sulphonamides, antibiotics, and tetanus immunization has now resulted in a high recovery rate.

Abdominal pain. The commonest type of abdominal pain is the griping pain of intestinal colic, generally due to the eating of unsuitable or indigestible food which sets up spasms of the bowel. A laxative produces rapid relief, and meantime the pain can be eased by application of hot-water bottles to the abdomen. Again pain in 'the pit of the stomach' may be due to constipation.

Other causes of pain are more serious. Pain beginning near the navel and then settling in the right lower part of the abdomen may well be appendicitis. Pain under the right ribs may be occasioned by inflammation of the gall bladder. Pain in the lower abdomen may be due to cystitis (bladder inflammation) or in women to inflammation of the ovaries or occasionally simply to menstruation. Pain in the upper abdomen, if associated with eating food, may be due to acidity or an ulcer. Pain, vomiting, and constipation, starting suddenly and causing collapse, suggest peritonitis or intestinal obstruction. Persistent pain, accompanied by wasting and frequent vomiting, may be due to cancer.

In general, unless there is an obvious minor cause for abdominal pain, the symptom should be deemed to need prompt medical attention.

abduct. To move a limb outwards, away from the mid-line of the body.

abortion. Expulsion of a foetus from the womb before it is able to live. It was formerly customary to describe the termination of pregnancy during the first three months as 'abortion' and later termination as 'miscarriage' (if the foetus was not far enough developed to survive) or 'premature delivery' (if the baby was viable, i.e., able to survive). However, the modern tendency is to restrict 'abortion' to artificially induced termination, while all spontaneous terminations before the age of viability are commonly termed MISCARRIAGE.

In countries where artificial termination of pregnancy is illegal, abortion can be very dangerous to the health and even the life of the woman. This applies whether it is conducted surreptitiously by an abortionist, using instruments often under conditions of doubtful cleanliness, or attempted by the woman, using either instruments or drugs. Various countries now deem abortion lawful if the birth would endanger the mother's health, or the health of the unborn child, or the health of other members of the family.

Carried out by a competent obstetrician under good conditions, abortion during the first three weeks of pregnancy is simple and almost without risk, but the danger of complications rises a very little in the fifth and sixth weeks.

Views on the ethics of abortion vary: at one end of the scale are those who hold that even the fertilized ovum is potentially alive and that induced abortion is therefore murder; in the middle are some who regard abortion as justifiable if childbirth would seriously harm the mother's physical or mental health, if the woman is a victim of rape or perhaps if the child is likely to be seriously deformed; and, at the other end, are those who consider an abortion preferable to an illegitimate or unwanted child or to a 'shot-gun' wedding and subsequent divorce.

Even in permissive societies the scales are a little weighted against abortion, because a woman has in a limited space of time to discover that she is pregnant, to decide that she wants an abortion, to find a doctor who will recommend her as suitable and an obstetrician who will carry out the termination. The position may change as a result of the development of prostaglandins which are in effect contraceptives that can be taken after sexual intercourse.

abrasion. The accidental rubbing off, as distinct from cutting, of the surface of the skin or of a mucous membrane. Although slight in itself, the injury can allow the entrance of germs and so lead to an abscess. For a skin abrasion the most effective treatment is to paint it immediately with an astringent and antiseptic fluid and then, if it is large, to cover it with a clean dressing.

abscess. A localized collection of pus, created by germs gaining access to a tissue from an injury or from disease in a neighbouring organ. As pus accumulates it produces reddening, heat, swelling, throbbing, and pain over the area due to pressure, and general symptoms such as headache and raised temperature. If untreated an abscess will finally burst, but pus formation can be accelerated by poultices or hot fomentations, and once there is evidence of pus the pressure can be relieved by lancing the abscess. Alternatively, an early-stage abscess can often be checked by injections of an appropriate antibiotic, such as penicillin.

abscess, cold. A chronic abscess which develops slowly over weeks or months, produces few symptoms, and is almost always due to tubercular infection. It occurs most frequently in glands, bones, and joints, but is nowadays becoming infrequent.

accidents. Man has always been subject to injuries as a result of inadvertent mishap but the rapid development of machinery and the increase in the complexity of living have converted accidents into the major epidemic of the twentieth century. In Britain there about 28,000 accidental deaths a year, and two million people receive medical treatment in consequence of accidents – roughly half following home accidents, and the other half following industrial and traffic accidents.

Domestic accidents. These are the leading cause of death in persons between 1 and 21 years of age and also a frequent cause of death or permanent disability to the elderly. Young children are at greatest risk to every type of domestic accident: one-quarter of all home accidents involve children aged 1 to 3 years and another quarter concern children aged 3 to 9 years.

Widowed, divorced and separated persons have a disproportionately high number of accidents, and although accidents occur in all socio-economic groups, there is a definite social gradient: the poorer the group, the higher the number of home accidents of all types.

While housing defects (e.g. outside steps without a handrail) and defects of furnishing or equipment (e.g. highly polished floors) are responsible for many accidents, by far the main cause is human – fatigue, anxiety, emotional upset, carelessness, or untidiness.

Here are a few simple rules for reduction of accidents. Ensure that the stair is well-lit and free from obstacles. Avoid slippery floors and loose rugs without non-slip surfaces. Replace toys and household utensils immediately after use. Keep handles of saucepans turned inwards. Keep hot water, knives, sharp tools, medicines and cleansing fluids out of reach of young children. Keep all medicines in distinctly marked containers. Keep all doors either closed or very fully open. Do not smoke in bed. Ensure that electric wires are in good condition and where practicable keep them short. Ensure that coal fires, gas fires, and electric heaters are adequately protected. Exercise particular care when tired, angry, or distressed.

For treatment of minor injuries received in the home, see First Aid section at the end of the book.

Industrial accidents. These fall broadly into two groups – those involving young workers who do not foresee the particular danger (education at entry to employment would perhaps reduce this group) and those among older workers who appreciate the risk but are unable to take sufficiently swift action to avoid the consequence. The second group might be reduced by adequate safety appliances and, where necessary, by transfer or early retirement of persons no longer agile enough to cope with an inevitable hazard. In both categories accidents to males greatly outnumber those to females.

smoking in bed

unanchored rugs and
highly polished floors

overladen sockets
with long trailing flexes

matches left in reach of a child;
handle of a saucepan left where
it can easily be knocked off the stove

using a rickety chair instead
of a firm step ladder

unsound and badly-lit stairs

Common causes of domestic accidents.

Traffic accidents. Despite the publicity that attends them, train and aircraft accidents are rarities. Motor accidents in Britain account for more than a dozen times the combined total of all rail and aeroplane deaths, and for every person killed in such accidents there are 37 injured.

Essentially there are three ways of reducing motor accidents. The first is by improving roads. Britain has for several decades kept its total of road deaths about level (despite constantly increasing numbers of vehicles) by providing better surfaces and wider roads, by marking danger points, by creating roundabouts to facilitate traffic flow at intersections, by establishing and seeking to enforce speed limits appropriate to particular roads and by separating adequately traffic moving in opposite directions (as on motorways). Some problems of road improvement remain to be tackled, e.g., giving motorists advance warning of sudden fog or ice, and the enforcement during the motorist's nightmare – freezing fog and black ice – of speed limits much lower than those normally applicable to the particular road.

The second method of reduction is improvement of vehicles. Four-wheel brakes, rear-view mirrors, windscreen wipers, and undamaged tyres can prevent many accidents; and most countries are increasingly making it a legal requirement that these should be in a state of efficiency before a car is taken on a public road. Seat belts have proved their value, as have crash helmets for motorcyclists. Other improvements, such as reinforced bumpers and padded and collapsible steering wheels, have been introduced.

The third and probably the most important method is educating the road user and preventing the ineducable road user from driving. In respect of drivers a great deal has already been done. The introduction of driving tests, although standards vary, was an enormous step forward, even though there is something strange in a person today taking a test in which he never exceeds the speed-limit for a built-up area and tomorrow being legally entitled to drive on a motorway. Attempts are being made to identify persons whose impaired health renders them a danger to themselves or others, but moderation seems necessary: for example it would seem an unwarrantable interference with the liberty of the individual to stop from driving a man of 76 who is fully aware of slowed reaction time and decreased vision, who deliberately avoids hazardous situations and has not been the cause of an accident.

In recent years much attention has been paid to alcohol: Sweden attempted – on negligible evidence, for a single whisky may actually improve a driver's efficiency and reaction time – to ban absolutely simultaneous drinking and driving, and in due course had to abandon the experiment;

Britain, perhaps more wisely, specified a permissible maximum of 80 mg. per 100 ml. of blood – a reasonable maximum for most people, but a few individuals could drive competently with 100 mg. while a few have impaired concentration and slowed reaction time with only 70 or 75 mg. Unfortunately, fatigue, anger, and distress are as hazardous as alcohol and less easily identifiable. Probably the most hopeful measure for reduction of errors by drivers is the policy – adopted by many insurance companies – of rewarding the accident-free driver by reducing his premium and correspondingly penalizing the driver who has had an accident. Yet, even if this policy were carried to the extent of taking the dangerous driver off the road, there are still no measures to cope with the dangerous pedestrian.

There are courses in schools in the U.S.A. designed to acquaint children with traffic conditions and regulations in the city and such instruction is being introduced into Britain. It could be a useful measure to teach all school children about the stopping distances of cars at various speeds and about the alterations in these distances when a road is wet or icy. Perhaps, too, pedestrians using roads at night should be encouraged – or even required by law – to wear or carry something of light colour. So far we have improved roads, we are improving vehicles, we are in process of improving drivers, but we have ignored pedestrians.

accident-proneness. A liability to road, home, or industrial accidents which is significantly greater than average. Most of us have increased predisposition to accidents at times, in particular when we are tired or emotionally disturbed or when we have consumed too much alcohol; but the term, accident-proneness, is generally reserved for persisting increased liability to accidents.

Defects of special senses clearly play a part: a person with impaired sight, hearing or smell has increased liability to various types of accident. Habitual preoccupation with other matters contributes: the well-known 'absent-minded professor' is a case in point and his equivalent can be found in many occupations. Also there is some evidence that many accident repeaters show more than average aggressiveness, impulsiveness, immaturity, and resentment of restrictions.

In most cases susceptible individuals cannot yet be identified in advance of their first accidents. Counselling of persons who have had one or more home or road accidents might help, and the relating of insurance premiums to previous driving records can discourage accident repeaters from driving.

accommodation. The faculty the human eye possesses of altering its refractive power so that rays of light, whether from far or near, are focused accurately on the retina. The alteration is achieved by means of the

The comparatively slim lens
required for distance vision

The increased convexity of the lens
required for near vision

Accommodation

elasticity of the lens within the EYE. See also EYESIGHT.

acetabulum. The cup-shaped socket on the PELVIS in which rests the head of the femur or thigh-bone, the two together forming the hip joint.

acetic acid. The active principle of vinegar. In strong solution it is a corrosive poison which is sometimes used to destroy warts or corns, the adjacent parts being protected with vaseline and the acid applied with a match, generally once daily for several days. In dilute solution, as in vinegar, it may be used as an antidote to poisoning by alkalis, such as ammonia or caustic soda.

acetone. A substance of sweet and sickly smell found in the urine and breath of persons suffering from various wasting diseases, including severe diabetes. It is the product of incomplete oxidation of fats during the digestive process.

Achilles tendon. The tendon behind the ankle formed from the soleus and gastrocnemius muscles and attached to the heel bone. It may be strained or torn during exercise so that walking and particularly running, become difficult or impossible. Treatment is by rest and possibly physiotherapy.

achlorhydria. Absence of hydrochloric acid from the gastric juice, with consequent lessening of the digestive capacity. This absence is found in pernicious anaemia and cancer of the stomach, but it is also found in about 5 per cent of healthy young adults and in about 10 per cent of healthy middle-aged people. Where no disease is found, no treatment is usually prescribed.

acholuric jaundice. A hereditary disease in which the red blood cells are abnormally

fragile, there is jaundice of the skin and mucous membranes, the spleen is enlarged, and symptoms and signs of anaemia are present, but no bile is present in the urine. Mild cases may need no treatment, but in severe cases removal of the spleen is necessary (because it acts as the destroyer of the fragile red blood corpuscles) and a blood transfusion may be required to enable the patient to withstand the operation. In general removal of the spleen appears to cure the condition, but if the operation is done in childhood it may increase the liability to infections.

achondroplasia. A hereditary abnormality of bone formation, inherited as a genetic dominant (see GENETICS), which produces the commonest form of dwarfism. The head becomes enlarged with bulging forehead, the trunk may be normal in length, but the arms and legs are grossly stunted. In very severe forms death in infancy is common, but in less severe forms survival into adult life is probable, with height seldom exceeding 120 cm. (4 ft.). There is no treatment. Appropriate contraceptive treatment and GENETIC COUNSELLING could eliminate the condition.

acid. A sour-tasting compound which can combine with an alkali to form a salt. While weak acids are sometimes used medicinally, most acids are strong corrosive poisons. Immediate treatment in acid poisoning is to give an alkali (such as milk of magnesia or baking soda in water) and to send for medical aid. An emetic to induce vomiting should not be given. External BURNS caused by acids should immediately have the acid gently washed off and should thereafter be treated like other burns.

acidity. A vague term generally denoting the burning sensation experienced in INDIGESTION and some stomach disorders. Essentially the symptom is due either to excess of hydrochloric acid in the gastric juice or to regurgitation of that juice.

acidosis. A state in which the blood would tend to become less alkaline but for the existence of bodily buffering mechanisms which provide (but use up) an alkali reserve. Acidosis may occur in severe diabetes, certain kidney diseases, and carbohydrate starvation.

In adults it is characterized by drowsiness, sighing respiration and presence of a sweet, sickly odour in the breath; it is prevented by adequate carbohydrate in the diet (a matter of fine judgment in diabetes, where excess carbohydrate is dangerous) and it is treated by giving glucose in solution.

In children it often starts with vomiting and high temperature (which have, of course, many other causes) and is most often caused by an excessive proportion of fat in the diet.

The immediate treatment consists of rest, ample fluid and glucose; and subsequent attacks can be prevented by adjustment of the diet, bearing in mind both the child's low fat tolerance and his need for sufficiency of the fat-soluble vitamins. In some cases emotional disturbances would appear to precipitate acidosis.

acne. A skin affection, occurring mostly between 12 and 25 years of age and characterized by pimples and 'blackheads' or comedones which are collections of dried grease in the openings of the sweat glands. They are found especially on the face and neck, caused by overactivity of the sweat glands and believed to be due to a temporary imbalance of the endocrine glands. Acne is difficult to treat, although sometimes helped by frequent washing with mildly antiseptic soap, avoidance of sweet-eating and inclusion of ample fruit and green vegetables in the diet. It usually disappears spontaneously about the age of 25.

acne rosacea. A skin condition in which blood vessels, especially of the nose and cheeks, become permanently enlarged, causing a purplish mottling. Possible causes include excess alcohol, chronic indigestion, and prolonged exposure to inclement weather. Provided the patient is willing to co-operate, treatment is possible and includes avoidance of the main cause, moderate use of sedatives, washing the face twice daily with toilet water, and nightly application of an appropriate ointment.

aconite poisoning. Poisoning by an alkaloid contained in the plant known as Wolf's Bane or Monk's Hood, the root of which looks like horseradish. Initial symptoms include tingling in the mouth and throat, followed by numbness. Treatment is by giving an emetic to induce vomiting, keeping warm, and if breathing becomes difficult applying artificial respiration.

acromegaly and gigantism. Related conditions caused by excessive secretion of the growth hormone of the pituitary gland and characterized by abnormal growth of bony and soft parts, especially of the face and limbs.

Gigantism. This condition begins in childhood, before ossification of bones is completed, and produces lengthening of the long bones so that there is an excessive overall height, with very long arms and increased size of feet, hands, and parts of the head.

Normal height varies with at least three sets of conditions: (1) racial inheritance, e.g., most Swedes and Zulus are tall by comparison with Spaniards; (2) personal inheritance, e.g., the child of tall parents is likely to be of greater height than the child of short parents; and (3) nutrition and exercise in childhood, e.g., the undernourished child of tall parents may reach 'normal' stature but in reality be stunted in that he has not reached his genetic potential, and the tall son of apparently 'average' parents may have reached his potential while his parents were really stunted.

Broadly speaking, for persons from Northern Europe, Canada and the U.S.A. a height of over 200 cm. (6 ft. 8in.) in men and 185 cm. (6 ft. 1 in.) in women is considered abnormal.

Acromegaly. Unlike gigantism, acromegaly starts after ossification is completed and therefore affects bones that can thicken but no longer lengthen. The face becomes enlarged with beetling brow and prominent jaw, and the hands and feet enlarge.

At first there is often increased muscular development in both conditions, and often sexual precocity, followed later by impotence. As the disease progresses headache, stiffness of the spine, and tingling of the extremities becomes common, visual disturbances are fairly frequent and about one-fifth of the cases develop diabetes. If untreated the patient normally dies at between 50 and 60 years from cerebral complications, diabetes, or heart failure. Treatment of the pituitary with x-rays enormously improves the outlook, although it cannot remove skeletal changes that have already taken place. If this irradiation fails, operative treatment is desirable.

acromion. The part of the scapula or shoulder blade that forms the tip of the shoulder.

ACTH. An abbreviation used for the adrenocorticotrophic hormone, nowadays most often shortened to corticotrophin. This is one of the hormones secreted by the front lobe of the pituitary gland, and it stimulates the cortex of another pair of endocrine glands, the adrenal glands, to produce other hormones in their turn. These include the corticosteroids, one of which is cortisone, which controls bodily usage of carbohydrate. By a curious 'feed-back' mechanism, deficiency of cortisone in the blood leads to increased production of ACTH, while increase – whether from over-activity of the adrenal cortex or from administration of cortisone – causes a lowering of ACTH.

Where a patient needs steroid therapy and his adrenals are efficient, ACTH can be given by injection – it is useless orally – as an alternative to cortisone, because the injected hormone stimulates the adrenal cortex to produce larger quantities of its own hormones.

Corticotrophin has been used in the treatment of rheumatic fever, rheumatoid arthritis, asthma and some other diseases. Essentially, however, it merely relieves symptoms but does not cure the underlying disease.

actinomycosis. A chronic suppurative disease, occurring mainly in cattle but rarely transmitted to man, and caused by the *Streptothrix actinomyces* or the ray fungus. The commonest site is the jaw, where a hard, tender swelling appears and is sometimes at first wrongly attributed to an infected tooth. Penicillin in high dosage is the drug of choice.

acupuncture. In China it has been claimed for at least 2,000 years that pain can be reduced by the insertion and vibration of solid needles into carefully chosen points which to Western investigators seem to have no particular relationship to the areas rendered painless. It is easy for sceptics to dismiss treatment of disease by acupuncture as 'quackery' and to explain any verified cures as due to spontaneous recovery, good nursing or psychological reaction. It is much less easy to explain away the use of acupuncture to produce analgesia during surgical operation, a method which Chinese doctors claim has the advantage of creating less blood loss than does operation under general anaesthesia. Yet such cases are definitely on record, although many attempts to repeat them in Europe and the U.S.A. have been unsuccessful.

A hint of possible explanatory significance may lie in the discovery that the brain in conditions of pain can produce opium-like substances (endorphin and encephalin). However, it is difficult to see exactly how the vibration of tiny needles stimulates the production of these substances, or to see why the needles have to be inserted at specific points which seem unrelated to the site of pain or to the nerves serving the affected area.

acute. A term indicating rapid onset and short duration, in contrast to 'chronic' which implies slower onset and longer duration. In medical usage 'acute' does not carry any implication of severity. A severe case of meningitis and a mild case of the common cold are both termed acute infections.

adder bite. See SNAKE BITE.

addiction. A condition characterized by craving for a particular drug, need for increasing quantities of it, increasing dependence on it and harmful effects. The craving is so strong that a person who cannot otherwise obtain the drug is driven to seek it by criminal means, such as breaking into a clinic or a chemist's shop or stealing to secure money to buy it. The decreasing effect caused by the drug means that the addict requires larger and larger doses. Dependence implies that if the drug is totally withdrawn suddenly the patient has severe withdrawal symptoms and may even die. The harmful effects include deterioration of the personality, inability to work, and ultimately impairment of physical health – largely because the person has neither the inclination to eat adequately nor the money to purchase sufficient food in addition to his drug.

Heroin and morphia are definite drugs of addiction: a couple of doses, many hours apart, as pain-killers, will not produce addiction, but regular dosage for several days almost definitely creates craving and later the other characteristics of addiction. Cocaine and LSD (although the latter is not normally classed as a drug of addiction)

lead to craving, increased tolerance and much deterioration of the personality, but rarely to severe withdrawal symptoms.

Alcohol cannot usually be called a drug of addiction since the vast majority of people do not show increasing tolerance but continue to drink the same amounts year after year and do not experience severe withdrawal symptoms if supplies are cut off. In a small minority of drinkers alcohol becomes a true drug of addiction.

The barbiturates are similarly seldom drugs of addiction, although in a few cases they lead to the four classic manifestations.

Tobacco, tea and coffee are not really drugs of addiction: not only do smokers and tea and coffee drinkers tend to consume the same amounts year after year (showing no signs of increased tolerance) but a heavy smoker or a heavy tea or coffee drinker, deprived of supplies, will not commit a crime to obtain them; and withdrawal symptoms are relatively slight.

Addison's disease. A disease caused by decreased or absent secretion of aldosterone by the suprarenal glands, and in most cases due to tuberculosis of these glands. The condition is characterized by slowly increasing general weakness, loss of weight, poor appetite, very low blood pressure and bronzed pigmentation of the exposed areas of skin. It was formerly fatal in one to three years, but cortisone and fluorohydrocortisone have completely altered the outlook. With efficient treatment, usually by mouth every second day, the patient slowly returns to normal weight, regains appetite, gradually loses pigmentation, and can live a reasonably normal life for many years. Since the treatment is replacement of a secretion – not a condition – it must be continued indefinitely.

adduct. To move a limb towards the mid-line of the body.

adenitis. Inflammation of a lymph gland.

adenoids. See TONSILS AND ADENOIDS.

adenoma. Tumour composed of glandular tissue. Adenomata may arise from any gland in the body, and their effect depends on their position and their growth. They do not give rise to secondary growths or involve neighbouring lymph glands, and unless they cause pressure symptoms or disfiguration they are harmless. If completely removed they do not recur.

adhesions. The uniting together, generally following inflammation or injury, of tissues which should normally be freely movable. They are relatively common after joint injuries, causing stiffness and restriction of movement and, unless prevented by massage and physical treatment while the injury is healing, they may have to be broken down by manipulation of the joint with the patient under an anaesthetic.

Adhesions are also liable to form in the abdomen after operations.

adhesive plaster. A dressing, sticky on the

inner side, employed to retain in position the primary dressing of a cut or wound. An adhesive plaster should not be applied directly to injured skin, and before it is applied to healthy skin the skin, if at all hairy, should be shaved. Adhesive plaster commercially prepared with an antiseptic pad is widely used for cuts and other small wounds.

adipose tissue. The technical term for the fat which is distributed under the skin and in the body cavities. It protects against cold, cushions internal organs, and forms a reserve store of food and energy. In starvation and in wasting diseases it rapidly decreases, as it may also do by strict adherence to a diet.

adiposity. Possession of excessive adipose tissue to the extent of OBESITY.

adolescence. The years of transition from childhood to adult life, the period in which the sex glands become active and many physical, emotional and intellectual changes take place.

The beginning and end of adolescence vary from person to person, and in general occur earlier in girls than in boys. Although there is some overlapping, adolescence may conveniently be divided into four phases.

1. The pre-puberty phase. This is the period roughly between the ages of 11 and 12 years. A boy grows appreciably, his shoulders broaden, his chest expands and his penis lengthens. A girl has a greater growth spurt, so that her height on average equals that of a boy of the same age and her weight slightly exceeds that of the boy, her hips broaden, her breasts start to develop, pubic hair begins to grow and in some cases menstruation commences. Both sexes become a little resentful of adult control and show more initiative than in earlier years, but are still essentially children.

2. The phase of puberty. At 13 to 15 years a boy's growth continues, pubic hair begins to develop, the voice breaks and he may have nocturnal discharges of seminal fluid ('wet dreams'). At 13 to 14 years a girl's growth spurt continues though slowing down, and menstruation becomes established. Both become interested in members of the opposite sex, very much aware of clothes and teenage fashions, increasingly resentful of the shackles of parental domination and control, although often seeking parental affection and support, and more and more distrustful of their own clumsiness and lack of poise, which are largely due to uneven growth of the arms, legs and neck.

3. Mid-adolescence. Boys of 16 to 18 experience a settling down or stabilization of physiological changes, they begin to need to shave, they start to 'go steady' with a particular girl, they become more independent and claim the right to form their own opinions and use their own judgments, and they have increased social consciousness and idealism with decreased interests in parents and home, although some boys adopt a very protective attitude to their mothers. Girls of 15 to 17 years experience a similar settling down and exhibit the same increased independence and social awareness. They become more self-assured and self-confident, and often have a number of boy-friends. Both sexes display increased curiosity, greater self-consciousness and very strong feelings of right and wrong, with a tendency to deep and distressing mental conflicts.

4. Late adolescence. The boy of 19 to 20 and the girl of 18 to 19 years have reached full physical maturity and have achieved their maximum intellectual capacities and their peaks for analytical thought and for imaginative creativity. While as yet having little experience of life, they are ready for life's responsibilities and are often prepared to 'put the world right'. They tend to be critical of the standards and beliefs of older people and severe in their judgments.

Since these stages overlap considerably, it is perhaps useful to summarize the main characteristics of the turbulent period of adolescence. There is a considerable increase in weight and height, so that an adolescent needs more food than an adult, and there are irregular alternations of energy and fatigue. Day dreaming and fantasy life loom large. There is a growing awareness of the physical self: clumsiness appears as a result of uneven growth and often causes embarrassment, and there tends to be anxiety about social occasions. A marked feature is resentment of parental control, frequently leading to family rows, and yet with the youngster who indignantly rejected parental domination yesterday expecting parental affection and support in the troubles of today. There is at times a desire for solitude. The longing for independence is strong and increases throughout adolescence. The period is characterized by idealism and a tendency to religious and political conversion. There is increasing awareness of the other sex and the phenomenon of falling in love, often with little appreciation of either the imperfections or the interests of the intended partner, and there is a tendency to sexual experimentation. Relationships with parents undergo a change or a series of changes: a capacity to argue develops and is a recognition of the fallibility of adults, sometimes carried to the point where it is assumed that what any adult says will probably be wrong. Understanding of environmental, social and political matters increases. There is a changed attitude to study – either much greater interest or a complete disinterest.

Yet, despite all these changes, many interests remain unaltered – the book-lover still visits the library and the cricketer still plays. Also the fundamental qualities of the personality do not alter, e.g., the introvert remains introverted.

Adolescence is an era of rapid mood swings, of alternation between dependence and independence and between surging hope and dark despair. Above all, it is an era of loneliness and anxiety. Few adolescents talk freely with adults, least of all with their parents, and many feel misunderstood, anxious, awkward, lonely or impure.

The main developmental tasks of adolescence include: the establishment of relationships with the opposite sex, the achievement of the physical and mental capacity to hold down a job which is recognized by the individual and his associates as worthwhile, the gaining of personal and financial independence and emancipation, and the finding of principles – moral, religious, political, philosophical or pragmatic – by which to live and by which to assess other people.

Success in these tasks and diminution of the turbulence of adolescence depend in considerable measure on three factors – the personality structure (itself conditioned partly by nature and partly by nurture), earlier parental and other relationships, and social and cultural pressures. For example, the development of a self-reliant individual who is no longer dependent on parents and friends is facilitated by security and a loving relationship in childhood, by opportunities to progress gradually and without stress from the safe relationships of the family to association with contemporaries, by friendliness of parents and teachers and by availability of appropriate social contacts. To take a converse example, future attitude to work can be damaged by over-ambitious parents never satisfied with their child's achievements (creating discontent and under-achievement), by parents preoccupied with status and prestige (sometimes producing the drop-out who rejects all traditional values and standards) and by parents who make all decisions, leaving the child with no experience in coping with problems.

Parents, youth leaders, teachers and others dealing with adolescents should remember that adolescents are as a rule easily led (e.g., by appeal to their idealism and sense of justice or by appeal to the reasoning power of which they are so proud) but that no other age-group is harder to drive.

Problems of adolescence. Hormones, intellectual development and emotional changes interact in the production of problems of adolescents, and no classification is really satisfactory. Some of the problems are considered below under four approximate headings – growth, regression, sex and rebellion.

1. Problems related to growth. The prolonged growth spurt means that an adolescent needs to eat more food than an adult and especially requires plenty of meat, fish, milk and green vegetables. So actual malnutrition may arise in an impoverished household or in one in which the parents do not understand the adolescent's needs. Obesity may be created through the satisfaction of hunger by consumption of carbohydrates in large amounts, especially if eating is also employed as a compensation for lack of affection. Under-nutrition may follow obesity as the youngster slims vigorously in an attempt to get rid of podginess and 'puppy-fat'. Uneven growth can create embarrassment over a gawky appearance and clumsy movements. An early or late growth spurt can cause the misery of the tall girl towering above her friends, or of the small boy, with unbroken voice, dwarfed by his classmates.

Most of these problems can be helped by a good diet and reassurance, but all too often parents and other relatives make matters worse by mocking the clumsiness, excessive height or apparent stunting, or by trying to insist that a child embarrassed by appearance nevertheless dons a swimsuit or pair of shorts.

2. Problems related to regression. One of the characteristics of the adolescent is temporary swings back towards the behaviour of childhood. A boy of 14 may at times show less sense of responsibility than displayed three years earlier, a class of 15-year-old girls may giggle in a way that they would not have done at 12, and a youngster of either sex may display a curiously juvenile sense of humour. Such happenings are best regarded as a sort of compensation for physical and intellectual growth by greater expression of childish emotions. If at all possible, the irresponsibility, giggling and juvenile pranks should be quietly tolerated, although this may be difficult in a school where two misbehaving children disturb the progress of an otherwise interested class.

3. Problems related to sex. Most girls nowadays are prepared for mammary development and the onset of menstruation, although the start of bleeding can be terrifying to a girl who has not had the necessary instruction. Boys, however, often receive no preparation for erections, nocturnal emissions and erotic fancies, and are initiated into the mysteries of sex by furtive conversations with other boys or incited to experiment by slightly more mature girls.

Masturbation, a common and usually harmless phenomenon, may give rise to deep guilt feelings.

While the underlying causes of sexual deviation mostly lie in earlier years, sexuality that has previously been repressed may appear at adolescence in deviant forms, e.g., as MASOCHISM or SADISM. Growth of sexual feelings before a child has ceased to be interested primarily in his own sex may create temporary homosexual relationships, usually only theoretical but occasionally physical.

Love for the opposite sex tends to be romanticized, with no awareness of the other person's imperfections and with exaggerated gloom when these are discovered. A couple may marry at 16 or 17 years without realizing that they have no interests in common, so that teenage marriages have a high rate of breakdown.

The conception of offspring by unmarried teenagers is in some cases a result of unplanned experimentation, in other cases a symbol of deliberate revolt against the standards of adults, and in yet other cases a consequence of belief in myths that are prevalent (e.g., that a girl cannot become pregnant until she has menstruated several times.)

To a very considerable extent, the sex problems of adolescents can be helped or avoided by adequate sex education in advance, such education including moral and aesthetic aspects as well as anatomy and physiology.

4. Problems related to rebellion. The adolescent is aware of his mental and physical maturity but feels shackled by inexplicable restrictions and regulations, e.g., he can legally marry as soon as he is 16 but he and his wife are legally obliged to attend school until a specified leaving date, and he cannot buy her a glass of beer. He sees some of life's injustices and cruelties, feels that he could put them right, but lacks even a vote. Not least, he is financially dependent.

Inevitably there tends to be conflict with authority, starting usually with small things in the home (such as the time of staying out or the wearing of make-up) but often progressing to a stage in which parents, teachers and policemen are banded together as 'enemies'. Adolescence is above all the period of rebellion and trial of strength, whether evidenced directly by delinquency (which may have its origins much earlier in an unhappy home, lack of love or parental domination) and open clash with authority, or shown indirectly, as when the son of a Conservative MP becomes a Socialist or the daughter of an Anglican clergyman becomes a Roman Catholic or humanist.

Many adolescents, however, achieve the transition from childhood to adult life without clashes with constituted authority and without too many family rows. Sympathetic and understanding parents and early introduction to participation in decision making, together with early training in the use of freedom and the substitution of self-discipline for externally imposed discipline, all play important parts in lessening the problems of adolescence.

adrenal glands. Alternatively known as suprarenal glands, these are important members of the system of ENDOCRINE GLANDS, producing the hormone adrenalin as their principal secretion.

adrenalin. The main hormone produced by the medulla of the suprarenal, or adrenal gland, which is one of the ENDOCRINE GLANDS, and also nowadays manufactured

synthetically by chemists. Whether secreted (as in rage and other emotional states) or injected, it raises the blood pressure, mobilizes energy in the form of sugar and dilates bronchial vessels allowing greater use of oxygen. As a natural secretion it is the body's response to fear. As an injected drug it can be life-saving in stimulating the heart muscle in collapse and shock, and is also very useful in acute attacks of asthma.

aerophagy and gastric flatulence. Aero-phagy or air-swallowing consists of air being gulped in and in a few seconds being belched out. It occurs mostly in nervous dyspepsia but is sometimes found in gastric and duodenal ulcer and in angina pectoris. Essentially the patient feels fullness or discomfort, attributes it to 'wind', tries unsuccessfully to belch, swallows air during the attempt and then belches. Treatment consists of explanation and of substituting sweet-sucking or water-sipping for the effort to disperse air. Gastric flatulence includes aerophagy but can also be caused by production of gas by fermentation of food in the stomach.

aetiology. Strictly the study of the causes of any particular disease, but often used loosely as a synonym for 'causes'.

affect. Essentially the effect of any emotion on the mind.

Psychologists often divide personalities into three main types: (1) the cognitive (the thinking, reasoning, logical type whose interests are in theories rather than application, the 'cold' personality whose response to a situation is usually intellectual rather than emotional); (2) the conative (interested in practical results and in active and purposeful activities); (3) the affective (concerned with his emotional reaction to events, and tending either to sympathize with others or to be actively hostile to them). Yet few of us belong solely to one of these types, although one may predominate.

In certain mental disorders the three main types become exaggerated. For instance the schizophrenic has very little affect, shows little affection for others and normally exhibits scant response to emotions: whereas the manic-depressive is dominated by his emotions, and swings rapidly from complete elation to utter dejection.

afterbirth. The name given to the placenta, cord and membranes which attach the unborn child to the mother's womb, and which are expelled shortly after the birth of the child. See CHILDBIRTH.

ageing. The gradual deterioration that occurs in all organized living creatures is occasioned in part by the wearing out of irreplaceable organs and structures. Hence it is inevitable: man is mortal. The deterioration is, however, to some extent a reflection of the life-long battle between the individual and the pressures of his environment, so that it is in part postponed by improvement of the quality of life.

Measured by such standards as 'reaching middle age' or 'becoming elderly' or the ultimate criterion of age at death, persons in a primitive community age more quickly than those in a highly developed society, and (despite the influence of the diseases of affluence, such as those caused by 'rich' diets and stress) the wealthy and the cultured tend to age more slowly than the underprivileged. Yet, within any one single group in any one community, inherited factors (or the influences of early life) are strong: the person whose parents were still physically and mentally active at 70 and whose grandparents were active at 68 is far more likely to be alert at 74 years than his neighbour whose parents were elderly at 60.

The common division into children, adolescents, young adults, the middle-aged, and the elderly (or Shakespeare's division into seven ages) is a loose generalization only. Apart from individual variations and the effects of environment, ageing of body and mind is far from uniform: eyesight and hearing are probably at their peak around 14 years, with slight deterioration thereafter; intelligence reaches its maximum around 16 years but its decrease over the next fifty years is very slight; lung capacity and cardiac output fall rapidly after the age of 30 while reaction time shows trivial reduction until after the age of 75. In general it is true to say that in most cases any physical or mental diminution is balanced in whole or in part by increased experience and skill. We might consider, for example, that a rifle-shooting marksman was 'getting beyond his best' at 26, that a boxer was nearing retirement at 34, that a statesman or an academic could reasonably be given a new post at 60, and that an otherwise healthy car-driver could safely have his licence renewed at 74.

The physical changes of ageing are, nevertheless, obvious – slight decrease in elasticity of skin and arteries beginning in the thirties, slower movements from the forties, in women the menopause in the late forties, and the muscle-shrinkage and bent backbone of old age. Mentally there are parallel, but rather later changes: a gradual decrease in tolerance, a slow narrowing of interests, and as ageing progresses some failure of recent memory and some exaggeration of the attitudes or prejudices held in earlier life. Simultaneously there comes an increased amount of susceptibility to illness and an increased number of medical consultations and hospital admissions.

Yet ageing is by no means all loss. The referee of 45 is neither less happy nor less useful than the sportsman of 30; the professor of 60 balances by greater knowledge and wider experience the slightly higher intelligence of his colleague of 40; and, just as the young adult is released from the turmoils and stresses of adolescence, the person of 'retirement age' comes to terms with life, has no more problems of ambition and promotion and, by the very narrowing of his interests, sometimes produces his best work.

Senility is a term employed for extreme old age accompanied by decay of mental and physical powers. There is no clear borderline between senility and normal old age, but the former is essentially a caricature or exaggeration of the latter. For instance, wrinkling of the skin, difficulty in standing upright, impaired vision, poor hearing and frequent passing of urine are all features of normal old age but are found to greater extent in senility; and mental deterioration, tedious repetition, loss of recent memory and lack of ability to concentrate, while all features of senility are to some extent found also in normal old age.

The truly senile person may collect rubbish, hide away money and food, wander outdoors in his night clothes, and become incontinent. Often, however, apparent senility is in some measure a result of poor nutrition, loneliness or lack of interests; and timely attention to these matters may prevent or postpone senility or may transform apparent senility into normal old age. Of particular importance in the apparently senile is attention to eyesight and hearing. Proper glasses and an efficient hearing aid may transform an apparently senile person into a reasonably normal senior citizen.

agglutination. The clumping together of bacteria by substances in the blood of persons who have – or have had – the relevant bacterial disease. The Widal test for typhoid is one of the many agglutination tests employed in modern medicine.

Apart from agglutination thus produced, similar clumping can occur when blood of different groups is mixed.

agoraphobia. A form of NEUROSIS characterized by morbid and irrational fear of open spaces.

agranulocytosis. A condition characterized by diminution of the granular white blood corpuscles, with high temperature, development of ulcers and a high death-rate. The main cause is an abnormally sensitive reaction to certain drugs, e.g., chlorpromazine, amidopyrine, antihistamines and sulphonamides. Manifestations include rigors, pains in the limbs and throat, prostration, high temperature and the formation of ulcers.

Prevention is achieved essentially by warning each patient receiving drugs associated with agranulocytosis to report immediately if any of the symptoms develop. Treatment consists of rapid withdrawal of the offending drug and injections of hydrocortisone or ACTH. About three-quarters of untreated cases die, but early treatment reduces the death-rate to about one-quarter. The risk of agranulocytosis is one of the reasons why certain non-addictive drugs remain available only on medical prescription.

air hunger. Difficulty in breathing, shown by gasping for breath, due to lack of oxygen in the blood and consequently in the tissues, known as ANOXIA. It occurs in various heart and kidney diseases and also in acidosis. Treatment with oxygen and carbon dioxide relieves the attack but recurrence is likely unless the underlying condition can be cured.

air swallowing. See AEROPHAGY.

albinism. A hereditary condition caused by absence of the enzyme required to form the pigment that is normally found in the skin, hair, and eyes. In albinos the hair is white, the skin very white and sensitive to sunlight, and the eyes pink owing to light shining through the colourless iris to the blood-vessels behind. Albinos often have to wear tinted spectacles and to avoid strong sunshine. The condition is inherited as a recessive character; see GENETICS.

albumin. The main protein contained in the blood. It helps to maintain the osmotic pressure of blood (see OSMOSIS). Where albumin is diminished – as in starvation, certain diseases of the liver (which normally manufactures albumin) and severe albuminuria – there is retention of fluid in the tissues and therefore oedema.

albuminuria. Presence of albumin in the urine. It occurs in most fevers and in various diseases of the heart and kidneys. Testing regularly for albuminuria is important in pregnancy because its presence may indicate disordered kidney function requiring skilled treatment.

alcohol. Any of a large group of organic hydroxides. The simplest chemically is methyl alcohol (wood spirit), a colourless, highly poisonous liquid distilled from wood. When drunk it produces unconsciousness without any preceding feeling of elation, it can create temporary or permanent blindness, and it may cause death. Methyl alcohol is not further considered in the paragraphs below.

Usually by 'alcohol' is meant the second simplest of the group, ethyl alcohol, a colourless liquid produced by fermentation of substances containing starch (e.g., barley, wheat, rye, potatoes) and used since history has been recorded to remove shyness or inhibitions and to induce a festive atmosphere. Simple fermentation produces a solution containing not more than about 12 per cent alcohol (e.g., beers and unfortified wines) because above that level the ferments become inactive. More concentrated solutions are prepared by distillation (e.g., whisky, brandy, gin, and vodka).

Since alcohol is very rapidly absorbed from an empty stomach it has value, taken in small quantities, as an immediate source of energy in some situations (although it should never be given to persons suffering from exposure on the hills), and since it promotes the flow of gastric juice it is commonly taken as an appetizer before or with meals. Normally, however, it is taken for its social and emotional effects. It induces a feeling of relaxation, lowers nervous tension and irritability, and reduces self-criticism. Other effects include a slight quickening of the heart beat and a dilating of blood vessels.

In appreciable quantity it impairs concentration, judgement, and self-control. The individual, while still apparently sober, may become – according to temperament – excitable, garrulous, quarrelsome or depressed; his reaction time is slowed and his manual skills and co-ordination of movements become less good. Larger amounts produce signs of drunkenness, including slurred speech and staggering gait, and often depression, while in still larger quantity, alcohol produces stupor and unconsciousness.

In general, absorption of alcohol is slowed by the presence of food in the stomach, especially milk or oil, hence the custom of eating oily hors d'oeuvres at the beginning of a meal. Absorbed alcohol is broken down at a fairly constant rate of 15 to 20 mg. per 100 ml. per hour (so that a man who had reached a level of 150 mg. would become legally fit to drive in about four or five hours). The effects of a given quantity of alcohol vary greatly with the individual (some people have 'no head for spirits' while others remain sober after large quantities) and with the person's previous familiarity or unfamiliarity with alcohol in general and with the particular variety of spirit consumed. Effervescence, as in whisky and soda, accelerates the effects, as does mixing of products of grain (e.g., whisky, vodka) and grape (e.g., brandy); so does cold air, so that the habit of 'one for the road' is to be deprecated.

While drinking is in general a controversial subject, its most controversial aspect is the relationship of alcohol to traffic accidents. Considering the speed at which cars are able to travel, anything that reduces a driver's reaction time or impairs his judgement is clearly liable to increase the danger of accidents. There is general agreement that the drunken driver is a menace and should be put off the road. Unfortunately there is no agreement as to what quantity of alcohol significantly impairs judgement or slows reaction time. Some workers claim that at around 25 mg. alcohol per 100 ml. blood (or very roughly the level produced in a man of average size by an ordinary single whisky) reaction time is actually improved, and that significant slowing does not appear until the level is about 100 mg.

The problem is extremely complicated because the blood level produced by a constant dose of alcohol varies with such factors as body size of the drinker, duration of period since drinking and stomach contents at time of drinking. Also, even if allowance is made for all known factors, there appears to be very considerable individual variation. For the safety of the public the permitted level of alcohol must clearly be low enough to allow for the reasonably worst combination of these various factors, but to set the level below that at which there was any possibility of reaction time being slowed would be merely repressive legislation.

While drunkenness is disgusting and alcoholism is a serious disease, the desirability or otherwise of moderate drinking is highly controversial. A few drinks can enliven a social occasion, and there is no indication that emotionally stable persons harm themselves by moderate indulgence. On the other hand, persons of unstable or inadequate personality may become utterly dependent on alcohol.

Alcohol and disease. Alcohol is useful in various conditions – to reduce fever by dilating the skin blood vessels and permitting easier access of air, to stimulate failing heart or respiration, to promote sleep at night, and to produce immediate warmth or relaxation of tension. It is definitely undesirable in cases of head injury and abdominal injury, is inadvisable in gastritis and gastric ulcer, and is considered by some experts to be detrimental in serious disease of the heart, cardiovascular system, or kidneys.

Since alcohol enlarges the small blood vessels in and near the skin and therefore increases heat loss from the body it should not be given to a person suffering from exposure to cold while he or she is still exposed.

In sudden excess it can cause intoxication, in the early stages of which the person may become aggressive and try to pick quarrels, or maudlin and tell his secrets to strangers, or over-generous and give away his possessions, or depressed and even attempt suicide, while in a later stage his speech is indistinct and his gait reeling. Unrepeated intoxication is not a disease. It is an episode, indicating that a youth has not discovered his limits, that an older person has over-used alcohol under abnormal stress, or that an individual has inadvertently mixed his drinks. Repeated intoxication is an indication that an individual cannot drink safely at all and is one form of ALCOHOLISM.

Even though not becoming an alcoholic, the habitual drinker, while deriving certain real or imagined benefits from his habit (such as personal pleasure, relief from worry and easing of social intercourse), runs certain risks. The first risk, often forgotten, is similar to that of the habitual eater of sweets or cakes - that of obesity, with consequent strain on heart and kidneys. Alcohol is a food, providing calories and energy; so that if alcohol does the work normally done by carbohydrates, the carbohydrates eaten are largely unused and deposited in the tissues as fat. Exact calorie values for any fixed quantity vary, being highest for spirits, less for

fortified wines, and lowest for light white wines and some varieties of beer. Roughly, 30 ml. (1 fluid oz.) of whisky contains 60 Calories, or about the same as three times that quantity of milk.

Alcohol, especially undiluted spirits, can cause inflammation of the lining of the stomach. Continued heavy drinking over a long period can produce cirrhosis of the liver, peripheral neuritis, and brain damage. Additionally, since alcohol consumes or inactivates vitamin B_1 prolonged high consumption of alcohol may cause symptoms of deficiency of that vitamin. A series of bouts of heavy drinking can lead to tremors of the hands, loss of appetite, and finally the hallucinations known scientifically as delirium tremens and colloquially as the blue devils.

Some workers suggest that a healthy man of average size can normally consume a daily ration of 50 ml. of whisky or a bottle of unfortified wine without damage to physical or mental health; but individual variation is considerable, and no dependable norm is possible.

alcoholism. Dependence upon alcohol to such extent as to interfere frequently or persistently with bodily or mental health, with interpersonal relations, or with working capacity. There are several types of which two will be mentioned here.

1. Episodic bouts of heavy drinking: the individual becomes completely drunk at intervals (e.g., about once a month), 'sleeps it off', perhaps wakes with a hangover but is sober in the considerable periods between bouts. Treatment of the episode involves letting the individual rest, sometimes giving a sedative to counteract restlessness, keeping him warm and offering adequate liquid, preferably with vitamins B_1 and C. Treatment of the condition is as indicated below, but - while far from easy - is less difficult than is that of the 'alcoholic who is never drunk'.

2. Persisting and increasing inability to abstain: the individual is perhaps never intoxicated, especially in the early years of his disease, but meets every fresh situation (from the emergence of a problem to the arrival of a visitor) with a drink, consumes gradually larger and larger quantities, and passes from heavy social drinking to secret drinking, e.g., having an extra glass before his guest arrives or after the guest leaves. Excessive expenditure on alcohol and a developing lack of interest in spouse and family often lead to marital unhappiness, causing in turn more drinking. Work begins to suffer, leading to lack of promotion and sometimes to unemployment, with further drinking as a compensatory mechanism. If untreated the individual steadily deteriorates over a number of years. It is important to note that, while he displays a poor memory, a lowered working capacity, and often garrulousness or irritability, he may never be intoxicated and may not be recognized

by neighbours and workmates as an alcoholic.

The wife (or occasionally the husband) of an alcoholic suffers enormous distress and is as much in need of help as the alcoholic. If, as often occurs in the second type mentioned above, the drink problem is unrecognized by relatives and neighbours the woman may be at her wits' end to know where to turn for aid. On the one hand she, more than anyone else, may be the person able to persuade her husband that he needs treatment and should seek either medical aid or the help of an organization such as Alcoholics Anonymous (branches of which now exist in about a hundred countries) and during treatment her help and support will be invaluable. On the other hand she may utterly fail to motivate her spouse, the situation may become increasingly intolerable, and for her own and her children's sake she may ultimately have to consider separation. Before taking such an extreme step and abandoning the husband as beyond redemption she should certainly discuss the situation with her doctor or with her health visitor or with an appropriate social worker: the mere airing of the situation will bring her a measure of relief, and an emotionally detached person with professional knowledge may be able to suggest to her a useful reorientation of her tactics to persuade her husband that he needs treatment.

Social patterns such as the spirit drinking of Scotland and Ireland play a part in the creation of alcoholics. So do ready availability – there is a high incidence in bar tenders – and loneliness, as illustrated in the alcoholism among men whose occupations necessitate frequent appreciable absence from their homes. Principally, however, alcoholism is a reflection of personality defect: the individual is unable to cope with life's problems and resorts to heavier and heavier drinking as an escape mechanism. The main hope for the long-term prevention of alcoholism probably lies in the fostering of good personality development in children – providing an atmosphere of security and demonstrated affection in which the child can develop but encouraging him in large measure to make his own decisions and experiments, with the result that he gradually acquires self-confidence and self-discipline.

Treatment of an alcoholic involves recognition – by the doctor, by other health and social workers, by the employer and especially by the spouse and family – that he is ill, not wicked, and needs help, not moralizing. Cure is impossible unless the patient actually desires to be cured. Where he has such a desire, he has to be 'sobered up' in a hospital or elsewhere and weaned completely from his drinking. Drugs like antabuse, which create unpleasant sensations if alcohol is subsequently consumed, may aid the weaning process but, if treatment is to succeed, the patient will require a great deal of help with his emotional and social problems. Short of providing that help over a long period, treatment of the alcoholism alone is merely seeking to remove his escape mechanism, and as such is likely to be doomed to failure, as alcoholics are notoriously cunning in outwitting their watchers. The patient, as in other personality problems, must be brought to recognize the underlying reason for his condition and encouraged either to overcome it by other means or to accept it.

aldersterone. A hormone, produced by the cortex of the adrenal gland (an ENDOCRINE GLAND) responsible for regulating the excretion of sodium and potassium by the kidneys. Diminished secretion is found in Addison's disease.

alimentary canal. The DIGESTIVE SYSTEM: the musculo-membraneous tube through which food enters the body, in which the food is digested, and from which the remains are excreted as faeces. The canal comprises mouth, pharynx, oesophagus (gullet), stomach, duodenum, small intestine, large intestine, rectum, and anus.

alimentary system. A term used to describe not only the alimentary canal but also the other organs concerned with digestion, e.g., salivary glands, pancreas and liver.

alkalaemia. Increase in the alkali reserve of the blood. It can occur through over-breathing in cases of hysteria or through ingestion of large quantities of alkali, as in cases of peptic ulcer. Symptoms include headache, nausea, vomiting, loss of appetite, and slow, shallow respiration. Immediate treatment is by acid sodium lactate, followed by treatment of the causal condition.

alkali. A substance that neutralizes acids, the general principle being that an acid and an alkali combine to form a salt and water. Strong alkalis, such as caustic soda, can produce severe burns. Milder alkalis, such as sodium bicarbonate, can effectively neutralize acids if given early enough.

The blood and digestive fluids are all slightly alkaline, with the exception of the acid gastric juice, and in the treatment of indigestion alkalis such as sodium bicarbonate (baking soda) are often used to neutralize the gastric hydrochloric acid.

alkaline poisoning. Strong alkalis such as caustic soda or potash are corrosive poisons, which can cause death but generally cause thirst, repeated vomiting, and symptoms of shock. Emetics should not be used because they bring the poison up to the throat. Treatment involves inducing the patient to swallow a weak solution of vinegar or lemon juice and counteracting shock by warmth.

allergen. A substance which can give rise to an allergic reaction.

allergy. An exaggerated susceptibility to certain foreign proteins. The individual, having become sensitized to a protein in a particular food or in a particular variety of pollen or in a particular dust, produces antibodies against it; and the combined presence of the protein and the antibodies causes release of histamine from the tissues – resulting, according to the tissues involved, in asthma, hay fever, nettlerash, migraine, or angioneurotic oedema. The symptoms – from the weal of nettlerash to the tightening of bronchioles in asthma – are essentially due to production of histamine.

Recent investigations show that not all the offending substances (allergens) are proteins. Some are simpler substances which combine with proteins in the body to form 'new' foreign proteins.

The causes of allergy are complex. In many cases a hereditary or familial factor is present but not necessarily related to any one allergic disease: e.g., the father suffers from hay fever and the son from asthma. Physical factors, in particular the presence of the allergen, are clearly important. Emotional factors, such as home tensions disturbing young people, may predispose the individual to an allergy, and in a high proportion of cases emotional factors also play a considerable part in precipitating attacks, sometimes even in the absence of the allergen; a person allergic to cats may develop an attack on seeing a picture of a cat. The typical victim of allergic diseases is described as intelligent, over-anxious, and highly strung. To add to the complexity, hypersensitivity may develop in the course of an infection: for instance, rheumatic fever, while initially due to streptococcal infection, is probably in part an allergic condition.

Where the allergen can be identified two courses of action are possible. First, where practicable the allergen and the patient can be separated: the man sensitive to eggs or feathers can stop eating eggs or exclude feather cushions from his house; and the person allergic to pollen can move from the country to a town. Secondly, the patient can be gradually desensitized by graded doses of the allergen.

Antihistamines are very effective in some allergic diseases (e.g., hay fever) but useless in others (e.g., asthma). Where the allergen cannot be identified and antihistamines are unsuccessful one can only provide symptomatic treatment and attend to the emotional factors. The latter may require anything from simple reassurance and explanation to full-scale psychotherapy.

alopecia. Loss of hair, BALDNESS.

altitude sickness. An unpleasant condition, sometimes serious and very occasionally fatal, occurring as a result of insufficient oxygen in the tissues as a consequence of the low atmospheric pressure of high altitudes.

As a result of the lowered concentration of oxygen in the mountain air, the red blood corpuscles cannot absorb enough oxygen in the lung-capillary exchange. Because of this deficiency, the breathing is quickened (to try to obtain more oxygen) and the amount of carbon dioxide in the blood is reduced. While there is much individual variation, common symptoms include breathlessness, lethargy, irritability, impaired judgement and muscular weakness.

Since modern aeroplanes are pressurized, the condition does not normally occur during flight, but quite often arises in people who have newly arrived at a high altitude, e.g., over 1500 metres (5000 ft.). Persons arriving at a place very considerably higher than that in which they previously resided are wise to refrain from all strenuous activity for the first forty-eight hours to give their bodies time to adjust to the new circumstances – and people with any disease of the heart should not travel to a high altitude without first seeking medical advice.

alveolus. A small cavity. The term is used both for the socket of a tooth and for the many tiny air-pockets in the lungs from which oxygen diffuses into the blood capillaries and carbon dioxide passes from the blood to the respiratory channels for excretion in the breath.

amaurotic family idiocy. A hereditary disease of infancy characterized by progressive diminution in sight (amaurosis), progressive bodily paralysis, and progressive mental impairment. The condition usually leads to death within three years.

ambivalence. Conflicting emotions, usually resulting in an alternation of affection and resentment.

To some extent this is a normal happening. At times most of us are angry and impatient with our closest relatives and best friends, with love temporarily replaced by irritation, and at these times we tend to be harsher towards them than we would be towards mere acquaintances who did exactly the same things to annoy us. This minor ambivalence is very common between children who are the best of friends today, not on speaking terms tomorrow and again close friends next week. Between adults with deep affection for each other it is generally tolerated, the person who is faced with unexpected anger either waiting patiently for the storm to pass or else 'clearing the air' with an open row followed by reconciliation. Where minor ambivalence between adults has serious results, such as the breakdown of a marriage, the consequence is not so much the result of temporary resentment as of human stubbornness, with neither party willing to say, 'The fault was mainly mine.'

Where minor ambivalence can be harmful is in the relationship between adults and their children. If a child is mildly rebuked for his behaviour on Monday, tries the same behaviour experimentally on Thursday and finds it tolerated, and is then severely punished for the identical behaviour on Saturday, simply because the parent is irritated and resentful, his sense of justice becomes confused, he may become suspicious of his parents and his personality development may be harmed. Yet probably not one parent in a hundred can honestly claim that he is always consistent and never lets resentment temporarily replace affection.

More serious ambivalence, such as frequent alternation of affection and concern for the well-being of a friend and jealousy of (and even hatred for) that friend, is not only detrimental to human relations but is also a common cause of neurosis, since it is an expression of unresolved conflict. Here psychiatric treatment often helps, but it may sometimes be necessary for the persons to sever their connections, giving up the companionship and solace of affection in order to be rid of the damaging effects of jealousy and hatred.

amblyopia. Loss of sight, partial or complete, without apparent disease of the eyes. It can occur after a stroke, or after poisoning by alcohol (especially methyl alcohol), lead, arsenic, or occasionally tobacco. It may also occur as a result of a squint when the sight of one eye is suppressed in order to prevent double vision. Depending on the cause, it may be temporary or permanent.

amenorrhoea. Absence of menstrual periods between puberty and the menopause. Primary amenorrhoea, where menstruation has never occurred, may be due to maldevelopment of the uterus or ovaries, or to anaemia, or – more rarely – to inflammation of the vulva or disturbance of the endocrine glands. Secondary amenorrhoea, in which menstruation ceases, is usually due to pregnancy but is sometimes caused by anaemia, shock following severe emotional upset, or premature menopause. Treatment depends on the cause.

amino-acid. A weak organic acid containing nitrogen and forming, with other amino-acids, the essential structure of PROTEINS. Human proteins contain some twenty-two different amino-acids, eight of which cannot be synthesized in the body and must therefore be provided in the diet.

ammonia. A colourless, pungent-smelling gas, generally used in watery solution for household purposes. If drunk accidentally it is a corrosive poison, best treated by giving a dilute solution of vinegar, lemon juice or orange juice, and by keeping the patient warm.

amnesia. Complete loss of memory in respect of a period of time. It may be current, i.e., an inability to retain new impressions, or retrograde, as in loss of memory for events leading up to a head injury. 'Middle-aged amnesia' is the term used colloquially for the gradual deterioration of memory that occurs as one ages. There is, as yet, no known

treatment, although some drugs are under trial.

amniocentesis. See PRENATAL DIAGNOSIS.

amnion. The membraneous bag which forms within the uterus to enclose the developing unborn child. The bag is filled with a clear fluid which protects the foetus and maintains it at an even temperature. See CHILDBIRTH.

amphetamines. A series of drugs which, in contrast to the barbiturates, stimulate the central nervous system, temporarily reduce fatigue, lessen appetite, and produce a sensation of well-being. Various amphetamines have been employed to create additional energy (e.g., in battle situations), as aids to slimming, and as treatment for depression and epilepsy. For all these purposes they have now been virtually abandoned as they are mildly but definitely habit-forming and, because of this risk of addiction, they are obtainable on prescription only. Almost the only remaining medical uses of amphetamines are for the treatment of barbiturate poisoning and in some mental diseases. Illegally, however, they still circulate and are known by such names as 'purple hearts', 'black bombers' and 'speed'.

Excess of amphetamine leads to excitement, tremor, euphoria, and dilated pupils, passing with larger doses to anxiety, hallucinations, and uncontrolled movements. In most cases the only immediate treatment required is rest and sometimes a mild sedative, but if the addiction is well established its cure may be difficult.

ampicillin. A synthetic derivative of penicillin which, unlike penicillin itself, is not inactivated by gastric juice and is therefore effective by mouth. It is effective against a wide range of organisms and is particularly useful in urinary infections and in typhoid and paratyphoid.

amputation. The surgical removal of a part of the body, such as a limb. Amputation becomes necessary when there is irremediable damage from a road, industrial or other accident, or from such conditions as gangrene, frost-bite, cancer or advanced arteriosclerosis.

amyl nitrite. A yellowish liquid, which will evaporate very rapidly, normally supplied in small capsules and inhaled after crushing in a handkerchief. By dilating the coronary arteries amyl nitrite relieves the pain of angina pectoris within seconds.

anaemia. Bloodlessness, and in particular shortage in the blood of haemoglobin, the oxygen-carrying pigment contained in the red blood corpuscles. The mass of disease known collectively as anaemia is most easily classified by cause.

1. Excessive loss of blood corpuscles. This occurs in severe haemorrhage, excessive menstruation and 'hidden' bleeding (e.g., into the stomach following consumption of too much aspirin). Here the blood cells and haemoglobin are at first reduced equally, but, as the bone

marrow vigorously produces replacement red blood corpuscles, these recover first – so that blood examination reveals an adequate number of corpuscles but with abnormally little pigment.

2. Excessive destruction of red blood corpuscles. In sickle-cell anaemia, an hereditary abnormality of the haemoglobin with an increased fragility of the cells, red blood corpuscles are shaped rather like sickles. Normally red blood corpuscles are destroyed and replaced about every four months, but in cases of excessive destruction they have a life of only one month and the bone marrow cannot manufacture new corpuscles speedily enough to keep pace with the destruction. Children suffering from the disease have signs and symptoms of anaemia, usually enlarged spleens, and bouts of fever and of pain in muscles and joints.

3. Iron deficiency. There is in this case insufficient iron in the diet for proper production of cells, so that the red blood corpuscles are small and the amount of haemoglobin in them is low. This anaemia of poverty and poor diet is by far the commonest anaemia in western countries. For instance, it affects fully 20 per cent of British women aged 20 to 50 years (i.e., roughly of menstruating age) and is also not uncommon in men and in children. It is preventable by proper diet.

4. Lack of vitamin B₁₂ in the diet or of folic acid. This variety, known as pernicious anaemia, was deemed inevitably fatal until 1926, when it was found to be treatable with large doses of raw liver, and has been relatively easy to treat since the isolation of vitamin B₁₂ in 1948.

5. Suppression of red blood cell formation by the bone marrow. This aplastic anaemia is rare but inevitably fatal unless the marrow recovers its ability to manufacture corpuscles; however, in order to afford a chance of such recovery the patient can be temporarily kept alive with blood transfusions.

6. Other types. These are such conditions as the anaemia that follows prolonged low-grade poisoning by lead, arsenic, or mercury, or the anaemia associated with various chronic diseases.

In general, irrespective of type, anaemia is characterized by signs and symptoms of oxygen lack. There is pallor of the skin, especially noticeable on the lips and eyelids, where the skin is thin; the patient feels tired and listless; the pulse is full and soft; both pulse rate and respiration rate increase unduly on very slight exertion, and ankles tend to swell. Some minor signs help to differentiate the types, e.g., the varieties caused by excessive destruction of blood corpuscles often show a yellowish, jaundiced appearance; for accurate differentiation, blood counts and haemoglobin estimations are essential.

Treatment varies according to the type.

In the commonest of all varieties – the iron deficiency anaemia of poverty or poor diet – it is necessary to treat the patient for months with a digestible iron salt (such as ferrous sulphate tablets, 200 mg. thrice daily after meals) and simultaneously – and afterwards – to ensure that he eats a good, mixed diet, including a sufficiency of meat and green vegetables.

anaesthesia. Generalized or localized insensibility to pain, induced by drugs. The main early anaesthetics were ether (used from 1844), nitrous oxide (1846), and chloroform (1847); but in recent decades anaesthesia has made vast progress and most modern general anaesthetics are given not by inhalation but by injection. The patient usually loses consciousness even before the syringe has been withdrawn from his arm, has no nausea or vomiting after the operation and is not unknown to enquire on wakening, 'When are you going to start the operation?' Sodium pentothal, cyclopropane and trichloroethylene are examples of modern general anaesthetics.

Local anaesthesia has also made enormous advances. It consists essentially of injecting – and temporarily deadening – the nerve which transmits sensation from the operation area to the brain, or temporarily abolishing sensation in the lower limbs by injection into the spine, or for very brief anaesthesia 'freezing' the surface of the skin. It is possible, for instance, to perform under local anaesthesia a cataract operation with the patient not only fully conscious but actually unaware of the operation taking place. Of many local anaesthetics administered by injection probably the best known is procaine hydrochloride (novocaine), and the spray most commonly used to 'freeze' the skin is ethyl chloride.

anal canal. The narrow muscular passage leading from the rectum to the exterior at the contracted orifice called the anus. It is about 3.5 cm. (1.5 in.) long, is lined with mucous membrane, and has a rich blood supply. Where a vein in the area becomes varicose it is termed a haemorrhoid or PILE.

anal fissure. An ulcer or abrasion at the lower end of the anal canal, causing sharp pain during and after defecation. In mild cases regulation of the bowels by laxatives and application of vaseline may effect a cure. In more severe cases a small surgical operation is required.

anal fistula. An unnatural channel from the anal canal to the exterior. It is generally caused by an abscess which, through pressure of pus, makes its way to the surface and is thereafter prevented from healing by constant reinfection of the raw surfaces by the passage of faeces. Treatment is surgical.

analgesia. Reducing or relieving pain by drugs. In the past, when complete suppression of pain was virtually impossible, the term was often used as synonymous with both general ANAESTHESIA (rendering the patient stuporous or unconscious) and local anaesthesia ('freezing' skin or temporarily paralysing appropriate nerves). Nowadays it is usually restricted to the use of pain-deadening drugs which neither cause sleep and stupor (as the narcotics do) nor the complete unconsciousness of general anaesthesia. The border between analgesics and narcotics is vague, however, because large doses of some analgesics create sleepiness and narcotics may relieve pain without actually causing sleep.

There is a vast number of pain-reducing drugs ranging from aspirin to heroin and some, such as opium, have been known and used for centuries. The analgesics in common use are derivatives of salicilic acid (e.g., aspirin), phenazone (e.g., amidopyrine), and phenacetin (e.g., paracetamol). These drugs provide temporary relief from pain and are extremely useful, but they do not themselves cure diseases.

In a terminal illness there seems no reason why the patient should be allowed to suffer, but in illnesses from which recovery is expected the stronger pain-killers have to be used with discretion. To let a patient endure prolonged agony is not only inhumane but very damaging to the sufferer, but to use strong drugs too frequently may produce addiction, and an overdose can cause death. For these reasons household supplies of such drugs should always be kept in a safe cupboard out of reach of children.

anal pruritis. Itching of the anus. In many cases the itching starts from a transitory cause and continues because of the patient's scratching. Other causes include threadworms, piles, and fistula, or fissure, dermatitis and more rarely disturbance of the intestinal bacteria following the use of an antibiotic. Cleanliness and careful but gentle drying sometimes effect a cure; and application of steroids is often helpful.

anal spasm. Painful contraction of the muscle controlling the orifice of the anal canal may arise from anal fissure, or fistula, or pruritus. Apart from attention to the cause, treatment usually involves keeping the motions soft by laxatives.

anaphylaxis. Abnormal sensitivity to a particular protein, an extreme form of allergy. This rare condition occurs mainly in relation to SERUM treatment. A person with this abnormal sensitivity who is given antitoxic serum may react very sharply to the protein contained in it, with bronchi going into complete spasm, and may even die unless given an immediate injection of adrenalin.

anastomosis. Linking of the branches of one blood vessel to another.

anatomy. The science concerned with the structure, form, arrangements and relationships of all parts of the body.

Accurate anatomical information is clearly essential for the surgeon, but knowledge of anatomy and of physiology (the science of how the parts of the body work) is also vital to the physician.

See individual entries for anatomical description of the various structures in the body.

androgen. A male sex hormone. Androgens include testerone, produced in the testicles, and several hormones produced by the cortex of each of the adrenals, two ENDOCRINE GLANDS. Androgens are also produced in small amounts in the ovaries of women.

Insufficient secretion of androgens in a boy prevents the development of such male characteristics as deepening of the voice, facial hair and enlargement of the sex organs. The condition can sometimes be helped by injection of androgens. Excessive secretion in boys, as occurs in certain tumours of the adrenals or the testes, causes precocious puberty.

Excessive secretion in females results in virilization, i.e., increased muscular development, growth of facial hair and enlargement of the clitoris, part of the female genital tract. Treatment varies with the cause.

anencephaly. Failure of the brain to develop while the unborn child is still in the uterus. The condition, while rare, is usually fatal.

aneurine. A name for vitamin B₁. See THIAMIN and VITAMINS.

aneurysm. A bulge in the wall of an artery. Aneurysms are often classified according to shape: fusiform, tapering towards the ends; saccular, forming a pouch; and dissecting, where the cavity develops between the coats of an artery. All types result from the combination of a weakening of the arterial wall and a rise of the blood pressure to a greater extent than the wall can resist.

Congenital aneurysms usually affect the arteries at the base of the brain. Traumatic aneurysms can result from any penetrating wound, such as a shotgun injury, and most often occur in the limbs. Syphilitic aneurysm, mostly of the aorta, was formerly quite common but has become extremely rare. So-called degenerative aneurysms develop mostly in early middle age in men who follow strenuous occupations such as dock labourers.

Where the bulge is in an accessible position the diagnosis is obvious: there is, in the line of an artery, a swelling which pulsates with each beat of the heart. Less accessible aneurysms can be shown by injecting a radio-opaque substance into the blood vessels in order to make them visible on x-ray in the process known as angiography.

Symptoms are generally due to pressure, e.g., an aortic aneurysm may press on the gullet, wind-pipe and laryngeal nerve, causing difficulty in swallowing, breathlessness and a barking cough. In untreated cases there is about a 50 per cent chance of rupture, when profuse haemorrhage may cause death.

Surgical treatment is sometimes practicable – tying off the aneurysm, or even tying the artery above and below it and then connecting the two parts of the artery by a tube. Sometimes, too, an attempt may be made to produce a clot which gradually increases until it fills the sac and prevents further growth. It has to be remembered, however, that an aneurysm in one artery often indicates that the arteries in general are in poor condition.

angina pectoris. Severe paroxysms of pain over the breast-bone, sometimes spreading down the left arm or occasionally both arms. The pain comes on during or immediately after exercise, bringing all activity to a sudden stop and tending to produce expectation of death. It usually passes off after a few minutes.

As a rule, angina is a condition of men rather than women, of middle age rather than of youth and of 'white-collar' workers rather than labourers. The agony, the consequent ashen-grey face and restrained breathing and the rapid relief after rest make the condition easily recognizable, although obviously other causes of chest pain should be considered when a diagnosis is being made.

Angina is a symptom, not a disease. It implies that the heart muscle is receiving insufficient oxygen (usually because of arteriosclerosis of the coronary arteries) and that the nerve-endings are being stimulated by the incomplete products of combustion of foods.

Treatment of individual attacks is by rest as soon as the first suggestion of pain appears, and by administration of drugs that rapidly dilate the coronary arteries. A 0.5 mg. tablet of glyceryl trinitrate chewed or sucked under the tongue will stop an attack within two minutes: and amyl nitrite capsules, broken into a handkerchief and inhaled, can be even quicker although in some people they produce other symptoms. A person subject to angina should always carry appropriate tablets or capsules, as prescribed by the doctor.

General management has to be adapted to the frequency and severity of the attacks, the patient's occupation and socio-economic status and even his temperament. Broadly, he should be encouraged to find a compromise and to limit his physical and mental activities to what he can do without producing an attack, but not to limit them more than is necessary. He should seek to avoid hurry, excitement and emotional tension and should, so far as is practicable, cultivate a philosophical attitude to life. Frequent small meals are usually better than occasional large ones, and while alcohol in moderation is not harmful, tobacco is inadvisable. Sedatives at night may be useful.

Prevention of angina is essentially prevention (ten or twenty years earlier) of the underlying coronary disease. Possible measures include taking of reasonable and moderate exercise; avoidance of obesity; limitation of sugar intake; and limitation or avoidance of tobacco. Avoidance wherever possible of abnormal emotional, mental and physical stress also contributes greatly to the prevention of angina.

angiography. A method of showing defects such as ANEURYSMS by x-rays.

angioneurotic oedema. A condition, probably hereditary, in which swellings appear on the skin and mucous membranes. The swellings – raised patches, usually hot and red but occasionally cold – occur chiefly on the face and hands and appear suddenly, most commonly after emotional disturbances. The swellings appear to be the result of dilation of capillaries and release from them of histamine or a histamine-like substance. The condition is related to allergy.

Where the underlying cause is physical a search for the allergen can be useful, with the idea of removing it from the individual or the individual from it. In psychosomatic cases sedatives (e.g., barbiturates or bromides) may be helpful. Irrespective of the cause, antihistamine drugs (e.g., anthisan) are valuable in attacks.

'heel' bone

'ankle' bone

articulating surfaces between leg and foot

fibula — tibia

The bone structure of the ankle joint

ankle. The joint formed by the lower ends of the tibia and fibula and the upper surface of the astragalus. The joint is of the hinge variety, permitting only two movements – flexion (bringing the foot nearer to the front of the leg) and extension or plantar flexion (straightening the ankle with the toes pointed downwards). The capsule of the joint is strengthened by several important ligaments.

The common injuries of the ankle are sprain and fracture.

Abrupt twisting of the ankle (as in a fall) tears the tendons and ligaments, causing a sprain, characterized by swelling and tenderness. A sprain is best treated by cold compresses followed by strapping for several days. Elastoplast perhaps gives more support to the injured ankle than does a crepe bandage.

Less common is the fracture-dislocation of the ankle known as Pott's fracture, in which the foot is twisted outwards, the fibula on the outer side of the leg is broken, and the tibia on the inner side may or may not be broken. The injury may occur from direct violence, as when a wheel passes over the leg, but is more often the result of indirect violence, e.g., stepping off a pavement without noticing. Symptoms include pain, partial loss of power in the leg, tenderness and swelling.

Differentiation between a fracture and a sprain is not easy, but in a sprain the foot is usually twisted inwards; any apparent sprain with pain and tenderness persisting for twenty-four hours should be x-rayed.

Splinting and bandaging of the leg are essential in cases of fracture, and in most cases the leg will need to be placed in plaster for some weeks, during which the patient will have to use crutches for walking.

ankylosis. Loss of movement of a joint through the joint surfaces becoming united by fibrous tissue, cartilage or bone. Fibrous ankylosis, occurring for example after prolonged immobilization of a joint in treatment of a fracture, can be treated by massage and movement. If these measures fail the fibrous adhesions can be broken down under general anaesthesia. Cartilaginous ankylosis, e.g., from fusion of two neighbouring cartilages in arthritis, and bony ankylosis, occurring where disease or operation has denuded a joint of cartilage, both produce complete immobility of the joint. They must either be left and the immobility accepted, or treated by surgical operation. Since a functionless joint is often preferable to a painful joint, ankylosis is sometimes deliberately produced by surgery to relieve persistent pain.

ankylostomiasis. See HOOKWORM DISEASE.

anodyne. An old name for any drug that relieves pain. See ANALGESIA.

anopheles. The generic name for a type of mosquito. One variety of the genus, *Anopheles maculipennis*, can transmit the parasite of MALARIA.

anorexia. The technical term for loss of APPETITE. It occurs temporarily in several acute fevers and toxaemic conditions, may be a result of certain anxiety states, or may also be the first sign of cancer of the stomach.

Anorexia nervosa. A dangerous condition of psychological origin, this chiefly occurs in women aged 15 to 25 years. It is a form of neurosis, characterized by extreme indifference to eating, restless energy, and increasing loss of weight. The condition is essentially a psychological refusal to accept adult life, with rejection of food serving as a symbolic rejection of adult sexuality. Treatment usually involves separating the woman from her relatives and providing skilled psychotherapy and appropriate drugs. Most cases recover after some months, but a considerable minority continue to have eating difficulties and about 10 per cent die, usually from infections due to lowered resistance.

anosmia. Loss of the sense of SMELL. Temporary forms are usually due to disease of the mucous membrane of the nose, e.g., partial anosmia occurs during a severe cold in the head. Anosmia of longer duration is generally a result of damage to the olfactory nerve (which carries sensations of smell from the nose to the brain) by, for instance, head injury or brain tumour. Our appreciation of different tastes is very dependent on the sense of smell so that the loss of that sensation also reduces our enjoyment of food. Heavy smoking is said to dull the sense of smell but not to the extent of causing anosmia.

anoxia. Insufficiency of oxygen in the blood. See ASPHYXIA.

antabuse. Antabuse or disulfiram is a drug used in the treatment of alcoholism. When it is present in the system consumption of alcohol produces nausea or actual vomiting. In extreme cases its use can be dangerous to life and it is, therefore, applied less often than in the past.

antacid. Any drug that neutralizes the acid of the gastric juice. See INDIGESTION.

antenatal care. See PREGNANCY, health in.

anthelmintics. Drugs employed to kill intestinal worms. Examples are male fern for tapeworm, oil of chenopodium for hookworm and santonin for roundworms.

anthracosis. A disease of the lungs and bronchi, caused by inhalation of coal dust and fairly common in miners. Repeated inhalation of coal dust causes excess fibrous tissue in the lungs, persistent bronchitis and ultimately emphysema. Treatment is very difficult and unsatisfactory. Prevention depends on suppression of dust, e.g., by water-drilling in mines and by hydro-blasting instead of shot-blasting.

anthrax. An infectious disease of farm animals sometimes called wool-sorter's disease, caused by a germ – the bacillus *anthracis*. It is very occasionally transmitted to man from the hair, wool, hide or flesh of infected animals and from manufactured products produced from infected raw material. In man the incubation period varies from one to seven days and this rare disease appears in one of two main forms: (1) the malignant pustule – a severe, localized and often painless inflammation generally at the site of a cut or abrasion through which the germ entered; this is the commoner form and is dangerous unless treated. (2) A fulminating pneumonia, when the germs have been inhaled or swallowed, which is generally fatal unless treated.

For treatment Schlavo's antiserum, in use for many years, is now superseded by a combination of penicillin and streptomycin. The patient, being highly infectious, is nursed in isolation, with the attendants wearing gloves and masks.

Preventive measures include identification, slaughter and either incineration or burial in lime of infected animals; immunization of animals deemed exposed to infection; thorough disinfection of effluents and trade wastes from premises in which contaminated hides or hair have lain; disinfection of hair and bristles from sources suspected of contamination; rapid identification and treatment of the disease in man; and isolation of the infected person until he has recovered.

anthrycide. A relatively new drug which cures several diseases caused by trypanosomes affecting cattle and horses and, sometimes, man. In addition to the curative effect, a single injection of the drug appears to confer an immunity lasting for several months.

antibiotics. Drugs produced from living organisms which prevent the growth and reproduction of other organisms. Thus the mould *Penicillium* prevents the growth of many bacteria, and penicillin is the drug manufactured from the mould. The inhibiting effect of the mould was noted by Alexander Fleming in 1928, and in 1941 H. W. Florey and E. B. Chain produced penicillin and used it on patients. Several different penicillins have since been prepared, some taken by mouth and others only by injection.

Other antibiotics include streptomycin (effective against the tubercle bacillus and in particular altering tuberculous meningitis from an invariably fatal to a curable disease), chloramphenicol (useful in typhoid) and terramycin (effective against the rickettsia of typhus).

While antibiotics are unquestionably life-saving drugs and while they have had an effect on mortality second only to vaccines and vitamins, three points should be noted. Firstly, many of them can have serious side-effects, e.g., streptomycin can cause permanent deafness and chloramphenicol can cause fatal aplastic anaemia. So antibiotics should not be needlessly used for minor infections that will yield to other treatment. Secondly, inadequate use of an antibiotic may create a resistant germ that has, in effect, developed an immunity. For instance, penicillin was at first completely effective against staphylococci (the commonest cause of septicaemia) and gonococci (the cause of the commonest of the venereal diseases), but sheer under-treatment of patients has produced many strains of staphylococci and gonococci resistant to

penicillin. Thirdly, while appropriate antibiotics can cope with most bacteria, spirochaetes and rickettsia, most of them appear to have no effect on viruses.

Strict control of their use is therefore of great importance and for that reason they are obtainable only on a doctor's prescription.

antibody. A protein formed in the body to counteract an invading foreign protein which has acted as an antigen. The antigen may be a bacterium, an allergen or an organ transplanted from another person.

For example, in diphtheria the toxin produced by the invading germs acts as the antigen, and the untreated person will die unless antibodies and antitoxin are produced in time to destroy the germs and toxin. In the serum treatment of diphtheria the defence mechanisms of the body are assisted by the injection of serum very rich in antitoxin: blood is drawn from the vein of a horse that has previously been immunized against diphtheria, and the serum is separated and concentrated. In immunization against diphtheria the body is 'tricked' into forming appropriate antibodies and antitoxin by injection of inactivated toxin. Thereafter the body, having learned the art of producing these, retains its capacity to produce them, so that if actual diphtheria germs later invade and start to produce toxin they are very promptly counteracted.

anticoagulant drugs. Drugs which reduce the natural tendency of the blood to clot, e.g., when the circulation is slow or the blood vessels narrowed. In coronary thrombosis, for instance, these drugs are often used to prevent further clotting in the blood vessels supplying the heart and the lungs.

antidote. A substance which neutralizes or counteracts the effect of a poison. Apart, however, from acids and alkalis, few poisons have specific antidotes.

antigen. A substance, usually a protein foreign to the body, which stimulates the production of ANTIBODIES. Thus a bacterium in addition to creating illness will stimulate the growth of antibodies and if these are produced quickly enough they may kill the invaders and end the disease, even without any treatment. Similarly the injection of killed bacteria, which are harmless but contain the same protein, causes production of antibodies which can destroy invading bacteria of the same type: this is essentially the mechanism used in immunization.

In allergic diseases pollens, fungi and dust particles may act as antigens and the antibodies produced cause physical reactions.

antihistamine. A substance acting against HISTAMINE, which is found in nettles and insect stings, and released when tissues are damaged, e.g., by burns. The released histamine causes narrowing of the bronchioles (and hence asthma), widening of small blood vessels with leakage into the tissues (and hence urticaria and inflammation) and various allergic manifestations. Antihistamine drugs combating these effects are very useful in nettlerash and hay fever, and also sometimes relieve travel sickness. They are less effective in asthma.

Antihistamines often cause drowsiness and therefore should not be taken shortly before driving a car. In excess they may produce excitement, tremors and convulsions, with some danger of choking, and very rarely they cause agranulocytosis.

antipyretic. The term applied to drugs which lower the temperature of the body in fevers.

antiscorbutic. Foods or chemical preparations containing vitamin c (ascorbic acid), the essential factor to prevent or cure SCURVY (also known as scorbutus). Among the richest natural antiscorbutics are lemons, oranges and blackcurrants. See VITAMINS.

antisepsis. Procedures designed to destroy bacteria or to prevent their growth. The pioneer of antisepsis was Joseph Lister who in the 1860s introduced the cleaning of surgical instruments with disinfectants, the spraying of operating theatres and wards, and the covering of wounds with carbolic dressings. These measures enormously reduced mortality from 'hospital gangrene', from puerperal fever (childbirth fever) and from wounds on the battlefield. Surgery had become painless following the introduction of anaesthetics about 1846; following the introduction of antisepsis it became relatively safe.

Yet under controlled conditions, such as those of an operating theatre, antisepsis was only a second best. In particular application to the tissues of too strong an antiseptic could damage them, while too weak an antiseptic might fail to kill some of the bacteria. Hence ASEPSIS, i.e., complete avoidance of all possible exposure to germs, gradually replaced antisepsis in surgery.

In uncontrolled conditions, as in the home, antisepsis still has a very important role. The ordinary procedure for treating an open wound is to remove dirt by gently washing with soap and water, and then to apply a mild antiseptic such as tincture of iodine or hydrogen peroxide. Babies' feeding bottles and other domestic implements are sterilized by well-recognized commercial antiseptics or, where appropriate, by boiling, and disinfectants are in common use in sick-rooms and lavatories, while minimal doses of specified antiseptics are used to preserve various foods.

Chemical antiseptics are essential for many purposes, but although heat is seldom effective unless the infected material can be boiled, the value of sunshine as an antiseptic should never be forgotten. Articles which would be damaged by boiling or by the use of strong chemical disinfectants can often be adequately sterilized by exposure to sunlight for a few hours.

antispasmodic drugs. Drugs which relieve spasm of a muscular organ. For instance, adrenalin and ephedrine relieve the spasm of the small bronchioles in asthma, and derivatives of opium reduce spasm of the intestine, kidney and ureter.

antitoxin. A substance formed in the blood, as a result of germ infection, for the purpose of neutralizing the toxin produced by the particular germ. An antitoxin is produced in the event of disease but may not be formed quickly enough to affect the outcome.

If a person or animal is given small, graduated doses of a known toxin, antitoxin is produced without the development of the disease. Not only is the person or animal rendered immune to the disease, but the blood serum of the immune individual can be used to provide a starting dose of antitoxin for somebody infected by the particular germ. This is the basis of the serum treatment of diphtheria, botulism and tetanus. A horse is usually selected, simply because it is a large animal which can supply a goodly quantity of blood; the horse is immunized with graded doses of toxin; when immunity has developed, blood is withdrawn, essentially as in the case of a person giving blood for a transfusion; the serum is separated off and concentrated; and the antitoxin is then ready for injection into a person suffering from the disease. Serum treatment has saved innumerable lives, although for many infections it has been replaced by treatment with appropriate antibiotics.

Part of the basis of active immunization against bacterial infections is injection into a healthy person of killed germs or inactivated toxin. The body is 'deceived' into manufacturing the appropriate antibody or antitoxin, so that the person becomes protected against the particular disease.

antrum. A cavity or air-cell in a bone. The term is especially used for the mastoid antrum, an air-cell in the bony process behind the ear. The cavity is connected with the middle ear by a small passage. Hence inflammation of the middle ear can develop into mastoid disease.

anus. The orifice at the lower end of the digestive system through which semi-solid waste matter (faeces) is discharged.

anxiety states. Intense and persisting fear or worry in the absence of obvious reason for anxiety. We all have momentary irrational fears and most of us have at times fears of longer duration but demonstrable cause; but the worry in an anxiety state not only lacks obvious cause (or persists with slight change of direction if the apparent cause is removed) but also dominates the person's whole existence. The sufferer has great difficulty in facing the ordinary stresses of life, lacks powers of concentration and effort, may be emotionally uncontrolled and may suffer from palpitations, breathlessness, loss of appetite, heart pains, sleeplessness and in some cases irregular beating of the heart. In other words, the anxiety state – which may apparently be related to work, to sexual relations, to physical health or simply to a deep, undefined dread – affects not only the mind but also the cardiovascular, digestive and nervous systems.

Anxiety states quite often occur in association with heart disease, asthma and peptic ulcer, and in women are sometimes associated with the menopause, but are also common in persons with no recognizable organic disease. The origin often lies, decades back, in insecurity or lack of affection in childhood. In other cases anxiety states arise from STRESS caused by overwhelming current financial problems or problems of personal relationships.

Simple reassurance is seldom effective. Tranquillizers and sedatives may be of some use in mild cases, and practical advice and help can be greatly beneficial in anxiety due to current problems. Where the main causes lie in childhood, however, it is necessary for a psychotherapist to unearth the basic fear or root conflict (which may well be hidden in the unconscious and quite unrealized by the patient) and to bring this to consciousness so that it can be discussed rationally. With adequate psychotherapy fairly rapid recovery is likely.

Anxiety states are not uncommon in children, where they may be accompanied by bed-wetting, nightmares, vomiting and diarrhoea. Investigation and treatment at a child guidance clinic are required.

Despite the enormously successful work of Freud and his successors, anxiety states are among the most under-treated of serious diseases. Too often the physician, having found no underlying organic disease, merely exhorts the patient to 'Pull yourself together', whereas in reality the patient is incapable of doing so until the root cause has been unearthed.

aorta. The main artery of the body, conducting oxygen-rich blood from the left side of the heart to all parts of the body. The aorta leaves the left ventricle where its opening is guarded by a semilunar valve; it then gives off two small branches, the coronary arteries, which supply blood to the heart muscle; after arching over the base of the heart, it gives off three branches from the arch, namely the innominate (which divides into the right common carotid and the right subclavian), the left common carotid and the left subclavian; it then runs downwards through the thorax and abdomen, giving off various branches to supply the viscera; and finally in front of the fourth lumbar vertebra, it divides into the right and left common iliac arteries (each of which

divides into an internal and an external branch).

Diseases of the aorta include arteriosclerosis (by far the commonest), aneurysm, and a congenital narrowing termed coarctation. Diseases of the semilunar valve are (1) aortic incompetence: deformity of the valve cusp with enlargement of the opening; and (2) aortic stenosis: narrowing of the valve cusp.

aperient. See LAXATIVE.

aphasia. Loss or impairment of the ability to speak. The commonest causes are cerebral haemorrhage, embolism, thrombosis and tumours, all of which can interfere with the areas in the left cerebral hemisphere of the BRAIN associated with speech. In motor aphasia, where the outgoing tract is damaged (i.e., the nerve transmitting the impulses which control the physical action of speech), the patient cannot speak but may understand and can sometimes write. In sensory aphasia, where the damage is to the incoming tract (i.e., the nerve transmitting the sensation of the sound of speech), the patient cannot understand speech but may retain the power of uttering words and even of reading aloud, but with no understanding of what he is reading.

Management must vary with the cause, but often there is some spontaneous recovery as the original condition subsides.

aphonia. Loss of voice, usually due to some disorder in the vocal cords. An acute form is found in laryngitis, and a more persisting but less complete variety is found in persons who habitually over-use their voices. Aphonia is also a common symptom in hysteria. For inflammatory aphonia rest of the voice is essential and steam inhalations of friar's balsam may help.

aphrodisiac. Any food, drink or drug believed to stimulate sexual desire or sexual activity. Over the centuries there have been extraordinary numbers of alleged aphrodisiacs, such as caviar, wheat-germ oil and celery, but none of these are of proved value, while cantharides simply acts by irritating the whole urinary system, and alcohol increases sexual desire but reduces sexual performance.

apomorphine. An alkaloid derived from morphia. When injected under the skin it rapidly induces vomiting so that it is useful in cases of non-corrosive poisoning.

apoplexy. A condition, colloquially called 'stroke' in England and 'shock' in Scotland, caused by interruption of the normal circulation in the brain. The three usual causes are: (1) cerebral haemorrhage, the bursting of a small blood vessel in the brain; (2) cerebral embolism, the blocking of a blood vessel by an obstruction, e.g., a fragment of a diseased heart valve; and (3) cerebral thrombosis, the blocking of a vessel by the formation of a clot.

The immediate treatment is to loosen

constrictive clothing (e.g., the collar) to turn the head to the side, reducing the danger of the patient choking, and to summon the doctor. See STROKE.

appendicectomy or **appendectomy.** Surgical removal of the appendix as in acute or chronic appendicitis.

appendicitis. Inflammation or abscess of the appendix, the commonest emergency of abdominal surgery. The condition, rare in primitive societies, seems to be associated with refined, low-residue diets. If bacteria and faeces enter the appendix, it – along with the adjacent peritoneum – becomes inflamed, and if the condition is untreated general peritonitis may follow with serious danger to life.

The main symptom of appendicitis is severe abdominal pain, usually at first generalized but settling in a position low on the right. There is marked local tenderness which is important in diagnosis, and nausea and vomiting may occur. Treatment is essentially by immediate surgical removal. This was considered a dangerous operation sixty years ago but is nowadays regarded as simple, straightforward and practically devoid of risk to life; persons unfit for operation sometimes respond to antibiotics.

Chronic appendicitis is a condition in which the diseased appendix causes vague and usually intermittent abdominal pain and tenderness. Diagnosis of a 'grumbling appendix' is not easy, but when it is made the obvious remedy is surgical removal.

appendix. A small blind tube, 7 to 10 cm. (3 to 4 in.) long, leading from the caecum at the junction of the small and large intestine. It has no known function and is probably a vestigial structure, i.e., a now needless organ left over in the course of evolution. It only becomes important when germs and faecal matter enter from the caecum and produce APPENDICITIS.

appetite. Desire for food and drink. Appetite should be differentiated from hunger. The latter, physical need for food, occurs when the stomach is empty and is accompanied by hunger pangs produced by contractions of the muscles of the stomach. By contrast, appetite can be present when the stomach is full and absent when it is empty although, fortunately, appetite and hunger normally coincide.

Appetite is in part created by sight: an interesting, well-cooked meal, pleasantly displayed and served in clean and cheerful surroundings, is more likely to stimulate appetite than a distasteful-looking food, badly served. In part it is created by the smell and taste of food: attractive food stimulates the secretion of salivary and gastric juices which are necessary for digestion. In part it is dependent on mental states: few of us have much desire for food when very angry or deeply grieved, although some people who feel unloved or bereaved develop a habit of eating in compensation for lack of affection.

Loss of appetite is most commonly a

The appendix

result of worry, apprehension or emotional upset, so disturbing and emotional topics should be avoided at meal-times and, where practicable, there should be a period of relaxation before a meal. Mental fatigue, physical exhaustion and impairment of the senses of smell and taste (as in the common cold) are other causes of poor appetite. Excessive smoking may also reduce appetite, as may eating between meals, too much alcohol, constipation, septic conditions of the gums and teeth, and various diseases of the stomach, liver and kidneys. Loss of appetite persisting for more than a few days requires medical attention. See also ANOREXIA.

Increased appetite may be found in cases of dilated stomach and in pregnancy, and, as already mentioned, it occurs in some people who are unhappy. It is also sometimes found in diabetes and hyperthyroidism, which results from goitre.

Perverted appetite, a desire to eat rare or strange things, is one of the symptoms of several mental diseases and also occasionally occurs in pregnancy.

arcus senilis. A white crescent appearing just below the upper margin (and later just above the lower margin) of the cornea of the eye. It is caused by fatty deposits in the corneal tissue. It does not increase and does not interfere with vision but is one of the recognized signs of advancing years.

arm. In ordinary speech the arm is the whole upper limb, but in descriptive anatomy the term is restricted to the part extending from the shoulder to the elbow (i.e., excluding the forearm). Its bone is the humerus, which joins with the scapula above, forming a swivel joint that can move in any direction, and with the radius and ulna below, forming a hinge joint. Its muscles are the deltoid over the shoulder, the biceps in front and the triceps behind; and its main blood supply is from the brachial artery.

armpit. The deep space, otherwise known as the axilla, between the upper chest wall and the upper part of the arm. It is enclosed by the pectoral muscles in front and the latissimus dorsi muscle behind. It contains the nerves and blood vessels for the upper limb and also a group of lymph glands; these can become inflamed from infection spreading upwards from the hand and may also be infected from the breast.

The axilla is well equipped with sweat glands and therefore needs frequent washing to remove perspiration and reduce odour.

arrhythmia. Any variation from the ordinary rhythm of the heart, which is normally regular in time and force. Arrhythmia is produced by any condition which interferes with the normal beating of the heart. Examples are: sinus arrhythmia (the normal variation caused by breathing, more rapid during inspiration and slower during expiration), extrasystoles (where there is an occasional premature beat followed by the missing of a normal beat), auricular fibrillation, auricular flutter, heart block and paroxysmal tachycardia.

arsenic. A crystalline metal, used from early times as a medicine and as a poison. In very small doses it has an alleged tonic effect, and an arsenical preparation, neoarsphenamine, was the standard treatment for syphilis until the era of antibiotics.

Arsenical poisoning causes vomiting and diarrhoea, numbness of the feet, muscular cramps and collapse. Until recently treatment consisted mainly of giving an emetic (to get rid of arsenic not yet absorbed) and keeping the patient warm, but a relatively new drug, BAL (British Anti-Lewisite or dimercaprol) has proved useful in poisoning by organic arsenical compounds.

Arsenic is used in insecticides and in the manufacture of glass and various pharmaceuticals, and accidental poisoning is largely from inhalation of dust. Preventive measures include (1) substitution, where practicable, of non-toxic substances, (2) exhaust ventilation, (3) use of protective clothing, including masks where appropriate, and (4) periodic medical examination to detect skin pigmentation and other early signs of chronic arsenical poisoning.

arteriosclerosis. Hardening and thickening of the coats of arteries, with consequent loss of the elasticity of the coats. This makes the arteries (1) narrower, so that increased pressure by the heart is needed to push the blood through, (2) brittle, and therefore liable to rupture, and (3) rough, with danger of blood clotting on the roughened surface.

Causes. The condition, the commonest vascular disease in developed countries, is primarily due to the deposit of minerals and fatty particles in the arterial walls, it both causes high blood pressure and is exacerbated by high blood pressure. The disease is frequent in persons whose diet is rich in foods containing large quantities of animal fats (e.g., fat meat, butter and cream) and it is thought that the saturated fatty acids in these foods raise the level of blood cholesterol and facilitate the depositing of fatty particles. Hence the partial substitution of foods containing unsaturated fatty acids (e.g., vegetable oils) should decrease arteriosclerosis. However, although the disease seldom produces symptoms until middle age, the substitution should be made much earlier, to prevent the early deposits which precede symptoms by many years.

Not all experts fully accept the cholesterol theory. Some maintain that excessive carbohydrates and resulting obesity are as potent factors, that heavy muscular work raises the blood pressure and throws strain on the vessel walls, that mental stress plays a considerable part probably by raising the blood pressure, and that heavy smoking is a factor. Others suggest that arteriosclerosis is simply a degenerative condition towards which some people inherit a tendency; but while the condition undoubtedly runs in families, the explanation may lie in family dietetic habits.

There are some associations between arteriosclerosis, coronary thrombosis, high blood pressure and chronic nephritis; almost certainly all four have several factors causing them, the main single one probably being high blood cholesterol.

Symptoms. Common early symptoms include loss of physical and mental vigour, giddiness, headache and attacks of breathlessness. Often, however, there are no specific symptoms until the arterial and blood pressure changes cause a major catastrophe, such as coronary thrombosis or cerebral thrombosis (STROKE).

Treatment. While a single, badly affected artery can be surgically repaired or replaced, there is no cure for generalized arterial thickening, but much can be done to check its advance and to prolong useful life. In particular, no extra strain – as from violent excitement or violent exercise – should be thrown on the heart and blood vessels, diet should be moderate, and alcohol and tobacco should be limited. Anticoagulant drugs may reduce the risk of clotting; and, although the body requires a fairly high blood

Artificial respiration: Schafer's method

pressure because of the narrowness of the vessels, drugs that reduce the pressure may be used in moderation.

Prevention. In the present state of knowledge the best preventive measures would appear to be: (1) avoidance of excessive animal fat from childhood or adolescence onwards, but bearing in mind the need for sufficient quantities of the fat soluble vitamins; (2) avoidance of excessive carbohydrates; (3) reasonable and regular exercise but avoidance of extreme muscular strain; (4) avoidance or limitation of smoking; and (5) avoidance of mental stress and emotional disturbance. Inevitably some people would consider that complete acceptance of these preventive measures would make life too dull and that a workable compromise is necessary to limit the risk of arteriosclerosis without damaging the quality of life.

artery. Any vessel carrying blood away from the heart. The pulmonary arteries convey blood to the lungs to receive oxygen. All other arteries carry oxygenated blood from the heart to the tissues.

The arterial system can be considered as resembling a tree with the aorta as its trunk; the carotids (to the head), subclavians (to the arms) and common iliacs (to the legs) as its main branches; thereafter it divides into smaller and smaller branches which end in numerous 'twigs' called arterioles. These in turn lead to a mesh of capillaries from which the oxygen and carbon dioxide exchange with the tissues takes place.

Each artery has an outer coat of connective tissue, a middle coat of elastic and muscular tissue, and an inner coat of fine cells which do not allow the blood to clot.

When cut across, arteries do not collapse, so that injury to an artery causes dangerous bleeding. Arterial bleeding is characterized by being bright red and spurting in jets coinciding with the heart-beat. Bleeding from a small artery can be stopped by applying pressure directly on the artery over the cut end nearer the heart. To stop bleeding from a large artery it is necessary to apply considerable pressure at a point where the artery lies close to a bone. See HAEMORRHAGE for arterial pressure points.

arthritis. Inflammation of a joint. It may be acute or chronic and due to many different causes, ranging from infection of joints and their related structures by identifiable organisms to the destruction of joints which occurs in certain diseases of the nervous system. Examples of infective forms are tubercular arthritis, gonococcal arthritis (arising from gonorrhoea), and streptococcal arthritis (resulting from infection from a wound) but antibiotic treatment has greatly reduced the risk of such diseases affecting the joints.

The term is most often used in reference to three common crippling diseases: rheumatoid arthritis, osteo-arthritis, and gout.

articulation. See JOINT.

artificial insemination. The introduction of male seminal fluid into the genital tract of the female by artificial means for the purpose of producing conception and pregnancy. The procedure is mainly used in veterinary practice for stock-breeding purposes.

Artificial insemination (which is carried out at the time of ovulation) has only a limited place in human reproduction. The semen of the husband can be used (artificial insemination-husband: AIH) when a husband is fertile but impotent, or semen of a donor (AID) when the husband is infertile. However, AID is fraught with medico-legal difficulties, for any offspring is technically illegitimate.

artificial pneumothorax. Artificial pneumothorax is the condition which results when air is deliberately introduced into the chest (pleural cavity) to produce collapse of one lung. The procedure is intended to put a diseased lung at rest in order to encourage healing, to promote the collapse and obliteration of infected cavities, and to minimize any tendency to bleeding from damaged areas.

artificial respiration. In cases of asphyxia from various causes such as drowning, suffocation, exposure to poisonous gases, narcotic poisoning, and electrocution, a patient's natural respiration may have

Mouth-to-mouth resuscitation

stopped but his heart and circulation and the vital processes of his central nervous system may not yet be incapable of recovery. If some form of 'breathing' can be contrived so that his blood receives a continuing supply of oxygen there is a chance that his life may be saved.

The various methods of doing this are known as 'artificial respiration' by which inspiration (breathing in) and expiration (breathing out) are artificially induced.

Although there are resuscitation appliances available for the maintenance of respiration, the nature of the emergency is such that it brooks of no delay. Treatment should be commenced forthwith and *must not be delayed* in anticipation of the arrival of skilled help and special equipment.

No matter which procedure is employed it is essential to make sure that there is a clear airway and that the upper part of the respiratory passages is not obstructed by a sagging jaw, by the tongue, or by dentures (which should always be looked for and removed). In cases of drowning it is essential as a first step to eliminate water from the air passages by tilting the patient's head downwards and compressing the chest.

The patient should also be treated in reasonably open surroundings where there is adequate fresh air, and it is advisable to take steps to conserve body heat by blankets or improvised additional covering.

Manual methods. These make use of the principle that some exchange of gases in the blood supply within the lungs can be achieved by alternate compression and relaxation of the chest wall.

The method which is probably most effective and least fatiguing for the operator is Schafer's. The patient is laid face downward with the head turned to one side. The operator kneels astride and with both hands and spread fingers placed on the back leans forward with his arms straight and compresses the chest by his weight (expiration). He then removes the pressure he is exerting and allows the chest to expand (inspiration).

In all these methods the movements should be repeated between ten and fifteen times per minute. If natural respiration shows signs of re-starting, the movements should be synchronized with the patient's efforts.

Eve's rocking stretcher. This is a very effective method which operates on a slightly different principle. It requires some equipment which may readily be improvised.

The patient is secured face-down by legs and arms to a stretcher or plank, which is then balanced at its mid-point on a trestle.

When tilted head down to 45 degrees the abdominal contents push on the diaphragm and compress the lungs (expiration). The stretcher is then tilted feet down to the same extent, the abdominal contents move downwards, drawing the diaphragm down also and air is drawn into the chest (inspiration).

Mouth-to-mouth resuscitation. This is the method popularly known as the 'kiss of life', and is really not so much mouth-to-mouth as mouth-to-nose. It is efficient and its use is indicated if there is any suspicion of fractures or other injuries.

After making sure that there is a clear airway and that the head is tilted back the operator holds the patient's mouth closed. He then applies his lips to the patient's nose and blows. The patient's chest rises with the insufflated air (inspiration), and is then allowed to relax again (expiration). As in the other methods this is repeated between ten and fifteen times a minute. The procedure may be made rather more aesthetic by the use of a simple plastic tube known as a Brook Airway which should form part of any First Aid kit.

Mechanical methods. A variety of special devices is available ranging from an airway with bellows to more elaborate mechanical equipment (e.g., iron lung) which may also be capable of supplying additional oxygen or oxygen and carbon dioxide mixtures. Most ambulances now carry such appliances as standard equipment but their safe and successful use requires some training and experience.

If natural respiration is not speedily restored the question then arises as to how long attempts at artificial respiration should be prolonged. In the absence of any professional advice it would be reasonable to assume that death had occurred if no response was obtained after one hour. In cases of poisoning from drugs, however, there may be severe depression of the respiratory centre and it would be wise to persist until the patient comes under hospital treatment.

artificial sweeteners. Synthetic compounds of no food value used to sweeten foods and drinks. Diabetics, who have to restrict their intake of sugar, either have to consume their food and drink unsweetened or to use artificial sweeteners. Persons who are overweight often employ these sweeteners as a convenient method of slightly reducing their calorie intake: for a person who drinks six cups of tea or coffee daily, with one teaspoonful of sugar in each cup, the substitution of a sweetener represents a reduction of about 150 Calories each day.

The most commonly used sweeteners are saccharin and the commercial preparations made from it. Another group of sweeteners, cyclamates, are now restricted in many countries because large amounts have been shown to have harmful effects on animals, although these effects have not been fully proved in man.

Ascheim-Zondek test. A test described in 1927 by two German gynaecologists for the early diagnosis of PREGNANCY.

ascites. The accumulation of free fluid within the abdominal cavity.

Causes. (1) Infections of the peritoneum (the membrane lining the abdominal cavity) such as tuberculosis or malignant diseases; (2) obstructions of the venous blood flow through the liver (the portal circulation) as in cirrhosis; (3) congestive cardiac failure; (4) chronic kidney disease, and (5) some types of severe anaemia.

Treatment. This is directed to the underlying disease, but the amount of accumulated fluid and the resultant abdominal distension may be very great and may produce symptoms such as difficulty in breathing with impairment of circulation and digestion in a purely mechanical way, because of the weight and pressure. When this occurs relief can be given by 'paracentesis', a simple operation for withdrawal of fluid through a hollow needle.

A salt-free diet and the administration of diuretics to increase the flow of urine from the kidneys may help to slow down the rate at which fluid re-accumulates.

ascorbic acid. Diets inadequate in fresh fruit and vegetables ultimately result in scurvy. This was recognized at least 150 years ago, and sailors were given a daily issue of lemon or lime juice to compensate for the lack of some unknown but obviously essential substance not provided by their sea-going rations. This substance was given the name vitamin C (see VITAMINS) and in 1937 research showed that it was ascorbic acid, a precise and relatively simple chemical compound.

Oranges, lemons, tomatoes, cabbages and other green vegetables are among the best natural sources of this vitamin but it is readily destroyed by overcooking, especially in the presence of air and of alkalis such as sodium bicarbonate.

In man the daily requirements of ascorbic acid are 1mg. per kg. body weight and about twice that amount for babies and pregnant women.

Vitamin C is not stored in the body and a higher intake is desirable during infective illness when the rate of utilization tends to increase. There is also a claim that doses of 1g. or more per day prevent or cure the common cold.

asepsis. The total exclusion of micro-organisms from the tissues during any surgical procedure.

Bacteria are to be found everywhere and during surgical operation there is a risk that they may gain access to a wound from the environment, from the person and clothing of the attendants, and from the surgical instruments and dressings. In an aseptic technique it is necessary that all these possible sources of bacterial infection should receive attention, and so operations are now carried out in specially designed operating theatres, which can be thoroughly cleaned and disinfected. The most modern also have arrangements for filtering or sterilizing the air. The surgeons and nurses change their outdoor clothing and after prolonged washing and scrubbing of their hands and arms array themselves in gowns, overboots, caps, masks, and rubber gloves, all of which have been previously sterilized and rendered germ free by autoclaving – a process of disinfection using steam at raised temperature and pressure.

Surgical instruments and dressings are usually similarly sterilized, although alternative methods may be used for instruments which could be damaged by heat. Increasing use is also being made of disposable small instruments, such as syringes and needles, which can be discarded after a single use. These are supplied commercially in sealed outer covers, having been sterilized after enclosure by the application of gamma radiation.

aspergillosis. A type of long-lasting chest infection due to invasion of the lung by fungi of the genus *Aspergillus.* The fungi grow in mouldy grain, and the disease is acquired either by chewing such grain or by inhaling its dust.

The disease mainly occurs amongst workers in grain stores, flour factories, malting floors and so on, and pigeon fanciers are traditionally liable because of the practice of feeding young birds by transferring grain from their own mouths.

Both from symptoms and x-ray the disease is liable to be confused with pulmonary tuberculosis but laboratory examination of the sputum should ensure a correct diagnosis. For treatment various antibiotics have been claimed to be helpful, steroids are sometimes used and an aspergillus vaccine is occasionally tried.

asphyxia. The condition which results when any interference with any stage of respiration denies the body tissues an adequate and continuous supply of oxygen.

Causes. 1. Obstruction to air-flow: smothering; obstruction by foreign body; throttling, strangulation, hanging; inhalation of vomit; fluid in the air passages as in drowning; injury and swelling of tissues from disease, burns, scalds, and corrosive poisons.

2. Quality of inspired air: irrespirable gases; rarefaction of the atmosphere as in mountaineering or high-altitude flying.

3. Failure of inspiratory effort: fixation of chest and abdomen by pressure as in burial by debris, crowd accidents, and overlaying of infants; penetrating wounds of chest causing pneumothorax; paralysis of voluntary muscles, as in poliomyelitis and injuries to the spinal cord.

4. Failure of respiratory exchange: disease of lung such as pneumonia; inadequate circulation as in heart failure; interference with oxygen-carrying

capacity of haemoglobin as in carbon monoxide poisoning.

5. Impairment of respiratory centre: narcotic poisons; head injuries; intracranial disease.

In acute asphyxia the patient struggles for breath, respiratory movements become violent, the face becomes livid and neck veins appear engorged. This first stage may last for about three minutes until unconsciousness occurs; respiration now ceases but the heart will continue to beat for a variable period and recovery may still be possible if the cause of the asphyxia can be removed and ARTIFICIAL RESPIRATION begun.

Some types of asphyxia require tracheotomy intubation and mechanical assistance with respiration.

In asphyxia of gradual onset due to disease the treatment is that of the underlying disease and the administration of oxygen may help.

Asphyxia of the new-born. Before birth the infant receives its oxygen supply from the maternal circulation. The oxygen is exchanged for carbon dioxide across the placenta, supplied on one side by maternal blood, and on the other by the infant's blood stream which reaches it and returns by the umbilical cord. At birth there is an abrupt change because this method of gaseous exchange ceases, the accumulation of carbon dioxide in the infant's blood then stimulates his respiratory centre, and he tries to breathe air in the normal manner.

If at any stage before delivery this process is initiated prematurely, the infant is born with a deficiency of oxygen and an accumulation of carbon dioxide in the blood stream and is thus in a state of asphyxia.

The chief causes of interference with the placental circulation before birth are prolonged labour, premature separation of the placenta, and pressure on the umbilical cord or its twisting or expulsion before the birth of the baby. The administration of drugs to the mother may impair the respiratory centre of the infant. However, even in the absence of any of these causes the premature infant may be born in an asphyxiated state because of the inherent feebleness of its circulation.

Asphyxia may also result from the inhalation of mucus or amniotic fluid during the infant's initial attempts to breathe, from brain damage during delivery, or from a failure of the lungs to expand properly.

aspiration. The act of sucking out fluids or gases from a vessel or cavity.

aspirin. Originally a proprietary name, 'Aspirin' is a synonym for acetylsalicylic acid, much used as a household remedy. It acts by allaying pain and diminishing fever and it is particularly helpful in rheumatic conditions.

A gastric irritant, it may cause indigestion or gastric haemorrhage, and in some sensitive persons it produces skin-rashes or asthma. It should not be given to infants and only with caution to small children. Household supplies of the drug should be kept out of reach of children owing to the substantial risk of accidental poisoning.

Symptoms of aspirin overdosage in a child include drowsiness, pallor and heavy breathing. In an older child or an adult these symptoms are often accompanied by dizziness and a sensation of alarm. Very rarely a rash appears on the skin. The immediate treatment of overdosage is to wash out the stomach with a 0.5 per cent solution of sodium bicarbonate (baking soda).

asthma. A respiratory disease characterized by recurrent paroxysmal attacks of difficulty in breathing, usually accompanied by wheezing, cough, and a sense of constriction of the chest. It may be associated with bronchitis but true bronchial asthma can occur quite independently.

It is due to spasm of the muscular fibres in the walls of the smaller air passages in the lungs (bronchioles). This reduces the size of the airway and impedes the respiratory air flow, particularly when breathing in. Activity of these muscle fibres is controlled by nervous impulses reaching them from the autonomic, or involuntary, part of the nervous system, particularly the vagus nerve.

Causes. The asthmatic attack is therefore brought about by factors which influence this nervous control. Amongst these are: (1) direct irritation of the bronchial mucous membrane; (2) reflex irritation from disease elsewhere, especially infection in the nose and throat; gastric irritation; intestinal infection; and (3) sensitivity or allergy: individual patients may be sensitive to a great variety of substances such as pollens, animal dandruff, hair and feathers, certain foods, moulds, house dust, and so on; house dust has frequently been shown to contain products of the house mite. Finally, (4) psychological factors such as sudden severe emotion, fear, anxiety, anger, and more deep-seated personality disorders undoubtedly play a part in precipitating some attacks.

Asthma may occur at any age but it is common in children, when it is often associated with eczematous dermatitis. It is more common in males. A hereditary tendency is well-recognized and often the patient's personality is of a definite type – highly strung and of general nervous instability.

Treatment. The acute attack usually responds quite dramatically to the administration of adrenalin, ephedrine, antihistamines, or the use of inhalations based on measured doses of newer drugs such as isoprenaline or cromoglycate; but the long-term treatment of the condition is difficult and unrewarding.

Skin tests should be used to detect any specific allergen and positive results followed up by desensitization. Any source of infection should be searched for and eradicated. Breathing exercises are sometimes helpful. Otherwise the indications are to attend to general health and hygiene and to provide drugs such as inhalant sprays for either routine use or relief of symptoms.

astigmatism. A defect of EYESIGHT in which the front of the eye is not curved uniformly so that the whole of an image cannot be brought into focus.

astringent. Substance which, when applied to skin or mucous membranes, contracts blood vessels and secretory ducts (so limiting haemorrhage or discharge) and which shrinks swollen membranes.

Those used to arrest superficial bleeding are given the special name of 'styptics' – e.g., alum and ferric salts.

Some astringents and where they act are: (1) on blood vessels – cold compresses; adrenalin; stypticin. (2) On skin ulceration – preparations of lead sub-acetate; silver nitrate; zinc sulphate (lotio rubra); calamine lotion. (3) On mucous membranes – alum; tannic acid. (4) On nose and throat – sprays of ephedrine. (5) On conjunctiva – zinc sulphate eye drops.

ataxia. Incoordination of voluntary movement characterized by an unsteady gait, lack of precision in hand and arm movements and inability to stand steady with the eyes closed (Romberg's sign).

There are three principal causes: (1) organic disease of the central nervous system affecting the cerebellum or the sensory pathways in the spinal cord (locomotor ataxia in the third stage of syphilis is the classic example of a disease affecting the spinal cord in this way), (2) disturbance of the balancing mechanism of the internal ear occurring in Ménière's disease and other types of vertigo, and (3) functional disorder of the nervous system due to the effect of alcohol or other drugs.

atelectasis. Incomplete expansion of one or both lungs. This is a relatively common cause of perinatal death, the infant failing to breathe properly and so to expand the lungs.

atheroma. Thickening and degeneration of the inner coat – and less often of the middle coat – of arteries, occasioned largely by wear and tear, and encountered mainly in old people and in persons with high blood pressure. Since the condition interferes with the passage of blood along the arteries it to some extent also creates high blood pressure and is one of the factors in causing ARTERIOSCLEROSIS.

atherosclerosis. See ARTERIOSCLEROSIS.

athlete's foot. A disease of the feet (and occasionally of the hands) characterized by white, sodden-looking skin on the inner surface of the foot with groups of blisters especially between the toes. The condition is an infection, due to a fungus closely allied to that of RINGWORM, and can spread wherever people mix in bare feet, e.g., at swimming baths. Excessive perspiration appears to render feet more susceptible.

Prevention includes adequate cleansing and disinfection of the surfaces liable to carry the infection. Daily applications of magenta paint are commonly recommended for treatment. The washing of sweaty feet both night and morning and the changing of socks daily assist both prevention and treatment.

atlas. The first cervical vertebra, i.e., the topmost of the bones forming the spinal column. It consists of a complete ring of bone, supports the head, and permits backward and forward movements of the head. Sideways movement of the head is really permitted by the second vertebra, the AXIS.

atrium. One of the muscular chambers of the HEART, often called an auricle.

atrophy. The shrinkage or wasting of any cell, tissue, limb, or organ.

Atrophy may be local or generalized and the latter in particular is part of the normal process of ageing. Some examples will illustrate the principles of other more specific causes.

1. Disuse atrophy: limbs which are splinted for long periods or immobilized by disease rapidly show muscular wasting.

2. Interference with nerve supply: damage within the brain (as in cerebral vascular disease such as cerebral haemorrhage) or in the spinal cord (as in poliomyelitis) causes paralysis and muscular atrophy. In other nervous and muscular diseases degeneration of spinal nerve cells produces a similar result.

3. Interference with blood supply: vascular disease can reduce blood flow to any part and impair its nutrition; this is especially important in the coronary vessels of the heart. Local pressure (as with a cervical rib) can act similarly.

4. Absorption of bone: old persons develop bone wasting leading to fractures from trivial causes and atrophy of jaw bones leads to loss of teeth.

5. Toxins: atrophy of optic nerve transmitting impulses of sight from the eye; acute yellow atrophy of the liver; inflammation of various nerves as in lead poisoning.

6. Infections: peripheral nerve lesions as in leprosy; degeneration of muscle in typhoid fever.

atropine. An alkaloid which is the active constituent of belladonna, a medicinal agent originally derived from the deadly nightshade plant although other sources are now used commercially.

Atropine is an important drug and its therapeutic effect is due to its selective action on the vagus nerve, which is inhibited. It is therefore employed to cause relaxation of involuntary muscle, i.e., the muscles of the body (mainly in the digestion system) which cannot be controlled at will. Atropine is particularly useful in such conditions as renal or intestinal colic, gastric ulcer and bronchial spasm associated with asthma. It is also prescribed before operation to reduce bronchial secretion and before certain eye examinations to dilate the pupil.

Undesirable side effects include increased pulse rate, dryness of the mouth, and inability to focus near objects.

It is a powerful and poisonous drug, effective in very small doses (0.3 to 0.6 mg.). Symptoms of overdose are alarming, with mental confusion, hallucinations, high temperature, blurred vision, a hot dry skin (due to inhibition of sweating) and sometimes a rash resembling scarlet fever. Treatment includes giving an emetic to induce vomiting, keeping the patient warm and providing ample hot fluids such as strong coffee.

aura. Any peculiar sensation or phenomenon preceding an attack of an illness such as epilepsy or migraine.

In the case of an epileptic fit, general symptoms such as headache, irritability, elation, or lethargy may be experienced some days before an attack, but usually the premonition is more immediate and takes the form of hallucinations of sensations such as visual images, strange noises and smells.

The aura which precedes attacks of migraine is very often visual, with flashes of dazzling light and dark and bright spots.

auricle. One of the muscular chambers of the HEART more correctly known as an atrium.

auricular fibrillation. A type of disordered heart action. The normal heart beat is a regular rhythmic contraction of the auricles followed by similar contraction of the ventricles. Impulses causing this originate in the 'pacemaker' of the HEART and pass in sequence to auricles and ventricles along a band of specialized muscle fibre. The rate and intensity of the impulses are determined by nervous and chemical stimuli influencing the pacemaker.

If this conducting band of specialized muscle is damaged by cardiac disease the regular coordinated contractions of the auricles become irregular, uncoordinated, and excessively fast. This is auricular fibrillation. The rate, rhythm, and force of ventricular contraction are also disordered by the imperfect impulses, causing the pulse to be weakened and irregular.

autism. A condition in which a child appears aloof and cut off from the world, with no apparent emotion (except occasional outbursts of rage), no indication of affection or response to affection, stereotyped mannerisms, an interest in toys rather than people and an avoidance of eye contact. Because the child does not listen to speech his speech is usually retarded and he is sometimes, wrongly, thought to be deaf; and in the past many autistic children have been falsely diagnosed as mentally defective, although, apart from speech problems, they show no indications of low intelligence.

As yet no adequate preventive measures exist, but with skilled management the outlook – formerly very bleak – can be greatly improved and an autistic child can often grow into an adult capable of earning his living and maintaining a reasonable existence.

automatism. A state of impaired consciousness in which a person acts in an apparently conscious manner but with no recollection afterwards of having done so. It occurs particularly after seizures of EPILEPSY and is of medico-legal importance when used as a defence against allegations of crime or indecency.

Somnambulism or 'sleep-walking' is another example of automatism; and likewise the true alcoholic after even a mild debauch may recover days later unaware of what he has done in the interval.

autonomic nervous system. See NERVOUS SYSTEM.

auto-suggestion. A form of self-hypnotism.

Certain psychosomatic diseases may be due to, or influenced by, psychic or emotional factors affecting the subconscious so that the patient experiences bodily symptoms which his conscious mind regards as 'real'. Auto-suggestion attempts to reverse this process by enforcing a conscious effort to appreciate the psychic or 'unreal' nature of the symptoms in the expectation that if the patient is really convinced at the level of conscious thought, the subconscious mind will accept that its apprehensions are unfounded. Conditions which may fall into this category include certain cases of gastric ulcer, asthma, migraine, and many skin diseases.

axilla. See ARMPIT.

axis. The second cervical vertebra, i.e., the second bone from the top in the spinal column. It has a small projection on its upper edge which lies in a hollow of the atlas (the first cervical vertebra). The skull and atlas can move around this, enabling the head to be turned to right and left.

B

baby. The human infant from birth until it begins to walk and becomes a 'toddler'.

A still-born baby is a child born dead after a pregnancy lasting long enough for viability – about twenty-eight weeks. Premature and post-mature babies respectively are those resulting from pregnancies shorter or longer than the normal period of about 280 days. A dysmature baby is one whose development at birth is less advanced than expected from its gestational age – the 'small-for-dates' baby.

See also articles on INFANCY, INFANT, POST-MATURITY and PREMATURITY.

bacilluria. The presence of bacilli in the urine.

bacillus. A term commonly used for any rod-shaped micro-organism or bacterium. See BACTERIA.

backache. Backache is a symptom and not a disease in itself. The term is used in a general way to describe pain and disability related to the spine and particularly the so-called 'low back pain' of the lumbar region and sacral part of the pelvis.

It is common in middle-aged and overweight women and is a major cause of industrial disability in manual workers. In the latter, because of the subjective nature of the complaint, it often causes difficulty in the certification of incapacity if there are inadequate physical signs.

Anatomy. Any rational discussion of the cause must be founded on the anatomical features and relationship of the parts involved, including the pelvis, the lumbar vertebrae, their ligaments and muscles, and the abdomino-pelvic organs which can cause 'referred pain' in the back.

The SPINAL COLUMN of this region is composed of the five lumbar vertebrae, the sacrum (which forms the rear wall of the pelvis and is attached to it by the sacro-iliac joint on each side) and the tail-piece or coccyx. Between the lumbar vertebrae lie the cartilaginous discs. The bony vertebral arch below the level of the first lumbar vertebra protects the nerve fibres coming from the spinal cord, and these emerge, pair by pair, between the vertebrae and from openings on the sacrum.

These bones are supported and laced together by fibrous ligaments and attached to this composite structure are the muscles which provide the power for voluntary movement – bending forwards (flexion), backwards (extension), and sideways (lateral bending) and also some rotation.

Accurate diagnosis by physical examination depends on an assessment of the effect of these movements supplemented by neurological tests and x-ray investigation. Movements are tested by voluntary action – the patient performing the action unaided – and by passive movement – the doctor moving the limb without the aid of the patient. There must also be a careful external inspection with the patient suitably undressed to detect any other feature such as skeletal asymmetry or muscle-wasting.

Causes. With these anatomical considerations in mind the following can be enumerated:

1. Lumbago. Fibrositis or 'muscular rheumatism' affecting the lumbar muscles.

2. Lumbar back-strain. A localized rupture of some of the lumbar muscle fibres. There is usually a point of tenderness and resistance to only some directions of passive movement, contrasting with the generalized pain and spasm of lumbago.

3. Lumbo-sacral strain. Damage to the ligaments supporting the lumbo-sacral joint with localized tenderness over the joint and general restriction of movement. It is usually due to lifting stresses, especially with a bent back, and it is the commonest cause of chronic disability in the overweight person.

4. Sacro-iliac strain. Similar causes affecting the joints between the sacrum and pelvis. Usually on one side only, the point of maximum tenderness is off-centre to the affected side; bending forward and to the affected side are painful and restricted. The condition is sometimes seen in people who have to work standing with their weight mainly on one leg, e.g., dentists, or in cases where the legs are of unequal length.

In the foregoing it is often possible to make a diagnosis on clinical grounds alone, but x-ray examination may show up the following:

5. Osteo-arthritis of the spine. The movements of the lumbar spine are limited, and x-ray shows some thinning and outgrowths.

6. Prolapsed intervertebral disc. (Commonly known as 'slipped disc'.) Excessive strain may rupture the fibro-cartilaginous pad between vertebrae, and portions of it may protrude to cause pressure on the related spinal nerves emerging between the vertebrae. This is also a common cause of pain radiating down the leg in the regions served by the sciatic nerve (sciatica).

7. Spondylolisthesis. In this condition there is developmental defect of a vertebra, usually the fifth lumbar, so that it does not retain its proper position in relation to the sacrum.

wrong

right

wrong

right

wrong

right

The right and wrong way of doing things

wrong

right

wrong

right

The right and wrong way of doing things (contd.)

8. Other bone disease. The spine is a common site of osseous tuberculosis, and in malignant disease secondary tumour deposits may be seen on x-ray examination.

9. Other causes. Any investigation must include search for causes in the abdominal and pelvic organs. The commonest abdominal causes are diseases, such as infection or abscess of the kidney and related tissues together with malignant disease of any organ.

In the female there may be pain, usually felt in the sacro-iliac joints, resulting from the laxity of ligaments which occurs during and after childbirth. Pain may also be felt in the back from pelvic infection, a displaced uterus, or tumours of the uterus and ovaries.

Treatment. This depends entirely on professional determination of the underlying cause and only some general principles can be stated. Lumbago generally responds rapidly to rest, analgesics, and local heat, although it is prone to recur. Lumbar back strain is dealt with similarly but lumbo-sacral and sacro-iliac strain will probably require some form of supportive corset.

Prolapsed disc can often be relieved by traction and subsequent support but some cases come to operation for removal of the damaged disc and surgical ankylosis.

Osteo-arthritis is an established chronic condition for which not a great deal can be done except to provide support to limit painful movement. Spondylolisthesis is treated by surgical ankylosis. Tuberculosis of the spine requires prolonged immobilization and anti-tubercular drugs.

Pelvic and abdominal conditions call for local treatment where this is possible.

Prevention. Since causes are numerous, prevention is highly complex. To take some examples, sacro-iliac strain can in large measure be avoided by teaching people who have to lift heavy weights how best to do so; the backache caused by a displaced uterus can be avoided by post-natal examination of the woman and attention being given to the displaced organ. Tuberculosis of the spine can be prevented by general measures for the prevention of tuberculosis, and osteo-arthritis can be made less common by attention to weight and posture.

backwardness in children. A child who fails to reach developmental status appropriate to chronological age is regarded as 'backward' or retarded. The term is conventionally restricted to delayed development of physical and intellectual skills. Retarded growth in itself is 'dwarfism' and delayed emotional progress is better referred to as 'IMMATURITY'.

In a child of school age 'backwardness' implies a limitation of intellectual ability or a retardation of educational progress likely to preclude education in a normal class. In general, 'backwardness' implies a retardation less marked than that indicated by 'MENTAL DEFICIENCY'.

Causes. Some cases are genetic in origin and the commonest of these is mongolism (or Down's syndrome). Others such as phenylketonuria, galactosaemia and hypothyroidism (cretinism) are due to faulty METABOLISM and relatively uncommon but it is important that they should be recognized early so that suitable treatment can be given before irreparable brain damage occurs. Most of these, if untreated or untreatable, really fall into the more extreme category of mental deficiency.

Many more cases of mental retardation are due to adverse influences such as toxaemia, infection and anoxia, which may affect the child before, during, or immediately after birth. The frequent association of physical defects such as congenital heart disease and brain or nerve damage confirm some such specific causation.

There is, however, a normal range of intelligence in the individuals of any community, from the dullards to the very clever, and some children regarded as backward are really within the normal intellectual range. They have potential within the lower levels of the normal range of intelligence but their progress may have been impaired by social deprivation or emotional difficulties. With appropriate and understanding care and education they have good prospects of improvement.

Another important group comprises children who have no intellectual defect whatever but have been held back by some physical handicap such as deafness, defective vision, or paralysis. They respond to appropriate treatment - once recognized. (In the past this has too often failed to happen.)

Developmental assessment. A suspicion of backwardness is aroused when either the mother or (in Britain) the health visitor notices that a child is failing to reach the 'milestones' of its development during infancy and pre-school years at the expected age for any particular achievement. Points to note are when the child starts to smile, sit, stand, walk, speak, feed himself, and become toilet trained. Other guidelines are his response to visual and auditory stimuli, his attention to sounds, the ability to follow with his eyes, his use of meaningful phrases and sentences, and his readiness to play with building bricks. Feeding difficulties, sleeping difficulties, irritability, or undue placidity also require consideration in forming an assessment of mental deficiency.

Although observations of this kind have a reasonable predictive value, a more formal plan of developmental assessment is desirable for all children, and well-organized child welfare schemes are providing this to an increasing extent.

bacteria. Minute living organisms of vegetable nature, bacteria are visible only microscopically.

Bacteria are found in air, water, soil, on the skin and hair of animals including man, and particularly in the intestinal tract, and they are found too wherever there is death or decomposition, and often in disease. They are responsible for the spoilage of food, and effects such as the souring of milk and the putrefaction of cheese and meat are everyday examples of their action. Some are associated with specific diseases and are called 'pathogenic bacteria'. Many of the bacteria found in man are harmless – or even beneficial – but others cause disease.

Bacteria are exceedingly small, single-celled plants without chlorophyll and of various shapes. Round ones are called 'cocci', straight or curved rods are respectively 'bacilli' and 'vibrios'. Spiral or undulatory forms are 'spirilli'. The latter are mobile but some of the rod-shaped forms have whip-like extrusions of their protoplasm, called flagellae, which also serve for propulsion.

Under favourable conditions of food supply, moisture, and temperature, bacteria multiply rapidly and their 'colonies' become visible to the naked eye. Most species require oxygen for their development (the aerobes) but some cannot tolerate oxygen and are classified as anaerobes. They reproduce by swelling and then simply dividing into two at intervals of about every two hours, so that one bacterium on Monday morning may have given rise to four thousand by Tuesday morning and to several millions by Wednesday morning. However, some also reproduce by spores, which are rounded bodies appearing at the end or in the middle of a bacterium.

Bacteria in nature. Bacteria obtain their food supply by breaking down organic matter, particularly the dead tissues and waste products of animals and plants, and by doing this the constituent elements are liberated to re-enter the cycle of growth and decay. The most vital of these is nitrogen. By bacterial action ammonia is released from dead protein and further oxidation forms the nitrates necessary for soil-fertility and plant growth.

Some bacteria can also extract nitrogen from the atmosphere. They grow in root nodules on certain plants, particularly the legumes and clovers. These plants can be grown on poor soils and ploughed in to improve fertility for better pastures and heavier food crops. All these soil bacteria are essential to cultivation and indeed (as a link in the 'nitrogen cycle') to life itself.

Bacteria in industry. Many traditional crafts and industrial processes depend on bacteria. Examples are the making of cheese and wine, brewing, the maturation of silage, the decomposition of pectin in plant tissues as in flax-retting, the manufacture of alcohol, glycerin, acetic acid, citric acid and lactic acid, the production of enzymes and antibiotics, and many others. The biological treatment of sewage is another of their indispensable uses.

Bacteria and disease. Harmful micro-organisms vary considerably. There are protozoa, fungi, and viruses in addition to bacteria which can invade the body and multiply within it to cause illness, and often death, by tissue destruction and the effects of their toxic products.

The list of bacterial diseases in man is a long one and the following merely indicates the variety of well-known conditions which have a bacterial origin:

1. Wound infections: local sepsis due to staphylococci or streptococci; septicaemia from the same organisms; tetanus; anthrax.

2. Cardiac infections: bacterial endocarditis.

3. Respiratory tract infections: scarlet fever; diphtheria; pneumonia; tuberculosis; whooping cough.

4. Intestinal infections: typhoid and paratyphoid fevers; cholera; bacillary dysentery.

5. Urinary tract infections: gonorrhoea; intestinal organisms.

6. Central nervous system: cerebro-spinal fever; other forms of septic meningitis.

7. Generalized infections: plague; glanders; undulant fever.

Infection. When bacterial invasion of the body tissues takes place the result is called 'infection' and the organism responsible is deemed 'pathogenic' or capable of producing disease.

But 'pathogenic' is not a rigid term as applied to a particular micro-organism. It is often only pathogenic to a particular animal species, and its capacity to cause disease, even in that animal, is determined by various factors such as its present virulence, the numbers of bacteria present in the infective matter, the path of infection, the local tissue resistance of the victim, and his state of immunity.

If an individual is in a healthy or resistant state even large quantities of virulent bacteria can be destroyed by the body defences before damage occurs.

If, however, the bacteria gain a foothold they exercise their harmful effects by means of their toxins which are of two kinds – exotoxins and endotoxins – and the difference is fundamental for treatment. Exotoxins, as in diphtheria or tetanus, can be neutralized by a suitable anti-toxin, but organisms producing harmful effects by endotoxins must themselves be attacked and the prospect of doing this successfully has been greatly improved for most common bacterial diseases by the development of ANTIBIOTIC drugs.

The manner in which the body overcomes infection by its own efforts or is protected from it artificially is dealt with in the article on IMMUNITY.

balance. The sense of balance is maintained mainly by the three semi-circular canals at right angles to each other in the inner EAR. Movement of the head in any direction causes movement of the fluid in one or more canals, from which nervous impulses are passed to the brain which then directs appropriate muscles to adjust the position of the body. Balance is also assisted by vision and by pressure of the soles on the ground, but in general any disturbance of the sense of balance is due to factors affecting the inner ear.

balanitis. An acute inflammatory condition affecting the mucous membrane of the

baldness

38

head of the penis and accompanied by pain, swelling, and purulent discharge. It is usually associated with gonorrhoea, but poor hygiene and a redundant or unretractable foreskin may pre-dispose to an infection caused by other pus-forming organisms.

baldness. The lack or loss of hair, known medically as alopecia. It occurs almost exclusively in males (although it appears in some women after the menopause) and may commence quite early in adult life with atrophy of the hair-follicles (see HAIR). No specific cause is known and a tendency to early loss of hair is merely an inborn characteristic of the individual. Sometimes, but by no means always, it is associated with seborrhoea in which inflammation around the follicle may hasten the process.

Baldness usually follows a familiar pattern, with thinning of the hair on the temples and top of the head gradually extending until the crown is quite hairless or covered only by downy growth while the sides and back remain comparatively normal. No known treatment has any real success.

Apart from classical baldness, a temporary or permanent hair-loss may occur from toxic influences e.g., acute infections such as typhoid fever and poisoning from arsenic or thallium. X-rays produce a similar result.

bandages and bandaging. Bandages are strips of material used for binding up any part of the body, and bandaging is the procedure of applying them in the proper manner.

Purposes of bandaging. (1) To maintain in position a dressing, splint, or other application; (2) to maintain a limb or other part of the body in a desired position; (3) to supply support or pressure, as in varicose veins; (4) to limit the collecting of tissue fluids after injury; and (5) to prevent or control haemorrhage.

Types of bandage. Bandages are of many types, materials, and sizes, adapted to the purpose for which they are required, and may be either inextensible or elastic. Those commonly employed in modern practice are (1) cotton bandages of varying densities of weave – gauze, muslin, and calico; (2) flannel or domette (cotton warp; woollen weft) bandages; (3) crepe bandages with natural elasticity from the nature of their weave; (4) elastic adhesive bandages; (5) rubber bandages – used for arrest of haemorrhage; (6) plaster-of-paris bandages used for supporting fractures; and (7) tubular gauze bandages which require a special applicator.

Bandages are now manufactured in metric sizes and the commercial range for ordinary cotton is 2.5 cm., 5.0 cm., 7.5 cm., and 10 cm. in width by 5.0 m. in length. They are supplied rolled ready for use and usually known as roller bandages.

Special bandages. (1) Triangular bandage – an isosceles triangle of calico

with base of 127 cm. and sides of 90 cm. It is versatile and is extensively used for first aid work. (2) Many-tailed bandage, for chest and abdomen. (3) Four-tailed bandage, for jaw. (4) T-bandage, for perineum. (5) Capelline bandage, a double-headed roller bandage used for the scalp.

Principles of bandaging. The availability of loosely-woven and extensible materials which readily conform to the shape of the body has greatly reduced the degree of skill which bandaging formerly required, but the correct application of an ordinary roller bandage is still something of an art which needs practice and some study of the technique employed. More detailed instructions can be found in any good First Aid manual.

There are, however, three standard bandaging procedures which can be readily adapted to various situations.

1. The spiral bandage. Stand facing the part to be bandaged with a bandage of suitable width in the hand nearest the outer side of the limb and with the unrolled part of the bandage uppermost so that it will unroll readily. Start from below and bandage from within outwards over the front of the limb. After fixing the tail of the bandage by two superimposed turns proceed up the limb covering two-thirds of the preceding turn. This procedure can be continued on a part of uniform girth but when the limb widens the bandage will not lie flat and it is then necessary to introduce 'reverses'. To do this the last turn is fixed by the thumb of the disengaged hand and the bandage is allowed to turn over so that it forms a fold with the edge against the thumb; the inner surface of the bandage thus becomes the outer. Another turn is taken and the process repeated, care being taken to keep the reverses in line. Finally the bandage is tied off by splitting the end and knotting or secured with a safety-pin.

2. The figure-of-eight bandage. This is used for ankle, knee and elbow joints. Starting with two turns round the joint the bandage is applied in widening loops alternately above and below the joint. The centre point of the '8' is kept in front of the elbow and ankle and behind the knee.

3. The spica bandage. A modified figure-of-eight bandage used for shoulder and hip and also for the thumb. For the shoulder start with spiral turns round the upper arm till the armpit is reached. Then carry the bandage over the shoulder, across the back, under the opposite armpit, across the chest, over the injured shoulder, under the armpit of the same side, and so back to the starting point. This procedure is repeated until the shoulder is covered. In other situations the figure-of-eight is made round thigh and pelvis or thumb and wrist.

Cautions. Never bandage a limb below the lower level of a splint and always on completion of a bandage inspect the extremities of a limb to see that the circulation is not impaired. By pressing on

Bandaging

the nails and then releasing the pressure it can be judged if blood flow is satisfactory.

barber's rash. An infective condition of the skin of the face affecting the 'beard region' where there are hair follicles. There are three main types according to the infecting organism. Streptococcal infection causes superficial crusting, as in impetigo, and ringworm of the beard *(Tinea barbae)* may be either scaly or suppurative. Sycosis barbae is usually due to infection with staphylococci often from the patient's own nostrils, and caused by minor injury during shaving. Papules and pustules appear in the beard area, often with reddening of the surrounding skin.

Treatment is by application of an appropriate antibiotic twice daily for about a fortnight with avoidance of shaving or the use of an electric razor. Hygienic precautions should include the use of personal towels and their disinfection before laundering. Most cases clear up readily. In the very occasional case that does not respond to treatment the patient may have to be advised to discontinue shaving and grow a beard.

barbiturates. A large and varied group of drugs which reduce the activity of the central nervous system. They are organic compounds derived from barbituric acid.

Types. Barbiturates may be classified according to their pharmacological action:

1. General anaesthetic agents. Preparations given intravenously to produce short term general anaesthesia. They are extensively used in dentistry and in minor surgical procedures. Examples are thiopentone sodium, hexobarbitone sodium, and thialbarbitone sodium marketed under various trade names.

2. Hypnotics and sedatives. The distinction between a hypnotic and a sedative is largely a matter of dosage. Hypnotic doses directly induce sleep but the same drug in lesser dosage may be prescribed simply to induce mental relaxation, lessen emotional tension, and decrease anxiety.

Barbiturates of this group also differ in their duration of action and this can be a factor in deciding which particular preparation should be given. (1) Long-acting: phenobarbitone and derivatives; (2) medium-acting: allobarbitone, butobarbitone and amylobarbitone; (3) short-acting: cyclobarbitone, quinalbarbitone, etc.

3. Tranquillizers. These are used when it is desired to calm anxiety without noticeable sedation or impairment of mental function but there are better drugs for this than the barbiturates.

Use. Barbiturates undoubtedly have a legitimate place in medical practice but their use needs careful consideration and control.

In some individuals they produce undesirable side-effects such as nausea, diarrhoea, lassitude, vertigo, and skin eruptions. In the elderly they often cause mental confusion. Their effect is enhanced by simultaneous consumption of alcohol, and this is not always appreciated by persons driving motor-vehicles.

Tolerance to their use is easily acquired and there is a temptation to employ increasing doses. They are also cumulative and carry a serious risk of accidental or suicidal overdosage. Poisoning by barbiturates leads to breathing becoming slower and also shallower and may lead to coma. These conditions require intensive and skilled treatment, but despite this many fatalities still occur.

In relation to drug dependence barbiturates now cause considerable concern. Psychic dependence is a continuing demand for the administration of a drug either for pleasure or for the avoidance of discomfort, and the very widespread use of barbiturates is in many instances an example of this.

The size of the problem can be seen from the fact that in Britain 6 per cent of the total number of prescriptions written is for drugs in the barbiturate group. It is also estimated that there are at least 600,000 regular users of barbiturates of whom 100,000 are dependent.

barium. In its pure state barium is a pale yellow metallic element.

Its soluble salts are poisonous and are not now employed pharmacologically. Barium sulphate has however an important medical use in diagnostic x-ray work as it provides the radio-opaque constituent of 'barium meals' and enemata. The gastro-intestinal tract is not itself opaque to x-ray, but the barium sulphate in the tract makes it visible on the x-ray plate.

basal metabolism. See METABOLISM.

battered baby. A child who has been subjected to violence from a parent. The frequency of such cases has been slow to gain recognition because of a natural reluctance to believe that any parents could maltreat their children, but it has been suggested that up to 10 per cent of cases of serious childhood injury reaching hospital may be due to this cause. The battered baby syndrome, however, includes lesser injury, and the child who shows frequent bruising, and who apparently fails to thrive at home may equally be a victim of parental abuse and neglect.

The parents of such children fall into three overlapping groups: some 4 to 5 per cent have been shown to have psychopathic personalities, a large number are emotionally inadequate or emotionally immature (often as a result of deprivation

in their own childhood) and many, while apparently normal and well-adjusted, are harrassed to the point of frenzy by abnormal local or domestic circumstances.

For recognizing children 'at risk' the British health visitor is in a key position: her nursing training is supplemented by her further training in psychology and social science; in addition she has unique knowledge of the families she is visiting and unrivalled access to their homes without being sent for. Unfortunately, however, many mothers who have struck or felt strongly tempted to strike their babies are overwhelmed by guilt feelings, considering their conduct (or contemplated conduct) monstrous and unnatural. So, instead of confiding their impulses to the health visitor in order to get support and help, they try to conceal their aggressive feelings and to hide minor violence, without realizing that the same circumstances that created the impulse to violence may recur, and on that later occasion they may seriously hurt the child.

Where a child is identified as being 'at risk', whether by the mother wisely confiding or by the health visitor observing signs of aggression or potential aggression, prevention is still far from easy. The harrassed parent of reasonable maturity can at least be given help and support during times of crisis and can sometimes be afforded considerable relief by the older children being admitted to a day nursery or nursery school; the less mature or inadequate parent can also be helped by these measures, by counselling by the health visitor, and sometimes by being given an address or phone number to contact in moments of despair; but it is difficult to aid a psychopath (or two psychopaths, since like tends to marry like) and removal of a child deemed to be 'at risk' is generally impracticable until there is clear evidence that child abuse has actually taken place.

Collaboration between health visitors, social workers and general medical practitioners is obviously desirable and can appreciably reduce baby battering, but two types are probably unpreventable: (1) where the parent has shown no previous signs of abnormal aggression and the child has no unexplained bruises, but sudden circumstances reduce the parent to such a state of harrassment that serious violence occurs; and (2) where a child is suspected to be 'at risk' but parents decline help, and evidence to justify removal is lacking.

BCG vaccination. The initials stand for Bacillus of Calmette (1863-1933) and Guérin (1816-95), French bacteriologist and surgeon respectively. The bacillus itself is derived from a culture of the bovine variety of the tubercle bacillus rendered harmless by prolonged breeding under laboratory conditions. The BCG vaccination is preventive; inoculation against TUBERCULOSIS uses a living suspension of this harmless organism.

To explain the procedure it is necessary to say something about the natural history of tuberculous infection. Under ordinary living conditions most individuals are likely sooner or later to acquire an infection caused by the tubercle bacillus. The first exposure to infection, although it produces a definite tissue reaction is not necessarily followed by disease and in most cases the 'primary complex', usually in the lung and associated lymph glands, heals without incident. Recovery is accompanied by a degree of immunity to re-infection and by development of allergy to 'tuberculin', a product of the tubercle bacillus.

The immunity although substantial is not absolute and if an individual is subsequently re-exposed to massive infection or if his resistance is lowered by other factors, re-infection may still occur. The disease process is then of a different pattern, determined by the pre-existing allergy and may cause local destruction of tissue without any spread along the lymphatic vessels.

BCG vaccination is an attempt to produce this relative immunity in a controlled fashion and at the most advantageous time, having regard to the risks of infection and the susceptibility of the subject.

Mention has been made of allergy or sensitivity to tuberculin, and the detection of this by means of the tuberculin test is an essential part of BCG vaccination, because it is both undesirable and unnecessary to vaccinate persons who have already been infected. The test also provides a means of checking that vaccination has been successful in inducing the altered reactivity associated with immunity.

There are several varieties of the tuberculin test based on pricking the skin (von Pirquet); application onto the skin (Moro 'patch' test); or injection into the skin (Mantoux, Heaf and modifications). The most reliable is the Mantoux test, in which a measured quantity of a standard concentration of tuberculin is injected into the skin of the front of the forearm and the result examined in seventy-two hours. An area of redness and thickening constitutes a positive result.

The detailed procedure for BCG vaccination is therefore as follows: (1) Mantoux test, (2) read result, (3) if positive – no further action, (4) if negative – give standard dose of vaccine, (5) six to eight weeks later repeat Mantoux test to determine whether the previously negative result has converted to positive, indicating acquirement of immunity.

There remains the question of whom to vaccinate. Clearly tuberculin negative contacts should be tested and also other persons at special risk, such as nurses and medical students. In addition most experts recommend routine vaccination of the pre-adolescent about the age of 14 to ensure good protection during the years of greatest susceptibility. On the other hand

some advocate vaccination of the infant at birth but the arguments against this are substantial and the reasons in favour have lessened as the level of community infection has declined.

In modern practice the procedure is now regarded as effective, safe, and practically trouble free.

actual size

Bedbug

bedbugs. Nocturnal insect parasites infesting unclean houses. The bedbug *(Cimex lectularius)* is 4 to 5 mm. long, reddish-brown in colour, broad and flat and has a prominent beak-like proboscis, which it uses to suck blood from its human hosts in bed at night. It lives in mattresses, in crevices of bedsteads, behind loose wall-paper and in cracked plaster; it prefers fairly warm conditions in the region of 10° to 21° C. (50° to 70° F.), and it has a characteristic musty smell.

Bedbugs can be eradicated by cleanliness and good standards of housekeeping combined with the use of a reliable insecticidal spray and powder based on pyrethrin/DDT.

bed sores. Sores or ulcers occurring in persons confined to bed for long periods and caused by continued pressure interfering with circulation of blood to the compressed tissues. Common sites are the back, buttocks, heels and elbows. Bed sores are in the main preventable by good nursing, including seeing that sheets are not crumpled, regular and frequent changes of the patient's position and careful washing and very gentle drying of the compressed areas. Further preventive measures are: gentle massage of these areas to stimulate blood circulation;

application of methylated spirit and zinc and boracic ointment; and, if reddening appears, cushioning of the part, e.g., by use of an air-ring or by air-beds or water-beds for long-term patients. Where bed sores have occurred, treatment is difficult; if there is no infection, spraying with a 5 per cent solution of tannic acid may help; and if infection is present, a penicillin cream may be useful.

bedwetting. Most children are dry at night by about the age of 2½ years. Substantial continuation of bedwetting, known medically as nocturnal enuresis, after that age, or reversion by a child previously dry, may indicate disease of the kidney or bladder, but is far more commonly of psychological origin. In such cases, the child is subconsciously seeking to return to the more protected life of babyhood, because he feels unprotected, insecure, or unloved often through no fault of the parents but because of such factors as the birth of a younger child or the mother's return to work.

Scolding and punishment merely aggravate the situation, and fluid restriction in the evening seldom helps. After the situation has been ignored for six months or so in the hope of spontaneous recovery, and after medical examination has excluded physical causes, the child may need expert psychological examination (e.g., at a child guidance clinic) so that his insecurities and frustrations can be identified and removed gradually.

bee sting. See BITES AND STINGS.

behaviour. The ways in which people (or animals) conduct themselves in relation to others or to their physical or social environment, and also the ways in which they react to stresses and to abnormal situations.

Sources of behaviour. It is only in recent decades that psychologists have begun to appreciate the enormous complexity of sources of behaviour.

The simplest theory of human behaviour is that it is normally rational: we do things initially as a matter of trial and error, and then persist in the actions that lead to satisfactory results. Obviously reasoning plays a substantial part in shaping our behaviour. We decline to trust a particular man because he has cheated us in the past and we infer that he might do so again, and we put on a raincoat because our experience suggests to us the likelihood of rain. Yet we do not necessarily take adequate exercise or cut down cigarette smoking despite knowing that the one is good or the other bad for us. Much of our behaviour is not based on reason.

The behaviourist school, led by Pavlov and later Watson, has shown that much behaviour can be traced to past training and experience; and indeed, if this were not so, our entire educational system would be valueless. Our religious and political philosophies, for example, are in most cases based either on views and attitudes acquired in childhood or, perhaps less frequently, on sharp revolt against those of childhood. Yet to attribute behaviour simply to an extension of conditioned reflexes is to ignore thought, feeling, emotion and virtually every creative impulse.

Freud and the psychoanalysts demonstrated that a considerable part of our behaviour is based on ideas and experiences that have been repressed into the unconscious. The existence of unconscious mental activity is revealed by the common practice of 'sleeping on a problem', and many of our likes, hates and fears are explicable only on the ground of influences below the level of consciousness.

Sociologists and social psychologists have stressed the large part played by cultures and sub-cultures. Even the person who prides himself on his independence is greatly influenced by the values and judgments of those with whom he is – or has been – associated.

Not least, our behaviour is influenced by the hormones produced by the endocrine glands. A woman of nervous type is more nervous during and immediately before menstruation and some women are capricious in the early months of pregnancy.

Also, just as mind influences body, body affects mind. When very tired we are irritable and may behave unreasonably. When recovering from influenza we tend to see the gloomy side of any situation.

Behaviour disorders. These are conditions in which behaviour is considered objectionable by a person's associates or by society at large. Examples are outbursts of destructiveness, stealing in a law-abiding community, and sexual conduct regarded as intolerable by the current standards of the district. The relationship to standards should be noted: for example, wife-beating is abnormal behaviour in most social groups today but not in all, and the whipping of erring servants was regarded as normal conduct in the eighteenth century.

As indicated above, a number of factors influence an individual's behaviour; these include standards learned in childhood, experiences of later life which have a psychological influence, and variations in psychological make-up – which, in turn, are governed by factors as widely differing as the daily alcohol intake and the functioning of the ENDOCRINE SYSTEM. In recent years it has been increasingly recognized that behaviour disorders may also be the outcome of social interactions.

In the past the tendency has been to account for behaviour disorders as being either the result of unusual chemico-physiological disturbances (such as are caused by alcohol or drugs) or of psychological problems such as repression or conflict, or of brain damage. To a great extent most cases of behaviour disorder probably spring from these causes (see FREUD, NEUROSIS and PERVERSION). However, nowadays a small additional group is recognized: in Russia people who hold unorthodox and inconvenient views are, by very definition, deemed mentally sick; and in the Western World it is far from unknown for families to reject an 'unacceptable' member by negotiating with the medical profession until an acceptable label of some form of mental illness is adopted.

The work of child guidance clinics has to some extent clarified abnormal behaviour in children, but - despite our increasing knowledge of hormones and the central nervous system on the one hand and of psychological and social interaction on the other - the appearance of extraordinary behaviour in a previously 'normal' adult is in many cases still something of a mystery.

belching. The sudden expulsion of wind from the stomach otherwise known as eructation. The gas may arise from fermentation within the stomach or from the swallowing of air.

belladonna. An extract from the deadly nightshade plant, containing ATROPINE.

Bell's palsy. See FACIAL PARALYSIS.

bends. See DECOMPRESSION DISEASE.

benign. Essentially harmless. A benign tumour neither invades adjacent organs nor gives rise to new tumours (secondaries) in other parts of the body. Any symptoms that it produces, e.g., from pressure, are purely the result of its size and position, and if it is removed the tumour is permanently cured.

benzedrine. A drug, amphetamine sulphate, occasionally used in the treatment of mild depressions and of behaviour disorders in children. It is also sometimes employed, in combination with menthol, for treatment of the common cold and of sinus inflammations. Because it has a mild tendency to cause ADDICTION it is tending to fall into medical disuse.

bereavement. The loss, through death, of a key figure in a person's life.

Personal aspects. When one is bereaved, grief and mourning are inevitable although varying with the closeness of the emotional relationship. There is often a withdrawal of interest from the ordinary affairs of life, a preoccupation with memories of the deceased person, a great feeling of loneliness and frequently weeping, sleeplessness and loss of appetite.

The feelings of unhappiness and even of desolation are natural, and no attempt should be made to hide grief. The grief has to be 'worked through'. In most cases the bereaved person will begin to take an interest in ordinary matters and return to a state of mental equilibrium in about a month, but it does no good to tell such a grief-stricken person that he will get over it. Quiet sympathy and kindness are helpful and, for those who are religious, visits by their clergyman are often useful. Where a husband or wife has died and the surviving spouse may have to move from their home, no immediate decision should be taken: the bereaved person is often in no condition to take decisions, and the sorrowing is sometimes less painful amid the memories - both pleasant and sad - stimulated by the previously shared home.

The visits of friends and relatives, important during the weeks of acute mourning, are no less important later, because the widowed person often finds a marked reduction in the number of friends - not only because some couples have been more interested in the partner who died but also because an unattached person can make an inconvenient number at a dinner table.

It is important to realize that, where the departed person has been much loved, grieving is psychologically necessary. The mourner has to do what has been called his 'grief-work' to enable him in due course to adapt to the loss and to fill the emotional gap.

The two types of mourner likely to need medical - or psychiatric - help (apart from the possible prescription of sedatives during the period of sleeplessness) are the person who shows no return towards normality after six or seven weeks, and the person who apparently utterly suppresses his grief, to all appearance simply coping with the problems of living without any remembrance of the departed loved one.

Social aspects. While the average age at death has increased the comparative advantage of women over men has not changed appreciably. Generally speaking, women tend to experience the consequences of bereavement for a longer period of time than is the case for men who lose their wives.

Used to living with one person for the majority of their adult life, in bereavement people are suddenly faced with the need to adjust to the circumstances and status of a single person. Western societies are erected upon the institution of marriage where occupational roles and social activities are built around the husband and wife as a complementary unit. When the husband dies income from his employment ceases and often a pension stops or falls sharply, and when the wife dies, the widower may have to employ domestic help at considerable cost. On top of this sudden crisis of income is the additional trauma of having to adjust to a single as opposed to a paired condition. However the widowed try to manage their situation, the circle of friendships and acquaintances is likely to diminish almost in spite of any attempt made to preserve them; many social activities and relationships are based on the assumption that two people will be involved, and a widow or widower becomes an awkward encumbrance in social arrangements. In addition to personal grief, financial insecurity, a loss of independence and a degree of social isolation are the frequent consequences of the loss of one's life partner.

The institution which is the major mechanism for handling the consequences of bereavement is still the family. While some relatively affluent couples may retire to 'pensioners' towns', such as Eastbourne, wives on the loss of their husbands frequently return to the families of their offspring. In working class communities the relationship between 'mum' and her married daughters is frequently very close and never severed by the marriage bond. In these circumstances the relationship continues throughout the life of the parents and that of the family or families of the younger generation which are formed as the children grow up and marry. Most widows and widowers are therefore cared for by their relatives, usually daughters and sons-in-law during the final stages of the life cycle.

Support services to families caring for old people are woefully inadequate and when the demands, in terms of time and effort, of providing for the elderly become too great they are removed to nursing homes or to hospital geriatric wards, often short-staffed and lacking in amenities. It is time western societies recognized this progression and increased the facilities available to care for the elderly.

beriberi. A disease of malnutrition due to deficiency of vitamin B_1. The disease is characterized by inflammation of the nerves, disturbed sensation, weakness of muscles, heart weakness, and shortness of breath. There is a 'dry' form with increasing weakness and pains, especially of the calf muscles, followed by muscle wasting. The 'wet' form shows oedema of the legs, breathlessness, rapid pulse rate and sometimes palpitations. There is also a 'mixed' form, combining these features.

It occurs mostly in countries in which the staple diet is polished rice, i.e., rice from which the husks (which contain vitamin B_1) have been removed. Prevention is by substituting unpolished for polished rice and by adding to the diet other foods rich in B_1. Treatment is similar, with additional B_1 for some days or weeks (according to severity) at first by injections and subsequently by mouth. A condition rather similar to beriberi is found in some alcoholics, both because they deprive themselves of adequate food and because alcohol to some extent destroys the vitamin.

biceps. Two headed. The term is commonly used as the name for the large muscle that lies superficially on the front of the upper arm, with two tendons to the scapula (or shoulder bone) and a single tendon at the other end attached to the radius. The muscle semi-rotates the forearm, bends the elbow, and helps to flex the shoulder joint.

bifocals. Spectacles in which each lens consists of a part for distant vision and a part for near vision. They are normally

the two heads of the muscle attached to the shoulder bone

The biceps

unnecessary where glasses are required for only one function, such as motoring or reading, but they can be extremely useful where rapid alternation of close and distant vision is needed, as for example in the case of a lecturer who requires both to see his notes and to see his students. A person wearing bifocals for the first time is liable to make occasional mistakes for a few days, inadvertently trying to use the distance lens for near vision or the close lens for distant vision. Some care is therefore desirable at first when descending stairs or crossing streets, but in almost all cases the difficulties disappear within a week.

bile. A yellowish-brown substance of bitter taste, secreted by the liver and collected and concentrated in the gall-bladder. It is utilized in the digestion of fats and the absorption of fat-soluble vitamins and also in the extraction of waste products from the liver. In certain conditions bile pigment is deposited in the skin, giving rise to the yellowish appearance known as jaundice.

bilharziasis. A disease, otherwise known as schistomiasis, caused by invasion of the body by parasites called fluke worms. The FLUKES have a complicated life cycle and, if swallowed by man, the adults settle in the bladder or intestine, and their spiked eggs irritate the organ before leaving the body in urine or faeces. The disease - common in Africa, the Far and Middle East, and South America - causes bleeding into the urine or symptoms of dysentery.

Eradication is possible by sanitation and health education, or by removing the snails which carry the flukes by chemical treatment of the water. Treatment of the disease is by antimony salts or lucanthone.

biliary colic. The intense pain which arises if a gall-stone is forced through the narrow bile duct towards the intestine. The pain persists until the stone either reaches the intestine or is surgically removed. The blocking of the duct may produce jaundice.

bilious attack. A vague term generally applied to the headache, discomfort, and vomiting that occur in inflammation of the stomach following dietetic indiscretions.

biopsy. Removal of a tiny piece of tissue from the living body for laboratory examination to determine, for example, the presence or absence of a particular disease or to decide whether a tumour is malignant or benign.

birds and disease. Birds eaten as food are neither safer nor more dangerous than other animals. Both can acquire the organisms that cause various diseases, and in both cases inadequate cooking can leave the germs alive. Because of their feeding habits ducks are alleged to be particularly common sources of intestinal infections. It is essential to thaw out frozen poultry for twenty-four hours before cooking, otherwise the cold will protect the germs in the meat. About 4 per cent of British wood pigeons suffer from an avian (or bird) form of tuberculosis: until recent years it was thought that humans were immune to this variety of tuberculosis, but it is now known not only that the avian form can occasionally infect man but also that the avian germ is particularly resistant to antibiotics.

The droppings and cage-dust of infected parrots can transmit psittacosis, a dangerous disease with symptoms like a mixture of typhoid and pneumonia, and various cage-birds can produce ornithosis, a severe form of pneumonia usually contracted by inhalation, e.g., of dust from a budgerigar's cage.

birth control. Deliberate prevention of the union of the sperm and the ovum within the body of a woman after sexual intercourse.

Contraceptive methods are probably as old as the earliest population explosions that produced an excess of people over food and resources. References are found in early Chinese, Indian, Jewish, Classical and Persian writings. Neither Mohammed nor Christ mentioned contraception, and the disapproval of some Christians stems from St. Augustine (who actually directed his attacks mainly on the use of the 'safe period') and St. Thomas Aquinas. The Church of England gave limited approval in 1930 and unqualified approval in 1958. The introduction of oral contraceptives in 1956 enormously simplified birth control.

Desirability. In respect of need or desirability birth control falls essentially into four groups: (1) family avoidance, e.g. in carriers of serious hereditary defects; (2) family postponement, e.g., in a young couple seeking to acquire some savings before having a child, or in unmarried people who seek to have intercourse without its consequences; (3) family spacing, e.g., to avoid the mother becoming exhausted or some members of a large family of young children becoming neglected; (4) family limitation, e.g., when a couple have had the number of children they desire, or when a still-birth or the birth of a deformed child has made them aware of a hereditary risk (though this does not imply that all still-births or all handicapped children are the result of genetic defects).

From a national or international point of view birth control should be encouraged because (1) world population is fast outstripping natural resources; (2) children with serious genetic defects (e.g., cases of spina bifida, schizophrenia, mongolism and phenylketonuria) survive in increasing numbers as antenatal care and obstetrics improve; they create enormous physical and emotional problems for the parents who have to care for them and constitute a growing burden on the community; and (3) the rearing of unwanted and neglected children again constitutes a heavy burden on society, while a child brought up in a nursery, orphanage or foster home is often psychologically disadvantaged. Most people appear to accept the general case for birth control, but some would restrict it to married couples (leaving the one-parent child to pay for the sins of his father and mother) and some (despite St. Augustine's attacks on the use of the 'safe period') would restrict the methods to those provided by nature.

In relation to family spacing and limitation it is important to get rid of the idea that a woman cannot become pregnant while breast-feeding a baby. Fertility is lessened in these circumstances but conception is perfectly possible. Perhaps the need for the mother to avoid pregnancy during breast-feeding and thereafter to have some months' rest is the most obvious example of the desirability of birth control in cases with neither hereditary defect nor excessive existing family.

'Natural' methods. 1. Continence (complete absence of intercourse) is obvious but is psychologically frustrating to a young and highly-sexed couple living together and can even cause nervous breakdown. It is practicable for unmarried persons 'going steady', but inhibitions are sometimes temporarily removed (e.g., by a combination of alcohol, opportunity and deep affection).

2. The 'safe period' or 'RHYTHM METHOD' is based on the idea that the female ovum is ripe for reception of a sperm between the tenth and the eighteenth day after the beginning of menstruation, so that the avoidance of intercourse during these nine days should prevent pregnancy. Unfortunately, not all menstrual cycles are at regular twenty-eight day intervals, and in some women the 'dangerous period'

extends from the sixth to the twentieth day after the start of menstruation (or roughly half the month). There are even recorded cases of conception before the sixth and after the twentieth day. Broadly use of the 'safe period', if carefully calculated in a regular woman, removes about three-quarters of the risk of pregnancy.

3. The 'temperature method' is an attempt to pin-point the time of ovulation (i.e., the beginning of the 'danger period') by noting a slight rise in temperature; but the rise is only about 1° C., and many other factors can cause or prevent such a small rise. This method, despite its scientific appearance, is no better than the use of the 'safe period'.

4. Withdrawal (coitus interruptus) of the penis before climax is reached is somewhat uncertain because some seminal fluid may be discharged before withdrawal. Also withdrawal may place considerable psychological strain on both partners.

Mechanical methods. 1. The condom or male SHEATH of appropriate size, rolled or slipped over the erect penis, is much more reliable than any 'natural' method. Provided the sheath is not torn, and provided spermicidal douches or creams are used if there is any suspicion of a leak, the method is 95 per cent effective. Curiously the condom is known in Britain as 'the French letter' and in France as 'la capote anglaise'.

2. The 'cap' pessary of rubber and the 'Dutch' or steel spring pessary, both inserted while the woman is in a squatting position, aim to shut off the vagina from the cervix of the uterus, thus preventing the sperm and the ovum from coming together. Pessaries are highly reliable, especially if used smeared with a spermicidal jelly or cream, and followed by douching, perhaps twelve hours after intercourse and before removal of the pessary. In some cases, however, they irritate the soft tissues.

3. Although invented as early as 1909 the INTRA-UTERINE DEVICE has for some reason little used until the second half of this century. It is generally inserted by a doctor (requiring considerable skill for insertion), can be left in for long periods, and is more reliable.

Oral contraceptives. In the last 25 years oral contraceptives, containing minute quantities of the female hormones oestrogen and progesterone, have come to dominate the field of birth control. They have a success rate of over 99 per cent, and in fact conception while using 'the pill' is almost always due to human error, e.g., forgetting to take a daily pill, although some modern varieties provide sufficient 'carry-over' to minimize the risk of a one-day omission. There are many varieties, so that side effects can be eliminated by giving each woman an oral contraceptive that suits her.

Oral contraceptives with relatively high oestrogen content were virtually abandoned before 1970, in which year a very large scale investigation showed that they had a danger to health approximating to one-tenth of the danger created by a pregnancy; by contrast the same investigation and later studies have not shown dangers in respect of the oral contraceptives in common use, although there are a few disease conditions which render these contraceptives undesirable for persons with these particular diseases. In highly developed countries (e.g., Western Europe and North America) millions of women have used oral contraceptives during the last twenty years, so that their effects are at least as well known as those of any other modern medicines.

Permanent methods. While oral contraceptives are ideal for family postponement or family spacing, it seems unfortunate that a woman who has completed her family by the age of 28 or so should have to take oral contraceptives for another eighteen years. So increasing attention is now being paid to the cutting or tying of the male or female tubes.

In the male, sterilization is carried out by the very minor and painless operation of vasectomy. Using a local anaesthetic the surgeon makes a small cut in the scrotum, either removes a tiny portion of the vas deferens or ties it with a ligature, and repeats the process on the other side. The whole operation, including the time waiting for the local anaesthetic to take effect, is over in fifteen to twenty minutes, the man normally leaves the clinic or hospital within an hour of entering it and is usually fit for work on the next day or sometimes even the same day. It takes two to three months for the spermatozoa already in circulation to die off, but thereafter the man is completely sterile. He can still feel sexual desire, have erections and ejaculate semen, but the semen contains no spermatozoa.

Vasectomy has the limitation that it is permanent (if a portion of the vas is removed) or difficult to reverse (if the vas is tied) but it is the simplest form of sterilization, much easier and more rapid than ligation of a woman's uterine tubes.

The operation is becoming increasingly popular with men who have fathered the number of children that they desire.

In the female, sterilization is carried out by cutting and tying – or in some other way closing off – the Fallopian tubes. The cutting and tying method requires abdominal operation but less complicated procedures now involve operating through a small stab-wound with the use of a laparoscope (a sort of periscope) to seal off the tubes either by diathermy or the application of special clips under direct vision. Both methods leave the woman with unaltered sexual feelings and menstrual periods but with the ova no longer able to travel to the womb. Other possible procedures are still on trial.

While some doctors themselves provide birth control advice and treatment, increasing numbers of individuals seek the expertise available at family planning clinics. These clinics of course provide both privacy and confidentiality. In the British cities with the most highly developed contraceptive services, and with parallel health education about these services, the birth rate has fallen by as much as 20 per cent, creating in these cities a stationary population.

birth marks. Congenital blemishes of the skin, falling into two types. The vascular naevus is a small cluster of tiny blood vessels. Of these the red 'strawberry mark' often fades after some years, while the purple 'port wine stain' usually remains. The pigmented naevus or mole is essentially a cluster of pigment cells.

Many, but not all, birthmarks decrease in size as the child grows older, but if they remain disfiguring plastic surgery or cautery treatment can be effective, although in many cases a cosmetic preparation can hide them. There is no foundation for the superstition that birth marks are caused by events which took place during pregnancy.

bites and stings. An insect which stings is acting malevolently in self-defence but one which bites is merely being a parasite and feeding on the blood or juices of a host which it is against its own interests to injure.

Insect bites. After puncturing the skin the insect injects a salivary secretion into the victim in order to assist the sucking process and this causes irritation and local swelling, even when there are no complications. However, the bites may become septic because of infection introduced from the mouth parts of the insect or by scratching. Bites should not be scratched; calamine lotion or antihistamine creams will allay irritation.

In tropical countries many insects harbour in their secretion organisms of serious disease which are thus inoculated into the host. Mosquitos, biting flies, fleas, lice and ticks are known carriers of a great variety of tropical diseases and so in tropical and sub-tropical areas the potential risks of insect bites should be appreciated and appropriate measures adopted to avoid being bitten. In addition, as a precautionary measure, drugs should be taken which will act against infection with malaria should this occur.

Animal bites. Unless there is a reason to suspect that the animal suffers from rabies, an animal bite should simply be thoroughly washed with a mild disinfectant solution, or – failing that – with soap and water, and thereafter treated like any other wound.

Stings. Stings (e.g. by bees, wasps and hornets) usually cause only sharp pain and local swelling or sepsis but can be dangerous in the mouth or at the top of the throat where swelling may cause difficulty in breathing. In such cases a doctor should be summoned urgently, since an injection of adrenalin or an intramuscular antihistamine or (in cases of extreme respiratory difficulty) a tracheotomy operation, may be life-saving. Occasionally signs of shock and collapse appear, in which case whisky or sal volatile should be given. It should however be emphasized that these are extreme rarities: nineteen stings out of twenty cause only minor irritation.

In most cases a bee sting is best treated by gently removing the sting (if it can be seen) and applying a mild alkali such as baking soda. Antihistamine drugs may also help to relieve the symptoms.

Like most insect stings wasp stings cause a release of histamine but, unlike most other insects, wasps inject an alkaline venom and therefore a mild acid, such as vinegar, should be applied.

Where a person is allergic to a sting venom and cannot change his residence to an area in which a sting is unlikely, a desensitization course may be required. See ALLERGY.

In sub-tropical and tropical countries the scorpion is feared. It holds on with its feet and stings with its pointed tail. It frequently kills children from resultant respiratory paralysis and even adults can be very ill. Local treatment employs ammonia with novocaine and adrenalin to relieve pain. A specific antivenene is available.

Other hazards are the giant centipede, and some tropical fish such as the sting-rays which have poisoned barbs in their dorsal fins. Jellyfish can give particularly painful stings; these are probably best relieved by mild acids such as vinegar. Skin irritation due to the stinging nettle is caused by formic acid and can be relieved by alkaline applications. See also SNAKE BITES.

Black Death. A particularly infectious and virulent form of PLAGUE that destroyed about a third of the world's population in 1346-51.

black eye. Darkening of the eyelids and surrounding skin and reddening of the conjunctiva of the eye following an injury. Essentially the mechanism is the same as in a bruise elsewhere, but there is much loose skin in the eyelids in which blood can easily accumulate. A cold, wet cloth applied to the eye is the best immediate treatment.

blackhead. Glands producing oil (sebum) to lubricate the skin release it through pores which sometimes become plugged by dried skin and other debris. The area around the gland becomes inflamed and the typical red spot with a black centre is produced.

black vomit. Black or dark-brown vomit, often described as 'coffee-grounds'; the indication is that blood has entered the stomach and been partially digested before being brought up. Possible causes include gastric and duodenal ulcer, acute gastritis, and - more rarely - cancer of the stomach.

blackwater fever. A rather infrequent but often fatal complication of MALARIA of the falciparum type. It is characterized by blackening of the urine through blood pigment which has passed through the kidney filters.

bladder. A flexible muscular bag that serves as a reservoir for the urine secreted by the kidneys. The bladder is connected to the kidneys by two tubes, the ureters, and to the exterior by a passage, the urethra, with the outlet from bladder to urethra guarded by a circular muscle, the sphincter. When empty, the bladder lies wholly in the pelvis, but as it becomes distended its upper end rises several inches into the abdomen. The adult bladder can hold almost half a litre (1 pint) of urine.

After the bladder has become appreciably distended from the continuous trickle of urine from the kidneys, the muscular walls begin to resist, producing the desire to pass urine. In a baby the subsequent relaxation of the sphincter is purely a reflex action, and the voiding of urine follows; but as a child ages this relaxation of the sphincter comes increasingly under control of the will. If the sphincter is deliberately not relaxed, the signal from the bladder muscles ceases but, as distension increases, is later renewed. If the signal of muscle resistance is repeatedly ignored, reflex emptying ultimately supersedes voluntary control.

Incontinence is loss of control over the sphincter muscle and it occurs when the bladder is irritated (e.g., by inflammation or stone or enlarged prostate) or when the sphincter is paralysed (e.g., in certain diseases of the spinal cord). Incontinence in children usually takes the form of bedwetting but the elderly may also experience an occasional involuntary voiding of urine.

Diseases. (1) Cystitis or inflammation - infection of the bladder, commoner in women than in men because the female urethra is shorter and so gives less protection against entrance of bacteria. The main symptoms are frequency of urination and some pain. (2) Stone from the kidneys or ureters; usually indicated by considerable pain, bleeding into the urine, and frequency. (3) Tumours, the most common being the benign papilloma, characterized by painless bleeding into the urine; cancer of the bladder, much less frequent, is initially hard to differentiate from papilloma. (4) Rupture of the bladder, generally as a result of violence.

bleeding. Any form of external or internal passage of blood from the arteries, veins, or capillaries. For immediate treatment see First Aid section at the end of the book. See also HAEMORRHAGE.

bleeding disease. See HAEMOPHILIA.

blepharitis. See EYELIDS, DISEASES OF.

blindness. Lack of sight in both eyes or in one. Perhaps the greatest triumph of health services has been the effective transfer of blindness from a condition of youth to one of old age. Some of the very numerous causes, listed here, fall into four principal categories.

Loss of vision from infancy. By far the commonest cause of blindness in children in developed countries until the last forty years was ophthalmia neonatorum, i.e., transmission of gonococcal infection from the mother to the baby during the birth process. Another cause of blindness in babies that has almost disappeared in the last twenty years is retrolental fibroplasia, created by giving excess oxygen to premature babies. Such few cases of blindness as are now found in young children in developed countries are mostly hereditary, such as hereditary cataract and amaurosis. These can be reduced by genetic guidance and family planning.

Gradual loss of vision in one or both eyes. In several less-developed countries the commonest cause of blindness is still trachoma, which affects all age groups but in developed countries impaired or absent vision is now primarily a condition of old age. Glaucoma is essentially a disease of the over-sixties, although its early stages are said to be present in about 5 per cent of persons aged 45 to 50 years: while it is not yet preventable, it can be controlled and usually blindness avoided. Cataract responds to surgical treatment, and amblyopia of the tobacco or the toxic variety responds to discontinuing the intake of the causing factor. Atrophy of the optic nerve and tumour of the pituitary gland also cause gradual loss of sight.

Sudden blindness of one eye. This may be caused by thrombosis of the vein draining the retina (the light-sensitive inner layer of the eye), embolism of the retinal artery or by detachment or degeneration of the retina.

Sudden blindness in both eyes. Sun-blinding is the result of looking directly at the sun - the intense brilliance of the light burns the area of the retina it shines on and the tissues can never recover. It is, therefore, extremely important always to shield the eyes with smoked glass if, for instance, watching an eclipse. Other causes of sudden blindness are uraemia, diabetes, and injury. In a very few cases of blindness, where the defect is caused by cornea (the transparent front covering of the eye) becoming opaque, sight may be restored by a corneal graft, replacing the damaged cornea with a clearly transparent cornea from a donor eye.

Social aspects. In the past partially-sighted or totally blind people were to be found in every age group but in the developed countries today blindness tends to occur chiefly among the elderly. Blindness, therefore, like other degenerative diseases, has to be discussed mainly in relation to the process of ageing and the various circumstances in which the elderly find themselves.

Expert medical advice and treatment can prevent blindness in many cases or limit it to partial loss of sight. Where the condition is unprevented or unpreventable it is important that the person, while still partially sighted, should learn to make full use of his other senses and also to be systematic, e.g., counting the steps as he walks down stairs, and placing his pipe and matches in a fixed and safe position where he can find them without using his eyes.

When blindness has developed he should promptly seek to become registered as a blind person, so as to gain such advantages as the chance of being trained for appropriate work and then helped to find a job, visits by experienced home workers for the blind whose advice can be very valuable, and in some countries free radio licences and reduced postage rates for embossed literature. If he is still relatively young and active, his mobility will be greatly improved by the acquisition of a guide dog, specially trained in the U.K. by the Guide Dogs for the Blind Association. Even if fairly old but mentally alert he should certainly be prepared to learn Braille in which many books are published.

The situation of people who lose their sight in old age is very different. Some degree of isolation, both physical and social, is often associated with growing old (see BEREAVEMENT). The loss of any of the senses is likely to increase the problem of social isolation, and the partial or total loss of vision may cause old people to withdraw even further into themselves. This may be particularly distressing since health and social services are not particularly well equipped to help the elderly blind person, and a person who is becoming sightless has usually no advance knowledge of blindness that he can use in trying to adapt.

The organizations, mostly voluntary, which exist to help blind people tend to place the elderly at the bottom of their lists of priorities. These organizations, while sometimes subsidized by public funds, are dependent largely upon voluntary contributions to continue their work. It is easier to persuade people to give money to a good cause if it is suggested that the afflicted can be helped and trained to fend for themselves and to make a positive contribution to the economic sector. Consequently organizations for the blind have tended to focus their efforts on the young person who can be trained in some economically productive role.

The elderly blind have greater needs which are more difficult to deal with without there being much possibility for helping such people to lead a socially 'useful' life. Their mobility may already be impaired so that the usefulness of guide dogs is limited, even assuming an old person is fully capable of caring for a dog. Like most elderly people the blind or partially sighted wish to remain in their own homes for as long as possible, which means that assistance has to be brought to them rather than their travelling to (or living in) a centrally based institution.

Gradually more resources are being devoted to the care of the elderly. In Britain retired people are contacted by HEALTH VISITORS although the case loads of these health and social workers are far too high for them to be able to provide a complete service. A vast expansion of resources devoted to the care of the elderly is needed and an increasingly important element in their work will be the care of the blind or partially sighted.

blister. A small area of the skin in which the surface layer is raised and contains fluid; it is caused by heat or friction. In general a blister is best left unbroken and treated by application of calamine lotion. Where it has broken it should be covered with lint spread with zinc or boracic ointment.

blood. The fluid, contained in arteries, capillaries and veins, which transmits oxygen and nutritive substances to the various tissues and conveys waste materials from the tissues to the lungs (in the case of carbon dioxide) and the excretory organs. Blood makes up approximately one-fourteenth of the weight of the body, or about 5 litres (8 pints) in the case of an average adult male.

Blood consists of a large number of red cells, and smaller numbers of white cells and of tiny bodies called platelets, all floating in a pale, yellowish, clear liquid, the plasma.

1. Plasma is the sticky, amber-coloured fluid which carries not only the blood corpuscles but also various raw materials and waste products. Plasma contains proteins – albumin, globulin and fibrinogen – which are formed mainly in the liver. These protein molecules are too large normally to pass through the walls of the capillaries. The presence of albumin is important to the function of OSMOSIS and deficiency leads to an accumulation of fluid in the tissues known as oedema. This occurs in certain diseases of the liver (where not enough is formed) and of the kidney (where albumin passes to the urine). Globulin is associated with immunity to certain infectious diseases. Fibrinogen is altered by a ferment released by the platelets when blood is shed. It forms threads of fibrin and these, entangling corpuscles in the network of threads, form a clot. (Serum is plasma which has no fibrinogen, i.e., it is the fluid which separates from a clot.)

2. Red blood corpuscles (erythrocytes) are circular, concave discs, normally about five million to each cubic millimetre of blood. They are manufactured in the bone marrow, and each corpuscle when worn out – after some three to four months – is destroyed by the spleen. Red blood corpuscles are essentially envelopes containing an iron compound, HAEMOGLOBIN, which combines with oxygen in the capillaries of the lungs and in due course gives up oxygen to the tissues.

Haemoglobin cannot be formed without an adequate supply of iron, and red blood corpuscles cannot mature without vitamin B_{12}. Red corpuscles are about a thousand times as numerous as white ones.

3. White blood corpuscles (leucocytes) are slightly larger and much less numerous than red cells, roughly about eight thousand to the cubic millimetre. They, like red corpuscles, are formed in the bone marrow and they constitute the main defence mechanism of the body. They gather rapidly at the site of infection by bacteria or invasion by a foreign body, and they have the power of surrounding bacteria and ultimately destroying them. Leucocytes are of two main types: granulocytes (which on being stained show small scattered granules in the cell) chiefly concerned with protection against bacteria; and lymphocytes (where on being stained the cell is seen to be largely occupied by a nucleus) which play a considerable role in resistance to virus diseases and also in chronic infections. Moderate increase in leucocytes is a healthy response to infection, and identification of such increase – by spreading a drop of suitably diluted blood thinly on a glass slide, staining appropriately and counting the cells – gives a useful clue to the presence of infection. Ungoverned over-production of white corpuscles is characteristic of a cancer-like disease, leukaemia.

4. Platelets (thrombocytes) are very much smaller than red or white corpuscles and are involved in the clotting of shed blood. They release a hormone which helps to convert fibrinogen to fibrin.

Blood tests. These fall into three main groups – haematological (or study of the state of the blood itself), chemical (or investigation of its contents) and bacteriological (or study for organisms or antibodies). Many tests require merely a single drop of blood, obtained by pricking the finger lightly with a needle. Others need several millilitres of blood, obtained by inserting the needle of a syringe into a vein.

Blood diseases. The various forms of insufficiency of red blood corpuscles are discussed under ANAEMIA. Polycythaemia, excess of red blood corpuscles, is thought to be due to excessive activity of bone marrow, and is hereditary in some cases. Excess of white corpuscles is considered under LEUKAEMIA, and hereditary tendency to uncontrollable bleeding is discussed under HAEMOPHILIA. For poisoning of the blood by germs or their toxins see SEPTICAEMIA and TOXAEMIA respectively.

See also CIRCULATION OF BLOOD and BLOOD GROUPS.

blood groups. Blood corpuscles contain two factors (agglutinogens), A and B, and these factors cause red blood corpuscles from a different sample of blood to clump together. These factors occur singly or together or are absent, and so four groups

are possible, A, B, AB or O. Serum from blood can be grouped in terms of agglutinins named anti-A and anti-B.

Group A, found in about 42 per cent of Western Europeans, will mix with blood containing A but will cause clotting if mixed with blood of group B; Group B, found in about 9 per cent, will similarly mix with B but will cause clotting if mixed with A. Group AB, the 'universal recipients', will accept without clotting blood from any group, and constitute about 3 per cent of the population, and Group O, the 'universal donors', can safely provide blood to any group and make up roughly 46 per cent of the population. Irrespective of these four main blood groups there is another variation, the RHESUS FACTOR; 83 per cent of the population are Rhesus positive (Rh+ve) and 17 per cent are Rhesus negative (Rh-ve).

A Rhesus negative person who has a transfusion of Rhesus positive blood, or more commonly a Rhesus negative woman who bears a Rhesus positive child (inheriting the factor from his father), is likely to form an antibody which reacts with a further contact with Rhesus positive blood, e.g., in a transfusion or a subsequent pregnancy.

Apart from implications both for blood transfusions and in obstetrics, the discovery of the four main types and the Rhesus sub-types is of considerable value in paternity cases, since a child inherits its blood grouping from either father or mother. To give two examples: if mother and child are both of group A, Rhesus +ve we have no evidence, because the child has inherited from the mother; but if the mother is of group A, Rhesus +ve and the child of group AB, Rhesus -ve, we have quite a bit of information about the father.

blood heat. The normal temperature of the blood is about 37.7° C. (100° F.) but the body temperature in health is about 36 to 37.2° C. (98 to 99° F.) and is conventionally taken as 36.7° C. (98.4° F.). The circulating blood maintains the body at very constant TEMPERATURE.

blood pressure. The pressure at which the heart pumps blood into the main arteries. The extent of this pressure depends principally on two factors – the force of the muscular pump of the heart, and the calibre, elasticity and resistance of the arteries. The blood pressure is normally measured at two points of time, namely that of maximum heart contraction (systolic pressure) and that of maximum relaxation (diastolic pressure).

Measurement. This is carried out on a SPHYGMOMANOMETER. An inflatable cuff is wrapped around the patient's arm and air pumped into it until it constricts the arm sufficiently for the pulse-beat to be stopped. This air pressure is meantime also raising a column of mercury against a scale and the blood pressure is recorded according to the height of the column of mercury. Thus in a healthy young adult at rest the average systolic pressure is equivalent to a column of 120 mm. of mercury, and the average diastolic pressure is equivalent to 80 mm. of mercury. There is, however, considerable individual variation, especially in respect of the systolic pressure. To an experienced examiner the PULSE can give an accurate assessment of the blood pressure.

High blood pressure. The pressure rises temporarily during exertion and in emotional disturbance. A sustained rise in blood pressure is perhaps the commonest pathological condition found in highly developed countries and is associated with excess worry and mental activity, over-eating and perhaps lack of physical exercise.

Causes of raised blood pressure include hardening of the arteries (arteriosclerosis) so that the heart has to work harder to pump in the same amount of blood, certain diseases of the kidneys with poorer blood flow through them, and occasionally increased stickiness of the blood (as in polycythaemia). Symptoms sometimes include headaches, giddiness and heart pains, but often a rising blood pressure is symptomless. A mild rise of pressure in middle-age is probably best ignored as merely a 'normal' feature of modern life: in millimetres of mercury the average systolic pressure is sometimes described as '100 plus number of years lived'.

Serious and increasing rise of pressure – and especially of diastolic pressure – indicates risk of a cerebrovascular incident, such as a stroke. Such continuing rise therefore demands a revision of life's routine to diminish both mental and physical strain, in the hope of stopping or slowing the increase. Certain drugs that act on the sympathetic nervous system (e.g. thiazide diuretics and methyldopa) can also be used in moderation to lower the pressure, but it has to be remembered that in general the pressure has risen because it is needed to force the blood into hardened arteries, and that too vigorous reduction of the pressure can do more harm than good.

Low blood pressure. A temporary fall in blood pressure can occur on suddenly standing up (because the reflexes have not yet adjusted to the changed posture and too much blood at first drains towards the feet) and is also found in shock. Permanently low blood pressure is characteristic of Addison's disease and also occurs in some prolonged debility states.

Blood pressure in pregnancy. During a normal pregnancy the blood pressure does not rise, and indeed a rise in blood pressure is an indication that a pregnancy is not proceeding normally and that skilled help is needed. During the actual labour the pressure rises but rapidly falls again after the birth.

blood spitting. See HAEMOPTYSIS.

blood tests. See BLOOD.

blood transfusion. The procedure by which blood from a donor is transfused to the circulatory system of a patient in order to restore loss of blood-volume resulting from haemorrhage and shock or to improve states of severe anaemia. In 'exchange-transfusions' all the blood of a patient is replaced by donated blood and this expedient is employed in new-born infants suffering from the effects of RHESUS incompatibility.

When blood is to be collected from a healthy donor an arm vein is usually made to stand out by the application of a tourniquet; a needle is inserted and blood allowed to run through the needle and a tube into a suitable receptacle where clotting is prevented by the addition of a small amount of sodium citrate. The citrated blood can be stored for several weeks at 3 to 4°C. (i.e., the temperature of an ordinary domestic refrigerator), and then when required can be run slowly into the vein of a person of similar BLOOD GROUP.

The discoveries first of the inherited blood group systems and then of the Rhesus factor have together removed the former dangers of blood transfusion. Freed from these dangers it is extremely useful – indeed life-saving – after accidents and injuries involving heavy loss of blood. Virtually all general hospitals now have 'blood banks', with stored blood of various groups available for immediate use when required

Very rarely (only, in fact, in the combination of a serious condition and an unusual blood group) is blood transferred directly from donor to recipient. The blood bank system is more suitable for the donor who can give his blood at a time convenient both for him and for the hospital staff; it is better for the staff, since when a transfusion is urgently needed they do not need to await the arrival of an appropriate donor; and if there is any doubt about the donor's health it allows time for investigation.

blood vessels. A collective name for the arteries (which carry blood from the heart), the veins (which return blood to the heart) and the capillaries (through which occurs interchange with the tissues of oxygen, nutrients and waste products). See CIRCULATION OF BLOOD.

blue baby. A new-born child with a bluish complexion, indicating unsatisfactory oxygenation of the blood in consequence of a congenital heart defect, e.g., a communication remaining between the right and left sides of the heart so that the oxygenated blood to be pumped around the body is contaminated by the deoxygenated blood which has returned from the body to the heart en route for the lungs. Modern surgical techniques can nowadays successfully cope with the abnormality.

blushing. Reddening of the skin, especially of the face and neck. In persons of nervous or excitable temperament any emotional disturbance – painful or pleasurable – may cause a dilation of the capillaries of the skin, resulting in production of a rosy colour. Of the many causes of flushing perhaps the commonest are: (1) temporary hormonal imbalance in adolescence; (2) similar imbalance at the menopause, and (3) anxiety states. In the first two cases the condition passes in time, and in the third the treatment is that of the underlying condition.

While not a serious condition and seldom unattractive, flushing places its victim in the position that the existence of strong emotion is revealed to the observer.

boils. Small abscesses commencing in a hair root and usually caused by a staphylococcus. A single boil is painful while the damaged tissues, leucocytes and bacteria are forming pus that is at first under tension. In due course the stretched skin breaks or the boil may be opened surgically to let the pus escape. The pus drains out and the lesion heals. Poultices may expedite the pus formation. Apart from lancing the boil when pus is definitely present, interference is undesirable. In particular, squeezing a boil not only damages the tissues but may send infectious material inwards.

A series of successive or simultaneous boils implies lowered vitality of the skin and suggests (1) chronic serious disease (e.g., of the kidneys), (2) extreme physical or mental exhaustion, or (3) faulty feeding. Apart from seeking for an underlying cause, building up the general health and attention to skin hygiene, the individual may benefit from injections of a suitable antibiotic.

bone. Bone is composed of two layers of tissue: externally, a dense, ivory-like shell of compact bone, traversed only by very narrow channels (the Haversian canals) in which run the nourishing blood vessels and lymphatics; and internally a spongy or porous network, the cancellous bone, rich in blood vessels and supporting the red bone marrow. A bone is surrounded by a tough, fibrous membrane called the periosteum. Sensation apparently from the bone really comes from the nerves in the periosteum.

Bones are classified into long, short, flat and irregular. A long bone (e.g., femur or thigh-bone) consists of a shaft and two expanded ends. Short bones (e.g., those of the wrist) consist of cancellous bone thinly encased by compact bone. Flat bones (e.g., those of the skull) are composed of outer and inner tables of compact bone with layers of cancellous bone sandwiched between. Irregular bones (e.g., the vertebrae) are simply those that do not conform to any classification.

Bones form the skeletal framework about which the body is moulded. They give protection to the vital organs, and they permit the body and limbs to be moved in various directions by the action of the muscles.

Formation. Bone tissue develops from cartilage and this begins early during pregnancy, but as late as the time of birth some bones are still entirely cartilaginous. Growth of the bone, which requires the availability of sufficient calcium (and also vitamin D to permit absorption of calcium) depends on the activity of cells called osteoblasts. These extract calcium phosphate from the blood.

In young children bones consist largely of cartilaginous tissue, and under strain they bend rather than break. With advancing years bones come to contain more and more calcium phosphate and become more brittle.

Disorders. Bone is subject to the same type of disorder as most other tissues, but it lacks nerve endings, so that (unless the periosteum is affected) bone diseases are painless.

Some of the commoner bone disorders are: fracture; periostitis (inflammation of the periosteum); osteomyelitis (inflammation of the bony substance itself), tuberculosis (now becoming rare); of the malignant tumours carcinoma is usually secondary to primary cancer elsewhere but sarcoma sometimes starts in bone. See also RICKETS, ACROMEGALY and OSTEOMALACIA. Abnormal fragility of bones is fairly common in old people (see OSTEOPOROSIS) and is occasionally found as a hereditary condition in children.

borborygmus. A rumbling noise arising in the bowel from intestinal indigestion.

Bornholm disease. A disease caused by a virus and characterized by high temperature, headache, severe pain in the muscles of the chest and abdomen, inflammation of the throat and sometimes pleurisy and mild meningitis. The condition generally clears up in two or three days but recurrence a few days later is quite common. Analgesics are needed to relieve the pain but there is no known specific treatment and no known method of prevention.

bottle feeding. Where the mother has an illness that renders breast feeding undesirable, e.g., heart disease or pulmonary tuberculosis, or produces inadequate milk, or has working commitments that prevent complete BREAST FEEDING, partial or total bottle feeding may be needed.

Modification of liquid cow's milk may be attempted at home – seeking to reduce the high protein and mineral content of cow's milk to about the levels of human milk (by addition of sterile water), to raise the low carbohydrate content (by addition of lactose) and to make the curd more digestible (by addition of sodium citrate), but proprietary dried milks (and in the U.K. National Dried Milk) make the required modifications more accurately and under conditions of guaranteed sterility. If the directions on the tin are strictly followed, and not varied except on the advice of a doctor or health visitor about the particular needs of an individual child, an infant can be very satisfactorily fed by bottle.

It is important that the baby be held in the arms while feeding, both for emotional stimulation and because it is dangerous to leave a baby sucking from a bottle attached to a pillow. The teat must of course be of the right size for the infant's mouth and the hole should be large enough for the milk to drop out when the bottle is inverted but not large enough for it to flow out. Bottles and teats should be carefully washed and scalded after each feed or else washed in a suitable disinfectant – all the various commercial preparations widely advertised for this purpose are satisfactory – and then rinsed in boiled water to remove traces of the disinfectant.

Vitamin supplements are needed, but to avoid risk of over-dosage of vitamin D the amount of that vitamin in any proprietary milk used should be known and taken into account.

The gradual introduction of other foods should be similar to that for breast-fed babies.

In the U.K. advice on bottle feeding (and breast feeding) and weaning is readily available from health visitors. See also BREAST FEEDING.

botulism. Food-poisoning caused by the micro-organism *Clostridium botulinus* and its toxin. It is often fatal but cases are extremely rare.

Botulism is mainly associated with food which has been inefficiently canned or bottled. The organism will survive to multiply and produce toxin if the temperature attained in the pack is not high enough to kill it. Because of this, home-canned produce is a special risk and should always be re-cooked before consumption.

Unlike other food-poisoning, gastro-intestinal symptoms are usually slight. Instead, botulinus toxin damages the nervous system. Onset occurs with dizziness, double vision, laryngeal paralysis, and loss of voice. The vital centres of the brain controlling the heart and respiration may be affected.

An antitoxin is available but unless the disease is promptly recognized opportunity for effective administration is easily lost. Treatment otherwise mainly consists in maintaining respiration and combating collapse.

bowel. The part of the digestive system which extends as a musculo-membranous tube from the lower opening of the stomach to the anus. It occupies most of the abdominal cavity and comprises the small and large intestines.

The small intestine comprises convolutions of some 1 m. (20 ft.) named successively duodenum, jejunum, and ileum. It digests fats and absorbs nutriments including those derived from earlier digestion in the stomach.

The large intestine is about 1.5 m. (5 ft.) in length and named successively as ascending, transverse, and descending colon and finally rectum. The junction between small and large intestines is the ileo-caecal valve.

The colon absorbs water from the fluid material reaching it from above and forms waste-matter into a semi-solid state suitable for evacuation as faeces.

Obstruction. Any hindrance to the normal onward progression of the foodstuffs passing through the intestine. This may be acute or chronic, and can occur at any point in the small or large bowel; the chronic type is always liable to become acute.

Causes include strangulated hernia; intussusception (part of the bowel becomes telescoped within a lower part); volvulus (the bowel becomes twisted); peritoneal bands and adhesions; impaction of foreign bodies; stricture (due to bowel disease); tumour (particularly carcinoma of the lower bowel), and, occasionally, congenital abnormalities.

Symptoms such as colicky pain, vomiting, shock, abdominal distension, tenderness and rigidity are suffered. The muscular efforts of the intestine, attempting to overcome the obstruction, may be seen on the abdominal surface as 'visible peristalsis'. Treatment is always surgical and acute obstruction calls for emergency relief.

bow legs. Lateral curvature of the legs so that the knees are widely separated when the ankles are in contact. The condition is due to rickets and is preventable by proper diet and adequate vitamin D.

In young children, cases generally improve under skilled supervision, combined with temporarily keeping the weight off the legs, and correction of dietary deficiencies. Adult cases in which permanent deformity has resulted from subsequent ossification may require surgical correction.

brachial. Relating to the arm.

bradycardia. Slowness of the heart beat. The usual pulse-rate is 72 beats per minute but a rate of 50 may be found in perfectly healthy athletic subjects, and old people often have slow pulse-rates.

Bradycardia may however indicate disease, especially 'heart-block', where heart-muscle damage causes irregularity of the impulses stimulating contraction of the ventricles. It occurs also in toxic conditions such as uraemia and jaundice; as an indication of heart complications in severe fevers, notably diphtheria and typhoid fever; in hypothyroidism; in poisoning by morphine and other depressant drugs; after excessive dosage of digitalis; and in increased intracranial tension.

brain. The complex mass of nervous tissue at the upper end of the spinal cord.

As animals evolved the simple reflex control provided by the spinal cord alone became inadequate for the needs of increasingly complicated organisms as

skull

cerebrum

mid brain

third ventricle

cerebellum

pons

fourth ventricle

medulla oblongata

spinal cord

Brain: anatomy

they adapted themselves to live more freely, more safely and more successfully within their environment.

In the nervous system this adaptation took place by the expansion of the upper end of the spinal cord in order to provide the additional nervous equipment needed to develop and maintain an independent and purposeful existence.

This upper expanded portion of the central nervous system is known as the encephalon or brain, and in man and all the vertebrates it is contained within the skull or cranial cavity. Its relative size in various animals is an indication of their status on the evolutionary scale and the human brain is by far the largest relative to body-size.

Inside the cranial cavity the brain is encased by three separate layers of membranes or meninges named, from the outside inwards, the dura mater, the arachnoid mater and the pia mater. The dura is tough and fibrous and represents the periosteum of the inner surface of the skull. It also provides four partitions (or septa) which extend into the cavity and form smaller spaces to accommodate and support the sub-divisions of the brain. The arachnoid is a more delicate membrane and between it and the pia (a layer containing blood vessels closely attached to the brain surface), is the sub-arachnoid space containing cerebro-spinal fluid. This fluid layer helps to cushion the brain against impact and sudden movement.

The substance of the brain is composed of grey matter and white matter with blood vessels and a small amount of connective tissue.

Grey matter is composed of nerve cells which originate and receive nerve impulses; white matter is made up of nerve fibres whose function is to transmit nerve impulses from point to point. The proportions and relationships of grey and white matter vary in different parts of the brain.

Parts of the brain. In a simplified description of the brain, the parts from below upwards are:

1. Medulla oblongata. Although continuous with the spinal cord below and only 3 cm. long its minute anatomy is very complex. Within it, nerve fibres from the right side of the fore-brain cross over to pass to the left side of the spinal cord and vice-versa. This is known as the pyramidal decussation and explains why damage to the fore-brain causes paralysis on the opposite side of the body. The medulla also contains the nuclei of the last eight cranial nerves.

2. Pons and cerebellum (or hind-brain). In front of the medulla is the pons, a broad, rounded mass of nerve fibres running transversely and connected below the medulla, above to the fore-brain and behind to the cerebellum which is an egg-shaped mass behind the medulla, and arranged in layers of both grey and white matter.

3. Mid-brain. This is a further short constricted section of the main axis. It is continuous below with the medulla but at its upper end it divides to form two large branches, the cerebral peduncles, which carry fibres to each of the cerebral hemispheres.

4. Cerebrum (the cerebral hemispheres

parietal lobe

frontal lobe

body movements

body sensations

memory

thought

speech

eye movements

taste smell sound

occipital lobe

sight

balance

cerebellum

temporal lobe

→ sensory impulses entering the brain

- - -> motor impulses leaving the brain

Brain: physiology

or fore-brain). This is much the largest part of the brain and occupies most of the cranial cavity. It is divided from front to back into two hemispherical masses of nervous tissue known as the right and left cerebral hemispheres and at the bottom of this central fissure is a broad band of communicating fibres, the corpus callosum.

Each hemisphere is in turn divided by grooves called sulci into four main lobes – frontal, temporal (at the side), parietal (on the top), and occipital (at the back).

The surface of the hemispheres or cerebral cortex is made up of grey matter and is arranged in a complicated pattern of ridges and furrows called respectively convolutions and gyri.

The cerebral hemispheres each contain a cavity, the lateral ventricle, occupied by the vascular choroid plexus which produces the clear CEREBRO-SPINAL FLUID. The lateral ventricles unite below as the third ventricle and the fluid passes down through a channel (Sylvian aqueduct) to the fourth ventricle behind the medulla and from there by an opening to the general sub-arachnoid space.

The PINEAL GLAND and the pituitary gland are both ENDOCRINE GLANDS which form part of the structure of the brain.

Functions of the brain. The individual areas of the brain all have very specific functions.

1. Cerebrum. Removal of the cerebral

lobes in an animal deprives it of volition and intelligence. All the higher functions of the brain can be referred to specific cortical areas and in very general terms the frontal lobes are concerned with memory and thought, the parietal with motor function and sensation, the temporal with taste, smell and hearing and the occipital with sight.

2. Mid-brain. In the region of the third ventricle are other important nerve centres, the thalamus, hypothalamus and basal ganglia. These are concerned with functions carried on automatically below the level of consciousness. The thalamus is the chief relay station of the sensory systems and receives impressions from cord, cerebellum, and cranial nerves; the hypothalamus regulates metabolism, stabilizes temperature and integrates the functions of the organs in the body, and the basal ganglia regulate muscle tone and co-ordinate voluntary movement.

3. Cerebellum. The cerebellum receives linking fibres from cerebrum, cord, and the vestibular part of the acoustic nerve and is concerned with reflex maintenance of balance and posture.

4. Medulla oblongata. Apart from its function as the main connection between the cord and the upper brain and as the site of the crossing of both motor and sensory fibres, the medulla is of supreme importance because it contains all the 'vital centres' and the nuclei of all but the

first four pairs of cranial nerves. These vital centres are concerned with respiration, blood pressure, and heart action.

Cranial nerves. Arising from the medulla and from the base of the brain are twelve pairs of cranial nerves all concerned with vital functions and sense-organs. Some are motor (i.e., stimulating muscles to act), others are sensory (i.e., transmitting sensations to the brain) and some contain both motor and sensory fibres. Within the brain their origins, terminations and connections with each other are complex, so that active co-ordination can occur. The nerves pass through openings in the skull.

By enumerating them from below upwards it can be seen that there is a pattern of increasingly specialized function parallelling the upward evolutionary expansion of the central nervous system:

Twelfth: hypoglossal – motor nerve of tongue

Eleventh: spinal accessory – movements of soft palate and head

Tenth: vagus – influences action of organs

Ninth: glosso-pharyngeal – sensory to tongue and assists swallowing

Eighth: acoustic – hearing and balance

Seventh: facial – motor nerve to muscles of face and mouth

Sixth: abducent – eye movements

Fifth: trigeminal – sensory to face and motor to muscle of mastication

Fourth: trochlear – eye movements

Third: oculomotor – eye movements

Second: optic – sight

First: olfactory – smell

Disease. Because of its complexity the brain is subject to many diseases and only some of the commonest are here mentioned.

1. Infections. Inflammation of the brain substance, encephalitis, may occur in various virus diseases, e.g., poliomyelitis, rabies and encephalitis lethargica (sleepy sickness). Inflammation of the surrounding membranes, meningitis, may be due to invasion by bacteria or viruses or, in the tropics, trypanosomes. All are serious but can be cured by modern treatment, mostly with antibiotics.

2. Arterial disease. There are three forms of stroke: cerebral haemorrhage, where a small artery (weakened by arteriosclerosis and overstressed by high blood pressure) ruptures causing bleeding into the brain substance; cerebral thrombosis where blood clots in a small vessel, depriving a part of the brain of nourishment; and cerebral embolism, where a particle (e.g., an air bubble) causes similar blockage. Again, rupture of a weak part of a blood vessel may cause bleeding between the layers of surrounding membrane (sub-arachnoid haemorrhage).

3. Tumours. Primary tumours, gliomas and meningiomas, are not uncommon, and secondary tumours may occur from spread

from elsewhere in the body. Whether actually destroying brain tissue or merely acting by pressure they cause many variable symptoms, e.g., headache, personality changes, fits, paralysis and blindness.

4. Degeneration and atrophy. Many poisons (e.g., lead) produce brain degeneration and a general atrophy of the brain occurs in senile dementia, chronic alcoholism, and advanced untreated syphilis.

5. Congenital abnormalities. Hydrocephalus is an example of a developmental anomaly.

6. Injuries. These are not uncommon, particularly in traffic accidents.

brain fever. An old-fashioned term signifying the delirium associated with infections of the brain and its enclosing membranes (meninges), or with toxaemia from acute fevers. See MENINGITIS.

breast. The breasts or mammae are glands accessory to the female reproductive system, producing milk for the nourishment of the infant. In the male they are rudimentary.

The weight and size of the breasts differ in individuals and at different periods of life. Developing as reproductive capacity is established, they enlarge during pregnancy and lactation, and atrophy in old age.

They consist of a glandular mass supported by fibrous tissue and rounded by fat. The gland tissue has many small lobes and from each arises a secretory duct known as a lactiferous tubule. There are between fifteen and twenty such ducts which open on the surface at the nipple, but within the nipple each has a small dilated section or ampulla, which serves as a milk-reservoir. The nipple is encircled by a coloured area of skin known as the areola.

When stimulated the nipple undergoes some erection so that it may be more readily grasped by a suckling's lips.

Diseases. Inflammatory conditions of the breast are mostly associated with lactation. Infection enters through a grazed nipple to cause either inflammation (acute mastitis) or mammary abscesses at various levels – sub-areolar, intra-mammary, or sub-mammary.

Chronic mastitis is related to the changes which occur in the breast after lactation and towards the end of reproductive life. Overgrowth of connective tissue constricts the glandular tissue and ducts and may give rise to cysts.

Tumours are frequent; if non-malignant they are mainly composed of glandular and connective tissue. The commonest malignant tumour is CANCER; it usually produces contraction and indrawing of the breast rather than enlargement. Paget's disease of the nipple is a cancer arising within the lactiferous ducts of the nipple.

breast bone. See STERNUM.

breast feeding. Although it was

unfashionable for a period, many mothers now breast feed their babies, and there are strong arguments in favour of breast feeding. The composition of human milk provides for the optimum nutrition of the human infant, and it is also sterile, conveniently available at the correct temperature as required, and free of cost. Also, the act of breast feeding forges a psychic bond between mother and infant which is beneficial to emotional development. In addition to this, although many children thrive completely satisfactorily on artificial feeding, there is a greater risk of malnutrition and infection through carelessness while preparing the bottles and filling them.

Lactation. Under hormonal influence, the breasts, soon after conception, prepare for subsequent lactation, but actual secretion of milk is inhibited until after the birth. The stimulus of suckling also encourages output. Immediately after childbirth the breast secretes only colostrum, a fluid especially rich in protein and not requiring digestion. This provides the infant's needs for the first two or three days until its digestive system is operative. It also provides temporary immunity to some infections as it contains substances from the mother's blood plasma. By the third day swelling of the breasts occurs and normal milk secretion begins.

Adequate lactation is conditioned by both physical and psychic factors. Good health, contentment, lack of fatigue, a liberal well-balanced diet with ample protein and a sufficient fluid intake are obvious requirements, but pleasure in nursing, determination and optimism are thought to influence by reflex the production by the pituitary gland of milk-forming hormone, while grief and worry inhibit this.

Methods of regime. Mothercraft lectures during pregnancy should encourage a determination to breast feed and should include instruction in the technique of nursing and the care of breast and nipples.

After washing the breasts and nipples the mother should sit comfortably in a low chair with her infant in the crook of the arm on the side being used. The breast is supported with the other hand and the skin above the nipple retracted by thumb to avoid obstruction of the infant's nostrils.

Hospitals and professional advisers favour their individual regimes but the following is typical:

Starting six to twelve hours after birth, three feeds of a few minutes at each breast are given each day during the first and second days, or until full lactation commences. During this period the infant obtains only small amounts of colostrum and its fluid requirements should be made up by sterile water from a spoon. When lactation is established the breasts provide about 425 g. (15 oz.) of milk per day, rising to 550 to 700 g. (20 to 25 oz.) at one month, 700 to 850 g. (25 to 30 oz.) at three months and 850 g. to 1 kg. (30 to 35 oz.) at six months. Thereafter the quantity declines.

There is difference of opinion about regular and 'on-demand' feeding, but regularity may be better both for emotional development and for the digestive tract. For the first two months three-hourly feeding is usual, (6 a.m., 9 a.m., 12 noon, 3 p.m., 6 p.m., 10 p.m.) changing to four-hourly at six to twelve weeks. One breast may be used alternately at each feed of about twenty minutes, or ten minutes given at each breast. The use of one breast is said to be preferable because the end-milk is richer in fat. The infant ingests air during suckling and should be 'posseted' - set upright and allowed to 'break wind'.

If there is fear of UNDERFEEDING, suggested perhaps by the infant failing to thrive, it is important to ascertain how much milk a breast-fed infant is actually getting. This is done by a 'test-feed' i.e., weighing the baby on an accurate scale before and after a feed. If needed, a 'complementary feed' can be given by bottle after each breast feed, or a 'supplementary feed' replacing one or more breast feeds.

Breast feeding is inadvisable if the mother is suffering from malnutrition, general illness, tuberculosis, chronic nephritis, severe heart disease or puerperal psychosis. It is equally inadvisable if the infant suffers from prematurity, brain damage or other mental abnormality, hare-lip or cleft palate.

If the mother does not wish to breast-feed, lactation may be checked by giving several doses of oestrogen. Without such help there may be swelling and pain in the breasts for a few days but, lacking in stimulus of suckling, the breasts gradually return to normal over several weeks.

breathlessness. Distressed respiration or dyspnoea, although temporary breathlessness after considerable exertion is a normal phenomenon and is therefore not dyspnoea. The basic cause of dyspnoea is over-stimulation of the respiratory centre in the brain by excess of carbonic acid in the blood. This implies that oxygen is not easily leaving the lungs (as in asthma), or is not being carried by the blood at sufficient rate (as in defective circulation), or is not being conveyed in adequate amounts by the blood (as in anaemia), or is limited in quantity (as occurs in high altitudes).

Respiratory distress may affect breathing in (inspiration) and breathing out (expiration) unequally. Obstructive causes tend to produce inspiration dyspnoea; lung damage mostly affects expiration. In other conditions there is no marked difference.

A complaint of breathlessness requires investigation, and appropriate treatment can only be decided after a precise diagnosis of its cause.

breath, offensive. A more formal term for offensive breath is halitosis. Common causes are septic conditions of the mouth, nose, or naso-pharynx – e.g., bad teeth, unhealthy gums with pyorrhoea, mouth ulceration, diseased tonsils, and certain chronic nasal conditions. Mild offensiveness is sometimes due to gastric disorder or constipation.

Excessively putrid breath occurs in such lung conditions as bronchiectasis or lung abscess. Some general diseases, such as uraemia or diabetes, may produce characteristic odours, as may certain drugs.

bronchi. The bronchi are part of the main air-passages and arise in mid-chest by subdivision of the trachea or windpipe.

The right bronchus divides into three branches which enter the root of the right lung and pass to the upper, middle, and lower lobes. The left bronchus divides into two main branches to enter the upper and lower lobes of the left lung. Within each lung, these main branches divide and subdivide throughout the whole organ to form the intrapulmonary bronchi or 'bronchial-tree', conveying air to all parts of the lungs, the fine terminal branches being known as bronchioles.

BRONCHITIS, or inflammation of the bronchi, is one of the commonest maladies, readily caused by a wide variety of physical agencies or infective processes.

bronchial cyst and fistula. See GILLS.

bronchiectasis. A lung condition in which the bronchi or larger air-passages become dilated, either in their length (cylindrical bronchiectasis), or irregularly to form cavities (sacculated bronchiectasis). It is due to two factors: weakening of the bronchial wall by chronic bronchitis; and forced inspiration after coughing, especially if peripheral parts of the lung are damaged by disease and cannot expand freely.

Purulent secretion accumulates in the dilated parts and this erodes and further weakens the bronchus, establishing a vicious circle. There is often offensive sputum and offensive breath due to decomposition of pus which has not been coughed out.

The treatment is that of chronic bronchitis. Postural coughing may help the evacuation of sputum, and pneumothorax or other surgical procedures are occasionally used in selected cases.

bronchitis. Inflammation of the bronchi. Acute bronchitis is very common, especially where winter conditions are inclement, and is sometimes called the 'English disease' and chronic bronchitis follows repeated attacks of the acute form. Acute bronchitis is due to infection by some bacterial or viral agent. The windpipe is generally affected as well and if infection extends downwards to the smaller air-passages the disease becomes indistinguishable from broncho-pneumonia. An attack usually begins suddenly with

malaise, fever, chest pain, breathlessness, and a dry ineffective cough. Sputum later becomes copious – moist and frothy at first but becoming pus-like. A typical attack without complications lasts about seven to ten days. Acute bronchitis may also be caused by inhalation of dust or of irritants such as smoke or chemical vapours.

Treatment is by bed rest and the administration of antibiotics. Poultices, cough-mixtures, and medicated inhalations, although rather old-fashioned, still give some relief from symptoms.

In chronic bronchitis, the bronchial walls become thickened and fibrotic, and the mucous glands and the cells lining the bronchi degenerate. Long-standing chronic bronchitis may lead to emphysema, pulmonary fibrosis, and bronchiectasis, which in turn affects the circulation to the lungs, so that a degree of right-sided heart failure (corpulmonale) may eventually develop.

The patient with chronic bronchitis complains of his 'chest' – persistent cough, expectoration, and breathlessness on exertion. The cough varies in severity, usually recurring each winter. Smoking is undoubtedly a contributory cause.

Treatment of established chronic bronchitis can only be precautionary and soothing. A mild winter climate, avoidance of chill and exposure, cessation of smoking, attention to diet and general regime, antibiotics or vaccines, may all help to prevent worsening of the condition. Attacks, when they occur, require treatment as acute bronchitis.

broncho-pneumonia. An inflammatory lung condition in which infection spreads from the terminal air-passages (bronchioles) to the air-sacs (alveoli) and thence to the surrounding tissue, producing a patchy type of consolidation (lobular pneumonia), in contrast to the massive consolidation of a whole lung lobe which occurs in ordinary lobar pneumonia. It can begin as a primary broncho-pneumonia, especially in children, but many cases are secondary to other disease such as whooping cough or measles.

Broncho-pneumonia is a common sequel to many debilitating diseases and often hastens death in the aged. Treatment nowadays is usually by antibiotics.

brucellosis. Undulant or Malta fever. An infection, caused by *Brucella abortus*, mainly from the milk of infected cattle, sheep and goats and characterized by continued or intermittent fever, headache, profuse sweating and joint pains, all of which may last for days, months or occasionally years. The disease is transmitted to man from the milk of infected animals, from contact with the tissues or discharges of such animals, and very infrequently by airborne spread. There is no evidence of the infection passing from man to man.

Diagnosis is difficult clinically because the symptoms are vague and intermittent so it usually depends either on blood tests which show a rise in antibodies or on laboratory isolation of the infectious agent.

Prevention depends finally on either (1) ascertainment of all infected animals by blood tests and elimination of these animals by segregation or by slaughter, or (2) immunization of all calves, etc., in any area in which the disease is present. Pending such measures imperative steps are pasteurization of milk and other dairy products from cows, sheep and goats, or boiling of milk if pasteurization is impracticable; great care should be taken by veterinary surgeons and meat inspectors to avoid infection.

Treatment prospects have improved in recent years: tetracycline, or another suitable antibiotic, usually cures the disease in about three months, but relapse occurs in quite a proportion of cases.

bruises. A bruise or contusion is a superficial injury caused by impact or other external violence without actually breaking the skin. This results in damage to tissue and blood-vessels immediately beneath the skin and blood infiltrates the area. If an actual rupture of the underlying tissues occurs, blood may accumulate in the resultant space to produce a haematoma.

The signs of a bruise are obvious, with discoloration and swelling, but the possibility of associated damage to underlying organs and other structures must always be considered.

The amount of subcutaneous bleeding and of swelling varies a great deal not only with the degree of violence, but also with the part of the body injured. Where the tissues are lax the amount of bleeding is correspondingly greater, and it may track along beneath the skin by the influence of gravity and according to the surrounding anatomical structures, so that the discoloration (or ecchymosis) may appear elsewhere than at the actual site of injury.

Bruises undergo changes in colour as the blood within them disintegrates and becomes re-absorbed. At first they are of a dark purplish-blue colour which gradually alters over a week or so to various shades of brown and green and then to a pale yellow before disappearing completely.

In the initial stages, bruises are best treated by cold compresses and firm bandaging in order to limit bleeding. Later on, when the bruise is no longer painful, the absorption of effused blood can be hastened by massage. A localized haematoma, which may remain tense and painful for some time, can be relieved by aseptic draining.

bubo. An inflammatory swelling of the lymphatic glands in the groin (inguinal lymphadenitis). The term is sometimes also applied (incorrectly) to a similar condition in the armpit.

Inguinal bubo is due to some infective condition in the related lymphatic drainage area. In the classical bubo of bubonic PLAGUE it is caused by the entry of the bacillus through bites from infected fleas. The common causes are more mundane, ranging from septic sores on feet and legs, to various forms of venereal disease. Certain tropical diseases such as filariasis and sleeping sickness produce similar swellings.

The treatment is that of the underlying condition but the bubo may form pus and require surgical drainage.

bubonic plague. A disease due to infection with *Pasteurella pestis*, the PLAGUE bacillus.

bunion. A condition, usually found over the joint at the base of the big toe, in which there is thickening both of the skin and of the head of the metatarsal bone. The main cause is the wearing of shoes which are too short or too narrow at the toes, so that the big toe is forced out of position towards the other toes. Prevention is essentially by wearing wide enough shoes. Where the condition has developed, treatment may include wearing socks like gloves with a compartment for each toe, or inserting every morning a piece of lint between the great toe and the next toe. In very severe cases operative treatment may be required.

burns and scalds. Exposure of any part of the body to excessive heat causes injury to the tissues. With flame or dry heat the result is a burn; hot liquids and hot moist vapours, such as steam, produce a scald. Burns may also be caused by acids, alkalis, electricity, friction, and exposure to sources of radiant energy, such as excessive sunlight, ultra-violet light, gamma-rays and x-rays.

Heat injury is described according to the severity of tissue reaction and damage. The classification of burns, ranging from 'first degree' to 'sixth degree', is still in current use, although to some extent the area of a burn is more important than its degree.

First degree: reddening and congestion of the skin; no tissue destruction.

Second degree: blistering of skin.

Third degree: cuticle and outer layer of the true skin is destroyed but the deeper papillae with nerve-endings survive. Since these are then left exposed, this grade of burn is very painful and causes considerable shock.

In these three degrees of burn, sufficient skin-cells survive to ensure healing by natural multiplication of cells without recourse to skin-grafting.

Fourth degree: the whole thickness of skin and subcutaneous tissue are destroyed.

Fifth degree: muscles are destroyed.

Sixth degree: a whole limb is charred or disorganized.

Clinical features. Apart from the tissue destruction described above, the immediate danger of a severe burn is the amount of constitutional upset. Shock and collapse are related more to the area of a burn than to its depth, and require immediate treatment. Later on there will be absorption of toxins from the burned areas, manifested by raised temperature and pulse-rate, and often delirium. Further complications may ensue, such as bronchopneumonia and suppression of urinary excretion.

In cases which survive, inflammation (usually accompanied by infection) gradually leads to separation of dead tissue as sloughs, leaving an ulcerated surface which eventually heals. If not skin-grafted, the resultant scarring may produce contractures and deformity.

Treatment. Local treatment depends on the severity of the burn and on its extent. The objects are to allay pain and to prevent secondary infection of the burned area.

Immediate treatment: separate the casualty from the danger, bathe the damaged part freely in cold water to reduce the pain and heat, and then apply a dressing and cover this with available soft materials, such as cotton-wool and a bandage.

For minor burns of small extent, initial cleaning with a mild antiseptic or normal saline (i.e., 1 teaspoon of salt to 0.5 l. (1 pt.) of water) followed by the application of medicated tulle, is simple and effective. The tulle is an open-weave gauze impregnated with soft paraffin and an antibiotic. If saline or antiseptic is not immediately available, the burned part may be held under cold running water for a few minutes. Any blister which may develop should not normally be drained.

In more severe burns, and in superficial burns involving large areas of skin, the immediate need is to initiate adequate treatment against SHOCK and possible complications. Such patients should be sent to hospital, and the first aid treatment is therefore just to cover the burned areas with a sterile, or at least clean, dressing. The dressing may be either dry or moistened with normal saline or a weak solution of sodium bicarbonate – say 2 teaspoonfuls to 0.5 l. (1 pt.) of water. Measures to combat shock should also be initiated by keeping the patient warm and giving hot sweet drinks.

In hospital it will probably be necessary to give intravenous infusions of saline or plasma. For local treatment, various centres have their own favourite regimes.

At a later stage, whole-skin destruction will necessitate skin-grafting.

Acid burns. Corrosive acids cause tissue damage with much the same effect as a burn by heat, but continue to act harmfully until removed or neutralized. Such injuries should therefore first be sluiced freely with clean or sterile water, saline, or a weak alkaline solution of sodium bicarbonate (2 teaspoonfuls to 0.5 l. (1 pt.) water). Thereafter a moist dressing can be applied using the same alkaline solution.

Alkali burns. Corrosive alkalis, such as caustic soda, also cause tissue damage with much the same effect as a burn by heat, and they too continue to act harmfully until removed or neutralized. Such injuries should therefore first be sluiced freely with clean or sterile water, saline, or a weak acid solution of vinegar (2 tablespoonfuls to 0.5 l. (1 pt.) water). Thereafter a moist dressing can be applied using saline or the vinegar solution.

Eye burns. Burns of the eye are always potentially serious since even small superficial injuries involving the cornea will impair subsequent vision. The eyelids automatically protect the eyes, which themselves often escape even in extensive facial burns, but a hot 'spark' may enter and cause injury. More common are the effects of splashes of caustic materials – acids, alkalis, quicklime, etc.

It is essential to wash out the harmful substance *immediately*: lay the patient down, hold the eyelids open, and pour plenty of plain water over the eye, or put the face in a basin of water and open and shut the eyelids while submerged. For acid injuries, a solution of 1 teaspoon of sodium bicarbonate to 0.5 l. (1 pt.) of water can be used for washing out, and for alkalis (including quicklime), a weak acid solution of 1 tablespoonful of vinegar to 0.5 l. (1 pt.) of water.

Speed is vital, and the value of immediate washing out with plain water outweighs delay in obtaining more precise antidotes. In all cases the subsequent first-aid treatment is to instil a drop of castor or olive oil, apply an occlusive pad and bandage, and send the patient to hospital.

bursa. A pouch, or sac-like cavity in the tissues, lined by synovial membrane (as in joint-capsules), and containing synovial fluid as a lubricant. Its purpose is to minimize friction of the tissues at points subject to pressure or movement. Bursae are found in many parts of the body as normal anatomical structures, between muscles and tendons, and between bony prominences and the skin.

Familiar examples are the bursae over the knee (pre-patellar bursa), the elbow (olecranon bursa), and over the bony points carrying one's weight when seated (ischial bursa). These frequently become inflamed in BURSITIS.

Repeated pressure and friction may also lead to the development of bursae not normally present, and therefore called 'adventitious bursae'. Examples include BUNIONS.

bursitis. Inflammation of a bursa. The sac of a bursa subjected to repeated small injuries may become inflamed and distended by an excessive development of the fluid within the bursa, usually mixed with blood. Deposits of fibrin from the blood produce a thickening of the bursal wall with a diminished capacity to re-absorb the excess fluid.

Swellings thus develop in familiar sites,

as 'housemaid's knee', 'miner's elbow' and bunions.

Initially these may respond to rest and draining of their contents but resistant cases will require removal of the sac. Bursae may become infected and develop pus, when they will also need surgical treatment.

Bursitis can also occur in general diseases such as gonorrhoea and syphilis, and in tuberculosis in proximity to infected joints.

byssinosis. A condition of diminished chest expansion and emphysema, characterized by paroxysmal cough and respiratory difficulty resembling that of asthma. It occurs among persons who have for long periods breathed the dust from cotton and cotton fabrics, and is ascribed to moulds present in these materials. Byssinosis is in part preventable by measures for the reduction of the dust, and regular medical examination of cotton workers can usually identify the disease in the early stages, when treatment is still relatively easy.

C

cachexia. A severe state of ill-health accompanied by constitutional disorder and serious malnutrition. It develops in chronic wasting diseases such as pulmonary tuberculosis, malignant conditions, prolonged sepsis and fevers, hyperthyroidism and other endocrine disorders, toxaemia from various causes, and some kinds of chronic poisoning.

caecum. A musculo-membraneous pouch situated down on the lower right of the abdomen and forming a cul-de-sac at the beginning of the large intestine. It receives the contents of the small intestine through the ileo-caecal valve before their onward passage through the colon. At its lower extremity it terminates as a tube of much reduced calibre which is the appendix.

caesarean section. Delivery of a child by an incision through the abdominal and uterine walls instead of by the natural passage.

Caesarean section is a routine and safe surgical procedure employed in obstetric situations where normal delivery might carry risk to mother or baby. It may be carried out if one or more of the following conditions apply: contracted pelvis; disproportionately large babies; obstructive position of the placenta (placenta praevia); ante-partum haemorrhage; toxaemia or other disease of the mother; rupture of the uterus; and more rarely, tumours or congenital abnormalities of the uterus interfering with the normal mechanism of labour.

caffeine. A white crystalline alkaloid substance contained in tea and coffee. A cerebral stimulant and mild diuretic, it is a common constituent of analgesic powders because of its reputed effect in relieving the migranous type of headache.

caisson disease. See DECOMPRESSION DISEASE.

calcification. The deposition of lime salts in body-tissues. Calcification is a normal process in the growth and development of bones and teeth when calcium salts, mainly phosphate and carbonate, are laid down in an orderly fashion. Calcium metabolism is controlled by activity of the parathyroid glands and by the availability of dietary vitamin D.

Calcification also occurs pathologically, and in general, dead or degenerating tissue tends to become impregnated by lime salts; this type differs from ossification since the lime salts are without definite structure and may produce harmful mechanical effects both to the tissue which they occupy and to its surroundings.

calcium. A hard, yellowish, metallic element, always found combined with another element, e.g. calcium carbonate or calcium sulphate. It is widely distributed in the soil and is a mineral constituent of all plants and animals.

The body requires calcium particularly for the formation of bones and teeth. Milk and vegetables are good sources but it is abundant in any ordinary diet. However, its proper utilization requires an adequate intake of vitamin D, otherwise children suffer from rickets and older persons develop osteomalacia. Calcium metabolism is also influenced by the parathyroid glands, over-activity of which decalcifies bone. Under-activity lowers serum calcium to produce the condition known as parathyroid tetany.

calculus. See STONE.

caliper. A caliper or walking-caliper splint consists of a padded ring which encircles the upper thigh and rests against the bony prominence in the lower buttock which is the ischial tuberosity of the pelvis. To this ring are attached two metal bars (usually adjustable in length), one on each side of the limb. Angled lower-ends fit into the heel of the patient's boot and thus his weight is transmitted through the caliper and not through the limb. Such a splint is used after fractures and joint disease so that walking is possible without crutches or risk of injury to diseased or healing parts. The same principles of caliper splintage or traction are used elsewhere. Digital fractures are an example.

callosity. A circumscribed thickening of the outer layer of the skin, occurring as a protective reaction to friction, pressure, or other chronic irritation. Callosities are commonly seen on the feet, on the hands of manual workers, on the shoulders of porters, and so on.

Callosities are generally painless, and require no treatment, but sometimes a sac, containing synovial fluid, develops beneath them to form an adventitious BURSA. A CORN is another type of painful callosity.

Calorie. For measuring quantities of heat the scientific unit is the gram-calorie; this is the amount of heat required to raise the temperature of one gram of water by one degree centigrade.

Food is the fuel which the body requires for its energy; since foods vary in the amount of energy which they liberate when 'burned' or metabolized, it is usual to express their food-value in this respect in units of heat. For this purpose the gram-calorie is an inconveniently small unit, so the heat-equivalent of foods is stated in Calories (capital C); these are kilogram-calories, equal to 1000 gram-calories. In the future a new unit of measurement, the KILOJOULE, will be used more frequently to measure food values.

Self examination for breast cancer. Lie down with a cushion under one
shoulder. Using the flat of the fingers rather than the tips, first check into the
armpits for any 'lump' and then work carefully round the breast, always
stroking from the edge towards the nipple. Change the cushion to the other
side and repeat the test.

Dietary needs in terms of Calories and
the Calorie values of individual foodstuffs
are explained in the articles on DIET and
NUTRITION.

cancer. Any malignant tumour or
unregulated growth of tissue is commonly
called 'cancer' but scientifically there are
three types according to the cells of the
tissue involved. The cells which cover the
outer surface of the body and line internal
passages and closed cavities are called
epithelial cells: malignancy in these cells is
known as carcinoma. In other body cells it
is sarcoma. Malignant proliferation of
certain blood cells is seen in leukaemia.

Cancer is essentially the unregulated
and unrestricted growth of new cells to
form tissue which lacks the useful function
of its parent tissue and serves no purpose;
which disorganizes the structure and
function of the part of the body where it
arises; which invades adjacent tissues; and
which tends to spread to other organs by
blood-borne metastases.

Cancer occurs in man and all vertebrate
animals. An incidence of about one in
twenty of the population is increasing
slowly, but the increase is probably more
apparent than real, due to better diagnosis
and because more persons now survive to
reach the older cancer-prone age-groups.

Causes. Although world-wide and
massive cancer research has so far failed
to demonstrate exactly why cells should
behave in this way, nevertheless much is
known about predisposing factors. Cancer
of the stomach has been shown to occur
more frequently in persons of certain
blood groups, but cancer is not hereditary
in the true sense and any hereditary
influence is apparently due to some
genetically determined variation in
resistance to environmental factors, whose
importance is undoubted. There are many
organic chemicals which tend to induce
carcinoma, for example: the polycyclic
hydrocarbons derived from tar;
benzyprene in cigarette smoke (which has
been incriminated as a cause of lung
cancer); and naphthylamine solvents used

in the rubber industry (which cause carcinoma of the bladder).

Mechanical and physical factors may also induce cancer: a jagged tooth or ill-fitting denture may produce a chronic mouth ulcer which refuses to heal and undergoes malignant change; and skin cancer can be due to prolonged x-ray exposure. It is known that virus material can induce malignant changes in animals. Recent evidence suggests that about half of all cancers may be related to diet, in particular deficiency of vitamin A.

Signs and symptoms. Because pain is a late feature, cancer is often neglected until the prospects of successful treatment are imperilled. In view of the importance of early treatment, attention may here be called to some warning signs, although it must be understood that there are other possible explanations of each sign listed below, so that, while indicating the desirability of skilled investigation, these signs do not necessarily indicate the existence of cancer.

On external surfaces any thickening of the tissues or any persisting sores and ulcers should arouse suspicion. Internal cancers are insidious but weight loss and anaemia in an older person need investigation, especially if accompanied by any of the following:

1. Breast: tumour; skin-puckering; retraction of, or bleeding from, the nipple.

2. Gastro-intestinal tract: persistent digestive symptoms; abdominal pain; constipation; 'tarry' stools indicating internal bleeding; fresh blood; alternation for an appreciable time between constipation and diarrhoea.

3. Respiratory system: cough; pain; breathlessness; blood-stained sputum; persistent hoarseness or difficulty in swallowing.

4. Bladder: blood in the urine.

5. Female genital tract: irregular bleeding or its persistence after the menopause.

Prevention. Known hazards, such as those noted above, should be avoided, adequate green and yellow vegetables should be eaten, and cigarette smoking should be abandoned; but in general the prospect of successful treatment depends on early detection.

Cancer detection clinics were pioneered by the American Cancer Society in 1920. The essentials are a careful clinical history and examination; x-ray of chest; blood examination of faeces for occult blood (i.e., blood that is not obvious on inspection). For the female, CERVICAL CYTOLOGY (the 'cyto-test'), when a smear is taken from the urine cervix for microscopic examination, is now widely available, and simple self-examination for breast cancer is carried out easily at home.

Treatment. The basic treatment for early accessible cancer is surgical removal with dissection of related lymph-glands. Deep x-ray therapy and radium application are used as alternative or auxiliary procedures.

Chemical methods are being developed. Such drugs may be antimetabolites (which inhibit nucleic acid synthesis), cytotoxins (which act on formed nucleic acid), radio-isotopes (for special tumours), steroids (which influence antibody response), antibiotics (e.g., actinomycin c in Hodgkin's disease) or other drugs such as methylhydrazine derivatives or vincristine sulphate.

cancrum oris. A very severe infective STOMATITIS with ulceration and gangrene of the lips and cheeks.

canine teeth. The single-cusped or pointed teeth of which there are two in each jaw situated on each side between the last incisor tooth and the first pre-molar tooth. In children they erupt at about the eighteenth month and their permanent replacements appear at the age of 11 years.

cannabis. A drug obtained from the Indian hemp plant (*Cannabis sativa*). The dried flowering tops contain a resin, cannabinol, and are used to make cigarettes (reefers). Cannabis is also called marihuana and another preparation using resin from the whole plant is known as hashish. The drug is taken to produce the pleasurable effects of a mild intoxication in which the user feels elated.

The possession and use of cannabis is now illegal in most countries and the United Nations Commission on Narcotic Drugs considers cannabis abuse a form of addiction likely to be a forerunner of dependence on more dangerous drugs. This view has been challenged on the grounds that cannabis is a less antisocial drug than alcohol. Nevertheless, the drug has powerful effects on the central nervous system and psychotic illness has been caused by its excessive use.

cantharides. The 'Spanish fly' is really a beetle, *Cantharis vesicatoria*, common in southern Europe. Their bodies contain a substance, cantharadin, a powerful irritant, which causes inflammation of the skin and blistering.

As a commercial undertaking, the beetles are collected and dried and various official pharmacopeial preparations – plasters, tinctures, and ointments, whose active ingredient is cantharadin – are made from the dried beetles for use in medicine.

Blistering is now an out-moded procedure, but these medicaments were once much used as counter-irritants. Acetum cantharadini is still employed to encourage hair-growth in baldness but its efficacy is doubtful, while its reputation as an aphrodisiac simply depends on irritation of the entire urinary system. When absorbed, cantharadin is an irritant poison with severe effects on the gastro-intestinal and urinary tracts. The use of its various preparations requires care.

capillaries. The minute blood-vessels which

→ blood fluid containing
nutriments

┄┄► body fluid containing
waste matter

The function of the capillaries

connect the terminal branches of the arteries (arterioles) to the small radicles of the venous system (venules) and which form a network in most parts of the body. The blood can thus circulate through the tissues to provide food and oxygen, arriving from the heart by the arterial system and returning through the veins.

Similar small vessels are found in the lymphatic system and are known as lymphatic capillaries.

capsule. Anatomically, a capsule is any fibrous or membraneous sac enclosing an organ or part of the body.

Capsules are also used in pharmacy to enclose various drugs. Amylnitrate is dispensed in thin-walled capsules (0.2 ml.) enclosed in absorbent fabric. They are crushed between finger and thumb and the vapour inhaled to relieve anginal pain. Officially these are called 'vitrellae' to distinguish them from gelatine capsules in which many medicines for oral use are now supplied, especially if they have a nauseating taste or are unsuitable for moulding into tablets. Somewhat similar are cachets made of two watch-glass shaped halves of soluble wafer-paper between which the drug is enclosed. These are used when a bulky dose is required (1 to 2 gm.).

Both gelatine capsules and cachets are intended to be held momentarily in the mouth till moistened and softened and then swallowed whole.

carbohydrate. An essential component of our food, carbohydrates are organic compounds containing carbon, hydrogen, and oxygen.

In terms of the diet, carbohydrates are the starches and sugars, almost entirely of vegetable origin, and they provide the greater part of the energy requirements of the body. In the process of digestion both the starches and the more complex sugars are broken down to glucose which is absorbed and stored in the liver and muscles until required as fuel by the tissues.

carbohydrate intolerance. Inability to digest and absorb carbohydrate. Signs and symptoms include flatulence and distension of the abdomen, watery diarrhoea, and in due course weakness, enlarged liver, and acidosis. The cause of the intolerance is either faulty secretion of the digestive juices which normally break down sugars and starches to simpler sugars (monosaccharides) for absorption, or inability of the digestive tract to absorb monosaccharides.

Treatment depends on the cause but may consist of supplying drugs to replace or stimulate the faulty digestive juices, of giving drugs which slow the movement of food in the digestive tract and so provide more time for absorption, or of removing ordinary starches and sugars from the diet and substituting the simplest of sugars, glucose.

carbolic acid. An organic compound distilled from coal-tar. Also known as phenol, it is a powerful antiseptic, disinfectant, and germicide. It has disadvantages in relation to toxicity and tissue damage and has largely been superseded by safer compounds.

carbon monoxide. A colourless gas, odourless, poisonous and lighter than air, produced by the combustion of carbon in a limited supply of oxygen. It is poisonous because it combines with the haemoglobin of the blood to form the stable, bright-red compound carboxy-haemoglobin which can no longer carry oxygen to the body tissues, and so death results from a form of asphyxia. A concentration of 10 per cent in the atmosphere is highly inflammable and a concentration of 1 per cent is definitely dangerous to breathe.

Carbon monoxide is a constituent of motor vehicle exhaust gas; defective exhaust systems or running engines in closed garages are therefore potential hazards.

Although in many places coal-gas is now being replaced by natural gas, which is mainly methane and relatively harmless except in high concentrations, domestic coal-gas contains carbon monoxide and it is therefore frequently a cause of accidental deaths resulting from carelessness or misuse, and is often used in suicide attempts.

In chronic, low-grade poisoning (as from a persisting small gas leak) the main signs are pallor, headaches and signs of anaemia. Acute poisoning is characterized by headache, nausea, vomiting, staggering gait, muscular weakness and mental confusion (a general picture resembling drunkenness), often continuing to coma and death.

In rescue work the wearing of a respirator, or failing that a wet cloth round the mouth and nose, is important: the intending rescuer may otherwise become a second victim.

On entering a room filled with coal-gas the rescuer should open the windows widely before doing anything else, and he should in no circumstances use a naked light. Having opened the windows and dealt with any immediate source of gas (such as a tap left on) he should get the victim into the open air, loosen clothing, especially round the neck, apply artifical respiration and send an available person for a doctor because administration of oxygen is likely to be necessary.

carbuncle. An area of localized infective gangrene resulting from invasion of the subcutaneous tissues by bacteria, most commonly *Staphylococcus aureus*.

This can appear anywhere but is most often seen on the back and over the back of the neck as an extension of a BOIL. A hard painful discoloured swelling develops, followed by the appearance of pus, sinus formation and sloughing of tissue. Constitutional symptoms may be severe and carbuncles of the face carry a special risk of venous thrombosis which may spread to blood-sinuses in the brain or cause generalized pyaemia. Debilitated and diabetic patients are particularly susceptible.

Treatment requires draining away the pus, removal of dead tissue and antiseptic packing with prompt administration of appropriate antibiotics. General health also needs consideration.

carcinogen. A substance liable to cause cancer.

carcinoma. The scientific term for CANCER, i.e. malignant disease arising from epithelial cells which form such tissues as skin, mucous membranes and secretory glands. Carcinomata may be further qualified to indicate the type of cell or organ involved, as for instance squamous (flattened cells) carcinoma, or bronchial carcinoma. Malignant change in supportive tissues is known generally as sarcoma.

cardiac. Concerning the heart.

cardio-vascular disease. Disease affecting the heart and blood vessels. The term is generally used in a more restricted sense to describe degenerative changes occurring in the arterial system and thus affecting the heart by increasing its work and diminishing its blood supply.

The arterial changes are mainly of two kinds. In sclerosis, high blood pressure leads to hardening, inelasticity, and narrowing of arteries. In atheroma, degeneration of the artery lining is followed by the appearance of deposits and accumulation of cholesterol, fatty substances and lime-salts, which narrow the vessel and may ultimately block it. The conditions may coexist and are of special importance in relation to coronary heart disease, which in the U.K. causes about one-quarter of all male deaths and a smaller but increasing proportion of female deaths.

It has been shown that a diet high in animal fat is associated with a high blood-cholesterol level and that the latter is in turn associated with increased numbers of deaths from coronary thrombosis. Many other contributory factors such as stress, obesity, cigarette-smoking, excessive sugar consumption and soft drinking water have also been incriminated to a greater or lesser degree.

However, it does appear to be worthwhile to advocate a diet relatively free from animal fats ('saturated fats') and low in cholesterol. Some of the unsaturated fatty acids, as found in margarine, and particularly linoleic acid, are 'essential fatty acids' (EFA). These are precursors of a newly-discovered class of hormones known as the prostaglandins. As these have some remarkable physiological effects, including reducing blood pressure and lessening the 'stickiness' of blood platelets, it may well be that the substantial replacement of animal fat by unsaturated fats of vegetable origin will in the long term reduce the incidence of cardio-vascular disease. Reduction of cigarette-smoking and obesity may also help.

caries. Usually this term refers to dental caries, which is the gradual dissolving and decay of the enamel and dentine of the teeth by acid substances in the mouth, a process prevented or reduced by dental hygiene (see TEETH).

Caries of bone is the decay and gradual disintegration of bone structure in the presence of chronic infection such as osteomyelitis or tuberculosis of bone.

carminatives. Drugs reputed to relieve flatulence by assisting the expulsion of gas from the stomach and intestines. Most of the usual carminatives contain volatile or 'essential' oils obtained from a variety of aromatic plants such as aniseed, peppermint and ginger.

carotid arteries. The principal arteries supplying blood to the head and neck.

carriers of disease. During an attack of infectious disease the organism responsible is present in the body of the sick person and can usually be detected by test during the illness. However, in some infections the germ can exist, or continue to exist, within the body of the host after recovery or without even producing obvious symptoms of disease. A person harbouring an organism in this way is a 'carrier', defined as being the apparently healthy host of a germ normally capable of causing disease.

Carriers are a risk to the community because the organisms they carry, although harmless to the carrier, may cause disease in other persons. The carrier state is particularly liable to occur in relation to diphtheria, typhoid fever, food-poisoning 'salmonellosis', bacillary dysentery, cholera, cerebrospinal fever and streptococcal infections of the respiratory tract.

The control of any epidemic of these

diseases should include a rigorous search for carriers amongst the contacts of known cases, and they too should be prevented from spreading the infection more widely.

Chronic carriers frequently present health authorities with a difficult problem, particularly in relation to typhoid fever and other salmonella infections. Such persons must be excluded from occupations involving food handling and must be instructed about their need for scrupulous personal hygiene.

Legal powers exist in many countries for the control of carriers likely to be a danger to the community.

cartilage. More familiarly known as gristle, cartilage is a firm, tough, elastic, translucent tissue devoid of blood vessels and nerves. In the body it is found in joints, in the discs between vertebrae, in the rib cartilages, in the larynx and trachea, and in the ears and tip of the nose. In general it increases flexibility.

There are several varieties of cartilage. Hyaline cartilage is mainly found in joints where the requirements are smoothness and resilience. White fibro-cartilage and yellow fibro-cartilage contain fibrous tissue in order to ensure additional toughness and elasticity.

The 'torn cartilage' which troubles footballers is one of the crescent-shaped structures of white fibro-cartilage which are present in the knee-joint. The 'slipped disc' of back injuries represents some form of damage to the pads of white fibro-cartilage, which lie between the vertebrae of the spine.

case-history. An account of previous illnesses and other major happenings in the life of the patient as an aid to the diagnosis and treatment of current physical, mental or psychosomatic illness.

castration. The procedure by which animals are deprived of their sex-glands (testes or ovaries) and so rendered sterile.

It is widely used in animal husbandry, particularly for male animals, to render them more manageable and more easily domesticated, and to improve and quicken their development as food animals for slaughter. The operation in the male is simple and the various methods employed are still fairly primitive and traditional. Female castration or 'spaying' is more difficult because of the position of the ovaries in the abdomen.

Human castration used to be extensively practised in Africa, Asia and under the Roman and Byzantine empires to provide eunuchs to look after harems. It was also employed in Italy until at least the eighteenth century to prevent breaking of the voice in boy singers since the range and timbre of a boy's voice allied to adult lung-power was particularly effective.

catabolism. See METABOLISM.

catalepsy. A nervous disorder producing a trance-like state in which the patient is unable to move or feel. Pulse and respiration are slowed and the body surface is cold and pale. The voluntary muscles are not paralysed: it is the will to move them that is lost. As a result limbs can be placed in unusual positions which will be rigidly maintained. Repeat attacks usually occur and the catatonic state may last from a few minutes to several days.

Catalepsy may occur as a manifestation either of hysteria or of schizophrenia. The differentiation of these two causes is often very difficult especially in the early stages of schizophrenia, and experienced psychiatric assessment is essential.

Catalepsy should not be confused with the very similar-sounding term cataplexy.

cataplexy. A condition in which there is a sudden loss of posture often as a result of some strong emotion. The muscles which control posture suddenly relax and the patient sinks limply to the ground fully conscious but unable to speak. Complete recovery ensues within a few minutes.

Cataplexy is usually classified with the minor epilepsies, but it is not generally agreed that it is a true epileptic phenomenon. It represents a sudden inhibition of brain function, whereas epilepsy results from a sudden and uncontrolled discharge of nervous energy.

Cataplexy should not be confused with the very similar-sounding term catalepsy.

cataract. An opacity of the crystalline lens of the eye, or of its capsule, causing blurring of vision and, if untreated, blindness.

In senile cataract opacity develops very slowly as a degenerative process in later life.

Infants may be born with congenital cataract which perhaps results from adverse antenatal influences. Traumatic cataract can follow bruising or penetrating injury; diabetic cataract may be a complication of severe untreated diabetes; glass-blower cataract is an industrial hazard of long exposure to excessive light and radiant heat, and occurs in such trades as glass manufacture and iron smelting.

The treatment is to remove the opaque lens surgically and compensate for the loss of focusing power by prescribing spectacles with a suitable convex lens to restore clear EYESIGHT.

A primitive operation known as 'couching' was formerly used in India and other tropical countries where cataract is common. The lens was merely displaced to the bottom of the eye by puncture and dislocation. In the classical operation the 'ripe' cataract is extracted through an incision at the edge of the cornea leaving the lens capsule behind. In the intracapsular operation lens and capsule are extracted together. This makes possible earlier operation but not without some additional risk of failure through loss of vitreous humour and a partial collapse of the eye. (See illustration on p. 68.)

catarrh. Inflammation of a mucous membrane usually accompanied by excess secretion of mucus.

Opacity of lens preventing
vision

Removal of lens enabling
only very blurred vision

Prescription of glasses
restoring sight.

Cataract

The term is most often used to mean inflammation of the upper respiratory tract which, as the 'common cold', runs its course in two stages. The mucous membrane is at first congested, swollen, hot and dry, and then subsequently produces a free mucoid or watery discharge, which may become purulent before drying up as the inflammation abates.

Repeated attacks may lead to a condition of chronic nasal catarrh often associated with some residual infection of the sinuses or with nasal polyps.

Other types of catarrh are hay fever, bronchial catarrh, gastric and intestinal catarrh and vesical catarrh – inflammation of the bladder.

Efficient nose-blowing, compressing each nostril in turn and vigorously expelling air through the other nostril, can sometimes prevent the development of nasal catarrh; and douching with a solution of bicarbonate of soda, common salt and borax is worth trying in early cases.

catgut. A cord-like material manufactured from sheep intestine and used in many operations as SUTURES for stitching wounds and tying-off blood vessels. Its advantage over other materials

such as nylon thread is that it is gradually absorbed by the tissues and therefore does not require removal.

cathartic. See LAXATIVE.

catheter. A tubular instrument designed to be passed into the urethra or external urinary passage in order to release urine from the bladder in cases of retention.

A female catheter is a short, straight, or slightly curved tube of glass or metal, but male catheters differ very much in design and material according to the needs of the particular case.

The term catheter has been extended to include tubes used for other surgical and medical purposes, for example, cardiac catheters are passed along veins to enter the heart for the investigation of cardiac abnormalities.

cat-scratch fever. A viral disease most commonly occurring as a complication of scratches from cats although other animals and insect-bites may also occasionally be responsible.

A minor inflammatory reaction around the scratch with swelling, erythema, ulceration, or papule formation appears at the site of the wound. The related lymph-glands become swollen and tender and may suppurate and there may be moderate fever of an undulating character. The condition usually subsides spontaneously in two or three weeks and it is not much influenced by treatment although it may be possible to alleviate constitutional symptoms.

It is an uncommon disease but on principle scratches should be properly cleaned and disinfected as a precaution. A skin test may be used to pin-point the diagnosis since cat injuries may also become infected, resulting in ulceration.

caul. Within the womb the unborn child is enclosed in the amniotic sac and surrounded by amniotic fluid. During labour the amniotic sac is forced downwards and helps to open the neck of the womb. After that the sac walls (membranes) rupture, the amniotic fluid escapes, the child is born, and the membranes and placenta follow during the third stage of labour. If the membranes fail to rupture, as occasionally happens, the child may be born still enclosed in membrane. This is being 'born with a caul', which is harmless.

cauliflower ear. A popular descriptive term for the final results of a neglected haematoma of the external ear ('auricle'). Blows on the ear may result in bruising which causes small veins to break so that blood escapes between the cartilaginous substructure of the ear and the over-lying skin. This blood is only slowly absorbed, and with softening of cartilage and subsequent fibrosis the ear becomes shrunken and twisted.

Immediate injury should be treated by cold compresses and a firm bandage to limit the bleeding, but any residual fluid swelling of effused blood should be drawn off to secure its removal before degeneration and contracture damage the shape of the ear.

causes of disease. Disease – lack of health of body or mind – is hard to define. It is fundamentally a condition in which the functioning of the body or of some of its parts or organs is disturbed or deranged. The causes of the derangement are very numerous, sometimes overlapping, sometimes poorly defined, and therefore difficult to classify.

Some diseases are essentially due to inheritance. Others that become manifest in later life are due to the biological processes of ageing and degeneration. Between these two extremes is a wide variety of other conditions which are caused by harmful agencies derived from 'the total environment', where this term is used in the widest possible way to include anything at all which adversely affects the normal functioning of the body.

Genetically-determined diseases. Genetic diseases and congenital abnormalities are becoming steadily more important. This is partly because of the successful control of many other diseases caused by external factors but also because, with improved recognition and treatment, many more cases of inherited disease survive to adult life. This has important implications for future generations, because these diseases are passed on in accordance with Mendel's principles of GENETICS. Briefly these are that defective genes may be dominant, recessive or sex-linked, affecting the influence they have on the developing embryo.

The list of diseases related to genes is now a large and growing one but some of the more common conditions include achondroplasia, Huntington's chorea, some types of muscular dystrophy, cystic fibrosis, familial mental defect associated with blindness, phenylketonuria, glycogen-storage disease, and haemophilia.

Partial or complex inherited factors can cause pyloric stenosis, spina bifida, hare-lip, cleft palate, congenital hip disease, some other congenital malformations, diabetes, schizophrenia and manic-depressive psychosis.

Chromosome abnormalities take the form of abnormalities of structure or number. The best known is the condition of mental deficiency known as mongolism, where there is an extra no. 21 chromosome (trisomy 21).

Exogenous diseases (external causes). These are the diseases brought about by harmful influences derived from 'the total environment'.

The group therefore includes the effects of parasites and infection by protozoa, fungi, bacteria, and viruses. It covers also conditions caused by dietary deficiency, unsuitability or excess, injurious atmospheric or climatic conditions, harmful living and working conditions, the action of poisonous substances, and the effects of injury.

The so-called psychosomatic or stress diseases are also primarily external in origin. The body normally reacts to stress in a physiological way. If it over-reacts, or reacts abnormally, or is forced to react excessively or for too long a period, its capacity for normal functioning is disturbed and the effects are shown in susceptible organs. The best known psychosomatic diseases are probably duodenal ulcer and migraine.

Degenerative diseases. Functioning is impaired as tissues age and change in character. So older persons become the victims of such chronic conditions as cardio-vascular degeneration, osteo-arthritis, malignant disease, and senile dementia.

It will be obvious that the sections of this classification are not mutually exclusive. To take an example, asthma is largely caused by allergy to a particular external substance but also has important psychosomatic elements and often runs in families. Cancer is perhaps another case in point. There is so far no evidence of it being hereditary but predisposition may have some genetic basis: we already know that certain types of cancer are common in persons of particular blood groups; environmental influences are certainly the main causes in such instances as the lung carcinoma of cigarette smokers and the bladder tumours of rubber-workers; and it is a matter of common knowledge and experience that malignant conditions occur predominantly in older persons.

Social diseases. So far, consideration has been restricted to conditions of disease in which there are demonstrable changes of some sort. Nevertheless society is becoming increasingly concerned with other departures from the normal.

The World Health Organization has defined health as 'a state of complete physical, mental and social well-being and not merely the absence of disease or infirmity'.

If absence of social well-being is thus being regarded as akin to disease any consideration of the causes of disease must also include some reference to our present basis of society. It would seem to be an inescapable conclusion that the manner in which it operates is responsible for the increasing proportion of its numbers who, as isolates, delinquents, neurotics and hypochondriacs, can certainly be regarded as socially sick although not physically ill.

cautery. Any instrument or device used to apply heat to the tissues in such intensity as to burn them.

Cauteries are sometimes employed to stimulate the healing of inactive ulcers but their main use is in the arrest of haemorrhage. Multiple small bleeding points which are difficult to reach or control can often be effectively dealt with by searing and so closing the vessels.

cell. The basic structural and functional unit of the living matter (protoplasm) which forms the tissues of animals and plants.

Like knowledge of bacteria, knowledge about cells and their characteristics has been largely dependent on advances in microscopy because most cells are of microscopic size. However, the yolks of birds' eggs are in fact single cells, and cell size actually ranges from less than one-thousandth of 1 mm. to the yolk of the ostrich egg.

Typical structure. Living cells, with only a few exceptions, have a standard fundamental structure. The main body of the cell consists of protoplasm, a sticky colloidal fluid known in this context as cytoplasm and contained within an outer wall, the cell membrane. Protoplasm consists of water, protein, fatty substances, starches and sugars, with various inorganic and organic salts.

Within the cell, and concerned with the regulation of cell activity, is a denser globular structure called the nucleus. This is made of chromatin, which holds the genetic information necessary to determine the specialized characters and function of the cell.

Chromatin is mainly made up of protein, deoxyribonucleic acid (DNA) and ribonucleic acid (RNA): DNA is a highly complex molecule and its structural arrangement is responsible for providing the 'code' which determines the hereditary characteristics and individuality of a cell and ensures that its regulated growth and function conform to an appropriate pattern.

Cell reproduction. In the animal body all tissues and organs originate from the female germ-cell (ovum) after it has been fertilized by a germ-cell from the male (spermatozoon). Thereafter the fertilized ovum multiplies by simple divisions into an enormous number of daughter cells which become modified in size, shape and other characteristics according to the sites and functions for which they are destined.

Before cell division the nucleus undergoes a complicated process known as mitosis in order to ensure that each daughter cell has an identical share of the chromatin material and especially of DNA by which its own invariability will be assured. In mitosis the nuclear material becomes divided into small pieces called chromosomes. These each divide into pairs which draw apart, and the nucleus and its surrounding protoplasm then divide into two. So each daughter cell is provided with the same number of chromosomes as the original cell.

A modification of this process is required before fertilization. It will be obvious that when two cells unite the resultant cell would have twice the proper number of chromosomes. The germ cells therefore undergo meiosis in which the number of chromosomes which each contributes is reduced to one half so that a

Cell mitosis

new sexually-reproduced cell has the proper number of chromosomes for the species; how this influences inheritance is the study of GENETICS.

Tissue formation. Cells are single units but they combine in multicellular organisms and become specialized for particular purposes.

A typical animal body contains a large variety of cells with particular characteristics all of which have arisen by repeated division from the original fertilized ovum.

They include epithelial and endothelial cells covering the outside and lining the inside surfaces of the body, cells for skeletal tissues such as bone and muscles, cells for the nervous system, and cells for all the diverse organs such as heart, lungs, blood, liver, kidney, glands and so on.

cellulitis. A spreading inflammation of the cellular tissues deep in the skin resulting from invasion by micro-organisms. It may proceed to suppuration, sloughing or gangrene.

It is particularly likely to occur with penetrating wounds, in lacerations where there is damaged tissue, and in patients whose general resistance is low as a result of other disease. The affected part is red, hot, tender and swollen and there is usually considerable constitutional upset.

The treatment is incision to secure adequate drainage of infected matter, the removal of damaged tissue, and the giving of appropriate antibiotics to combat the infection.

central nervous system. The brain and spinal cord. See NERVOUS SYSTEM.

cerebellum. The part of the brain lying within the lower rear part of the skull. It consists of a central and two lateral lobes, and is concerned with balance and the maintenance of posture.

cerebral embolism, haemorrhage and thrombosis. See STROKE.

cerebrospinal fever. A serious disease due to infection of the membranes of the brain which is alternatively known as meningococcal MENINGITIS.

cerebrospinal fluid. The fluid which surrounds the brain and spinal cord forming a water bed for their protection. Its function is to cushion the brain and cord against sudden movement and to equalize changes in pressure.

In various diseases such as meningitis, poliomyelitis, and syphilis, changes occur in the chemical nature of the fluid, white blood cells appear, and fluid pressure increases. These alterations are of diagnostic importance and can be demonstrated in a specimen of fluid obtained by lumbar puncture.

Obstruction of the flow of cerebrospinal fluid may cause hydrocephalus. See also BRAIN, diseases of.

cerebrovascular. Concerning the blood vessels which supply the brain.

cerebrum. The upper and largest part of the BRAIN occupying most of the cranial cavity, and larger and more complex in man than in other mammals.

cervical. Concerning the neck, or concerning a neck-like structure, e.g., the neck of the uterus.

cervical cytology. A rapid and easy method of detecting the very beginning of cancer of the cervix of the uterus long before the condition is dangerous.

Essentially where cancer of the cervix is developing the cells become abnormal in appearance and only later become cancerous.

In cervical cytology the doctor or nurse takes, absolutely painlessly, a tiny scraping – called a cervical smear – from the mucous membrane of the cervix. The specimen so obtained is stained and then examined under a microscope. In the overwhelming majority of cases the cells so examined are normal, but in a tiny proportion of cases they show abnormality and therefore render operation desirable before the cells actually become cancerous.

In most countries the examination is now advised for women every three years.

Cervical cancer is commonest in mothers of several children and especially in women of the lowest socio-economic groups; but unfortunately these are the very people least likely to respond to invitations to visit clinics or doctors' consulting rooms for cervical smears. So in large measure the reduction of cervical cancer depends on person-to-person persuasion by health workers.

cervical rib. An abnormal extra rib arising in relation to the seventh cervical vertebra.

It is often not discovered until the age of puberty but at that age the ribs, which are

cartilage in childhood, become hard and bony, and the bones of the shoulder may be pulled down by breast development so that symptoms ensue from pressure on the artery and nerve supplying the arm.

The pulse is weakened and the arm may become cold, blue, and swollen with fluid from interference with its circulation. Effects on the nerves include neuralgic pain, tingling and numbness, with weakness and wasting of the muscles of the hand.

The only effective treatment is surgical removal of the rib.

cervix. The lower segment of the uterus or womb.

It is about 2.5 cm. (1 in.) long with a central canal, and it projects downwards into the vagina as a narrow cylinder with a rounded end.

The cervix is frequently the site of disease.

Chronic cervicitis may result from the infection of a tear occurring during childbirth and may persist to cause shallow ulcerated areas (known as cervical erosions) producing discharge and discomfort.

The lining cells of the lower part of the cervix are very susceptible to malignant change, so carcinoma of the cervix is also not uncommon. Regular examination of the characteristics of these cells by means of CERVICAL CYTOLOGY provides a means of detecting potentially dangerous developments in time to ensure successful treatment.

chafing. Abrasion and superficial inflammation of the skin produced by friction. This can occur in various ways and the chafing produced by rough wet clothing at points of movement such as the neck or wrists is a matter of common experience.

Less obvious however are the effects of rubbing between opposed skin surfaces as sometimes seen in obese persons where rolls of flesh overlap, beneath heavy and pendulous breasts, and in the groins of babies. In such circumstances the skin secretions are prevented from drying so that the superficial cells become softened; this increases the friction and aggravates its effect.

Chafing also occurs over 'pressure points' especially the heels and sacrum, of persons confined to bed, and may be the first stage of an ultimate bed sore.

Treatment is really a matter of proper hygiene. The areas affected should first be carefully washed and dried to get rid of debris which would otherwise form a lodging for micro-organisms. Subsequent application of a skin lotion to dry and harden the skin can be followed by the use of a dusting powder to minimize friction.

For the patient in bed suitable pads should be used to provide protection from the effects of pressure and friction.

chancre. The primary sore resulting from infection with the organism which causes

SYPHILIS. In acquired syphilis the initial site of infection in both men and women is usually in the genital area, but chancres are occasionally also seen on the lips, breasts, fingers and indeed any part of the body. The risk of infection by contact is considerable.

chancroid. A venereal disease, sometimes called soft sore, which is much less common than gonorrhoea and less well known than syphilis. Infection is almost always through sexual intercourse and, after an incubation period of one to five days, a red papule appears in the genital area; this breaks down to form a painful ulcer and the lymph glands of the groin become swollen. The discharge of pus may infect the surrounding skin to produce further chancroids. There is often general disturbance and a raised temperature.

The disease responds well to sulphonamides and to streptomycin. After treatment there should be blood tests at intervals for three months because syphilis may also have been contracted at the same time, but its presence masked by the chancroid.

change of life. A colloquial expression for the MENOPAUSE.

chapped skin. A superficial disorder of the skin characterized by the occurrence of cracks and fissures of its outer horny layer. It affects exposed areas, especially the fingers, hands, forearms and face.

External irritants such as friction, cold, dust and injurious chemicals cause thickening of the horny layer. Because of its inelastic nature this readily cracks to produce fissures which are painful because the sensitive lower layers of the skin are exposed.

When the condition is extensive it may be due to ichthyosis or to a form of dermatitis (eczema), but many persons have 'chaps' in cold weather without these being regarded as due to specific skin disease.

Treatment involves protection of the skin from any irritant including cold and application of a glycerin-based lotion of which many examples are available commercially. Greasy applications are less suitable.

chemotherapy. The treatment of infection by using chemicals to kill the organisms that are causing it. The term is used especially in respect of the groups of chemicals that now dominate the treatment of infections, namely SULPHONAMIDES and ANTIBIOTICS.

Chemotherapy, while enormously important, is not a complete form of treatment. The patient's own resistance must be sustained by rest, diet and fluids, by the neutralization of toxins and the correction of metabolic deficiencies, and sometimes by surgical removal of damaged tissue. Lack of attention to these points courts failure, as do faulty dosage schedules, inaccessibility of the seat of infection, and ending the treatment too early.

Chemotherapy should be used with discrimination. Many mild infections are probably best treated only by reducing the symptoms, and not by immediately deploying the full panoply of the chemotherapeutic armoury.

chest. A familiar name for the thorax, the bony cage of the upper part of the body containing the heart and lungs. It is formed behind by the twelve thoracic vertebrae of the spine from which twelve pairs of ribs sweep round to join the sternum or breastbone in front. Its narrow upper opening is occupied by the structures of the neck and it is closed below by the diaphragm which forms its floor.

Its shape may be altered in disease and various deformities are characteristic of rickets; in emphysema the chest is enlarged, a condition known as 'barrel-chest'.

The chest is an essential part of the mechanism of the RESPIRATORY SYSTEM.

Cheyne-Stokes respiration. A pattern of breathing in which there is a regular cycle of variation in volume. In each cycle, the breathing increases in depth until it becomes noisy and distressed. Respiration then gradually diminishes until for thirty seconds or more there is a pause, followed again by gradual increase. Various modifications of this pattern are also loosely referred to by the same term.

Cheyne-Stokes breathing occurs in cases of coma, head-injury, 'stroke', increased intracranial tension, hyperpyrexia, and in many heart, lung and kidney diseases as death approaches. It is due to disturbance of the part of the brain which controls respiration, and it is always of grave significance.

chickenpox. The common name for varicella, a mild but highly infectious disease mainly affecting children and caused by the varicella virus. The same virus is found in shingles (herpes zoster) and in some cases of encephalitis.

Chickenpox is world-wide in distribution and endemic in all large populations. Epidemic outbreaks occur at irregular intervals with greatest prevalence in the autumn. Infants are rarely affected, because of temporary inherited maternal immunity, and most cases occur in children under 10 years. Adult cases are uncommon but tend to be more severe.

Infectivity. In its early stages chickenpox is very infectious, spread occurring from case to case by inhalation of 'droplet' respiratory spray. Dried crusts of skin are also regarded as infective. Patients are infectious from about one day before the appearance of the first vesicles to a week later.

The incubation period of the disease is normally a fortnight with extremes of eleven and twenty-three days, and isolation should be maintained until all the crusts from the pustules have separated.

Childbirth: normal

Clinical features. Older children may initially have some malaise and rise of temperature with a pinkish general rash for twenty-four hours, but usually the disease is simply heralded by appearance of the typical skin eruption. This appears as 'crops' of clear vesicles (blebs) which become pustular and then dry up to form scabs. The crops appear on successive days for about three days, usually on the back, chest and abdomen, face, scalp and limbs in that order.

In most cases there is little or no general disturbance and children make an uneventful recovery but complications, although rare, are not unknown especially if the patient was already not well.

In varicella haemorrhagica there is haemorrhage not only into the vesicles but also into the skin and mucous membranes, and this type is often fatal. The same is true of varicella gangrenosa where secondary infection of the vesicles causes ulceration and intense toxaemia. Encephalitis is also rare and the outlook for recovery is generally favourable.

Treatment. The ordinary case requires little active treatment. Application of an antiseptic paint may help to prevent secondary infection of the vesicles. If there is any suspicion that this is occurring antibiotics are given.

chilblains. An inflammatory condition of the skin generally occurring on exposed parts of the hands and feet as a reaction to cold.

It is a disturbance akin to Raynaud's disease in which the arterioles are constricted while blood stagnates in the dilated capillaries to the detriment of skin nutrition. The affected parts are swollen, reddened, shiny, itchy or painful, and superficial ulceration may ultimately occur.

Effective management is essentially preventive: susceptible areas should be adequately clothed in cold weather. There is no specific internal treatment but calcium lactate or gluconate with additional vitamin D or vitamin K is commonly prescribed. Treatment of the affected area which is designed to improve blood flow is sometimes helpful. Friction, infra-red radiation, paraffin-wax baths, diathermy, counter-irritation with tincture of iodine, and exposure to ultra-violet light all have their advocates. The distressing irritation from chilblains may be relieved by painting them with compound tincture of benzoin to which menthol has been added.

Patients with chilblains are often anaemic as well and this possibility should be investigated and corrected if necessary.

childbirth. The process of parturition, i.e., the act of giving birth to a living child. Delivery of a dead child whose intra-uterine development has continued long enough for viability (6½ months) is known as a still birth; expulsion of a less mature foetus is an abortion or miscarriage.

Childbirth occurs as the climax of PREGNANCY. The whole products of conception and pregnancy – foetus, amniotic fluid, placenta, and membranes – are normally expelled and separated from the uterus by the physiological processes of labour affecting the mother. The course of events from the onset of labour until the mother is able to resume her normal activities is generally referred to as her CONFINEMENT.

Onset of labour. Labour occurs spontaneously after a gestation period of about 280 days. The exact causes of onset are still imperfectly understood. Older theories postulated the influence of reflex irritability of uterine muscle, uterine distension at term, and degenerative changes in the placenta which stimulates uterine muscle. While these factors may be relevant, it is now considered that the onset of labour is largely due to hormones.

Course of labour. It is usual to divide labour into three stages: (1) dilatation – from the onset of true labour pains to full dilatation of the cervix (twelve to eighteen hours); (2) expulsion – from full dilatation to expulsion of the child (two or three hours with a first child; often much shorter in later pregnancies); (3) delivery – from birth of child to expulsion of placenta or 'afterbirth' (half to one hour).

First stage: The mother experiences periodic pains due to contractions of the uterus. The contractions bring about dilatation of the neck of the womb as the amniotic fluid within its membraneous sac is forced down to act as a fluid wedge. Dilatation is usually accompanied by a slight discharge of blood-stained mucus known as the 'show'. When full dilatation is achieved the amniotic sac ruptures leading to a gush of amniotic fluid – the escape of the 'forewaters'. Premature rupture of the membranes may occur if the position of the baby is abnormal (e.g., in breech presentation).

Childbirth: breech presentation

Second stage: After rupture of the membranes labour pains often cease temporarily but then begin again with greater force and frequency and develop a 'down-bearing character'. The abdominal muscles begin to play a part.

In a normal delivery the child is born as a 'head down' or vertex presentation and with its face directed backwards in relation to the mother. In this position its head passes most easily along the birth canal formed by the pelvis and the associated soft tissues.

The final obstacle to the child's delivery is the perineum or area of tissue between the anus and vaginal opening. The perineum gradually thins out and stretches. It may tear or require to be divided surgically, the operation of episiotomy.

As soon as the head is born, the shoulders, trunk and limbs follow without great difficulty and the actual birth is concluded by tying and cutting the umbilical cord.

Third stage: After the birth of the child there is a short cessation of pains but the uterus soon begins to contract again and can be felt through the abdominal wall as a hard and solid mass. Its contractions ultimately expel the placenta and the remains of the ruptured amniotic sac (otherwise known as the 'membranes').

Management of childbirth. The conduct of labour is a matter for the professional expertise of the attendants. In most advanced countries the great majority of mothers are now being confined in hospital where the necessary skill and facilities are assured.

The two essentials for safe childbirth are the recognition of abnormalities in time to deal with them in the most appropriate manner and the maintenance of a strict technique to avoid the risk of infection reaching the birth canal or uterus.

Much can be done to minimize the actual pains of labour. Anaesthesia in childbirth was pioneered by Sir James Y. Simpson, the discoverer of chloroform, but this substance because of its inherent risks is now seldom employed. Scopolamine-morphine narcosis or 'twilight sleep' enjoyed a vogue for some time but the favoured methods of obstetric analgesia now rely on inhalation procedures employing automatic devices suitable for unskilled use. The first of these inhalers supplied nitrous oxide gas as the anaesthetic agent but a more compact apparatus which has largely superseded it relies on the vaporization of tri-chloro-ethylene (Trilene).

The use of inhalation analgesia in this way under patient-control and with supervision by the midwife has greatly served to minimize the immemorial pangs of childbirth. See also CAESAREAN SECTION.

Diseases. These include the factors complicating labour and certain other conditions arising between the start of labour and the end of the puerperium.

The first group is usually sub-divided into faults in 'the powers', in 'the passages' and in 'the passenger'.

Successful labour depends essentially on the expulsive force exerted by the uterus with assistance from the abdominal muscles. This may be inadequate (primary uterine inertia) in nervous women because of the inhibitory effects of fear, in cases of malpresentation where the normal stimulus of the descending head is lacking, or in over-distension of the uterus as in hydramnios (when there is excessive amniotic fluid), or in cases of twin pregnancy. Secondary uterine inertia occurs in a uterus exhausted by prolonged effort to overcome some obstructive difficulty.

Faults in the birth canal are numerous. The most common is some form of contracted pelvis but malposition of the uterus, rigidity of the cervix and other soft parts, and tumours of the uterus may all cause difficulty in childbirth.

In the present context the 'passenger' is the child and its surrounding amniotic sac filled with amniotic fluid. The amniotic sac or 'membranes' may be unduly adherent to the uterus, sometimes as a result of previous inflammation of the lining of that organ, or of earlier haemorrhage; or the sac may rupture prematurely. Both conditions may delay labour but disproportionate size or faulty positioning of the child are more usual causes. Other complications related to the child are congenital abnormalities and prolapse of the umbilical cord.

Childbirth: forceps delivery

Apart from faults in the powers, the passages or the passenger, the most serious complication of labour is haemorrhage occurring either during labour or immediately after. Haemorrhage during the birth usually occurs because the placenta is so situated that it is ruptured during the delivery. Haemorrhage after the birth occurs at the end of labour from an exhausted uterus or as a result of damage to the soft tissues.

After delivery the most serious risk is infection of the raw surface of the genital tract to cause puerperal pyrexia or puerperal fever.

Eclampsia is more properly a disease of pregnancy but may first show itself during the puerperium. Another condition, fortunately rare, is puerperal insanity which though usually short-lived can be very distressing. Sudden deaths are occasionally recorded from pulmonary embolism where air or amniotic fluid has entered the venous blood stream from the open uterus sinuses.

No attempt has been made here to deal with the treatment of any of the conditions described. With adequate prenatal care and skilled professional attendance at the delivery the aim should be to avoid or at least anticipate the difficulties.

child guidance. Many children suffer from disorders of personality and conduct which influence their attitude to everyday life and prevent them from making a satisfactory and acceptable adjustment to the demands of the society in which they live. There is a great variety of indications of such personal maladjustment.

The young child may develop undesirable habits such as thumb-sucking, nail-biting, bedwetting, masturbation, eccentricities of movement, or whims about food, and may show abnormal personal characteristics in the form of excessive shyness or aggression, oversensitiveness or obstinacy, seclusiveness or quarrelsomeness, laziness or restlessness, timidity and exaggerated fears – to name only a few.

The school age child may similarly come to notice because of 'school phobia', truancy, lying, stealing, destructiveness, bullying, temper-tantrums, rebellious outbursts or sexual misbehaviour.

Child guidance is a service, still in a developing and evolutionary phase, which recognizes that many of the difficulties of the maladjusted adult have their roots in infancy and childhood. It therefore seeks to identify those children with abnormalities of attitude and behaviour, who – at home, at school, or in the community – are in some sort of conflict with their environment. It also owes a great deal to the concepts of psychology elaborated by Sigmund Freud (1856-1939).

In some instances problem children may in fact be suffering from mental illness or mental defect, but these are the province of the psychiatrist or mental deficiency specialist. Child guidance is primarily concerned with children who are capable of more or less normal development.

Child guidance clinics. Most of the work of these clinics is with children of school age. For the behaviour problems of the infant and pre-school child useful advice is in most places readily available from an ordinary child health clinic where there will be a doctor experienced in paediatrics and health visitors with the opportunity and insight to appreciate the family background, and with the ability and knowledge to explain to mothers the needs of their offspring for love, talk, play, company, consistency, and the avoidance of over-protection, over-dependency, over-strictness, or over-indulgence.

It is generally older children with behaviour difficulties related more to the outside world who eventually reach the child guidance clinic, brought by parents or referred by teachers, probation officers, church and social agencies, or sent more formally from the courts or children's panels.

Team work. In child guidance every child who comes to notice has to be considered not in isolation but in relation to the setting or situation in which he lives. It is unhelpful to label a child as a thief, truant or coward without undertaking a thorough study of the social and psychological factors which have made him what he appears to be.

Child guidance therefore requires to be a team effort in which the paediatrician, the child psychiatrist, the psychologist and especially the social case-worker all play their respective parts, with the health visitor and the general practitioner also involved.

Diagnosis. A physical examination is an essential part of the investigation because mood and behaviour are influenced by health. The fatigue of chronic illness is different in quality from that of an anxiety state; the restlessness of chorea can be confused with the overactivity of mental stress; apathy and dejection may be created by hormone imbalance as well as by psychological factors; allergies may indicate psychosomatic instability; bodily conformation has been shown to be correlated with mental make-up.

A full history of the child should include an account of his medical, developmental, psychological and educational progress from his earliest years.

These medical aspects of the case require to be supplemented by the investigations of the social case-worker, by school reports, and by the views of the psychologist who has at his disposal a wide range of scientific techniques for the investigation of intellectual capacity and personality.

Treatment. A linking together of all the investigations, either by consideration of reports by a case conference, or more usually by informal discussions between members of the team, will enable a diagnosis to be made and a plan of treatment decided. The diagnosis will normally fall into three categories; (1) that the problem is purely intellectual and that the remedy lies in remedial educational measures with the assistance of the psychologist and his facilities for continuous constructive help; (2) that some environmental adjustment and parental enlightenment can be undertaken by the social worker or health visitor, or (3) that an established neurosis exists which will require psychotherapy from the psychiatrist.

In this context psychotherapy can range from play therapy, either alone or in groups, through simple talks, suggestion, re-education and reinforcement of the personality, to the more advanced forms of analysis which seek to explore the unconscious mechanisms of conduct and behaviour.

child health services. Services provided with the aim of safeguarding and improving the physical and mental health of children, monitoring their development, guiding parents as to requirements for good development and identifying and rectifying diseases and disabilities.

Broadly the services are centred on the home in the early years of childhood and on the school in later years. In the pre-school period there are two key figures: (1) a qualified nurse with subsequent training in psychology, human development, sociology and health teaching, known in the U.K., South Africa and Nigeria as a HEALTH VISITOR and elsewhere identifiable under other names; and (2) a qualified doctor, often specialized in preventive paediatrics, but sometimes an unspecialized general practitioner, and in all these cases usually seeing the child in health centre, clinic or consulting room. In the school period the key figures are the school doctor and school nurse who may be the same people as in the pre-school stage or may specialize entirely in children of school age.

In some areas the health visitor sees the parents in the prenatal period, sharing with the midwife guidance on the hygiene of pregnancy, advising the prospective parents about the child's future physical and emotional needs, persuading them to attend an appropriate health class or discussion group, discussing the preparation of any older child for the baby's arrival, and tactfully inducing the mother to think (when she has more time than after the birth) about such relevant matters as the avoidance of home accidents, the value of immunization and the question of spacing of children. In other areas these important educational opportunities are lost, and the health visitor pays her first call after mother and child have left the maternity hospital.

At the first visit and to some extent at later visits she examines the baby carefully for abnormalities and, gearing her teaching to the apparent needs and capacities of the mother, begins systematic guidance as well as answering questions raised by the mother. She also encourages the parents to attend the appropriate health centre or clinic for medical examination and for immunizations, to take advantage of any relevant health discussion group provided in the neighbourhood and, if she has found any signs of disease or abnormality, to seek treatment promptly.

The doctor undertakes comprehensive developmental assessment of the child at periodical intervals, gives or arranges for appropriate immunizations and tries to ensure that any physical or mental abnormality or any sensory defect (e.g., impaired hearing) receives remedial or supportive treatment. If he is specialized in healthy children he does not himself undertake treatment but refers the child to the appropriate general practitioner or to a paediatric physician, paediatric surgeon, child psychiatrist or child psychologist.

After the child enters school there is usually a routine medical overhaul to detect abnormalities missed earlier or recently developed, and one or more routine medical examinations later, together with specially arranged examination on request by parent, teacher or school nurse. Additionally there are periodical dental inspections by a dental officer or dental hygienist and general health surveys from time to time by the school nurse or school health visitor. There are frequent discussions between doctor and nurse on the one hand and teacher on the other to ensure that the educational provisions are matched to the health and capacity of the child: to give a simple example, to ensure that a short-sighted child is encouraged to wear his glasses and is not seated at the back of the classroom. Both the nurse, especially if she is a qualified health visitor, and to a smaller extent the doctor are likely to be involved in health education in the school, and they have obvious roles in relation to school hygiene and the control of infectious diseases.

childhood, psychology of. The personality, character and mental health of a child, and of the adult which he becomes, are influenced profoundly by parental attitudes during the formative years from birth onwards and also by the relationships which he makes with brothers, sisters and playmates. The mother, or failing her some permanent mother substitute, has the greatest opportunity of moulding and influencing its psychical development. She is best situated from the very beginning to provide the comfort and security required. Some of the psychological factors affecting infant development are dealt with in the article INFANCY, PSYCHOLOGY OF but between the ages of 1 and 5 years the child begins to emerge as an individual, and character formation can be significantly affected for good or ill by the pattern of his upbringing. Faulty physical development from malnutrition or neglect is now relatively rare but it is just as important that parental care should help children to develop with healthy minds and balanced personalities. The adult who has grown up with undesirable social attitudes – such as hostility, aggressiveness, self-assertion or timidity, inability to work reliably and conscientiously or to accept responsibility, lack of initiative or unwillingness to face new experiences with resolution, resource and adaptability – is as a rule showing the end-results of misunderstanding or mis-management in childhood.

Behaviour problems. Many mothers are troubled by what they regard as wilfully deviant behaviour by their children. Destructiveness, temper-tantrums, persistent disobedience, lying, bullying or stealing are symptoms of basic unhappiness. Punishment is usually of little avail. Compliance may be enforced by pain or fear but only at the cost of inducing an attitude of mind which may show as withdrawal, an increasing sense of inferiority, a reluctance to think and act independently, a fear of criticism or ridicule, or a readiness to deny before accusal. It is necessary therefore to seek for the real causes of misbehaviour. A child may be resentful over displacement in favour of a new baby or over-excessive parental discipline or from being bullied and teased by elder brothers and sisters. He may not have adequate outlets for his growing curiosity and sense of exploration or he may not have the scope for play and the play-material appropriate to his age. On the other hand he may be so over-protected and over-indulged that he feels his lack of independence. Physically he may be getting too little rest or be subjected to too much excitement.

Jealousy. The toddler sees a new baby as a threat to his security and may seek to regain attention by unconsciously trying to become a baby himself again. He will refuse to play, cling to mother, develop food-fads or refuse to eat, suck his thumb or become incontinent. Punishment does not help; it only reinforces his conviction that he is unloved. Verbal reassurance is equally unsuccessful; active demonstrations are required. He should be involved in the new family situation and encouraged to help with the new baby as for instance in bathing and feeding. Jealousy also promotes quarrels between children and one child should never be held up as a model to the others. This only increases antagonisms and conversely makes the model vain and self-righteous.

Fear. Children should be helped to face life with courage. Basically they are rather fearless and the mother who over-protects is undermining this attribute and will induce either resentment of domination or inability to face life without help. It is right to safeguard them unobtrusively from real dangers but constant admonishments to take care and the encouragement of fear-reactions to objective situations such as lightning, dogs, policemen or doctors only causes harm. The consistently timid child has subjective fears. He lacks self-confidence because in some way his sense of security has been destroyed often by parental treatment where impatience, anger, criticism and constant correction have engendered a feeling that whatever he does cannot gain for him the approval or love which he craves.

Negativism. This may be defined as contrariness or behaviour in which requests or commands are bluntly refused.

Around the age of 2½ years negativism is not naughtiness but a normal stage of development. The previously docile and dependent child has begun to realize that he has a choice. Where previously he obeyed instructions without thought, he now delights in saying 'I won't'.

Punishment is undesirable and struggles of will between parent and child are harmful to both. The wise parent, recognizing the beginnings of the stage, will make life more tolerable for himself by minimal interference with the child's activities, and, where a request must be made, by framing it in such a way that there is a choice: e.g., instead of 'Put your toys away now', asking 'Which one do you want to put away first?' Where the parent receives an actual refusal, the best plan is to ignore it and to divert the child to another topic.

When an older child reverts to a negativistic stage, parents and teachers, before seeking psychological help, should ask themselves, 'Am I creating this by inadvertently ordering almost every detail of the child's life?'

Play. Play is not just a childish method of passing the time. It is fundamental to a child's exploration of his environment, and playthings matched to his growing capacities help him to do this. Up to 9 months or so a baby enjoys rattles or bright dangling objects and soon after he will achieve satisfaction by hammering with a spoon, banging blocks together, or playing with soft toys. By 15 to 18 months he is ready for peg-boards, a posting-box, or insert cutouts. The toddler needs pushing and pulling toys, blocks to build, a sand-box and tins or floating toys and water-play. There is a need for vigorous movements and large toys, and modern housing often makes this difficult. Confinement to a play-pen frustrates the need for adventure and exploration. Throwing out toys expresses resentment of restriction or conversely the reaction may be one of sulkiness, withdrawal and lack of interest.

Constructional toys and painting books are needed by the 4-year-old child, and he should be allowed to carry out his own plans in order to encourage independence. Help should be given only if asked for and must not become interference. Too much passive amusement submerges the creative urge which expresses itself in childhood as imaginative play, and life becomes boring and meaningless.

General. The understanding mother will find many other ways of influencing her child's development: by involving him in household activities such as shopping, by teaching table-manners and skills, by conversation and stories, and by encouraging questions and providing patient and accurate answers. Pets are another good idea. They satisfy two very strong natural tendencies – the desire for possession and the desire to protect – and they also inculcate a sense of responsibility.

Preparation for the change from home (where the child is very central) to school (where he is one of a group) is also important.

Apart from formal education a school should strive to encourage a sense of duty and responsibility and should foster feelings of accomplishment. Particular care is necessary with several types of child, e.g., the unintellectual and unathletic child who may feel a failure, the very bright child who may become bored, and the child with a minor disability, such as obesity, who may be mocked by his mates.

Parents should be on their guard about over-forcing a child and about making him feel a failure by expressions of dissatisfaction with his progress. The child who feels a failure may react with hostility to both school and parents, and may develop antisocial tendencies in an attempt to gain recognition. See also INFANCY, PSYCHOLOGY OF.

children, behaviour disorders. A diverse group of socially unacceptable behaviour patterns in children. Causes may be of a social and/or psychological nature, while other, co-existing, physical or mental handicaps may contribute and complicate the situation. See BEHAVIOUR.

children, diseases of. Disorders usually only encountered in infancy or childhood. They include all classes of illness, from infections to tumours. Many of the infectious diseases which used often to be fatal are now preventable by routine immunization in infancy, and have thus been virtually eliminated from developed countries; these include whooping cough, diphtheria, and poliomyelitis. Less serious complaints, however, such as chickenpox, still cause widespread illness, while some less common diseases, such as leukaemia, still generally lead to death.

It is also recognized that many 'adult' diseases often run a quite different course in children and should properly be regarded as children's diseases, needing treatment employing paediatric skills.

chill. A sensation of cold accompanied by involuntary shivering or shaking, and skin pallor. When associated with an elevation of temperature in the interior of the body, it may indicate the invasion of the blood by toxins, signifying the early stages of an infectious disease. Chill in this sense is especially characteristic of malaria and pneumonococcal pneumonia.

Preventive measures include the wearing of protective clothing against the elements and the suppression of malaria with drugs. Specific treatment depends on the identification of the cause, and might therefore include the use of anti-malarial or antibiotic drugs, as well as general measures of rest, appropriate fluid intake, and diet.

In popular usage a chill also implies a respiratory (or sometimes a gastric or urinary tract) disorder, held to be caused by exposure to cold and damp. Hence the term includes a host of complaints.

chiropodist. A person specialized in the care and treatment of minor foot disorders.

Besides dealing with conditions that affect the soft tissues of the feet (e.g., corns) and the nails (e.g., ingrowing toenails), matters of little medical significance, a chiropodist is also involved in the treatment of (1) foot disabilities directly associated with general medical and surgical states; (2) structural and functional disturbances of more importance, such as club foot, abnormalities of the arch of the foot and deformities of the toes; and (3) infections resulting from sepsis, foot warts and ringworm.

choking. Partial or complete suffocation. It may be caused by (1) mechanical obstruction, through inhalation of a foreign body or from external pressure on the larynx or trachea; (2) spasm of the larynx caused by an irritating gas or liquid; or (3) excessive secretions from the inner surface of the lungs, which accompanies acute left heart failure.

Relief of choking is directed at removal or treatment of the specific cause. In cases of immediate obstruction a hard slap between the shoulders may dislodge the obstruction. In severe cases emergency measures such as tracheotomy or artificial respiration are sometimes required

cholecystitis. Inflammation of the gall-bladder. There are two main types: (1) acute: usually caused by impaction of a gallstone in the duct of the gall-bladder or, occasionally, by infection, and (2) chronic: usually caused by long-standing presence of gallstones within the gall-bladder.

Acute cholecystitis is usually treated by general medical measures involving bed rest, adequate fluid intake, and analgesics, while chronic cholecystitis generally necessitates surgical removal of the gall-bladder.

cholera. An acute infectious disease of man, caused by cholera bacteria, and occurring in epidemics chiefly in Asia. It is characterized by a profuse watery diarrhoea and a state of collapse, and is rapidly fatal if untreated. Spread occurs by faecal contamination. Recent spread to Europe and Africa has accompanied the arrival of mass air travel.

Preventive measures include the control of people's movement to and from infected areas, measures of personal hygiene, and the use of anti-cholera vaccines. Prompt treatment with bed rest and adequate fluid replacement usually leads to complete recovery.

cholesterol. A naturally occurring substance found in all animal fats and oils including the blood and most bodily tissues. It plays an important part in metabolism, being related to the bile acids, the sex hormones, and vitamin D.

Its level in the blood plasma is fairly constant for each individual, but shows wide variation between individuals. There are characteristic changes of level in certain diseases: it is low, for example, in hyperthyroidism, and high in hypothyroidism and untreated diabetes mellitus. The association of raised plasma cholesterol levels with an increased incidence of heart diseases and arteriosclerosis has led to

their treatment with specific cholesterol-lowering drugs, as well as to the increasing adoption of low cholesterol diets. These include the use of unsaturated fats (as in margarine and corn oil) rather than animal fats.

chorea. A disorder characterized by irregular, involuntary, twitching movements of the limbs or facial muscles.

Sydenham's chorea, also called St. Vitus' dance, is an acute, toxic or infective disorder of the nervous system, usually associated with acute rheumatic fever. The characteristic movements of the face and fingers often spread to the limbs and trunk, and there is weakness and incoordination of voluntary movements, and emotional instability. The disease chiefly affects children aged 5 to 15, and girls twice as frequently as boys. It disappears in sleep and responds to treatment of the underlying cause, including rest in bed, skilled nursing and, usually, tranquillizers.

A completely different disease, HUNTINGTON'S CHOREA, is an inherited chronic disorder.

choroid. The middle coat of the EYE, lying between the sclera and the retina, and composed of arteries, veins and capillaries.

choroiditis. Inflammation of part or all of the CHOROID, usually affecting the underlying retina. The effects depend on the area involved, and may sometimes involve partial or complete loss of vision. Choroiditis may be associated with an infective or non-infective general disorder, or with other eye disease or injury.

Treatment consists of eradicating the underlying cause, if known, and employing drugs to restrict inflammation, relieve pain, and control any infection. Prolonged rest is occasionally required.

chromosome. One of a number of small, rod-shaped bodies present in each cell of the body and carrying certain genes which determine a person's inherited characteristics. In human beings every cell except the ovum and sperm contains twenty-three pairs of chromosomes: a woman's cells contain twenty-two pairs of ordinary chromosomes (autosomes) and one pair of sizeable sex-chromosomes commonly called x-chromosomes; and a man's cells contain twenty-two pairs of autosomes, a single x-chromosome and a much smaller chromosome called the Y-chromosome.

In preparation for reproduction the pairs of chromosomes divide. The ovum contains twenty-two autosomes and one x-chromosome. The sperm contains twenty-two autosomes and either an x-or a Y-chromosome. When the ovum is fertilized by a sperm, if the sperm happens to contain an x-chromosome, the result will be a girl (twenty-two pairs of autosomes, one of each pair from each parent, and two x-chromosomes, one from each parent). If on the other hand the sperm contains a Y-chromosome, the result will be a boy (twenty-two pairs of autosomes, one x-chromosome from the mother and one y-chromosome from the father).

From the genes, situated along the chromosomes, derive the inheritance of all predetermined characteristics, e.g., colour of hair and blood group.

Dominant inheritance occurs where a stronger gene (e.g., for achondroplasia, Huntington's chorea or diabetes insipidus) is inherited from one parent and a weaker gene (e.g., for normality in respect of the particular condition) is inherited from the other. The child will show the effects of the stronger gene, i.e., suffer from the disease. If the affected child reaches adult life, clearly half his sperms will contain the dominant (stronger, abnormal) gene and half will contain the recessive (weaker, normal) gene. So, if he marries a normal person, on average half his children will be affected (inheriting the dominant gene from him and a normal gene from the other parent) and the other half will be unaffected (inheriting normal genes from both parents).

In the case of recessive inheritance a weaker gene (e.g., for cystic fibrosis, phenylketonuria or deaf mutism) is inherited from one parent and a stronger gene (e.g., for normality) is inherited from the other. The child will appear normal, but if he reaches adult life half his sperms will contain the weaker (recessive, abnormal) gene and half will contain the normal (dominant) gene. So, if he marries a normal person, on average half the children will be normal (with normal gene from each parent) and the other half will appear normal but be capable of transmitting the condition (having normal gene from one parent and recessive gene from the other). If the apparently normal person (with normal and recessive gene) marries a similar person, it is likely on average that a quarter of their children will be normal (inheriting normal gene from each parent), half will appear normal but be capable of transmitting the condition (inheriting a dominant normal gene from one parent and a recessive abnormal gene from the other) and a quarter will suffer from the disease (inheriting the abnormal gene from both parents). Dominant and recessive inheritance are rather more fully considered in GENETICS.

X-chromosome. As indicated above, a girl inherits one x-chromosome from each parent, and a boy inherits an x-chromosome from his mother and a y-chromosome from his father. Where one of the mother's two x-chromosomes is recessive for a disease (e.g., haemophilia) the girl inherits a normal (dominant) x-chromosome from her father (and therefore will not show the disease) but has a 50 per cent chance of inheriting a normal or recessive x-chromosome from her mother. In adult life the ovum of the girl who had normal inheritance from both parents will clearly contain either a normal x from the father or a normal x from the mother, but the ovum of the girl who inherited the recessive x-chromosome from her mother has equal chances of passing to her ovum a normal x-chromosome (from her father) or the dangerous x-chromosome (from her mother). In other words the daughter of a mother who is a carrier of haemophilia has a one in four chance of being a carrier in turn; but, since a female has two x-chromosomes of which the normal one is dominant, neither she nor her daughters will themselves show the disease.

On the other hand, if the mother is a carrier (with one normal and dominant x-chromosome and one recessive abnormal x-chromosome), on average half the sons will inherit y-chromosome from the father and the normal x-chromosome from the mother (and therefore be normal) and the other half will inherit y-chromosome from the father and the abnormal x-chromosome from the mother (and therefore suffer from the disease). This situation in which a quarter of the daughters are carriers and half of the sons are sufferers is what is termed sex-linked inheritance. Where the father is a sufferer from haemophilia, his sons will be normal (inheriting y-chromosomes from the father) but his daughters will be carriers (inheriting the abnormal x-chromosome from the father and a dominant normal x-chromosome from the mother).

Y-chromosome. As mentioned above, the male sperm is of two types, one containing twenty-two autosomes and a sizeable x-chromosome (leading on fertilization of the ovum to a female child) and the other containing twenty-two autosomes and a small y-chromosome (leading on fertilization to a male child). So sex is determined at the moment of conception and depends solely on which of the father's sperms reaches the ovum.

Unlike the larger x-chromosome, the y-chromosome is not notably associated with transmission of hereditary disease.

Spermatozoa containing the y-chromosome of maleness are a shade lighter and more motile than those containing the x-chromosome. So on average something like 110 to 120 boys are conceived for every 100 girls. Males, however, are the weaker sex even before birth. Male babies are slightly more subject to miscarriages and stillbirths than are female babies. At birth the ratio is about 104 boys per 100 girls. In the long era of high baby and child mortality more boys died than girls, the sexes became about equal in numbers by 15 or 16 years and from about 20 years there were more women than men. In the improved preventive and curative services of today there are still more deaths of boys than of girls but there are far fewer deaths, so that males are more numerous than females up to the age of 40.

This change in the sex-ratio has important implications. For instance, 'surplus' females are no longer available to staff such professions as nursing and teaching or to provide maid-servants for the wealthy; a child today is more likely to have a bachelor uncle than a maiden aunt; there are increasingly fewer unmarried daughters to care for elderly parents; and, just as male deaths in 1914-18 resulted in increased numbers of women entering formerly male occupations (e.g., as doctors, lawyers and secretaries), so the relative fall in the numbers of young women is causing the appearance of men in previously female occupations (e.g., as nurses, primary school teachers, etc.).

chronic. A longstanding condition. The term relates to duration only and does not imply that the condition is permanent or incurable.

chyle. A form of LYMPH, found in the lymph vessels of the small intestine after the absorption of fat from foodstuffs. Milky-white in appearance owing to the presence of emulsified fat, chyle passes into the veins by the way of the thoracic duct.

chyme. Food, partly digested in the stomach, liquid in form, and brown or grey in appearance, passing into the intestines for the completion of digestion.

cigarettes. See SMOKING.

circulation of the blood. From the heart the blood makes a double circuit. Venous blood, containing carbon dioxide and other waste products and coloured dark because of the interaction of carbon dioxide and haemoglobin is brought to the right auricle from the superior vena cava (which drains venous blood from the head and arms) and the inferior vena cava (which drains from the rest of the body). It passes to the right ventricle and then travels by the pulmonary artery and its branches (the only arteries containing venous blood) to the lungs. In the capillaries of the lungs there is an interchange of gases: carbon dioxide passes out to the alveoli of the lungs and is subsequently breathed out, and oxygen passes in, inter-acting with the haemoglobin and giving the oxygenated blood (arterial blood) its bright red colour.

The oxygenated blood is carried by the pulmonary veins (the only veins containing arterial blood) to the left auricle, passes to the left ventricle and is from there pumped into the AORTA, the main artery of the body. From branches and sub-branches of the aorta the arterial blood passes to capillaries in the various muscles and tissues of the body. From the capillaries the oxygen is removed to supply the needs of tissues and organs, and carbon dioxide and other waste products enter the capillaries, so that the blood becomes venous blood. The capillaries carrying venous blood unite into small veins and these into larger veins which in due course empty into the superior and inferior vena cava.

So for the transport of oxygen and

Diagrammatic scheme showing continuous blood flow round the circulatory system.

carbon dioxide there are really two circulations: venous blood travelling from the right side of the heart to the lungs, gaining oxygen and returning as arterial blood to the left side of the heart; and arterial blood pumped from the left side of the heart to the tissues, losing oxygen and travelling as venous blood to the right side of the heart. (See illustration on p. 82.)

There is also a third circulation. Blood from the stomach, pancreas, spleen and intestines travels by veins to the liver. In the capillaries of the liver glycogen is extracted from the blood for storage or returned to the blood for use in the tissues, and the blood with its glycogen adjusted to balance needs is returned by the hepatic veins to the inferior vena cava. This third circulation is termed the PORTAL CIRCULATION.

circumcision. The operation of cutting away part or all of the foreskin (prepuce) of the penis. The origin of this practice is probably very ancient, circumcision having been practised as a ritual in diverse cultures, performed before or at puberty. Its practitioners attach profound religious significance to the ritual. The Ethiopians, the Jews, and a few other peoples practise it at birth; when performed at puberty it

subclavian

common carotid

aorta

phrenics
to
diaphragm

renal arteries
to kidneys

coeliac
artery
to liver
and
stomach

superior mesenteric
to intestine

spermatic or ovarian
to reproductive organs

inferior mesenteric
to intestine

femoral

internal iliacs
to pelvic organs

The circulatory system, showing the main arteries

represents the beginning of initiation into manhood.

It has been widely practised in some countries (e.g., the U.S.A.) as a hygienic measure, the circumcised seldom suffering from inflammation of the glans penis or from carcinoma of the penis. The other possible benefit (protection against carcinoma of the cervix of the uterus among women who consort only with circumcised men) is unproven and the subject of considerable current research.

cirrhosis. A progressive liver disease in which normal liver tissue is partially destroyed and replaced by non-functional tissue. It leads to impaired liver function, frequently resulting in jaundice and other complications. Its most frequent cause is alcoholism, though it is uncertain whether alcoholism leads to cirrhosis through a direct effect on liver tissue or because of an associated nutritional deficiency. It is also caused by obstruction of the bile ducts and is an occasional late effect of infective hepatitis.

Prevention depends mainly upon control of alcohol intake. Alcohol avoidance and vitamin supplementation form the basis of treatment.

claudication, intermittent. Attacks of lameness and pain, especially in the calf muscles, brought on by walking. The symptoms increase as walking proceeds until further progress is impossible, but after a short rest, during which the symptoms cease, walking becomes possible again. Intermittent claudication is caused by limitation of blood supply to the leg muscles due to narrowing, by ARTERIOSCLEROSIS, of the arteries of the legs. It is the commonest symptom of a process involving the whole arterial system, and is therefore commonly found in people suffering from heart disease and cerebrovascular disease. No specific treatment exists, though weight control may be helpful, and cigarette smoking is particularly discouraged.

claustrophobia. An irrational dread of being within walls, or of being shut in a room or confined space. Like other obsessional neuroses it generally starts in early adult life. In Britain, treatment is usually by psychotherapy and tranquillizers, though treatment by psychoanalysis, by hypnosis, and by behaviour therapy is also practised. About 70 per cent of patients recover or become much better within a year or two, whatever treatment is given; the outcome seems to depend more on the duration of the illness and the previous personality and circumstances of the patient than on the form of treatment employed.

clavicle. See COLLAR-BONE.

cleft palate. See HARE-LIP AND CLEFT PALATE.

clergyman's throat. Prolonged hoarseness and tickling cough, usually due to excessive voice strain, as is liable to occur in public speakers, clergymen, teachers and others who frequently have to address large groups, but also occasionally caused by excessive use of tobacco or over-indulgence in alcohol. See PHARYNX, DISEASES OF.

climacteric. As far as women are concerned, this is a synonym for the menopause (see MENOPAUSE).

A similar crisis affects most men in middle life, generally between 45 and 60 years of age, resulting from their increasing realization of their own mortality in association with a waning of their physical powers. The appreciation that he can never hope to achieve all that he had once dreamt of doing, together with the prospect of an apparently steady decline of his faculties, precipitates depression or unexpected uncharacteristic behaviour in a few seemingly well-adjusted individuals. For some men the crisis provides the incentive for a sensible re-planning of their lives: most just muddle through.

Reproductive ability is not lost at the male climacteric as it is in women; in common with women, men suffer no diminution of sexual drive at this time unless psychological disorders supervene.

climax, sexual. See ORGASM.

clitoris. Part of the female genitalia: the small, highly sensitive mound of tissue lying at the front of the vulva. Its stimulation is an important part of love-play, eventually leading to orgasm.

club foot. Technically called talipes equino-varus. A deformity of the foot long known to be due to faulty development before birth and nowadays recognized as being hereditary in origin. The deformity, which occurs rather more frequently in boys than in girls, consists in the sole of the foot being turned inwards and the heel drawn up, so that the person walks on the outer border of the foot on which corns tend to develop.

If the condition is identified early it can sometimes be cured by manipulation, splinting and massage. If it is not identified for a couple of years or so, surgical reconstruction of the joints of the foot may be required, and even after the operation special footwear may be needed. If untreated it causes life-long deformity.

coal gas poisoning. See CARBON MONOXIDE.

coal miner's lung. A disease of the lungs and bronchi arising from prolonged inhalation of fine particles of coal dust, creating breathlessness and chronic bronchitis. Preventive measures include ventilation of mines and wet-drilling. Where the condition is identified in an early stage a change of occupation is desirable.

cocaine. An alkaloid, derived originally from the leaves of the coca plant in Bolivia and Peru, sometimes used in ophthalmology, dentistry and nose and throat surgery to produce local anaesthesia, but seldom employed internally because of the great danger of addiction. Habitual use of cocaine causes temporary feelings of elation, severe craving, and ultimately complete deterioration of the personality.

coccus. A micro-organism of spherical shape. Cocci are microscopically small (often about one-thousandth of a millimetre in diameter) and they have characteristic patterns of growth, appearing as pairs (diplococci), clumps (staphylococci), or long chains (streptococci).

Various species are responsible for numerous important diseases. Certain diplococci cause pneumonia, gonorrhoea, and cerebrospinal fever. Superficial infections of the skin and subcutaneous tissues, and localized deep infections of bones, joints, and internal organs, are usually due to staphylococci. Streptococci are associated with scarlet fever, tonsillitis, respiratory tract infections, endocarditis, wound infections, postnatal infections, and spreading septicaemic conditions generally.

coccydinia. See COCCYX.

coccyx. The lower end of the spinal column. It is a triangular bone beyond the sacrum and consists developmentally of four tiny vertebrae that are fused together. It is all that remains in man of the tail of animals.

Coccydinia, which is pain in the area of the coccyx, is sometimes the result of injury, e.g., a fall, but is more often a neuralgia of the nerves in that neighbourhood. In some cases it is a neurotic symptom. Treatment varies with the cause and no single treatment is of guaranteed efficiency. Surgical removal of the coccyx is a last resort which should not be used until less dramatic remedies have proved unsuccessful.

cochlea. The true organ of hearing (organ of Corti). It consists of a spiral tube resembling a snail-shell and forms part of the inner EAR.

codeine. A white crystalline compound, derived from morphia but not possessing its addictive qualities, much used in tablet form to relieve mild pain and in cough mixtures to reduce unproductive coughing. However it also slows the movements of the muscles of the intestine and so may cause constipation, and it often tends to cause slight drowsiness.

cod-liver oil. A pale yellow liquid of fishy odour and unpleasant taste obtained from the fresh liver of cod fish. It is a very rich source of vitamins A and D, and was formerly much employed for the prevention of rickets and – perhaps less effectively – for the treatment of children suffering from bronchitis, tuberculosis and various other diseases. Because of its unpalatable taste it was often given combined with malt or orange juice, or as an emulsion. In general cod-liver oil has now been replaced by purer, more concentrated preparations of fat-soluble vitamins.

coeliac disease. A wasting disease of childhood in which the lining of the intestine is damaged by gluten (a protein found in wheat, barley and some other cereals) so that it fails to absorb fats and calcium properly. The condition appears between the ages of 6 and 24 months; the child loses appetite and ceases to thrive, and diarrhoea develops with large, pale, offensive stools containing much unabsorbed fat. If the disease is untreated signs of vitamin deficiency and anaemia appear; there is considerable emaciation and the abdomen becomes very distended. A minority of cases die but the majority ultimately recover although they may be permanently stunted in consequence of having had a year or so of malnutrition during what should have been an important growth period. Such stunting is also common if treatment is started late.

Early treatment with a gluten-free diet, which means eating cereals only when the gluten portion has been removed, and

some attention to vitamin supplements together with restriction in the amount of fat eaten, usually result in complete recovery with ultimate ability to assimilate ordinary food. The required duration of treatment varies from under six months to over two years and is best estimated by trying the child every few weeks with a little ordinary flour and watching the state of the stools.

coitus. Sexual intercourse, or the act of sexual union. Intercourse is preceded by arousal, a stage of sexual excitation, during which the penis of the male, by engorgement with blood, becomes enlarged, erect, and capable of penetrating into the vagina. In the female similar engorgement causes the thick folds of skin at the entrance to the vagina to swell and turn outwards, so that the opening is exposed; there is also an increased secretion of mucus which lubricates the parts and facilitates penetration. Since female arousal is generally less immediate, preliminary 'love-play' (e.g. caressing of breasts, thighs and genitals) will ensure mutual readiness.

After penetration, rhythmic movements by both partners increase excitation until the culmination of orgasm is reached. In the man this is accompanied by reflex ejaculation of semen, and in the woman by pleasurable muscular spasms, primarily in the genital area but sometimes spreading more widely.

Ideal coitus should aim at achievement of simultaneous orgasm and this calls for forbearance and an understanding approach by the man, since female orgasm is generally attained less rapidly. Prolongation of arousal, with variations in position and technique, will help to ensure the mutual release from tension, and the pleasurable feelings of relaxation and refreshment which should follow.

coitus interruptus. An unreliable non-medical method of CONTRACEPTION. At intercourse the penis is withdrawn as ejaculation is about to occur, so that semen is discharged well outside the vagina. It requires considerable self-control on the part of the man 'being careful', and tends to diminish sexual satisfaction in both partners.

There is a substantial failure-rate, variously quoted as 5 to 20 per cent, because motile sperms may be present in the man's mucus even before climax; or because ejaculation may have been gradual and not appreciated as a well-defined climax; or finally because sperm deposited at the vaginal entrance may still succeed in ascending to the cervix by their own motility.

Coitus interruptus may also be psychologically harmful by increasing feelings of emotional insecurity and contributing to frigidity and failure of female orgasm.

cold, the common. Technically termed coryza. A catarrhal inflammation of the nose and upper respiratory passages, characterized by a feeling of chilliness, watering nose, sneezing, watering eyes and general discomfort. A cold usually lasts three to five days.

Most cases of coryza are due to a virus and therefore infectious, so that the sufferer should remain at home in the interests of others as well as for his own comfort. It appears, however, that some colds are allergic in nature and not infectious.

Frequent colds may arise as a result of debility, lowered general resistance, adenoids or minor deformities of the nose or throat. Certain families have more than their average share of colds, whether from poorer nutrition or from similarities in their nasal passages. By contrast some people appear to have a high natural immunity.

Aspirin tablets and warm drinks promote perspiration and make the patient feel a little better, and cough medicines may be required when the catarrh reaches the larynx and bronchi. Anti-coryzal vaccines are under trial but the outlook is not very hopeful since coryza itself does not confer any lengthy immunity and since infectious colds may well be due not to one virus but to a series of broadly similar viruses. Decongestant nasal sprays may also give relief but proprietary medicines to be taken by mouth often contain drugs which interact with alcohol - a popular remedy - so that alcohol should be avoided if these are taken.

cold, effects of. A cold environment causes the blood vessels near the surface of the skin to contract thus decreasing the loss of body heat; it also reduces the conducting capacity of nerves so that the cold portion of the body becomes numb. If the cold is extreme the fingers, toes and ears may become damaged by FROSTBITE. Raynaud's disease (pallor and purpling of the fingers and toes) and chilblains (patches of itching, bluish-red, cold skin) are precipitated in susceptible persons by cold.

A cold environment also causes increased secretion of the thyroid hormone and of adrenaline, which in turn increases heat production by combustion of carbohydrate and fat - as if the body were attempting to compensate by deliberately raising its heat. Shivering is essentially a result of this increased heat production. Body hair becomes erect with the appearance of 'goose-pimples' in an attempt to trap still air in the spaces thus formed next to the skin and, as air is a poor conductor of heat, this prevents heat-loss from the body.

If severe cold continues, the body's balancing attempts ultimately cease, the whole body begins to cool (hypothermia), the person usually falls asleep, and he is likely to die when his temperature falls below 20 °C. (68 °F.).

Inability to withstand cold, and thus the risk of HYPOTHERMIA, is particularly marked - and particularly dangerous - in babies and old people. Sensible use of clothing and DIET are important.

cold feet. A source of considerable discomfort, cold feet are also a frequent cause of chilblains. The essential underlying cause is poor circulation either of blood or of lymph. This poor circulation is less often due to cardio-vascular disease than to the impeding of the circulation by tight belts at the waist, tight garters on the legs or constricting shoes. Treatment consists principally in removing the cause, but additionally vigorous exercise and a diet containing adequacy of calcium and vitamin D are thought to help.

cold sores. See HERPES.

colic. Irregular, painful and spasmodic contractions of the muscular tissue in hollow organs, most commonly in the intestine. Intestinal colic is usually due either to inflammation from an irritant or to pressure from indigestible material in the bowel, but is occasionally caused by poisoning of the nerves (as in lead poisoning) and is sometimes a symptom of other conditions such as appendicitis and intussusception. The degree of pain varies from slight spasms of little more than discomfort to almost intolerable paroxysms.

Treatment varies with the cause. In cases due to an irritant a fairly mild laxative may suffice to remove it, and meantime hot fomentations may help to reduce the pain. Repeated attacks of colic call for medical advice.

Colic may also arise in the gall bladder, the stomach and the kidneys.

colitis. Inflammation of the colon, characterized by uneasy feelings in the lower abdomen accompanied by occasional sharp pains. Colitis may be acute - a result of bacterial or other food poisoning - in which case acute diarrhoea is a symptom; or it may be chronic, associated with chronic constipation or over-use of laxatives.

Prevention of acute colitis is mainly a matter of good hygiene on the part of all persons handling food. The treatment is obvious - temporary cessation of solid food, supply of ample fluids to prevent dehydration, a laxative to remove the irritant and in severe cases of bacterial origin an appropriate antibiotic which is not easily absorbed from the intestine.

Since the chronic variety of colitis often occurs in nervous, over-anxious, obsessional persons, psychological treatment is necessary in many cases. Additional possibilities in treatment include antispasmodic drugs such as hyoscyamus and bromides, colonic lavage with alkaline fluids, and mild laxatives.

colitis, ulcerative. A severe persistent inflammation of the intestine, occurring mostly in women aged 25 to 40 years, and thought to be due primarily to bacterial infection although the bacteria appear to invade mucous membranes already damaged by some unknown process. There may be an allergic factor involved, and many experts believe that an emotional factor plays a part in the cause, although it is equally true that the symptoms can cause emotional upset.

Symptoms – lasting over many months – include irregular bouts of high temperature, and long continued diarrhoea and painful motions, with blood, pus and mucus in the stools. If the condition is untreated the diarrhoea leads to dehydration and emaciation and the continued small loss of blood leads to anaemia.

Treatment is difficult but includes a period of rest in bed with warmth, an easily digested diet with little indigestible residue, colonic lavage, antibiotics to combat infection and in some cases corticosteroids. Occasionally surgical treatment is needed.

collagen diseases. Collagen is a protein and is the main constituent of the connective tissue found in ligaments, tendons and capsules of joints. The molecules of the protein are structurally like three-stranded ropes.

Disorganization of the collagen fibres is in some cases a hereditary condition, in others a sequel to inflammation and in yet others perhaps simply a result of ageing; and the diseases caused by the disorganization are numerous and vary with the age of the patient and with the parts of the body affected. Marfan's syndrome, characterized by excessive growth of the length of fingers and toes and to a lesser extent of the length of arms and legs, is an example of a collagen disease inherited as a Mendelian dominant (see GENETICS), and so is gargoylism, in which the patient has an abnormally large head and a saddle-shaped nose. Lupus erythematosus, manifested by raised temperature, skin eruptions and joint changes resembling those of arthritis, is a collagen disease of inflammatory origin. Some forms of rheumatism are thought to be associated with degeneration of the collagen fibres.

In general CORTICOSTEROIDS suppress symptoms in the collagen diseases but do not cure the underlying conditions.

collar-bone. A long, doubly curved bone otherwise known as the clavicle that forms part of the shoulder girdle. It is affected by two particular types of injury resulting from a fall on the shoulder – dislocation at its joint with the sternum in adults, and fracture in children or adolescents. Fracture may also be caused by a fall on the outstretched hand. Treatment of dislocation is rarely required but treatment of fracture requires the application of a figure-of-eight bandage for about a month.

Colles' fracture. The term is now usually applied to the fracture of the radius about half an inch above the wrist joint,

generally due to a fall on the outstretched hand. The fracture is usually transverse, and the small fragment of the radius that is broken off is displaced backwards, rotated and tilted.

If no doctor is at hand padded splints should be applied to the inside and outside of the wrist and an arm-sling used to support the forearm. Early manipulation is, however, important to place the broken fragments in a position in which they can heal without deformity. Thereafter the wrist is normally placed in plaster for a few weeks.

colon. The large bowel – that part of the DIGESTIVE SYSTEM into which the small bowel opens and in which the waste products of the bowel become transformed from a fluid into a solid or semi-solid stool by the absorption of water. It is a large tube which starts in the lower right hand side of the abdomen, passes up under the rib cage on the right (the ascending colon), crosses from right to left in the upper part of the abdomen (the transverse colon), travels down on the left hand side of the abdomen (the descending colon) into the pelvis where it becomes the pelvic colon and ends by becoming continuous with the rectum.

colostomy. The operation of making an artificial opening into the intestine to permit evacuation of faeces. This operation is usually performed when an obstruction in the large bowel prevents the normal passage of waste products through the anus. It may be a temporary measure in an acute obstruction but in some patients has to be permanent. In the latter event there is a wide range of appliances – belts, bags etc. – which minimize the inconvenience of what is essentially an abdominal anus.

Persons with a colostomy can lead a normal life but require moral support while learning to cope with what is, for them, an entirely new method of waste disposal. Such support can be obtained from others who have had and adapted to the operation and also from voluntary organizations.

colostrom. The first milk produced by the mother after the birth of her child. It differs from all subsequent milk in that it has a higher protein content and less sugar. In some animals, probably including humans, it appears to be of major importance in that the mother transfers antibodies to her offspring in this 'milk', in effect providing temporary immunization to diseases to which the mother has acquired a resistance.

colour blindness. A visual defect in which the sufferer cannot distinguish between different colours or perceives them differently from the normal person. About 8 per cent of men and 0.4 per cent of women have some defect of colour vision. The rarest type is the person totally unable to distinguish colour, but most colour blind persons can differentiate some shades.

complex

Red-green colour blindness is the commonest type. In this condition sufferers have very little colour discrimination at the red end of the spectrum and thus are unable to distinguish between red, green and brown. More rare is the 'blue blind' person who cannot distinguish blue from green but has normal discrimination at the end of the spectrum. In contrast with the other forms, blue blindness is as common in women as in men, but other forms may be recessive sex-linked characteristics (see GENETICS) carried on the x-chromosome and consequently are more likely to be found in men; a woman only suffers if she had a carrier mother and an affected father.

colour vision. There are many theories of colour vision which can shed light on the nature of colour blindness. Specific cells in the retina of the EYE (the cones) appear to contain pigments sensitive to colour. There are three types of these, those sensitive to red, those to green, and those to blue. Red-green colour blindness is due to lack of the red or green sensitive pigments while lack of the blue gives rise to blue-green blindness. Persons who perceive colours differently from normal individuals are thought to have abnormal amounts of pigment in the colour sensitive cones.

coma. A state of deep unconsciousness in which the individual is unresponsive to any form of stimulus. It can arise as a result of illness, severe intoxication by drugs or drink, or serious head injury. It frequently occurs just prior to death in patients who have been ill for a long time.

comedo. A BLACKHEAD.

community health services. The term has several different meanings.

1. Where 'health' is interpreted in its positive sense, i.e., as good health in contrast with both absence of health and actual disease, community health services are the services provided within and by a community for the purpose of safeguarding and promoting health. These often include health education (of individuals and groups and also by use of mass media), antenatal care, maternity services, health visiting of mothers and children (and sometimes of other groups), infant and pre-school health services (such as child health clinics), immunization and vaccination, school health services, family planning services, 'well women clinics' and cervical cytology, control of infectious diseases, port health services, environmental health services and services to maintain the health of the elderly (e.g., pre-retirement courses, advice by dieticians, counselling by health visitors and other health workers, chiropody services, etc).

2. Quite often 'community health' is understood as including both the promoting and safeguarding of good health and the treating and supporting in their own homes of people in bad health. In such circumstances the term 'community

health services' comes to include, in addition to the preventive services mentioned above, such items as home nursing services, ambulance services and the services of non-hospital medical and dental practitioners.

3. All the services falling under the jurisdiction of the health authority for a particular district, often with a sizeable general hospital as its focal point.

complex. A system of repressed and usually unconscious feelings and ideas, often derived from experiences in early childhood, giving rise to patterns of behaviour at variance with those that would be expected from the person's cultural background and social circumstances. A very simple example may be given first: an intelligent and inquisitive 3-year-old enters a dark cellar, the door swings shut behind him, he cannot open it and for a time his cries are unheard; thirty years later he has completely forgotten that half hour of terror but he has a persisting and apparently irrational fear of the dark. Other examples are the man who habitually shrinks from responsibilities for which his education and experience would seem to fit him, the woman who becomes panic-stricken in a thunderstorm, the person who has an irrational hatred of members of a particular race and the person who obtains sexual pleasure in an abnormal way.

Essentially complexes are an antisocial or pathological equivalent of sentiments and dispositions. When the mind of the child is still being shaped he acquires various dispositions and sentiments (e.g., a disposition to be fair-minded and a sentiment of loyalty to his family) and is later unaware that he has acquired these through a mixture of example, precept and personal experience. Simultaneously he may acquire abnormal or pathological dispositions – complexes – which create tendencies to anxieties, phobias and other types of unacceptable behaviour.

Clearly we can to some extent prevent the development of complexes by seeking to avoid in children the type of happening that gives rise to them, by being careful to minimize (rather than accentuate) any infirmity or deficiency of a child, and by trying in the presence of children to avoid showing exaggerated reactions of anger, fear or depression; but probably very few adults have had such perfect childhoods that they have absolutely no complexes. Indeed, some complexes probably arise simply as a result of physical defects or infirmities, e.g., very small people are often unduly aggressive.

In many cases a complex creates abnormal behaviour only during periods in which it is precipitated by unusual circumstances. In these cases we can try to avoid or minimize the particular circumstances. The person terrified of trains can avoid travelling by rail and the person afraid of responsibility can take a routine job.

Where a complex creates seriously abnormal behaviour or deep personal unhappiness elaborate psychological treatment is required. Changing the physical or social environment will not alter a sexual deviation or a persisting depression or an irrational hatred of a particular religion. To change these attitudes we have to search for the long-forgotten causes of the complex and then to attempt the difficult task of eradicating these causes.

compression of the brain. Pressure on the brain as a result of a fall, blow or other head injury, so that a depressed piece of bone or a clot of blood from a torn blood-vessel presses on the delicate brain tissue. There are sometimes no symptoms for several hours while the pressure is building up, but in due course the patient becomes deeply unconscious, with heavy breathing, full and slow pulse, and unequal pupils. In such cases operation is urgently necessary to relieve the pressure and to stop any bleeding inside the skull.

The condition has to be differentiated from CONCUSSION. In concussion there is a commotion of the brain cells, leading to a dazed state or unconsciousness, but often responding to the patient being simply put to bed in a darkened room with ice-bags, if available, applied to his head. In compression the pressure on the brain goes on building up and in the absence of urgent surgical relief the patient is likely to die.

From these points it follows that a person who has sustained any severe injury to the head should, even if he is conscious and lucid immediately after the injury, be kept under observation for several hours, preferably in a hospital with facilities for brain surgery.

conception. The union of the sperm and the ovum within the body of a woman, whereby she becomes pregnant.

If intercourse has taken place only once in the relevant weeks the date of conception is generally presumed to be that of the intercourse, but there can actually be a period of several days between the two events. After intercourse the spermatozoon propels itself upwards at a speed of 2 to 3 mm. per minute. If the ovum is already in the uterus the sperm may push its way into the ovum within an hour of the sexual act. On the other hand, if the ovum has not yet reached the uterus – and the process of ovulation occurs only once a month starting thirteen to fifteen days after the end of menstruation – the sperm can remain alive for several days and can still fertilize the ovum.

The ovum during its journey to the uterus has divided, losing half of its chromosomes. So at the moment of conception the sperm has twenty-two somatic chromosomes and either a single male or a single female sex chromosome,

and the ovum has twenty-two somatic chromosomes and one female sex chromosome. So there is no possibility of continuing life of the ovum or sperm alone.

The sperm is about one-twentieth of a millimetre long and the ovum is a sphere of about one-fifth of a millimetre in diameter. It is a matter of philosophical rather than medical argument whether life can be considered to begin when the head of the sperm enters the ovum; or two months later when the embryo is about 25 mm. long, the head is assuming a human shape and the tail of the embryo is beginning to disappear; or after five months when the foetus is 200 mm. long and might possibly survive if separated from the mother.

concussion. A shaking of the brain cells, e.g., as a result of a blow or a fall. In slight concussion there may be a dazed feeling or a short period of unconsciousness, the victim may have no recollection of the injury and he may act automatically for some hours afterwards. In severe concussion there may be deep and prolonged unconsciousness.

Rest, quiet and, if available, application of icebags to the head may be all that is needed; but the person should be kept under observation for several hours because of the possibility that he is also suffering from COMPRESSION OF THE BRAIN.

condom. See SHEATH.

condylomata. Rounded, fleshy-like swellings of mucous membrane, occurring in the secondary stage of SYPHILIS.

confinement. The period during which a woman is in bed through giving birth to a child. The term is often used as synonymous with labour but strictly should include not only the period of the actual labour but also the days of restoration of strength after the birth of the child.

Calculation of the probable date of the start of confinement is best done by reckoning from the first day of the last menstrual period, a date which the patient may remember. Allowing 5 days for menstruation, a further 2 days as an average time before coitus occurs and 273 days for the normal development of the unborn child, we can estimate that labour will probably start about 280 days after the beginning of the last menstrual period; but this is only an approximate date and is liable to considerable alteration. Labour may occur several days earlier than expected, or up to three weeks later, the explanation of the second feature being that conception occurred not soon after the last period but shortly before the first period missed. As pregnancy progresses rough checks may be attempted by measuring the height of the top of the uterus or by trying to count from the date of quickening, but in general these do not give more accurate results than simply calculating from the last period.

Health education, improved antenatal care, anaesthesia and improved obstetrics have during the present century enormously reduced the dangers and the discomforts of confinement. It can be regarded as a normal physiological event provided (1) that GENETIC GUIDANCE, if needed, has made inherited abnormality unlikely, (2) that several pregnancies do not follow each other in successive years, (3) that the woman is reasonably healthy and aged under 40, (4) that medical and obstetric supervision are satisfactory.

conflict. The distressing situation where a person's strong desires are in opposition either to the codes of the society in which he lives or to deep-rooted parts of his own personality.

The first of these is easily understood. For instance, in time of war a man who has either an intense disbelief in the violent taking of life or a strong instinct of self-preservation finds himself in conflict with the general wave of patriotic enthusiasm, and usually resolves the conflict in one of three ways – by resisting the opinions of his associates (and becoming a conscientious objector), by submitting to them (and reluctantly joining the army) or by escaping (retaining his pacifist views without publicly expressing them and contriving to find a job which will exempt him from military service). Another example might be where a woman whose religion forbids divorce strongly wishes to marry a divorced man; she usually either resists the dictates of her religion or sadly abandons the idea of the marriage. These external conflicts occasionally remain unresolved and can lead to illness, but in the vast majority of cases one or other of the opposing forces gains the victory, so that the conflict ends, the person becoming either a conformist or a rebel.

Rather less easy to understand is the purely internal conflict. To take an example, when Shakespeare's Lady Macbeth tells Macbeth that she would have slain the sleeping Duncan but for the fact that he looked like her own father, she is exhibiting an internal conflict, the conflict that ultimately drives her mad.

Few people go through life without conflicts. Many a highly sexed man of high moral principles has at some point in time felt a strong desire to make love to a woman other than his wife; many a normally honest person has been under deep temptation after finding a note-filled wallet in the street. However, in most cases the conflict ends fairly quickly with the submission of one side or the other. The person either bows to the codes of his associates or the laws of the community or the sentiments and moral views that he has developed from childhood, or else he resists these and follows the dictates of the strong emotion. In submission he may ease his frustration by a transfer mechanism: for example, the man whose strong power-drive has urged him to seize an opportunity to damage his immediate

superior may, after resisting that impulse as contrary to his whole ethical code, ease his frustrated power-drive by bullying his subordinates or his children.

Where neither side submits he may use an escape mechanism. He may succeed in repressing from his conscious mind the forbidden desire, though it may sometimes emerge in distorted forms in dreams. Alternatively he may seek to escape the conflict – by physically removing himself from the circumstances (as with the person who suddenly throws away a good job and leaves the district), by hysteria or psychosomatic illness, by day-dreaming and fantasy, by over-indulgence in alcohol, or more usefully by transfer of his energies to an absorbing hobby. Clearly the use of an escape mechanism can be either helpful or harmful, and in relation to the conflict itself it can be successful or unsuccessful.

The most dangerous situation, however, is where there is neither submission of one side or the other nor any successful escape mechanism but continuation of the unresolved conflict, for instance the woman with aged and dependent parents and a fiancé who has accepted a promotion post a hundred miles away, who neither accepts nor rejects marriage and change of residence but remains undecided, worried and miserable; or the teacher who decides that he has become dull, uninspiring and disliked by his pupils but who neither makes up his mind to try to change his job or his methods nor faces the fact that not all teachers are brilliant and that he must be content to be a rather poor member of his profession; instead he just broods constantly, with increasing feelings of guilt and unworthiness. Such continuation of conflict is the commonest cause of anxiety neurosis and indeed of other forms of psychoneurosis.

Where a stable personality has been formed in childhood – by influences such as physical and emotional security, demonstrated affection, consistency, adequate opportunity to explore and investigate, opportunities to take decisions, kindly and not excessive discipline, suitable playthings and playmates, and plenty of praise and encouragement – the conflicts that arise later are likely to be satisfactorily resolved, whether by submission of one side or by successful use of an escape mechanism.

If a conflict remains unresolved, discussion either with a trusted friend or with a professional worker of known integrity (e.g., a health visitor or a social worker) sometimes helps, both by bringing the issues clearly into the victim's consciousness and because the dispassionate listener may be able to indicate additional aspects sufficient to tilt the victim's mind towards resolution of the conflict in one direction. Unfortunately, however, in many cases of unresolved conflict the roots lie deep, so that extensive psychological or psychiatric treatment is needed.

confusional psychosis. Clouding of consciousness with disorder of memory and of sense of time and place, difficulty in recognizing people and places and (frequently) hallucinations, all in consequence of poisoned or exhausted brain cells.

congenital. A term applied to disease and deformities existing from birth. In general the word covers three kinds of disorder of differing origin: (1) the enormous number of hereditary (i.e., inherited) conditions, e.g., spina bifida, phenylketonuria and deaf mutism; (2) conditions acquired during the mother's pregnancy, e.g., the various defects that are associated with the mother suffering from German measles (rubella) during the early months of pregnancy; and (3) conditions acquired during the actual passage of the child through the birth canal, e.g., ophthalmia neonatorum acquired from a mother suffering from gonorrhoea.

conjunctivitis. Inflammation of the conjunctiva, i.e., the membrane which covers the front of the eye. The conjunctiva, although exposed to many sources of irritation and inflammation, is well protected, first by the mobile action of the eyelids which close very rapidly in hostile environments such as a cloud of dust, and second by the secretion of tears, by which foreign matter is quickly removed from the front of the eye to the tear duct. Nevertheless, conjunctivitis is not infrequent, especially in the young and especially during the dry sunny months.

The causes are numerous, perhaps the commonest being measles, in which conjunctivitis is really part of the disease.

In the most usual form of conjunctivitis, sometimes called the catarrhal type, the symptoms include smarting of the eye, a sensation of grit beneath the eyelid, reddening of the eyeball and excessive watering or flow of tears. Where the pain is appreciable or where the condition does not clear up without treatment in a couple of days medical advice should be sought.

constipation. Failure to pass solid waste matter known as stools or faeces. Causes can be grouped into those resulting from dietary deficiencies, from mechanical obstruction to the passage of food along the bowel, or from faulty bowel habits.

The waste is the indigestible part of food and if the diet is high in foodstuffs which can be absorbed and low in vegetable fibre (such as is found in fruits, bran and vegetables), which cannot, there may be insufficient bulk of waste in the bowel to form more than the occcasional stool. Starvation also causes constipation for obvious reasons.

Mechanical obstruction can occur from narrowing of the bowel by inflammation, tumour or compression from fibrous bands. It can also occur from the

accumulation of hard lumps of waste in the bowel.

Faulty bowel habits are the main cause of constipation in Western society. A mythology has persisted about the desirability of evacuation of excrement with daily regularity. However, metabolisms and diets differ. Preoccupation with a daily performance causes some people to resort to laxatives. The most harmless of these increase the bulk of the stool, for instance, bran or mineral salts are not absorbed by the bowel and ensure a copious stool because they require water to dissolve them. Others, such as senna and cascara, increase the physical movement of the bowel causing it to hurry along the reluctant faeces. This 'flogging' of a bowel that is functioning normally can give rise to a vicious circle because a bowel that has been stimulated unnecessarily relaxes after the stimulus disappears and, as the faeces due 'tomorrow' were passed 'yesterday', there is, naturally, a pause in bowel activity. But this produces the anxiety that led to the use of the laxative in the first place and so a repeat dose is taken.

Children. The commonest cause in infancy is insufficient food. It can occur in both breast-fed and bottle-fed infants receiving an adequate diet for different reasons. In breast-fed children, because human milk is a minimum roughage diet, it is perfectly reasonable for a child to go for a week without passing a stool. Cow's milk, the basic source of nutrition for bottle-fed children, contains more protein and calcium than human milk. These consituents are less well coped with by the infant bowel and can lead to hard stools that the child cannot pass.

In older children constipation can occur because they are too preoccupied to go to the toilet: if the stimulus of a full rectum is ignored, such neglect can become increasingly easy because the muscle of a loaded rectum becomes sluggish. If the child finds it painful to defecate (as can occur with a tear in the skin of the anus), postponement leads to chronic constipation. Such tears commonly result from the passage of hard stools. Therefore, to prevent habitual constipation, children should be encouraged to respond promptly when nature calls.

consumption. See TUBERCULOSIS.

contact lenses. Transparent structures that are applied close to the eye to correct defective vision. Because of their close contact with the surface of the eye they can be uncomfortable to wear, but 80 per cent of users can wear them for twelve to eighteen hours without discomfort.

Contact lenses have the advantages that they are almost invisible and can be used in occupations and sports in which spectacles would be cumbersome.

contagious diseases. A category of infectious illnesses transmitted mainly by direct physical contact with an infected person; consequently they are usually diseases of the skin (with the exception of venereal diseases). The types of infectious organism that can be spread by touch include viruses (e.g., warts), bacteria (e.g., impetigo, erysipelas), funguses (e.g., ringworm, or athlete's foot) and free living animals (such as the mites that give rise to scabies and the lice producing infestations of the hair on the head and body).

Contagious disease is much less common than it used to be, because of greatly improved living standards, better personal hygiene, and more effective specific treatments.

contraception. The deliberate prevention of fertilization of the egg cell. See BIRTH CONTROL.

contusion. See BRUISE.

convalescence. The period after an illness or operation during which the patient recovers strength. With the increasing tendency towards active rehabilitation after illness, rather than waiting passively for recovery, and the increasing recognition of the dangers of prolonged bed rest there has been a steady fall in the period of time allotted by doctors for convalescence for nearly all illnesses. Also the increased availability of effective therapies, e.g., penicillin for pneumonia, and better pre-operative and post-operative treatments, means that patients are less debilitated and so will require less time to recover.

convulsion. Violent uncontrolled movement of a muscle or group of muscles or even all the muscles in the body; it may be accompanied by loss of consciousness as in the case of major epilepsy.

Children, and particularly infants, are much more liable to convulse than adults. If they are feverish they may have a convulsion, and the onset of an acute infection may be heralded by a convulsion, but these feverish convulsions become less frequent as the child grows older and generally do not recur in adulthood. Less frequently convulsions can occur because the blood calcium is low (as in rickets) or as the result of breath-holding attacks.

When alterations in the level of consciousness occur, the convulsions are usually caused by brain damage of some sort, either (1) physical such as after injury or (2) biochemical, as can occur when the body accumulates large amounts of toxic products of metabolism because of failure of the kidney or liver to function properly. Convulsions can also occur without loss of consciousness because of increased muscular activity, such as shivering, or increased nervous excitability, as can be seen in tetanus.

Care. The important points in looking after someone who is unconscious and convulsing are to make sure that he does not strike any sharp object or edge, does not choke, and does not bite through his tongue. The patient is best lain on side or face and a gag put between his teeth. Fingers are unsuitable for gags and a spoon covered with a handkerchief is an adequate emergency substitute.

corn. A localized, thickened area of skin caused by the pressure of tight or ill-fitting shoes. It can be hard or soft but the hard ones are much commoner.

Hard corns are usually formed over the outer parts of the little or big toe. Pressure causes hardening of the skin till eventually a horny cone is formed with its flat base on the outside and its apex pointing inwards. This apex will cause pain whenever any pressure is put upon it and if infection of the corn occurs such pain can be excruciating.

It is possible to remove corns by paring them with a knife after softening by immersion of the foot in warm water for a period. Pain can also be relieved by placing a ring of felt around the base of the corn so as to prevent pressure from being applied to its centre.

Soft corns occur between the toes and probably do not result from increased pressure. The overgrowing skin is white and sodden because of the presence of sweat and their removal is best undertaken by a chiropodist.

Corns are better avoided than treated, and the best means of prevention is to wear appropriately fitting shoes that do not rub against the toes.

cornea. The curved transparent structure, through which we see, covering the iris and pupil of the EYE.

coronary thrombosis. The blocking of the arteries supplying the heart muscles so that they receive insufficient blood. The condition may occur gradually in one vessel in which case dilatation of others can maintain a satisfactory blood flow, but it usually causes ischaemic heart disease, i.e., the disability arising from reduction of blood supply. Coronary thrombosis is now the largest single cause of death in men in Western society. Over one-third of all male deaths between the ages of 35 and 65 years are from ischaemic heart disease, and, while it is more common in men than women under the age of 45 years, after the menopause the rate of disease in women begins to equate with that of men. It is a dangerous disease, being fatal in 10 per cent of heart attacks occurring in persons under the age of 40 years, in 30 per cent of attacks between 40 and 70 years, and in 50 per cent of attacks in persons over 70 years of age.

How it occurs. The basic degenerative process is atherosclerosis, a hardening and internal narrowing of the arteries because of the accumulation of cholesterol (a compound derived from fat) under the internal lining of the arteries and the deposition of successive layers of other blood constituents on top of this to form a plaque. Eventually such raised plaques are to be found under the lining of all the larger blood vessels. This process of atherosclerosis is a gradual one and it occurs to some extent in all men and most women over the age of 20 in Western society.

Unfortunately the coronary arteries are peculiarly liable to plaque formation because they are subjected to much physical movement on account of the regular contraction of the heart. Slight physical injury to the lining may be one of the stimuli to cholesterol, and disturbances of flow through increased turbulence help the process of plaque formation. The blood flow in the coronary arteries is uniquely turbulent because it is very much reduced during the contraction of the heart muscle.

Ultimately deposition of further layers of the assortment of cellular and fatty substances results in increasing 'silting up' of the artery and reduction of its internal diameter so that insufficient blood can get through to provide adequate nutrition for the heart muscle. If this narrowing is a gradual process the sufferer will notice pain only when he taxes his heart by physical effort. Typically, on exertion he will feel a dull tightness over the front of his chest, perhaps spreading up into the neck and chin or down into the arms, and this pain will disappear soon after the exertion stops. This pain is called angina. Such 'early warning' pain is useful in that it allows the sufferer to know what amount of effort his heart muscle can tolerate. Drugs that dilate the coronary blood vessels will also give relief from this pain, and the most commonly used are nitroglycerine derivatives.

Sudden narrowing can occur without warning and usually results in severe pain and distress in the sufferer, although it is not uncommon for 'silent' heart attacks to occur in which the patient feels no discomfort. With the cutting off of blood flow to a part of the heart muscle the deprived muscle dies (becomes infarcted) although a certain amount of blood supply may persist because of links between the smaller blood vessels supplied by different branches of the main arteries. The dead muscle tissue is replaced with fibrous tissue which cannot contract and extend; consequently the remaining heart muscle must work harder to maintain an adequate cardiac output. There is some reserve in the myocardium and, provided the amount of killed tissue is not too great, the individual may recover to such an extent that his physical capabilities are as good as before the attack. However a very severe first attack may cause so much damage as to leave a heart that cannot cope without the use of drugs (such as digitalis) and leave the sufferer severely incapacitated.

The acute attack. This can be a terrifying experience in which the sufferer feels agonizing pain or tightness across the chest and sometimes in the arms and neck. He is pale, sweating, and short of breath with a weak rapid pulse. He should be made to sit down (not lie down), be reassured as much as possible and kept warm. Spirits may be given in moderation and a doctor should be sent for immediately. Because the myocardium is damaged it may be very irritable and contract irregularly or stop altogether. If the person becomes suddenly unconscious, stops breathing and is pulseless (the weak pulse is best felt in the neck) he should immediately be laid on his back on a hard surface, with care during this process not to bang or jerk the head. The head should be turned to one side, and a sharp hard blow struck on the bottom part of the breast bone just above the hollow between the lower edges of the rib cage. If no pulse is felt after this, then cardiac massage must be started. If there is only one person present, he should try both cardiac massage and mouth-to-mouth resuscitation at about ten beats to one breath.

Cardiac massage is accomplished by the masseur kneeling by the side of the patient with both arms fully extended placing the heel of one hand on top of the other on the lower left hand side of the breast bone and then putting his full weight on his extended arms at a rate of 70 to 100 beats per minute. This pushes down the breast bone and compresses the heart, forcing blood from it into the general circulation. If two people are present one can feel for a pulse in the root of the neck and, if this is felt, the massage is effective. If not, the hands should be moved to a position in which pressure produces a pulse. The other person should also be inflating the lungs of the patient by mouth-to-mouth breathing. See ARTIFICIAL RESPIRATION.

Such measures should be continued until the patient's pulse is felt and he begins to breathe. Should he become pulseless again, the same procedures must be resumed. If the patient fails to respond after twenty-five minutes there is little likelihood that he will revive.

Prevention. One of the basic steps in the production of atherosclerosis is the deposition of cholesterol. Measures to diminish the level of cholesterol in the blood of the population (e.g., by reduction of animal fat eaten) may be tried, but are not easy because they demand substantial changes in dietary habits and because some people with different metabolisms can keep blood cholesterol low in spite of a high fat intake. Nevertheless, raised blood levels of cholesterol and other fatty compounds indicate a predisposition to heart disease, and these levels can be lowered by diet and certain drugs.

Diets that diminish blood cholesterol and fat levels are those which are low in animal fats and high in unsaturated vegetable oils. Their value in the prevention of heart disease is still arguable though studies indicate that the frequency of ischaemic heart disease is diminished in groups on such diets. It is of course essential to ensure that a person on such a diet receives sufficient quantities of the fat-soluble vitamins.

Smoking, particularly in the younger age groups, is associated with an increased likelihood of heart disease, so abstaining from smoking should diminish the chance of a heart attack.

The incidence of heart disease is higher in districts with a soft water supply than those with harder water but the nature of the link between hardness of water and freedom from thrombosis is not yet established.

High blood pressure and obesity are associated with many increased health risks. As obesity may be an indicator of indolence and consumption of atheroma-causing foodstuffs it would seem logical to recommend that weight loss be suggested to the overweight, while the control of high blood pressure certainly reduces the likelihood of strokes (which arise from diseased blood vessels in the brain) and may have a similar influence on the coronary vessels.

It seems likely that lack of exercise predisposes to coronary thrombosis, and the taking of exercise by the customarily sedentary is to be encouraged. Brief periods of taxing exercise are probably to be preferred to the sustained gentle sort such as is provided by jogging, etc., but should not be undertaken until the flabby subject has been restored to some degree of fitness.

Excessive mental stress plays a big part in causing the disease. It occurs largely in persons working overhard in an effort to secure promotion, or under constant tension through holding jobs beyond their capacities, or suffering from domestic or marital difficulties; features like over-smoking and over-eating are perhaps merely compensatory mechanisms. Preventive measures should include the fostering of good emotional health and personality development in childhood (so that the person becomes able to withstand life's normal stresses) and emphasis on the importance both of healthy exercise and of leisure interests. The early years are also the best time to start prevention of obesity (since fat children become fat adults) and discouragement of cigarette smoking.

To summarize, prevention can be considered under two heads. Long-term prevention, or keeping a healthy heart healthy, involves attention to the whole pattern of living. It includes, for example, measures to foster development of a personality that can cope with normal stresses, to encourage development of eating habits that neither create obesity nor raise the blood cholesterol and to dissuade the taking up of cigarette smoking. More commonly prevention is applied to the person who already has a raised blood pressure or anginal pain on effort. Here it induces attempts to modify stress factors, cultivation of a philosophical attitude to life, reduction of obesity, limitation of animal fat in the diet, curtailing or cessation of smoking, and the giving of appropriate drugs to reduce blood pressure and to decrease the risk of clotting.

corpuscles. The small round cells of the BLOOD.

corrosive. A chemical which destroys the substance of the tissues. Medically, the term is usually applied to a group of poisons which act by burning into the tissue; they may be splashed or spilt upon the body and occasionally they are swallowed – more often by accident than intent because their effects cause intense pain. Strong acids, such as nitric, hydrochloric and sulphuric acid, alkalis, such as caustic soda or potash, and salts, such as mercury chloride or sodium hypochlorite (bleach), are the commonest corrosive substances. Caustic soda is particularly dangerous if it is splashed into the eye. It should immediately be washed out with clean water and medical aid sought. If such substances are swallowed the person should be given liberal amounts of water immediately and egg white in milk if available. He should not be made to vomit and medical attention should be sought at once.

The late result of swallowing corrosives may be severe scarring of the throat and gullet. In view of the damage done to tissues both immediately and in the long term by such substances, prevention is important and eminently possible by the wearing of appropriate goggles or clothing when working with corrosive substances, by storing them only in distinctively marked containers, and above all by making sure that they are inaccessible (particularly to children) when not in use.

cortex. The outer layer or part of an organ. The term is commonly applied to the brain, the kidney and the adrenal gland. In the brain it is applied to the convoluted folds that form the outer part of the brain as distinct from the more central larger concentrations of grey matter. In the kidney the term is applied to the paler outer part of the kidney and similarly in the adrenal gland.

corticosteroids. A group of chemical substances (hormones) produced by the outer part (the cortex) of the adrenal gland. They are liberated on occasions of stress and controlled by ACTH from another of the ENDOCRINE GLANDS, the pituitary. In general, they suppress inflammatory response and reduce allergy: they also increase resistance to stress and affect the state of the mind.

Some corticosteroids have an effect on the excretion of salt by the kidney and can be produced in excess in such conditions as tumours of the adrenal gland. Yet others affect the sexual characteristics and if they become unbalanced they can lead to virilization of women with the appearance of beards and deepening of the voice, while others can cause the reverse process in men with the appearance of breasts and loss of facial and body hair.

Besides being necessary as replacement therapy in Addison's disease, they are used in the treatment of some inflammatory diseases such as rheumatoid arthritis and the collagen diseases; in acute allergic states such as asthma, drug reactions and serum sensitivity; in some skin disease, leukaemia and other blood disorders, Hodgkin's disease, ulcerative colitis, and acute gout. Their effect is also of value in organ-transplantation, in that they suppress the response of the body to foreign tissue.

Cortisone. This corticosteroid and its derivatives are powerful drugs and prescribing them involves risks which must be taken into account when deciding on their use. Their many unwelcome side-effects include decreased resistance to infection which may reactivate old disease (e.g., tuberculosis); osteoporosis; other tissue changes which may aggravate peptic ulceration; retention of water and sodium with weight-gain and hypertension; changes in fat deposits in the body with development of 'moon-face' and 'buffalo-hump'; mental changes; and sex-hormone effects such as the appearance of facial hair in women, acne, loss of sexual desire and cessation of menstruation. They also weaken natural adrenal gland activity so that treatment once established can only safely be withdrawn very gradually.

In carefully-selected conditions, corticosteroids are undoubtedly of great benefit in a variety of distressing and disabling states but prolonged treatment requires that the balance of advantage and disadvantage should be well considered and that patients should be made aware of potential risks. They should also carry Steroid Warning Cards to guard against the risks of sudden withdrawal of treatment in any accidental circumstances.

corticotrophin. See ACTH.

cortisone. See CORTICOSTEROIDS.

coryza. The common COLD.

cough. A sudden noisy expulsion of air from the lungs. Its purpose is protection, to expel any inhaled foreign matter or secretions that are produced in response to infection. A cough that is accompanied by the production of phlegm is achieving this purpose and generally should be encouraged, while one that produces nothing is a dry cough resulting from laryngeal irritation.

Cough is a prominent symptom of any disorder of the lungs, particularly infections such as bronchitis or tuberculosis. The linings of the tubes respond to infection by increased production of mucus which is swept upwards from the smallest bronchial tubes into the windpipe and then into the larynx. Presence of this mucus in the larger tubes, particularly the larynx, stimulates the cough. In this the pressure in the chest is suddenly increased while part of the throat, the glottis, remains closed and then suddenly opens so that air moves very rapidly through the upper part of the airway carrying mucus and other debris with it. Such coughing is desirable in the acute stage of any chest infection.

Any irritation of the larynx can produce coughing. This occurs most commonly with colds and infections of the upper respiratory tract and, of course, smoking. The coughing thus produced is usually of a dry barking nature and, if severe (as can occur in whooping cough), is best suppressed. Suppression of the cough reflex is produced by various drugs such as codeine and morphia. Most proprietary cough mixtures contain such substances or their derivatives in addition to soothing substances that reduce the congestion of inflamed membranes.

The early morning 'smoker's cough' is one of the earliest features of chronic bronchitis and is a sign that the linings of the respiratory passages have been damaged. Smoke irritates the lining cells so that excess mucus is produced. This is not cleared from the tubes during the night because the cough reflex is slightly depressed in sleep. The accumulated mucus is cleared by coughing on awakening, and the frequent repeated coughing may contribute to the degenerative processes that occur in chronic bronchitis.

The plugging of small tubes by mucus causes air to be trapped in the small air sacs (alveoli) of the lung. Coughing increases the pressure inside the chest and because air cannot be expelled from blocked alveoli, they become stretched and the membranes between adjacent alveoli break down, thus making fewer but larger air sacs which are less efficient for the gaseous exchange upon which life depends. See EMPHYSEMA.

counter-irritation. The relief of pain or symptoms in one locality by inducing irritation in another. This was the reasoning behind the application of mustard plasters to the chest in pneumonia: it was believed that the application of such an irritant to the skin would cause congestion there, redirecting the excess blood flow and fluid from the lung to the site of new irritation. Counter-irritants are still in use, particularly as liniments for the relief of muscular pain. However, the massage and the belief in their efficacy are more likely to contribute to symptom relief than the constituents of such an application.

coxalgia. Pain in the hip. Any disturbance of the alignment of the hip joint usually results in pain; the commonest causes are arthritis and fractures of the hip joint, particularly fracture of the neck of the thigh bone or femur.

cracked lips. Painful fissures in the lips as a result of exposure to cold, windy or dry atmospheres. The skin of the lips is very thin and has a plentiful blood supply, so evaporation constantly occurs. There are oil-producing glands in the lips to provide lubrication, but they need to be kept moist as excessive drying causes cracking. Ordinarily licking the lips provides adequate moisture, but in conditions producing rapid evaporation cracking may occur. This is prevented by the application of vaseline or some cosmetic face cream.

cracked nipple. See NIPPLE.

cramp. A painful spasm of the muscles. There are essentially three main varieties.

1. Cramp can arise from excessive loss of salt under conditions of great heat. Ships' stokers, for example, not infrequently suffer from cramp in the calves, arms and abdomen, sometimes accompanied by fall in blood pressure and by vomiting. Treatment consists of rest, plus restoration of salt balance by adequate salt in drinks and soups. Salt tablets, useful in some other conditions, should be avoided here because they are not always absorbed.

2. Bathers' cramp is thought to be due to the effects of cold on the nervous system. Simultaneous immersion of the whole body is said to be less likely to create cramp than is gradually walking into deeper water. Since cramp may, prevent movement of the affected limbs and so cause drowning, sea-bathing, especially in cold weather, should be undertaken only in the company of swimmers who can use life-saving methods if one of them develops cramp, and never immediately after a meal.

3. Ordinary cramp, most frequently occasioned by sitting or lying with pressure on nerves, but occasionally produced by muscular stretching which again puts pressure on nerves. Brisk rubbing of the affected part generally ends the spasm and relieves the pain.

cranial nerves. The twelve pairs of nerves which arise in the BRAIN (in the case of motor fibres conveying impulses outwards) or terminate there (in the case of sensory fibres).

cranium. The part of the skull enclosing the brain.

crepitus. This term has two meanings:

1. The grating sound heard when the broken ends of a bone are moved and scrape on each other. The sound indicates a fracture, but fracture may be present without the sound being audible.

2. The term is also applied – more usually as 'crepitations' – to a bubbling sound heard through a stethoscope when there is moisture in the lungs or respiratory tracts.

cretinism. A condition resulting from under-functioning of the thyroid gland, which is one of the ENDOCRINE glands, before birth or in early infancy. If it remains untreated growth is stunted, the face looks prematurely aged, the skin is thickened and coarse, the hair is scanty, the abdomen is protuberant, development of the sexual organs is delayed and the

victim is mentally retarded. The condition occurs in areas of severe iodine deficiency (with the thyroid gland unable to function properly through lack of iodine) and less frequently as a hereditary disorder. In districts where simple goitre is prevalent, indicating deficiency of iodine, cretinism can often be prevented by administration of iodine during pregnancy.

Where cretinism is diagnosed very early and treatment with thyroxine is instituted to replace the inadequate functioning of the thyroid, the outlook both physically and mentally is very good, but the treatment has to continue for life. Where treatment is not started until the child is 4 or 5 years old much improvement is possible but there is little chance of full recovery from the handicap imposed by several years of faulty skeletal and mental development.

croup. A general name for a harsh, stifling cough and strained, noisy breathing, occurring in children and caused by any inflammation or spasm of the larynx.

cryptorchism. See TESTICLE, UNDESCENDED.

curare. A South American Indian arrow poison extracted from various plants and causing rapid paralysis of muscles. Death from curare poisoning can often be prevented by applying artificial respiration until the effects of the poison wear off.

curettage. Scraping the interior wall of the uterus with a spoonlike instrument called a curette. The operation is performed in three sets of circumstances: (1) along with dilatation of the cervix in women who are having difficulty in conceiving a child; (2) after a miscarriage, to remove any remaining fragments of membrane; and (3) in some cases of chronic inflammation of the uterus.

curvature of the spine. Viewed from the side the spine has four normal curves: (1) the cervical curve in the neck, convex forwards; (2) the thoracic curve, convex backwards; (3) the lumbar curve, convex forwards; and (4) the pelvic curve, convex backwards. The two backward curves are present before birth and are sometimes termed primary curves. The cervical curve develops as the child begins to control movements of the head, and the lumbar curve appears later, as the child begins to walk.

Abnormal curvatures of the backbone may arise as exaggerations of normal curves or by the formation of new curves.

Kyphosis is the term applied to the exaggeration of the thoracic curve known in severe cases as 'hunchback' and in mild cases as 'round shoulders'. It often arises from faulty posture, or from the peering forward associated with bad sight. Disease or injury to the spine (e.g., tuberculosis or fracture dislocation) may also cause it. Treatment varies with the cause.

Lordosis or abnormal 'hollow back' occurs from severe muscle weakness and in congenital dislocation of the hip. Owing to the combined weight of the foetus and of the liquid surrounding it, some temporary normal   kyphosis

lordosis   scoliosis

Curvature of the spine

lordosis occurs in pregnancy. Treatment is not necessary unless symptoms develop.

Scoliosis is sideways or lateral curvature of the spine; there are various types: (1) congenital scoliosis, seen in babies and due to defective vertebral development; (2) rickety scoliosis due to the effects of rickets, in which the bones are softened by vitamin deprivation; (3) compensatory scoliosis due to asymmetry of the legs, usually resulting from disease or injury; (4) paralytic scoliosis from paralysis of the trunk muscles on one side; and (5) postural scoliosis – the commonest type, occurring in children and delicate adolescents from bad posture at desks, sometimes in those who ride side-saddle, and in workers who mostly have to use one leg at their trade.

In the early stages the spine can be seen to straighten when the patient hangs by his arms and at this stage treatment is by exercises and, sometimes, traction, which pulls the spine straight by the use of weights. Later on the curvature of the spine becomes fixed and the person may require a supportive spinal jacket.

cuticle. The epidermis or outer layer of the skin. This layer, which does not contain blood vessels, is thick and horny on the palms and soles but thinner elsewhere. The term is applied more specifically to the layer of skin which grows round the bases of the nails.

cuts. Among domestic accidents serious enough to receive medical treatment cuts rank second only to falls. There is, however, a curious age difference: both cuts and falls are commonest among children, especially children under seven years, but in adults cuts are most frequent before middle age while falls occur mainly in middle-aged or elderly persons.

Treatment. Even where the cut has been created by a clean instrument a break in the skin provides a possible entrance for bacteria and should therefore be taken seriously. In general the wound should be cleansed with warm, boiled water, gently dried, and swabbed with a mild disinfectant (e.g., tincture of iodine), after which a gauze or lint dressing should be firmly bandaged on and left undisturbed for some days. If, however, the wound throbs or surrounding parts become inflamed, indicating that germs have penetrated to the tissues, medical aid should be promptly sought and antibiotics given.

cyanides. The salts of prussic acid, the most rapidly acting of all poisons. They are used in industry and for fumigation. The inhaled fumes of prussic acid kill almost instantaneously, while swallowed cyanides kill within minutes. In cases of poisoning an emetic should be given to induce vomiting, artificial respiration applied and medical aid summoned at once. A victim who survives for the first half hour is likely to recover.

cyanocobalamine. The chemical name for VITAMIN B$_{12}$.

cyanosis. The bluish coloration of the skin which arises from inadequate oxygenation of the blood. It may be due to insufficient intake of oxygen from the lungs (as in pneumonia or suffocation) or to stagnation or inadequate circulation of the blood (as in various diseases of the heart). Localized cyanosis of the lips occurs in debilitated and rheumatic persons in cold weather, and localized cyanosis of the fingers occurs in Raynaud's disease.

Treatment depends on the cause, and in addition the administration of oxygen is usually necessary in severe cases.

cyst. An abnormal swelling containing fluid. Cysts are found most frequently in the skin (usually from blocked sweat glands) and in the ovaries (in which they may grow to enormous sizes unless removed).

cystic fibrosis. A very serious hereditary condition (alternatively called fibrocystic disease of the pancreas) characterized by pathological changes in the pancreas, lungs, intestines and most mucus-secreting glands. The disease is inherited as a Mendelian recessive which means, in GENETIC terms, that both parents carry the genes but do not show signs of the disease.

Clinical features which appear in the early weeks of life include failure to thrive (because of absence of pancreatic juices to digest food), distended abdomen (a characteristic of all forms of malnutrition), diarrhoea with offensive stools (from failure to digest fat) and a cough which often heralds bronchopneumonia. Diagnosis may be confirmed by examination of stools for fat and absence of pancreatic juices, or by examination of sweat for increased salt content.

A high protein diet with vitamin supplements is useful; pancreatic extract may partially replace the absent hormones; extra salt is required because of the high salt loss; and antibiotics are needed for the respiratory condition. Despite treatment a high proportion of patients die.

cystitis. Inflammation of the bladder, usually due to bacterial infection. The condition is commoner in women because of their shorter urethras, but also occurs in men, especially where enlargement of the prostate causes narrowing of the urethra and some retention of urine. Symptoms include pain in the lower abdomen, frequency of urination and a scalding sensation on passing urine. Treatment includes rest, mild alkalis especially sodium citrate, and usually sulphonamides or antibiotics.

Occasionally an acute attack which has been inadequately treated passes into a chronic cystitis with persisting frequency of urination, feeling of weight in the lower abdomen and a danger of the infection ascending to the kidneys. Treatment depends on the particular germ concerned.

cystoscope. An instrument for viewing the interior of the bladder. It consists of a narrow tube containing a sort of telescope, with an electric light at the end and an appropriate mirror in which the highly illuminated bladder surface is reflected.

D

dactylitis. Inflammation of a finger or toe.

dandruff. A scaly condition of the scalp in which small flakes of dead skin form and are shed. See HAIR.

dangerous drugs. In ordinary speech the term is generally used for the so-called 'hard' drugs, i.e., those that are definitely liable to lead to addiction, in particular (1) morphia, (2) some of its derivatives, such as heroin, and (3) cocaine.

Legally, however, dangerous drugs are those specified by legislation in a particular country. In the U.K. a Dangerous Drugs Act includes various drugs other than those mentioned above, e.g., Indian hemp (cannabis); it also restricts possession of these drugs to certain 'authorized persons' such as medical practitioners; requires that the drugs be kept under lock and key with an exact record maintained of their use; and specifies requirements for medical prescriptions containing these drugs. See DRUGS and ADDICTION.

day dreaming. A form of thinking in which free rein is given to the imagination. Day dreaming is unrelated to constructive planning and is essentially the elaboration of fantasies, often of a wish fulfilment nature, with the dreamer as hero or, less often, as suffering martyr. Fantasy life is strong in most young children, dwindles in older children and increases again in adolescence before reducing once more during the twenties. Excessive day dreaming sometimes indicates the beginning of withdrawal from the problems of real life, as in early schizophrenia.

day hospital. An institution which provides treatment for patients who are able to live at home. It is differentiated from an out patients clinic by the fact that the patient attends for a substantial part of each day. The service varies, according to the type of patient, from active medical treatment, often including physiotherapy and occupational therapy, to merely providing a meeting place for persons with chronic disease.

As contrasted with care in the patient's own home, a day hospital gives a period of relief to overburdened relatives and can offer treatment facilities not normally available at home. As contrasted with an ordinary hospital, it gives the patient some continuation of home life and saves the cost of night staff.

day nursery. A form of day care for pre-school children. Unlike a nursery school it is open for sufficiently long hours to enable the mother to undertake a full day's work and it has no lower age limit for

acceptance of children. The matron is usually a qualified nurse and there are specified standards of staffing and accommodation.

For unsupported women who have to earn a living, and in times of illness and family stress, nurseries perform a valuable function, and they often improve the nutrition, physical development and habits of children; but for children under 2½ years daily separation from the mother can harm emotional development.

DDT. Diclor-diphenyl-tetrachlorethane. As an insecticide it is harmless to mammals but lethal to mosquitoes, house flies bluebottles, fleas and lice. A 5 per cent spray destroys mosquitoes, house flies and their larvae and the solution if sprayed on walls and windows remains effective for several weeks.

For lice and fleas a 5 per cent DDT dust can be applied from a compression gun, enabling large numbers of people to be disinfected without removing their clothes. This advantage, trivial when one is considering a single infected family, is enormous when a typhus outbreak makes necessary the disinfection of thousands of potentially infected persons.

deaf aids. See HEARING AIDS

deaf mutism. A condition in which a person is unable to hear and therefore has not learned to speak articulately. In most cases the deafness is of hereditary origin although it can also occur through the mother suffering from German measles during early pregnancy or from various conditions occurring soon after birth. If a baby does not respond to sounds within the first three months the advice of a doctor or health visitor should be sought, because there may be some disease of the ear which can be corrected with treatment.

Hereditary deafness on the other hand is incurable, but the child should be sent to a special school where he will be taught to speak by lip reading and by the sense of touch. Training a completely deaf child to speak sufficiently clearly to convey his meaning is an arduous task but the results are worthwhile.

deafness. Complete or partial absence of hearing can result from any impairment of the chain of communication from the outer EAR to the brain.

1. Outer ear. The skin of the outer ear secretes wax from modified sweat glands. Entry of water during washing causes the wax to swell, blocking the passage, and this is by far the commonest cause of temporary deafness. It is easily cured: the wax should be softened by inserting a few

drops of oil and, a day later, gently syringed out.

2. Middle ear. (1) Infection (otitis media) causes deafness and usually earache. Most cases respond to suitable antibiotics. (2) Inflammation of the Eustachian tube, which often occurs in conditions like the common cold, disturbs the middle ear and may cause temporary diminution of hearing. (3) Blockage of the Eustachian tubes by large adenoids may have a similar but more lasting effect. Treatment consists of surgical removal of the adenoids. (4) Otosclerosis, or formation of excess bone in the middle ear, ultimately creates complete deafness. It is a condition of unknown cause, tending to occur in relatively young adults; surgical reconstruction – the operation of fenestration – is often highly successful.

3. Inner ear and auditory nerve. (1) The commonest cause of deafness from birth is a hereditary defect, causing DEAF MUTISM. (2) Maternal rubella (German measles) and possibly other virus diseases during pregnancy can also cause deafness from birth. (3) Continual exposure to loud noise, as in the case of boilermakers and riveters, damages the auditory nerve. (4) Various poisons and drugs can affect the nerve. (5) As life advances the efficiency of the nerve decreases.

In general disorders of the outer and middle ear can be successfully treated while disorders of the inner ear and nerve are as yet incurable. Where deafness is incurable the patient may be given a HEARING AID, but in nerve deafness it may be ineffective.

Deafness in children. Suspected cases are normally tested with a pure tone audiometer which emits a note of any chosen frequency (pitch) and volume (loudness), so that the child's ability to hear high and low notes can be ascertained; this investigation is generally undertaken by an audiologist. For educational purposes children with defective hearing are placed in three groups: (1) those with deafness so slight that it need merely be kept under observation but will not interfere with their education; (2) those who need special facilities (ranging from special places in class to hearing aids and special classes) but can be taught as hearing children; and (3) those whose hearing is so defective that they must be educated as deaf children, e.g., by lip reading.

Impaired hearing in the elderly. Insensitivity to high notes is the main symptom. This increasing loss of sensitivity is for the most part a normal process: children can hear the high-pitched cry of a bat, but few people over 25 years can hear it. Many elderly people can hear low-pitched voices but have difficulty with high-pitched voices and particular difficulty in distinguishing consonants which are higher pitched than most vowels.

The handicap of deafness. It is often said that to be deaf from birth is a greater handicap than to be blind, but that in later life loss of hearing is perhaps less serious than loss of sight. Both are obviously grave disabilities. Yet hearing and sighted people tend to react differently to the two handicaps: the blind man is offered sympathy, understanding and help; the deaf man is too often the subject of ridicule, and becomes isolated socially because of the comparative difficulty of communicating with him.

death. If we defer for later consideration the rare cases in which the circulation of the blood is maintained through the use of an artificial respirator, death can be defined as the process which takes place when the circulation finally ceases and breathing stops. Breathing alone may cease for a number of minutes and be restored by artificial respiration. Cessation of heart action may arise during anaesthesia and in other circumstances but cardiac action can often be restored by massaging the heart. However, the outside limit for cessation of circulation is about four minutes. Any longer interruption of the circulation usually leads to irreparable damage of the brain.

Death can be ascertained by listening for the heart beat (or seeking to feel the pulse) and by holding a mirror over the mouth and nostrils and noting whether it becomes hazy with exhaled breath.

Under normal climatic circumstances the body cools at a definite rate after death, and this enables the time of death to be ascertained with some precision. Rigidity of the muscles (rigor mortis) sets in within a few hours while bruise-like marks on the parts lying lowest and post mortem lividity set in later. If the time of the last meal is known, a study of the degree of digestion of the food in the stomach also provides useful information about the time of death.

In recent years, however, problems have arisen that involve not simply the hour of death but the minute. The first of these problems relates to the transplant of organs. If one patient is likely to die soon unless he receives a transplant of an organ (e.g., heart) to replace his damaged one, and if another patient who is willing to act as a donor in the event of his death is dying (e.g., from a traffic accident), it is clearly vital for the well-being and even the life of the intended recipient that the organ be removed and the transplant started as soon after the death of the other patient as is practicable; but the idea of over-early presumption of death of the donor is ethically completely repugnant. In general, however, the donor is in hospital and under observation when death occurs, and it is possible to begin the transplant only minutes after death has taken place.

The second problem concerns patients whose circulation has been maintained by the use of a mechanical respirator. In the ordinary case, where a person dies at home or in the street or in hospital without a respirator in position, no problem arises: even if a respirator were immediately available it takes a little time to connect it up and start it, and as indicated above death is absolute within four minutes of the cessation of circulation. A problem can arise, however, with a patient who has been linked to a mechanical respirator because of failing circulation. If the patient's own circulation fails to recover, the circulation can be maintained artifically for hours or even days after the brain has become permanently inactive, and there exist a full range of neurological tests to establish whether the brain has ceased to have any activity. From a strictly medical aspect, although the use of the respirator may be continued for a few additional hours for absolute certainty, there is no point in continuing artificial circulation after the brain has become permanently inactive. There is, however, an unsolved legal problem: if a person is attacked and almost killed, is taken to hospital, has failing circulation maintained by a respirator, fails to recover, and finally has the respirator disconnected after indications of brain death, can the death be deemed murder or can it be argued – on the old definition of death occurring with cessation of blood circulation – that the immediate cause of death was the switching off of the respirator? No court decision has yet been given, but most lawyers hold that death in such circumstances would be regarded as murder, the disconnecting of the respirator being merely a recognition that death had occurred.

death certificate. A document, stating the cause of death and giving various other particulars, required before burial or cremation, and of which a copy is often required for the claiming of life insurance or the claiming of death grants and pensions for dependants. The document is completed by the physician who attended the patient in his last illness and saw him after death and is passed, usually by the undertaker, to the registrar of births, deaths and marriages.

Where no doctor has been attending during the final illness, or where the doctor is uncertain of the cause of death, the doctor who certifies that death has occurred has to comply with certain legal requirements (e.g., notification of the coroner in England and Wales) and in circumstances of suspicion or uncertainty a post mortem examination may be ordered.

debility. A vague term used popularly to describe a low state of health, a lack of vitality and an inability to withstand the normal stresses and demands of life.

decompression disease. A condition, characterized mainly by pains in the limbs and sometimes by changes in bones and joints, caused by excessive retention of nitrogen in the blood as a result of over rapid return to normal atmospheric pressure after breathing under high pressure. It occurs therefore in diving tunnel construction, and anywhere a caisson or diving bell is used, and is alternatively called the bends or caisson disease.

The severity of symptoms varies with the working pressure, the length of exposure, and the rapidity of return to normal pressure. Effects are due to the fact that the nitrogen in air is soluble in the fluids and tissues of the body, and especially in the fat. This solubility varies directly with the pressure and, when pressure is released, nitrogen bubbles form in the tissues. These bubbles are most liable to occur in the white matter of the nervous system, causing paralysis, and in the joints to produce pain and disability.

The condition can be avoided completely by slow decompression, and approved diving technique provides a code of rules specifying the stages and pauses necessary in raising a diver from various depths after various times of exposure. When cases actually occur through carelessness or accident, the victims must be immediately re-compressed and then decompressed slowly in accordance with the code of practice.

defective vision. See EYESIGHT.

defence mechanism. Measures adopted unconsciously as a protection against an emotionally painful subject. For example a father unwilling to face the fact that his child is mentally subnormal may react by refusing to use the offered diagnostic services or by expressing hostility to doctors and nurses; in so acting he is behaving quite honestly because his conscious mind does not appreciate that he is unwilling to accept a diagnosis of mental handicap.

deficiency diseases. Strictly, a deficiency disease is an illness arising from prolonged inadequacy of any essential constituent of the DIET, e.g., shortage of first class protein, calcium or iodine. Increasingly, however, the term is becoming restricted to illnesses occasioned by the diet containing less than the required minimum of one of the VITAMINS, while more general deficiency is termed MALNUTRITION.

The main deficiency diseases are:
1. From inadequacy of fat-soluble vitamin A. Night blindness, xerophthalmia, hyperkeratosis (a thickening of the outer lining of the respiratory system and of the skin), and perhaps cancer.
2. From inadequacy of fat-soluble vitamin D (in the absence of enough sunshine to synthesize the vitamin). Rickets in the growing child, and osteomalacia in adults, especially pregnant women.
3. From inadequacy of fat-soluble vitamin E. Sterility, proved in rats fed on a deficient diet but not definitely established in humans.

4. From inadequacy of fat-soluble vitamin κ. Spontaneous haemorrhage, a result of low prothrombin content of the blood; haemorrhagic disease of the newborn.

5. From inadequacy of water-soluble vitamin B_1. Beriberi and infantile beriberi.

6. From inadequacy of water-soluble compounds collectively termed vitamin B_2. Pellagra, which is due to deficiency of nicotinic acid (sometimes called the pellagra-preventing factor), and seborrhoeic dermatitis, especially of the skin of the nose, mouth, scrotum or vulva. This is due to deficiency of riboflavine, but a similar condition can arise from deficiency of pyridoxone, sometimes called vitamin B_6.

7. From inadequacy of water-soluble vitamin B_{12}. Pernicious anaemia, and anaemia following operations to the stomach.

8. From inadequacy of water-soluble vitamin c. Scurvy and infantile scurvy, which broadly resembles the adult form.

9. From inadequacy of water-soluble vitamin p (if indeed this exists separately from vitamin c). Spontaneous haemorrhages and delayed healing of wounds.

10. Certain other conditions, e.g., failure of a child to grow and increased susceptibility to infections, are associated with deficiencies of almost any of the vitamins, with A and c perhaps most heavily involved.

All the diseases mentioned above are preventable by an adequate and properly balanced diet, and, unless identified in terminal phases or after irreversible damage has occurred, can be cured by administration of the appropriate vitamin. However, overdosage of vitamins A, B_1 and D can occur, and some vitamins are effective only in the presence of adequate quantities of other substances.

Deficiency diseases are still very prevalent in underdeveloped countries. In highly developed countries they were until fairly recently second only to infections as causes of illness, and their virtual eradication is one of the greatest triumphs of the preventive services. The conditions should still be looked for in the very young, the very old, the very poor and persons with unusual dietetic habits.

deformities. By far the commonest deformities are those present at birth which are inherited. Examples include – hare lip, cleft palate, spina bifida (unclosed spinal canal), imperfect genital organs, club foot and dislocation of the hip. Prevention in these circumstances is largely a matter of studying the GENETICS of a family with a deformed child to assess the chance of that particular couple producing another. After this assessment the decision must rest with the parents.

Other deformities present at birth are due to illness or some other abnormal condition of the mother during pregnancy. A seriously malnourished mother has an increased chance of producing a deformed child, as has a mother suffering from various diseases. Prevention of this group of deformities is normally possible with adequate antenatal care.

Yet a third group of deformities present at birth are caused by the taking of drugs which affect the foetus. Thalidomide, an apparently harmless tranquillizer, previously tested on animals and human volunteers (not including expectant mothers) was widely used in several countries and resulted in the birth of babies with absent or shortened arms or legs.

Because of the frequency of deformities present at birth, every baby should be carefully examined during the first weeks of life, so that corrective treatment can be started where necessary.

There is absolutely no truth in the common superstition that deformities which arise before birth are the result of the mother suffering from some emotional shock or seeing some distressing sight.

Deformities arising subsequent to birth are the result of diseases or injuries of bones, joints or nerves, e.g., those occasioned by the faulty union of broken bones that have been badly set, or the knock knees, bowed legs, deformed chest and narrowed pelvis associated with rickets, or the round shoulders associated with persistent bad posture.

dehydration. Depletion of WATER arising from inadequate replacement of fluid loss from the body.

In temperate climates adults excrete about 3 litres (5 pints) of water daily, in urine, breath, perspiration and faeces; and a considerable amount of salt is lost along with the water. In warm climates the loss of water and salt is correspondingly greater. Since the body fluids and tissues consist largely of water, the body needs an equivalent intake, including of course the water contained in food, e.g., potatoes are slightly more than one-half water.

Dehydration occurs (1) in persons deprived of adequate fresh-water intake, as when stranded in a desert or adrift at sea; (2) in conditions associated with prolonged and profuse perspiration not balanced by water intake, e.g., various fevers (especially if the victim is unable to drink) and working in very hot weather with water not readily available; and (3) in conditions associated with excessive urination (e.g., after large doses of diuretics), excessive passing of watery motions (e.g., cholera and dysentery) and occasionally excessive vomiting.

The symptoms include extreme thirst, fatigue, giddiness and ultimately delirium, coma, and death.

The remedy where available is obvious – adequate intake of water and (especially in cases associated with heavy perspiration) of salt: most forms of heat exhaustion are more the result of salt deficiency than of water deficiency.

Persons with high temperatures should be given ample cool drinks of water, fruit juice and other liquids. If the patient can eat solid food the necessary salt may be more acceptable when sprinkled on food than if added to drinks.

Where there are symptoms of dehydration and the patient is unable to drink, the injection of sterile water by a doctor or nurse may well save his life, and if there is any possibility of salt depletion as well as water depletion the injected fluid should contain a teaspoonful of salt per tumblerful of water.

déjà vu. Literally 'already seen'. The technical term for the feeling that one has already experienced a situation identical with the present one. The phenomenon is common and its explanation is disputed. One theory is that the two eyes on occasion focus separately, so that impulses from the second eye seem familiar to the brain when they reach it.

delinquency. Although often loosely applied to youthful aberrations in general, delinquency is strictly conduct in a person between the ages of 8 and 17 years that is so at variance with the accepted pattern that the offender has been dealt with by a court.

Useful information for investigating the causes and prevention of delinquency is very hard to obtain – because delinquency is a legal rather than a scientific term and has no precise and uniform definition, because standards of unacceptable conduct change from time to time and vary from place to place, because offenders who are brought to court and thereafter classed as delinquents are only such of the offenders as are caught, and because most classifications of delinquents relate only to the type of offence.

On the whole, delinquents tend to come from large rather than small families; many of them are from broken homes or affectionless homes with parents of a cold, punitive type; they are largely – but by no means wholly – from the lower and more impoverished socio-economic classes; they often have histories of truancy and bad reputations at school; and often other members of their families have been in trouble with the law.

One classification is into delinquency of gradual or sudden onset. In the former group (numerically by far the larger) personality or behaviour difficulties have appeared from the toddler stage; the child has been troublesome and naughty at home and in school; the difficulties have increased as he becomes older; and he steadily becomes more offensive to the community. This type can be subdivided into four subtypes, although in some measure these types overlap.

1. Predatory, i.e., aggressive and acquisitive, stealing or destroying. Possible causal factors include poor home conditions, parental neglect or indifference, lack of moral training and

lack of opportunity for wholesome recreation.

2. Neurotic, e.g., the girl who commits sexual offences through an inordinate desire for affection. Possible causal factors include a broken home, a lack of affection at home, parental disharmony, and over-strictness and domination at home and school.

3. Inadequate personality. The child becomes delinquent essentially because he cannot do even reasonably well either in school subjects or in games. All the causes mentioned in (1) and (2) above may operate, but an additional cause is over-ambitious parents who are never satisfied with the child's achievement.

4. Psychotic type, which is very rare.

Secondly (and much less commonly) there is delinquency of sudden onset, the previously 'good' child who kicks over the traces in adolescence. Here again it is possible to divide into subtypes.

1. Genuine delinquency. This is caused sometimes by over-strict discipline and repression. Instead of external discipline being gradually replaced by self-discipline, the child has to conform too closely to over-strict rules for too long, and finally reacts against dominating parents or teachers by 'sowing his wild oats'. Or it may be the result of over-forcing: the child finds that he cannot measure up to the standards expected, he becomes frustrated, feels a failure and uses delinquency as an outlet. Again this sudden, genuine delinquency may be the result of boredom at school, in the child who is much brighter or much duller than his classmates.

2. Apparent delinquency. Here the endocrine imbalance at adolescence, increased freedom and lack of maturity may combine to produce an apparent delinquency which is simply an exaggeration of normal high spirits.

In most cases of delinquency over-strict or affectionless or over-ambitious or bickering or separated parents are probably the main cause, though economic and environmental factors also play a part.

delirium. A disturbance of the brain, occasioned by injury, fever or poisoning, and characterized by incoherent talk, confusion, delusions and poorly regulated muscular actions.

delirium tremens. A disordered state of mind, usually including terrifying hallucinations, affecting heavy drinkers and occurring mostly after an unusually heavy bout of drinking or after injury or sudden illness following heavy intake of alcohol. Symptoms include hallucinations of the eyes (e.g., pink elephants) and of the skin (e.g., sensations of snakes or spiders crawling over it), intense anxiety and fear, restlessness and complete sleeplessness. Although recovery is usual, in about one case in twenty the condition is fatal. Immediate treatment consists of rest in bed (not always easily accepted by the patient) and the giving of adequate fluids with addition of glucose and vitamin B₁. Subsequent treatment is that of ALCOHOLISM.

deltoid. The larger triangular muscle covering the shoulder. The apex of the triangle is on the outer side of the humerus, and the base is a broad attachment to the clavicle and scapula. The deltoid is the main muscle used in raising the arm sideways.

delusion. An unshakeable false belief. It is easy to define a delusion as a belief that continues when logic and experience have proved it false, but there is no clear demarcation between mild delusion and simple error. For example, a man whose employer repeatedly passes him without a greeting has the delusion that the employer dislikes him, whereas the employer may really be short-sighted or preoccupied.

Most delusions are harmless unless they render a person's conduct antisocial, but some delusions are dangerous. Thus a sufferer from paranoia who thinks he is being persecuted may decide to kill some of his persecuters. In paranoia such delusions of persecution are common, in schizophrenia the victim tends to live in an unreal dream world and in some forms of psychoses delusions of grandeur occur. Delusions, like HALLUCINATIONS, can occur in mentally normal people who are exhausted or under great emotional strain.

dementia. Serious disorder of mental capacity, usually accompanied by disturbances in emotion and behaviour. In most cases the onset is gradual, with recently acquired memories soonest lost, decreasing ability to reason and to judge, and increasing display of emotion over trivial matters.

Senile or pre-senile dementia – a tendency to become dotards in old age – is in part familial (seen in successive generations of a family) in part occasioned by sudden stresses (like death of a spouse or loss of occupation) and in part due to arteriosclerosis and insufficient blood supply to the brain.

Dementia of cerebral arterial disease, mainly due to arteriosclerosis of the blood vessels of the brain, is very similar, as is the dementia of cerebral syphilis (dementia paralytica) and the dementia sometimes found in cases of cerebral tumour.

A person suffering from dementia needs help. Complete cure is rare, but tranquillizers and other drugs can do much to lessen the symptoms and to improve the patient's sense of well-being. Occupational therapy can also be useful. Where the sufferer is treated at home his relatives have to cultivate patience and tolerance of irrational behaviour and emotional outbursts; but it has to be remembered that the necessity to exercise continuing understanding, tolerance and patience for months or years under the relatives under considerable mental strain.

dengue fever. A tropical disease caused by a virus transmitted by a mosquito.

dental caries. Tooth decay, the commonest disease of highly developed countries and the main cause of toothache. See TEETH.

dentine. The hard, enamel-like exterior surface of the teeth.

dentist. A practitioner of the science of preventing and treating diseases of the teeth. Dental surgeon is an alternative or synonymous term.

Dentistry is now a full profession, completely separate from medicine, and with its own specialists, such as those in orthodontics (correction of deformities of the teeth). Cooperation between doctors and dentists is already very good, but perhaps the next big advance in dentistry will be emphasis on its hitherto neglected preventive aspects, involving collaboration between dentists on the one hand and health education officers and health visitors on the other.

dentition. The kind, number and arrangement of TEETH. See also DEVELOPMENT.

dentures. Artificial or false teeth may be partial, replacing only a number of teeth, or complete, replacing all the teeth in a jaw. Their provision is essential to allow a person who has lost teeth to chew properly, and they also prevent the face of such a person from developing a sunk-in appearance.

After dentures have been inserted soft foods may have to be eaten for a couple of days until the patient becomes used to the dentures. A return visit to the dentist is often necessary as false teeth may press at one or two places and require adjustment. It is important to wear the dentures on the day before visiting the dentist, so that he can see the reddened areas and thus identify the exact points of pressure. Speech may be slightly indistinct for the first two or three days after starting to wear dentures.

The care of artificial teeth includes rinsing or brushing them after meals and placing them overnight in water containing salt or denture cleaner.

deodorants. Chemical substances which remove or mitigate objectionable smells. Some, such as eucalyptus, oil of cloves or turpentine simply mask the unpleasant odour. Others, such as hydrogen peroxide and potassium permanganate act by giving up oxygen, converting objectionable substances into acceptable ones. Some deodorants such as carbolic acid and creosote are also disinfectants and are used to purify water closets, drains, etc. In general the best method of removing body odour is frequent use of soap and water.

deoxyribonucleic acid. Commonly referred to as DNA; see CELL.

depilation. Removal of superfluous hair from the body. Various chemicals are quite effective (e.g., a barium sulphide paste, containing one part barium sulphide, three parts zinc oxide and four parts starch), but the hair grows again in a few weeks. Electrolysis, or destruction of the hair root by electricity, is more permanently effective, but it is a slow and expensive process.

depression. A lowering of spirits greater in duration and in degree than one would expect in the particular person under the circumstances present. Ordinary grief and mental suffering after bereavement is not depression, nor is the subdued mood of the person of a normally melancholy temperament. Again, we all have fluctuations of mood, and to be dejected for a day without obvious cause is not depression. Depression as an illness implies a considerable and persisting change of mood, out of all proportion to the factors that may have triggered it off.

A depressed person has a bleak and pessimistic attitude to the future, is uninterested in activities that he previously enjoyed, often complains of various physical symptoms for which no organic cause can be found, and may either lose interest in food or compulsively over-eat. In extreme cases suicide may be attempted.

Depression occurs most commonly at critical or unsettled periods of life – in adolescence, after childbirth, at the menopause or at retirement from work. It is also common, but usually fairly transient, after certain illnesses such as severe influenza.

Simple reassurance and exhortation are useless: a depressed person can no more 'pull himself together' than can a person with a hormone deficiency produce more of the hormone. Psychotherapy (to bring difficulties below the level of consciousness to the conscious understanding so that the patient can deal with them) and electric shock therapy are both sometimes used, but have largely been replaced by drugs called monoamine-oxidase inhibitors. These destroy the enzyme monoamine-oxidase, which if produced in excess causes depression.

dermal. Pertaining to the deeper layer of the skin, as contrasted with 'cutaneous' which refers to the superficial layer.

dermatitis. Alternatively known as eczema, this is an inflammation of the skin. It may occur in any part of the body, and takes the form of reddening of skin, the development of blisters and, if the condition becomes chronic, a thickening of the skin. External irritants are a common cause. Workers in certain trades – gardeners, bakers, french polishers and others who handle potentially irritating substances – often suffer from dermatitis on exposed parts of the body; but many people handle these substances without ill-effect, and in affected people the dermatitis often persists long after contact with the irritant has ceased. In other words, dermatitis depends on the existence both of an internal factor leading to the sensitivity and of contact with an irritant.

There is also probably a strong emotional factor.

Local treatment consists mainly of the application of soothing ointments. General treatment involves either separation of the person from the irritant or an attempt at desensitization by gradually increasing injections of the offending irritant.

The term dermatitis probably covers several diseases that are not yet clearly differentiated but that are mostly related to ALLERGY.

dermographia. See SKIN WRITING.

desquamation. The shedding of superficial layers of the skin. This may occur after some local injury such as sunburn or in the healing of a slight burn from other causes.

The skin rashes which occur in a variety of infective fevers or as a result of sensitivity to certain drugs are an indication of general toxic damage to the skin which eventually sheds its injured cells either in a powdery fashion or as large flakes.

The desquamation which follows scarlet fever is a particularly well known example of this.

Desquamation is also the principal feature of the primary skin disease pityriasis or dermatitis exfoliativa.

development. Human development begins when a female germ-cell or ovum is fertilized by a male germ-cell or spermatozoon and proceeds by stages until the full adult status is achieved. The first 40 weeks of this progression are the period of intra-uterine development during which the fertilized ovum gradually grows from a single cell no more than 0.1 mm. in diameter to the fully-formed infant with an average length of 50 cm. (20 in.) and an average weight of 3.4 kg. (7.5 lb.).

At birth. The infant has the appearance of a miniature adult but its head is relatively larger than in the adult and the face (owing to the small size of the jaws, nasal cavity and air sinuses) forms only one-eighth of the size of the head compared with one-half in maturity. Its abdomen is also relatively larger because of the increased relative size of the liver. Its skeleton is also different since most of its 'bones' are still mainly cartilaginous, the skull bones in particular are only partially ossified and are incompletely joined together so that gaps may be felt in the skull. These gaps are known as fontanelles and the largest is the anterior fontanelle easily located in the centre or the crown of the head. It gradually diminishes in size and will generally be completely closed by 18 months.

Physical growth. The child continues to grow and to increase in size and weight from birth until about 18 years of age but the progress is not uniform. Broadly a child reaches a weight of 9 to 11 kg. (20 to 24 lbs.) by 1 year, doubles that weight by 5 years and then increases by 1.5 to 2.5 kg. (4 to 6 lb.) each year until the growth spurt at around 11 years in girls and 12 years in boys, with larger increases for the next few years. Ideally an adult should neither gain nor lose weight after the age of about 25 years, although most of us gain a little in middle age. See HEIGHT AND WEIGHT.

Tables of heights and weights of children are much used but of fairly limited value. Firstly, the tables represent averages, not optimum weights: in the first half of this century malnutrition was common in Britain so that tables of average weights were distorted by considerable numbers of undernourished children.

Secondly, a table of average heights and weights must show three variables, not two, with the third variable – age – acquiring increasing importance as the child grows older; thus we can perhaps say that an average child of either sex measuring 106 cm. (42 in.) weighs around 19 kg. (42 lb.) irrespective of whether he or she is a fairly tall child of 5 years or a small child of 7 years; but while tall girls of 7 years measuring 134 cm. (53 in.) might average 30.3 kg. (67 lb.), small girls of 12 years measuring the same 134 cm. would average about 32.6 kg. (72 lb.). The average weights of 11 year old and 17 year old girls both of 152 cm. (60 in.) show a still more marked difference, the younger child weighing 45 kg. (100 lb.) while the older child is 4.5 kg. (10 lb.) heavier.

Average weights, even when adjusted for height and age, have little meaning when one is considering an individual child: the big-boned son of large parents may be both taller and heavier than the average and yet be undernourished; and the child of small frame and slender bones may be adequately nourished although below the normal for his age and height. The important question is not how the child compares with a rather artificial average, but how he compares with his past performance. Is his weight gain balancing his height increase, or too little, or too much?

Dentition. Two sets of teeth are developed during growth. The first, temporary, or milk teeth totalling twenty, appear as follows:

2 lower central incisors
      6 to 8 months
4 upper incisors
      8 to 10 months
2 lower lateral incisors
      12 to 14 months
2 upper front molars
      12 to 14 months
2 lower front molars
      12 to 14 months
4 canines
      18 to 20 months
4 posterior molars
      2 years to 2½ years

These times are subject to considerable variation. The temporary teeth are then followed by the permanent dentition (32 teeth).

4 first molars	6 years
4 central incisors	7 years
4 lateral incisors	8 years
4 anterior pre-molars	9 years
4 posterior pre-molars	10 years
4 canines	11 to 12 years
4 second molars	12 to 15 years
4 third molars	17 to 25 years

Puberty and sexual development. Puberty is the age at which reproductive organs begin to become functionally active and ushers in the period of adolescence.

In girls this may be between 10 and 14 years of age but extremes in either direction are not unusual. In boys it is slightly later. There is said to be a tendency at present for puberty to occur at earlier ages, the average onset falling by two months every decade. Possibly this is a temporary trend due to better general standards of nutrition.

The changes of puberty are brought about by the fact that the sex glands, the ovaries in girls and the testes in boys, have become mature. The internal secretions which these produce stimulate the development of secondary sex-characteristics. In girls there is pubic hair, breast development and the onset of menstruation; in boys the external sex-organs enlarge, there is growth of body and facial hair, the larynx and vocal cords enlarge and the voice 'breaks'. In both sexes, psychological changes occur. Boys become more aggressive, adventurous and addicted to active pursuits. Girls usually become more appealing and seductive. Both tend to cast off the former associates of their own sex and form friendships with members of the opposite sex.

Mental development. Intellectual capacity depends on a combination of basic inherited intelligence and its enhancement by experience. Mental development during the formative years is therefore influenced to a considerable extent by the opportunities for contact with the realities of the outside world.

At birth an infant responds to external stimuli in a primitive protective fashion by reflex actions. As the functional capacity of his brain develops, external stimuli are received with increasing discrimination of their significance and produce increasingly purposeful and accurate responses. The rate and extent of progress are thus affected very much by the opportunities for gaining experience; see INFANCY, PSYCHOLOGY OF.

In the very young child these are provided by contact with his mother and by being talked to and played with. As he grows he becomes influenced successively by his home surroundings, by his brothers and sisters, by his play with other children and still later by his schools, his teachers and his work and by all the other opportunities which daily life affords.

The progress of the child under 5 years of age is now generally assessed by a

Age (years)	BOYS Height in cm. (in.)	Weight in kg. (lb.)	GIRLS Height in cm. (in.)	Weight in kg. (lb.)
1	73.6 to 76.9 (29.0 to 30.3)	9.5 to 10.8 (20.9 to 23.8)	72.3 to 75.9 (28.5 to 29.9)	9.0 to 10.4 (19.8 to 23.0)
2	85.8 to 89.4 (33.8 to 35.2)	11.9 to 13.5 (26.3 to 29.7)	84.5 to 88.9 (33.3 to 35.0)	11.5 to 13.2 (25.3 to 29.2)
3	93.9 to 98.5 (37.0 to 38.8)	13.7 to 15.6 (30.3 to 34.5)	93.4 to 98.0 (36.8 to 38.6)	13.4 to 15.7 (29.6 to 34.6)
4	100.8 to 106.4 (39.7 to 41.9)	15.4 to 17.7 (34.0 to 39.0)	100.3 to 105.6 (39.5 to 41.6)	15.2 to 18.0 (33.5 to 39.6)
5	107.1 to 113.2 (42.2 to 44.6)	17.5 to 20.5 (38.6 to 45.3)	106.4 to 112.2 (41.9 to 44.2)	17.2 to 20.2 (38.0 to 44.5)
6	114.0 to 120.9 (44.9 to 47.6)	20.1 to 23.6 (44.4 to 52.1)	113.2 to 119.3 (44.6 to 47.0)	19.4 to 22.8 (42.9 to 50.2)
7	120.3 to 127.5 (47.4 to 50.2)	22.5 to 26.6 (49.7 to 58.7)	119.1 to 125.9 (46.9 to 49.6)	21.8 to 25.5 (48.1 to 56.3)
8	126.4 to 134.1 (49.8 to 52.8)	25.1 to 29.7 (55.5 to 65.5)	124.7 to 131.5 (49.1 to 51.8)	24.1 to 28.7 (53.1 to 63.3)
9	131.5 to 139.7 (51.8 to 55.0)	27.7 to 32.7 (61.1 to 72.3)	129.7 to 137.1 (51.1 to 54.0)	26.2 to 32.0 (57.9 to 70.5)
10	136.3 to 144.2 (53.7 to 56.8)	30.0 to 36.1 (66.3 to 79.6)	134.6 to 142.4 (53.0 to 56.1)	28.5 to 35.9 (62.8 to 79.1)
11	140.4 to 149.0 (55.3 to 58.7)	32.5 to 39.5 (71.6 to 87.2)	140.2 to 149.0 (55.2 to 58.7)	31.7 to 40.4 (69.9 to 89.1)
12	145.2 to 153.4 (57.2 to 60.4)	35.2 to 43.5 (77.5 to 96.0)	145.7 to 156.4 (57.4 to 61.6)	35.4 to 44.8 (78.0 to 98.8)
13	149.6 to 160.7 (58.9 to 63.3)	38.0 to 48.9 (83.7 to 107.9)	152.6 to 161.5 (60.1 to 63.6)	40.5 to 50.3 (89.4 to 111.0)
14	156.4 to 168.4 (61.6 to 66.3)	43.3 to 55.8 (95.5 to 123.1)	156.2 to 163.5 (61.5 to 64.4)	45.3 to 54.3 (99.8 to 119.7)
15	162.3 to 172.9 (63.9 to 68.1)	49.0 to 61.2 (108.2 to 135.0)	157.7 to 164.8 (62.1 to 64.9)	47.7 to 56.2 (105.1 to 123.9)
16	167.1 to 176.5 (65.8 to 69.5)	53.9 to 65.5 (118.7 to 144.4)	158.4 to 165.6 (62.4 to 65.2)	49.2 to 57.7 (108.4 to 127.2)

Children – Heights and Weights at Various Ages (Median 50 per cent of
population)

consideration of his success in reaching certain 'milestones' of development. These are based on criteria related to (1) posture and large movements (2) vision and fine movements (3) hearing and speech (4) social behaviour and play.

Basic intelligence can be tested by standard intelligence tests. These permit the determination of an Intelligence Quotient which is calculated as one hundred times the mental age divided by the chronological age.

Full mental development however must aim at something more than mere ability to achieve a respectable score in standard tests of intelligence. The emphasis in modern education is towards the enhancement of creative ability. Learning by rote is no longer sufficient for the demands of modern life, and the stimuli provided by music making, dancing, claywork, picturemaking, constructional equipment and 'projects' are designed to provide the more comprehensive experience which is now required to foster the development of the abilities and competence necessary for success in an increasingly competitive and challenging environment. See also BACKWARDNESS IN CHILDREN.

dextrocardia. An unusual condition, probably always congenital, in which the position of the heart and associated blood vessels is the mirror-image of the normal, so that the heart lies slighty to the right (not the left) of the centre of the chest. As a rule the condition – diagnosed only accidentally on radiological or clinical examination – causes no harmful effects.

diabetes insipidus. A disturbance of the water-balancing mechanism of the body characterized by an enormous output of low specific gravity urine and a correspondingly great thirst for water. 'Insipidus' means 'tasteless' and marks the distinction from the ordinary type of diabetes (d. mellitus) in which the urine contains sugar and tastes sweet.

Diabetes insipidus is due to a deficient secretion of hormones by the posterior lobe of the pituitary, which is one of the ENDOCRINE GLANDS, and requires to be treated by replacement of the deficient hormone either by nasal insufflation or by injection. The treatment continues for life.

diabetes mellitus. An endocrine disease producing chronic disorder in the usage of starches and sugars. The pancreas contains special tissue known as the Islets of Langerhans which are ENDOCRINE GLANDS and produce insulin, which passes straight into the blood stream. An insufficiency of insulin damages the ability of the body to store and utilize glucose so that it remains in the blood (hyperglycaemia) and there is a loss of sugar in the urine (glycosuria). The disease is characterized by thirst, increased urinary output, emaciation and a tendency to coma.

Diabetes is an important disease. Its incidence in the community is increasing and is probably now about 1.5 per cent; about half of the cases go unrecognized until the symptoms become sufficiently noticeable to make the patient seek advice, often because of a complication such as impaired eyesight. It occurs in both sexes and at any age but it is more common after middle age.

There is an undoubted hereditary factor and diabetic tendency is inherited as a Mendelian recessive according to the laws of genetics. Obesity, over-eating and worry are also regarded as contributory factors.

The hereditary nature of the disease and its increasing incidence give rise to speculation as to what may happen in future generations. Before there was effective treatment about 70 per cent of adult cases died within ten years and the outlook was even worse for children. Nowadays most diabetics can be well-controlled and enabled to lead a fairly normal life. The implications of this are obvious.

Diabetic coma and other complications. In severe untreated diabetes the inability of the body to store and utilize sugar means that it has to derive its energy needs from other sources. Use of protein leads to tissue wasting and the abnormal use of fat causes the accumulation of poisonous substances in the blood and these produce diabetic coma.

Other complications of diabetes are increased susceptibility to infections, neuritis, cataract and retinitis, gastric and renal disorder, myocarditis, and vascular disease sometimes causing gangrene of the extremities.

Treatment. Mild diabetics may often be controlled by dietary measures alone. The aim is to give a balanced but adequate diet and restrict carbohydrate foods to the minimum. If sugar loss in the urine cannot be prevented by this means, it will be necessary to give a suitable dose of insulin by injection. The development of slow-release types of insulin has reduced the number of injections required to one or two per day.

Until about 1954 insulin was the only effective treatment for diabetes but since then certain drugs have become available which may be taken by mouth. The first of these were compounds of sulphonylurea which acted by stimulating remnants of functioning pancreatic tissue to produce more insulin.

Others drugs have subsequently been developed. Their mode of action is less well understood but they appear to increase the activity on cells of any insulin still being produced by the pancreas. These drugs are mainly of use in certain cases of mild diabetes of late onset. Their success is dependent on the continued presence of at least some functioning insulin-producing tissue.

Insulin coma (Hypoglycaemia). Overdosage of insulin, or delay in taking food after an injection, or excessive exercise, may lead to a serious fall in blood sugar with symptoms of weakness, muscular tremors, drowsiness and ultimately coma. The swallowing of sugar leads to rapid recovery and well-instructed diabetics who are taking insulin will be made aware of the condition and the appropriate emergency action. In other circumstances the differentiation between diabetic coma and insulin coma may be difficult.

'Renal diabetes'. Not all cases of glycosuria are due to diabetes mellitus. In certain individuals the kidney has a lowered 'leak-point' for the elimination of sugar so that sugar appears in the urine even with a normal blood sugar level. This is an individual idiosyncrasy; it causes no symptoms and requires no treatment.

Community surveys. Since there are at least as many unrecognized diabetics as those which have been diagnosed, and since the treatment is fully understood and very successful, there is great scope for organized measures of detection. Populations can be asked to provide urine samples which are simply and easily tested for glycosuria. Those who show a positive reaction are then given further tests to differentiate between renal glycosuria and true diabetes; the patient eats a known amount of glucose and the urine is tested every half hour to see how the body is dealing with it.

diagnosis. The term is used in two senses. Primarily it refers to the procedure, partly an art but increasingly a science, which a physician employs to assess the symptoms and signs presented by a patient and to identify the disease from which he is suffering. It can also refer to the actual disease as, for instance, in answer to the question 'What is the diagnosis?'

Diagnosis as a procedure is fundamental to the effective practice of medicine and surgery and on its accuracy depends the best hope of rational and effective treatment.

Before the advent of supplementary aids to diagnosis a physician had to depend on what he could learn by questioning the patient and on the signs which he could recognize during the actual examination.

The interrogation or case-history is of great importance and should cover general matters such as age, occupation, marital status, family history, personal history (environment and habits) and previous health. This is then supplemented by more detailed enquiry regarding the actual symptoms. The nature and scope of these further questions will be governed by a provisional assessment of which particular system of the body is at fault.

Even before proceeding to physical examination the skilled diagnostician will have taken note of the general appearance, demeanour and behaviour of his patient since these may often afford valuable clues. Complexion, attitude (standing or in bed), voice, restlessness,

development, nutrition and gait should all be noted.

In the physical examination much can be learned by a systematic visual survey supplemented by careful feeling with an educated sense of touch. A sharp tap on the surface of the body elicits a sound which is either resonant or dull according to the nature or condition of the underlying structures. This is known as percussion, and by this means the borders of organs can be mapped out and an opinion formed as to their condition. Auscultation is the procedure by which the physician listens to what is going on within the body and this can afford helpful information about the state of the heart and its valves, of the lungs, and sometimes of the digestive tract.

In relation to the nervous system physical examination entails an assessment of the patient's special senses, touch, taste, sight, hearing, balance and co-ordination, together with an examination of both voluntary and reflex movements.

Aids to diagnosis. So far the procedures described have been dependent entirely on the physician making use of his own unaided senses guided by experience and knowledge. The development of more precise diagnosis has followed the development of ever more sophisticated items of equipment.

The first of these was the clinical thermometer, since elevation of the body temperature is an important indication of fever due to some infection. Direct auscultation was a difficult and unsatisfactory procedure until Laennec's invention of the stethoscope (1819), which transmitted sound to the doctor's ears from a sound-piece which could be applied to the body. Blood pressure estimations were made possible by the invention of the sphygmomanometer and availability of small battery-operated light sources led to the development of various instruments which extended the scope of examination of the eyes and body orifices. The variety, complexity, capacity and performance of such instruments continues to extend.

Perhaps the greatest single advance was the discovery of x-rays by Roentgen in 1895 and x-ray apparatus of increasing power and capabilities, assisted by the use of appropriate contrast media, now facilitates the examination of almost every part of the body. Electrocardiographs and electroencephalographs record the electrical activity of heart and brain and provide a visual 'trace' which records their functional condition. Other appliances are used to measure respiratory condition and metabolism and even radio-isotopes and ultra-sound are used for other types of investigation.

Laboratory aids. Laboratory investigations are dependent on the work of the bacteriologist, the histologist, and the biochemist who deal respectively with the presence or effects of bacteria and other invaders, the changes in tissue brought about by disease, and abnormalities of body chemistry.

The information provided by appropriate tests is often essential, not only to confirm a tentative diagnosis but to assess the progress of treatment and its likelihood of success.

Community diagnosis. The procedures previously outlined have been concerned with the management of an individual patient but many diseases may be present in latent form before they give rise to symptoms. Pre-diagnostic screening of sections of the population holds prospects of detecting latent conditions before they give rise to actual disease so that appropriate early treatment can be instituted.

The first great successes of such a concept were the mass radiography campaigns of the detection of tuberculosis, but screening procedures are now used for a variety of other diseases such as diabetes and cancer of the uterine cervix, and more elaborate forms of 'health-check' are being pioneered or being employed in the care of selected groups with special risks.

Diaphoretics. Drugs which increase the amount of perspiration; they can act either on the central nervous system or on the blood vessels in the skin. Diaphoretics are given either to bring down a feverish temperature by increased evaporation of sweat, or to compensate for failing urinary secretion. However, better drugs are now available for both purposes and specific use of traditional diaphoretics has greatly declined.

Diaphragm. The dome-shaped musculo-fibrous partition which separates the abdominal cavity below from the cavities of the chest above. The diaphragm is the principal muscle of RESPIRATION. It is attached below to the lumbar vertebrae, sternum and lower ribs.

Occasionally, part of the diaphragm is congenitally deficient or weak allowing some of the abdominal contents to protrude into the lower part of the chest cavity. This is known as a diaphragmatic or hiatus hernia which requires surgical treatment if it gives rise to serious symptoms.

Diaphysis. See EPIPHYSIS.

Diarrhoea. A disorder of bowel function characterized by the frequent evacuation of loose, fluid or semi-fluid stools. Severe cases may be accompanied by the passage of blood and mucus or by tenesmus which is a painful and ineffectual straining in the attempt to pass stools.

Causes. Diarrhoea is common at all ages (in fact INFANTILE DIARRHOEA is a significant cause of death during the first year) and its possible causes are both numerous and diverse. Normally the entry of food into an empty stomach produces a reflex which results in the pelvic colon being emptied once a day after breakfast but an over-active reflex may cause loose stools after every meal. This is post-prandial or

when breathing out

chest cavity
diaphragm

chest wall   diaphragm
raised   depressed

when breathing in

The diaphragm

lienteric diarrhoea, and in a somewhat similar fashion a sudden fright or emotional stress may cause nervous diarrhoea.

Apart from infections the commonest cause of diarrhoea is excessive or unsuitable food, such as eating unripe fruit, which irritates the intestine.

If there is a lack of hydrochloric acid in the stomach (achlorhydria) insufficiently digested food may be passed on from there to the intestine to set up irritation both mechanically and by fermentation. Excessive use of laxatives is another possibility, and many poisonous substances may irritate the bowel.

Diarrhoea also often accompanies disease of the bowel or of its associated digestive glands. Chronic peritonitis, tuberculosis, mucous and ulcerative colitis, cancer and pancreatic and biliary insufficiency are examples.

It may occur too in general diseases of the heart, lungs or liver where there is interference with the general venous or portal circulation, or in kidney disease with uraemia where toxins usually excreted in the urine pass through the bowel and upset its normal function.

Infection, however, is by far the commonest cause and the agents responsible include viruses, the organisms causing dysentery (both bacillary and amoebic), food poisoning, typhoid fever, and cholera.

Accurate diagnosis depends on bacteriological, chemical and microscopic examination of the stool with perhaps the aid of x-ray or examination of the bowel if organic disease is suspected.

Treatment. This largely depends upon the cause but attacks of acute diarrhoea should be regarded as infective until proved otherwise and precautions taken to protect other persons.

The routine treatment of simple cases of diarrhoea suspected of being infective is usually based on a kaolin or chalk mixture which absorbs toxins and allays intestinal irritation, and on the administration of antibiotics. Since there is fluid loss in the stools adequate fluids should be given. Sweetened drinks such as barley water with 1 teaspoonful of salt added to every litre (2 pints) are useful.

In severe diarrhoea a danger is dehydration from excessive loss of fluid and this is especially so in infants who rapidly collapse from this cause. The same is true of cases of cholera. Because of the extreme diarrhoea fluid replacement by mouth is usually ineffectual and intravenous infusions of a suitable solution will be required.

diastole. See SYSTOLE.

diet. An individual's customary daily intake of FOOD and drink.

The body requires food for several purposes: as fuel for the production of body-heat and muscular energy, as raw material for the growth, replacement, and repair of tissue, and as a source of the mineral salts, vitamins, and liquid necessary for the vital processes of the cells.

Since foods differ in composition they provide for these needs to different extents, so that a person requires not only an adequate total amount of food but a proper balance of the basic nutrients.

Proteins. These are needed for growth and repair of tissues. An adult of average size requires about 90 g. (3 oz.) of protein daily, of which at least half should be of animal origin. As explained under PROTEIN no vegetable protein contains all the essential amino-acids, so a complete vegetarian needs about 150 g. (5 oz.) of well mixed plant proteins. In proportion to size children need two or three times as much protein as adults, with at least 60 per cent of animal origin (including, of course, protein from milk, eggs, cheese and fish as well as meat).

No foods consists wholly, or even mainly, of protein. Most cheeses, the foods of highest protein content, are roughly one-third protein, one-third fat, and one-third water. An egg is about 12 per cent protein, so that a hen's egg weighing 50 g. provides 6 g. of protein. Lean bacon and lean beef are about 25 per cent protein. Milk is about

3.5 per cent protein, so 300 g. (10 oz.) of milk provide about 10 g. of animal protein. In an affluent society we can get three-quarters of our daily requirements of animal protein from a breakfast egg, a generous helping (60 g.) of bacon and about 300 g. of milk during the day, and a fairly small helping of meat, fish or cheese later in the day will complete our requirements. Alternatively, if we prefer a cereal breakfast 160 g. of meat (5½ oz.) and the same amount of milk will meet our needs.

As for plant protein, bread is about 6.5 per cent protein, potatoes about 2.2 per cent, broad beans and dried peas approximately 20 per cent protein (although not wholly absorbed in digestion) and most vegetables and fruits contain a little protein.

In affluent communities protein deficiency is rare. Apart from a few food cranks, people who can afford sufficient animal protein usually have plenty of protein in their diet. Excess protein is less likely to cause obesity than is excess of other foods, because the unrequired protein is largely excreted, in cases of great excess causing diarrhoea. Poor people often have diets inadequate in animal protein and are sometimes unaware of the importance and relative cheapness (in some countries at least) of milk, cheese and eggs. In underdeveloped countries insufficiency of protein is a widespread, major nutritional problem.

Fats. Although it is sometimes said that the average adult in a temperate climate needs about 90 g. of FAT daily – or about the same as his protein requirement – there is little scientific evidence of minimum need, except that the diet requires to contain sufficient fat to supply adequate quantities of the fat-soluble vitamins. Butter and margarine are about 80 per cent fat, and other rich sources are meat fat, fatty fish and cheese. The burning up of fat takes place only in the presence of sufficient carbohydrate, and consumption of fat to an amount disproportionate to carbohydrate leads to indigestion. On the other hand persons living in extremely cold climates appear to be able to consume enormous amounts of fats.

Apart from being needed for their vitamin content, fats are required to prevent the diet from becoming too bulky. Not only does an ounce of fat provide more Calories than an ounce of protein and an ounce of carbohydrate together, but most protein foods and starchy foods contain very considerable amounts of water. A fat-free diet of 3,000 Calories daily would involve enormous meals.

In recent years it has been suggested that too much animal fat (e.g., from butter cheese and meat fat) raises the blood cholesterol level and may predispose to coronary thrombosis, and that about half of the total intake of fat should be obtained from vegetable oils.

MEAL 1 (containing 740 calories)
70g. (2.5 oz.) roast beef
170g. (6 oz.) boiled potatoes
110g. (4 oz.) cabbage
85g. (3 oz.) raisin suet pudding
55g. (2 oz.) custard sauce
0.25 litres (0.5 pt.) tea
(food values on chart shown ▬)

MEAL 2 (containing 790 Calories)
100g. (3.5 oz.) bread or rolls
15g. (0.5 oz.) butter
55g. (2 oz.) cheese
0.25 litres (0.5 pt.) milk
an orange
(food values on chart shown ▨)

MEAL 3 (containing 436 Calories)
100g. (3.5 oz.) bun
15g. (0.5 oz.) butter
0.25 litres (0.5 pt.) tea
(food values on chart shown ▨)

Diet: three meals, showing the food value of each

Excess deposition of fat in parts of the body is generally caused not by over-eating of fats but by over-eating of carbohydrates. The body stores excess of sugar, or of starch which is converted to sugar, as fat.

Carbohydrates. These are the starches and sugars, all eventually broken down by digestion to glucose and then stored mainly in the liver and muscles as the polysaccharide glycogen. When required, glycogen is reconstituted as glucose and oxidized to provide muscular energy and heat.

Sugar is of course entirely carbohydrate except for a trace of moisture; flour varies from 70 to 75 per cent carbohydrate; potatoes are approximately 20 per cent carbohydrate; the proportion in fruits varies from nearly 20 per cent in bananas to just under 3 per cent in tomatoes; and in common vegetables the proportion ranges from 10 per cent in carrots to about 5 per cent in turnips.

Excessive carbohydrate is converted into fat in the body and stored as fat in the tissues. During periods in which food intake is insufficient, to balance energy requirements the fat stores are reconverted into carbohydrate and then utilized for energy.

In developed countries 50 to 70 per cent of the total Calories are usually derived from carbohydrates; and the carbohydrate foods consumed in greatest quantities include wheat, corn, rice, barley, potatoes and other vegetables and fruits. Increased usage of cane and beet sugar, white flour and polished rice produces risk of obesity and also risk of nutritional hazards from decreased intake of minerals and vitamins.

If the common dietetic danger of the poor is protein deficiency, that of those not on the poverty line is carbohydrate excess leading to obesity.

Vitamins. These comprise certain organic substances necessary for normal metabolism and variously present in many foodstuffs. They do not form a chemically related class of compounds and they range from the relatively simple ascorbic acid (vitamin c) to much more complicated molecules.

An adult requires about five thousand international units of vitamin A daily, about 1.5 mg. of aneurin (vitamin B_1), approximately 2 mg. of riboflavine and 15 mg. of nicotinic acid (components of the vitamin B_2 complex), about 55 mg. of ascorbic acid (vitamin c) and about 100 international units of vitamin D. Vitamin excess can occur with vitamins A and D. Vitamin deficiency is, even in developed countries, still relatively common in children and old people. See VITAMINS.

Minerals. The body requires a variety of MINERAL SALTS. Sodium, potassium, magnesium, and phosphorus are present in adequate amounts in any ordinary diet and need no special attention. There may, however, be deficiencies of calcium, iron, or iodine. Calcium is required for bones and teeth; children should have at least 1 g. per day and the best source is milk. Iron is essential for the synthesis of haemoglobin and insufficiency leads to anaemia. The daily requirement is 15 to 20 mg. and the best sources are meat, eggs and certain vegetables, especially spinach. Iodine is needed for the production of thyroid hormone and deficiency leads to goitre. Sea foods are the chief natural source but many brands of ordinary table salt contain added sodium iodine (1 in 100,000) and provide for the small daily requirement of 15 micrograms.

Other 'trace-elements' needed are cobalt, manganese and copper but they are rarely lacking from human diets although some are of importance in animal husbandry. Special interest also attaches to the element fluorine, lack of which reduces the resistance of tooth enamel to decay.

Roughage or fibre. The indigestible residues of diet are mainly fibrous material derived from vegetable food. Until recently little attention has been paid to the role of ROUGHAGE in the diet but it is becoming clear that it is important in maintaining the bulk and plasticity of faeces and that modern low-residue diets are a main cause of constipation which in turn is associated with varicose veins, haemorrhoids, and various diseases of the colon.

Amount of food. Heat production and muscular activity are forms of energy derived by the body from the METABOLISM or 'burning' of its food, and the amount of food eaten must be sufficient to provide for an individual's energy requirements.

The energy value of any foodstuff is measured in CALORIES which are units of heat. A person at rest in a normal environment expends a certain amount of energy merely to maintain his temperature, circulation, respiration and other vital functions. This basic demand for fuel is his basal metabolism, quite easily measured physiologically by recording oxygen consumption.

The basal metabolism of the average man calls for about 1100 Calories per day but in addition provision must be made for the energy expended daily in his normal life. This varies widely according to environmental temperature and the amount of exercise taken.

Heat is an expensive form of energy – more so than exercise. Eskimos and polar explorers need a large Calorie intake. This can be illustrated by the fact that 1000 watts of electrical energy used by a one-bar electric fire is equivalent to more than 1 horse-power.

The average total Calorie requirement in various circumstances can be stated approximately as follows: sedentary life: 2,200 Calories; light work 2,300 to 2,900 Calories; moderate work 3,000 to 3,500 Calories; heavy work 3,600 to 6,000 Calories.

It should be noted that it is not necessary to have a large, elaborately-prepared meal to ensure the best food value, as is clearly demonstrated by the example on p. 111 of three possible meals, showing the Calorie content and the important food values of each.

Energy balance. The laws of the conservation of energy demand that an organism must obtain an amount of energy, in utilizable form, equal to the amount which it expends.

Animals, including man, carry a body reserve of energy in the form of fat, stored mainly in the subcutaneous tissues where it also provides thermal insulation, mechanical protection and a cosmetic function. This store is both large and variable. An average male may have 16 per cent of his body weight as fat and this represents a reserve of perhaps 100,000 Calories, very adequate in relation to his daily turnover of (say) 3,000 Calories, but an obese person may be 65 per cent fat which is grossly excessive. Fluctuations in the daily intake-output balance are compensated for by this reserve.

However since adults may eat as much as half-a-ton of food per year some mechanism is required to ensure that small daily excesses do not build up in an impossible extent. This is dependent on appetite, at least partially indicative of the body's need for food, and controlled by centres in the mid-brain. The effectiveness of this control can be affected by over-indulgence in attractive foods or by using food as a solace for psychological stresses. In these circumstances obesity results and there is also evidence that over-feeding in infancy increases the number and capacity of fat cells so that they store fat more readily in adult life.

Civilization leads to an increased intake of readily available food and to reduced energy output as we replace internal production of heat by a controlled environment (e.g., central heating) and substitute transport and machinery for walking and manual labour.

All these are factors which tend to increase obesity – perhaps the major dietary problem of the age.

iets, special. The treatment of various diseases may sometimes be influenced beneficially by dietary adjustments designed to add or exclude certain factors. Diets specifically so prescribed are known as special diets and although many may only reflect a current fashion or the personal fad of a particular physician there are at least some basic regimes based on recognized physiological principles.

Light or milk diet. Commonly prescribed for any invalid or convalescent or in the treatment of gastric or duodenal ulceration, gastritis, or other disorders of the gastro-intestinal tract. The basic constituent is usually milk with the addition of easily digested foods, such as eggs, chicken, fish and potatoes. Milk diets or modified milk diets given at short intervals are frequently used in the treatment of acute gastric ulcer with the intention of continuously neutralizing gastric juice.

In general, foods with indigestible residues, spices and fried dishes are excluded. Supplements of vitamins and minerals should be added.

Salt-free diet. It is difficult to exclude salt entirely but low salt diets are recommended for kidney disease and hypertension. Bacon, ham, salted butter, cheese and bread should be avoided, and no salt used in cooking or at table.

Low-protein diet. Some varieties of chronic kidney disease lead to nitrogen retention, the forerunner of uraemia. Nitrogen is derived from protein and so meat, fish, eggs, milk and cheese are restricted.

High-protein diet. In kidney disease with marked albuminuria, excessive protein loss occurs and this is compensated for by allowing up to 0.5 kg. (1 lb.) per day of meat or fish. It is also desirable to reduce fats and therefore eggs and full cream milk are unsuitable.

Extra protein is also indicated in certain liver diseases and during recovery from wasting conditions.

Low-carbohydrate diet. Used in the reduction of obesity; bread, cakes, confectionery, sugar, potatoes and cereals are eliminated or reduced in this diet.

High-fat or ketogenic diet. Formerly this diet was used in treatment of epilepsy. It had been noted that epileptics had fewer fits if they were starved and became acidotic and since excess fats cause acidosis due to incomplete metabolism producing ketone bodies, such a ketogenic diet enjoyed a vogue as a means of treatment. It is now largely out-moded by modern anti-convulsant drugs.

Low-fat diet. Recommended for gall-stones and other disorders of liver and gall-bladder as well as for arteriosclerosis, in which fatty deposits collect on the artery walls. Butter, cheese, milk, fatty and fried foods are excluded. In arteriosclerosis it is particularly desirable to exclude the saturated fats of animal origin.

Gluten-free diet. In abdominal disease patients cannot digest gluten, a protein found mainly in wheat products. Gluten-free bread (from which the gluten part of the cereal has been removed) is obtainable and other carbohydrates such as rice and tapioca are permissible.

Diabetic diet. Diabetic patients require restriction of carbohydrate intake. A specific regime requires to be worked out for individual patients.

High-calcium diet. Pregnant and nursing mothers require to double their intake of calcium, and this is best supplied in the form of additional milk and cheese. See also VEGETARIAN DIET.

digestion. The process by which the alimentary tract breaks down the elements of food and prepares them for absorption into the blood stream so that they may be utilized by the body in its vital functions; see METABOLISM. Digestion combines both mechanical action – chewing, swallowing and movement by the stomach and intestines – and chemical action by ferments and similar substances.

The constituents of FOOD requiring digestion are proteins, carbohydrates and fats: the parts of the DIGESTIVE SYSTEM concerned in dealing with them in varying degrees are the mouth, stomach and small intestine.

Proteins. Protein molecules consist of linked chains of amino-acids. In the stomach, hydrochloric acid and pepsin break protein down into proteoses and peptones, and another ferment, rennin, coagulates milk for subsequent attack by pepsin. Further protein digestion occurs in the small intestine where the ferment trypsin breaks down the proteoses and peptones from the stomach into successively smaller groups of amino-acids (polypeptids and peptids), and finally, by the action of erepsin, into individual amino-acids suitable for assimilation. Trypsin and amylopsin are secreted in the pancreatic juice; erepsin is present in the intestinal secretion.

Absorption of the amino-acids occurs mainly in the small intestine, where they pass into the body through fine projections known as villi.

Carbohydrates. These are the starches and sugars. The ferment ptyalin in the saliva acts upon starches converting them to the di-saccharide maltose. Further digestion of starches and sugars then occurs in the small intestine where the pancreatic ferment amylopsin and the intestinal ferments sucrase, maltase and lactase finally convert them to glucose ready for absorption.

Some absorption of simple sugars takes place in the stomach, which is the reason why sugar is given when energy is required quickly, the only food rapidly absorbed being alcohol. Most carbohydrates, however, are - like proteins - absorbed in the small intestine.

Fats. Fats are almost entirely dealt with by the small intestine. A ferment lipase, acting upon fats, is secreted by the stomach but, except in infants, its action is weak. In the intestine fats are emulsified by bile and then split by the pancreatic ferment lipase. The products of fat digestion are fatty acids and glycerin. These are absorbed by the epithelial cells of the intestine and reconstituted as neutral fats. Only a small fraction of these synthesized fats passes directly into the portal blood stream. The rest is taken up by the lymphatic system and then reaches the main blood stream via the main lymphatic channel (thoracic duct) which discharges into the venous system at the junction of the left subclavian and left internal jugular veins.

digestive system. In order to maintain life and provide for all its vital activities the body requires FOOD but it cannot utilize the ordinary substances of a normal diet until these are broken down into simpler elements capable of absorption into the blood stream for subsequent distribution to the tissues. The process by which food is thus broken down is known as DIGESTION, and this process, as well as absorption, is carried out by the digestive system, a term which comprehensively includes the several parts of the food canal together with associated organs such as the salivary glands, pancreas and liver.

The first part of the system is the mouth equipped with jaws and teeth. Teeth are of two basic types: incisors or cutting tools serving to bite off convenient portions of food, and molars designed to grind it down into smaller particles. The teeth are set in the upper and lower jaws which are fixed

The digestive system

and moveable respectively so that the grinding action can take place by muscular action.

Food taken into the mouth is said to be ingested and the function of the mouth jaws and teeth is to chew small quantities of food and, in breaking it down, to mix it with saliva, a digestive ferment supplied by three pairs of salivary glands known as the parotid, submaxillary and sublingual glands. Saliva also assists in the formation of the food into a slippery mass or bolus of a size suitable for swallowing (deglutition).

When prepared in this way the bolus enters the pharynx which is a cavity common to both the air-and food-passages and which provides arrangements for ensuring that the food does not get into the larynx but instead correctly enters the oesophagus or gullet, a muscular tube traversing the chest in its downward passage to the stomach.

In the stomach, which acts as a reservoir, food is delayed for some four hours while it undergoes preliminary digestion. The stomach walls contain cells which provide hydrochloric acid and the ferments rennin, pepsin and lipase.

The lower opening of the stomach is controlled by a muscular ring or sphincter known as the pylorus. Food released from the stomach next traverses the small intestine, a convoluted musculomembranous tube some 6 m. (20 ft.) in length. The intestine is lined with mucous membrane which is not smooth but composed of innumerable fine projections known as villi disposed like the pile of a piece of velvet.

The intestine secretes a digestive fluid, the succus entericus, produced by glands whose mouths open into the intestinal lumen at the bases of the villi.

The parts of the small intestine are known successively as duodenum, jejunum and ileum and in the upper duodenum is an opening, the ampulla of Vater, which represents the junction of the common bile-duct with the pancreatic duct and through which bile from the liver and pancreatic juice from the pancreas enter the intestine. Bile serves to emulsify fats and pancreatic juice provides certain ferments; together they help to complete digestion initiated in the stomach.

Food is moved along the intestine by waves of muscular contraction - peristalsis - and ultimately reaches the lower end of the ileum. From there it passes by the ileo-caecal valve into the caecum and thence to the large intestine. The material reaching the large intestine is food which has been fully digested and stripped of its nutriments by absorption in the small intestine.

The large intestine, which comprises successively the ascending, transverse and descending colon and finally the rectum is some 1.5 m. (5 ft.) in length. It absorbs water from the fluid material reaching it from above and forms waste matter into a semi-solid state suitable for evacuation through the anus as faeces.

The functioning of the digestive tract as a whole is under both nervous control from the sympathetic and autonomic nervous systems, and chemical control by the hormones, (gastrin, secretin, cholecystokinin, and entero-gastrone) secreted by ductless glands in the walls of the stomach and small intestine.

Diseases. Diseases affecting the tract from the mouth to the anus may include those due to general causes such as infections and malignant change, but some conditions are peculiar to the stomach and intestines.

Of these the commonest is ulceration which may be either gastric or duodenal. In this condition the lining of these organs is itself locally digested by the digestive ferments, which produces ulceration. This is particularly apt to occur in tense and nervous persons and is recognized as a typical psychosomatic disease. The ulceration may cause haemorrhage or perforation and then requires emergency treatment. Chronic gastritis results usually from over-eating or over-indulgence in alcohol.

The colon is subject to two types of chronic disease: simple colitis usually caused by excessive dependence on laxatives, and ulcerative colitis, mainly affecting the lower end of the colon. In the latter there is abdominal pain and often severe diarrhoea with the evacuation of blood and mucus. A potential risk is perforation which requires emergency treatment.

digitalis. A drug, originally obtained from the powdered leaf of the foxglove, with a specific action on heart muscle: slowing its rate of contraction and increasing the strength of contractions.

It was, and to some extent still is, given in the form of a tincture, i.e., essentially a solution of the powder in alcohol, and it is valuable in various heart diseases, especially auricular fibrillation. To a considerable degree, however, it is now replaced by drugs derived from it, such as digitalin in which the exact strength is more easily measured and the derived drug is usually given by injection.

Digitalis is not useful in all forms of heart disease: where the heart muscle is exhausted to give digitalis is equivalent to whipping a tired horse. Also the drug is not easily destroyed or excreted by the body and therefore can have a cumulative action. So it should be used only under strict medical supervision.

Poisoning or overdosage is suggested by failure of appetite, going on to nausea and vomiting, and by some irregularities of the pulse. Unless there is considerable vomiting an emetic may help, followed by strong tea or coffee, but the most important measure is temporarily stopping the doses of digitalis.

diphtheria. An infectious disease caused by the diphtheria bacillus (*Corynebacterium diphtheria*) and characterized by inflammation of the fauces or larynx with a typical fibrinous exudate ('wash-leather' exudate) and often by severe general symptoms produced by the effect of toxins on the heart muscle and the peripheral nerves.

It was formerly a common endemic disease of children usually causing a long, serious, and tedious illness which often ended in death, but since about 1940 a general policy of active immunization has resulted in its virtual eradication from all countries with an adequate health service.

Laryngeal diphtheria causes special difficulties because of obstruction to respiration and may require tracheotomy. Otherwise the treatment is by complete bed rest and the administration of diphtheria antitoxin and penicillin.

Active immunization involves a course of usually three suitably-spaced injections of diphtheria toxoid starting at about 4 months of age. Further 'booster' doses are usually given at school entry and again at about 9 years of age. Diphtheria toxoid is a component of 'triple antigen' which provides simultaneous protection against diphtheria, whooping cough and tetanus.

The carrier state is common in diphtheria epidemics and such people must be sought for and isolated. The bacillus is also occasionally found in unusual situations e.g., in rhinitis, conjunctivitis, or in infected wounds.

diplopia. A disorder of vision in which the

patient sees single objects as double.

Each eye forms a separate image on its own retina and for these images to become fused in accurate binocular vision the visual axes of both eyes must be truly directed at the object or 'point of fixation'.

If any of the muscles moving the eyeballs are paralysed, weakened, or uncoordinated, this will not be achieved and the patient then 'sees' two objects.

This is binocular diplopia and the double vision disappears on closing one eye.

In monocular diplopia, which is much less common, two images are formed on the retina of one eye and this can result from irregular refraction, early cataract, dislocated lens or the congenital condition of double pupil.

dipsomania. An intermittent craving for alcohol which is then taken in excess to the point of severe intoxication. It is a compulsion neurosis usually related to conditions of mental stress or depression. The frequency of attacks varies with circumstances.

A chronic alcoholic has come to be dependent on alcohol as a drug of addiction but the dipsomaniac between bouts may appear to be quite normal. Nevertheless the condition is an indication of a manic-depressive personality, and proper psychiatric supervision is desirable.

disabling diseases. Almost any chronic disease can produce some measure of disablement. In a child disablement is some condition which precludes his education in a normal school. An adult of employable age is disabled if, on account of injury, disease or congenital deformity, he is substantially handicapped in obtaining or keeping employment. After pensionable age a severely disabled person is someone who by reason of physical or mental disability requires continual supervision and attention.

A broad classification is as follows: (1) disease of the heart and circulation; (2) diseases of the lungs and respiratory system; (3) diseases of digestion and assimilation; (4) diseases of the nervous system such as epilepsy, and disseminated sclerosis; (5) mental deficiency and mental illness; (6) diseases and injuries of the skeletal and locomotory system such as osteo-arthritis or loss of limbs; (7) endocrine disorders, and obesity; (8) chronic nephritis; (9) defects of the special senses, especially blindness, partial sightedness and deafness.

discharging ears. See EAR.

disease. Definitions range from any departure from complete physical, mental and social well-being to any malfunctioning of body or mind sufficient to produce pain, disability or abnormal behaviour.

For classification of diseases, see CAUSES OF DISEASE.

Measures against disease can be taken at two levels. Clinical medicine (including surgery and psychiatry) seeks to treat the person who is already ill, while community medicine (or public health) seeks to eradicate or reduce the causes of disease. Clearly both types are needed, but until about a hundred years ago emphasis was almost entirely on treatment, whereas in recent decades there has been gradual increase in awareness of the importance of prevention, e.g., stress on HEALTH EDUCATION, development of IMMUNIZATION, concern with NUTRITION, and the beginnings of GENETIC GUIDANCE.

disinfection. The destruction by artificial means of disease-producing organisms and particularly those from an infectious patient. Disinfection implies something less than sterilization (the extinction of all life) but more than antisepsis (the prevention or retardation of bacterial growth).

Disinfectants include liquid or gaseous chemicals and the physical effects of heat, as hot air or steam. Air and sunlight dry and oxidize bacteria and destroy them by ultra-violet light, and the purifying influence of plain soap and water is also of disinfectant value in relation to many diseases not calling for more drastic measures.

The measures which may be taken to disinfect the sick room and its furnishings at the conclusion of a case are now regarded as comparatively unimportant, and ritual fumigation, spraying and steam sterilization of mattresses has largely been given up in recognition that only the patient presents any real danger. However, there should be an immediate disinfection of discharges and excreta and of inanimate objects as soon as they are infected during the course of an illness.

Disinfection by heat. Swabs and dressings should be burned. Most textiles except blankets can be boiled, which kills non-sporing organisms immediately; if maintained for one hour it kills most spores. Steam disinfection requires a special pressure chamber.

Liquid disinfectants. The standard solutions employed are 5 per cent carbolic acid, 2 per cent cresol ('lysol'), 5 per cent chlorinated lime, or one of the proprietary disinfectants. Formalin solution (1 per cent) is used in sprays.

Gaseous disinfectants. Formaldehyde gas is now standard, liberated by heat-vaporization of solid formaldehyde or by the action of potassium permanganate on formalin (a 40 per cent solution of formaldehyde).

The following represents an effective code of practice:

1. Nasal discharges etc. – received on paper handkerchiefs subsequently burned.

2. Sputum – received into container with 5 per cent carbolic acid; paper sputum containers which can be burned are available.

3. Faeces and vomit – mixed with 5 per cent carbolic, 2 per cent cresol, or 5 per cent chlorinated lime and allowed to stand

2 hours before disposal to drains.

4. Urine – mixed with equal volume of similar disinfectant solutions and allowed to stand for two hours before disposal.

5. Textiles – soaked in 2 per cent cresol for twelve hours before being boiled and washed. If boiled before soaking any discharges will cause staining. Blankets and most synthetic fabrics should not be boiled.

6. Cutlery, crockery etc. – kept for individual use: sterilized by boiling; food residues burned.

7. Nursing equipment – boiled or treated with above disinfectant solutions: thermometers, toothbrush etc., kept in 2 per cent proprietary disinfectant.

8. Hands – 5 per cent commercial preparation for two minutes.

9. Person – protected by overalls kept in sick room; use of mask if appropriate.

head of the humerus dislocated from its socket

Dislocated shoulder

dislocations. A dislocation is a displacement or separation of the bony surfaces which form a joint.

It is accompanied by rupture of the supporting ligaments and of the joint capsule. Subluxation is a partial dislocation.

Dislocations commonly occur in the joints at the ends of the long bones when indirect violence levers the joint beyond its normal range (traumatic dislocation), but a joint may become displaced through bone disease (pathological dislocation), or be unstable at birth through developmental abnormality especially in the hip joint (congenital dislocation).

The knee cap, jaw, and shoulder are quite often liable to dislocate through muscular action alone, without any external violence.

Dislocations usually occur in active mature adults. The bones of the elderly will fracture rather than dislocate and in young children a separation of the growing end of the bone is more likely to occur.

Signs of dislocation. There is usually deformity, loss of function, rigidity, and swelling with pain both at the site of injury and referred down the limb through pressure on nerves by the displaced structures. This may also produce numbness.

Treatment. Traumatic dislocations are restored (or 'reduced') by manipulation, usually under a general anaesthetic. Some dislocations, especially of shoulder and jaw, are very liable to recur and in many such instances the patient may become quite adept at reducing them himself.

In congenital dislocation of the hip, reduction is obtained by moving the leg from its natural position, and rotating it. This posture is maintained by some form of splintage until the joint surfaces develop sufficiently to ensure stability.

disseminated sclerosis. See MULTIPLE SCLEROSIS.

distension. The swelling and enlargement of a body cavity or of a hollow organ by its retained and accumulating contents.

Abdominal distension may be due to ascites (i.e. free fluid which accumulates in the abdominal cavity) or to the accumulation of gastro-intestinal fluid and gas within the stomach and bowel, usually as the result of digestive disorder, infective processes or obstruction.

Distension of the bladder occurs when there is obstruction to its outflow as from stricture of the urethra or prostatic enlargement.

diuretic. Any drug which increases the quantity of urine excreted by the kidneys. Diuretics act either on the circulation to increase blood flow through the kidney, or directly on the renal cells to increase their action.

The most important of the former group is digitalis which regulates the rate and rhythm of heart action, and reinforces ventricular contraction.

Of the numerous old-style drugs reputed to act directly on the kidney probably only caffeine and potassium citrate are now of much importance. The place of the others has been taken by new synthetic compounds of much greater effectiveness most of which act by interfering with enzyme control of the kidney tubules so that more fluid is excreted.

Prolonged use of powerful diuretics leads to potassium depletion in the body and this requires correction.

Diuretics are given to relieve oedema – the accumulation of fluid in the tissue spaces of the body – usually resulting from chronic cardiac or renal disease.

diverticulitis. Inflammation of a

diverticulum which is a small protrusion of mucous membrane bulging out through a weak part of the bowel wall.

Diverticulosis tends to occur in older persons with a long history of constipation. The diverticula are usually numerous and they become filled with stagnant faecal matter which may cause infection and inflammation of the surrounding tissue. When this occurs symptoms are produced very similar to those of acute appendicitis but on the left side of the lower abdomen.

Acute diverticulitis may proceed to abscess formation or peritonitis and requires prompt surgical treatment.

Chronic diverticulitis requires investigation to exclude the possibility of other conditions. X-ray examination following a barium enema will show evidence of the pocket-like diverticula. If the condition is extensive, of long standing and perhaps giving rise to symptoms of obstruction it is often best dealt with by removing the affected area of bowel.

divorce. A formal breaking of the legal tie of marriage by a decree of an appropriate court or other authority.

While the exact grounds on which divorce is permissible vary from country to country the general trend in legislation has been able to move away from the idea of proving 'guilt' (such as adultery, cruelty or desertion) towards that of simply establishing that a marriage has irretrievably broken down.

Because of changes in the grounds for divorce and because of decreases in the costs of obtaining a divorce the proportion of marriages ending in dissolution is increasing in many countries. The rising divorce rate is sometimes quoted as an indication of increased permissiveness or of lowered moral standards. It is not really such an indication. Indications can reasonably be sought in such things as the number of extramarital conceptions or the number of cases of venereal diseases, but the main explanation of the increasing divorce rate is that in many western countries divorce is now available to an incompatible couple without proving 'guilt' (which may not exist) and at much lower cost than in the past.

Couples who find themselves in continuing disharmony often seek to delay divorce until the children are 'old enough to stand it'. Where a couple who have lost affection for each other can contrive to live in the same house without bickering, having their separate interests and going their separate ways but showing the same courtesy and toleration that they would give to strangers with whom they happened to be sharing lodgings, the delay is probably beneficial to the children. On the other hand, if the domestic situation is one of constant stress and frequent quarrels, the delay may well be harmful to the children. In at least some cases, however, a couple who earlier had enough mutual affection and community of interest to marry may have temporarily irritated each other, so that an agreed short period of separation – e.g., for six weeks with the question of permanence considered after the trial period – may remove the need or desire for divorce.

dizziness. A feeling of unsteadiness in relation to the surroundings; 'giddiness' is an alternative term but 'vertigo' more properly denotes a sensation of spinning.

Dizziness results from two distinct groups of causes. The function of nerve cells in the brain can be disturbed by disorders of the circulation, toxins of various kinds, and conditions affecting intracranial tension. Examples of these are high blood pressure; disease of the heart valves; heart failure; low blood pressure such as occurs in certain diseases of the endocrine glands; in acute infections and in anaemia, cachexia and malnutrition; toxins such as alcohol and carbon monoxide; brain tumours and other intracranial conditions such as epilepsy. The brief giddiness when standing up suddenly or after a very hot bath is due to temporary changes in the blood supply to the brain.

The second group is related to the balancing mechanism or vestibule contained in the inner ear which may be damaged by infection or by some vascular disorder. Symptoms produced in this way are usually known as Ménière's disease often characterized by true vertigo. Disorders leading to double vision may cause similar feelings of instability because of the lack of co-ordination between visual and balancing sensations. The giddiness of travel sickness is probably due to vestibular effects.

Giddiness in a young person is generally of small significance. It is related to fainting which commonly results from an unduly sensitive vaso-motor mechanism. In older persons it requires investigation to discover the underlying cause.

DNA. See CELL.

doctor. In Britain 'doctor' has two completely separate meanings: (1) A person possessing a higher or postgraduate degree from a university, e.g., as a doctor of science, doctor of philosophy or doctor of medicine. Only a minority of medical practitioners are doctors in this sense. (2) As a courtesy title, any medical practitioner who holds a bachelor's degree in medicine and surgery from a university or a similar licence from a recognized college. The picture is further confused by the fact that, while a clinical medical consultant, a community medicine specialist and a general medical practitioner are called 'doctor' irrespective of whether they possess a higher qualification in medicine, a surgeon – who must hold a medical practitioner's bachelor's degree or college licence – is traditionally addressed as 'Mister'. About half the medical practitioners in Britain work in hospitals (roughly 12,000 full consultants and 19,000 junior doctors). Most of the others are general practitioners, while about 2500 are specialists in Community medicine, and some work in occupational health services and in the Forces.

domiciliary. Pertaining to a person's home. A domiciliary visit implies that the doctor, health visitor or nurse travels to the person's house, as contrasted with the person travelling to hospital or clinic.

dominant. The term is frequently used in the sense of influential or ruling: for instance, 'In that family the wife is the dominant partner'.

In genetics the word is used specifically in respect of one gene (dominant) over-ruling another (recessive). See GENETICS.

dose. The quantity of a medicine to be taken at one time. The official or standard dose, as set out in the pharmacopoeia, is usually given as a range, e.g., 50 to 100 mg. Within this range lie the doses suitable for most adults. The right dose for a particular adult depends partly on size and body-weight and partly on individual tolerance or susceptibility. Where a patient's reaction to a medicine is unknown - ,because the patient is new to the doctor or because the drug is new to the patient - it is generally considered good practice to start with a dose near the lower end of the range and subsequently increase if necessary.

For a child the dose of any medicine is always less than for an adult, but the broad rule of proportion - e.g., a child of one-quarter the weight of his father requires a quarter of the adult dose - has many exceptions. For instance the dose of morphia for a child is considerably less than in proportion to weight.

double personality. A disordered state of mind in which the patient appears alternately to lead two lives with neither personality being aware of the memories and experiences of the other.

In the majority of cases it is a hysterical phenomenon. Hysterical persons over-react to any situation either to fulfil subconscious wishes or to evade difficulties.

A later stage of this behaviour is the development of hysterical 'fugue' or flight from reality, which is a narrowing rather than a clouding of consciousness, with dissociation of existing memory.

The patient can thus live out some fantasy or more commonly simply pass into a state of amnesia where he does not know who or where he is.

Double personality is only a fragmentation of a single personality with different aspects predominating from time to time.

double vision. See DIPLOPIA.

Down's syndrome. See MONGOLISM.

drain. In a medical context, a piece of rubber tubing, corrugated rubber, gauze-wick or other device inserted into a wound to facilitate the discharge of fluid or pus and so helps to promote healing.

dreams. Sequences of thought, fancy, and imagery occurring during sleep and impinging on consciousness to a variable degree.

In common with many other animals, human physiology provides for a daily cycle of being awake and being asleep. The depth of intensity of the state of sleep fluctuates considerably. A relatively simple way of measuring this is to subject a sleeper to a progressively louder sound until he awakes but a great deal more about the inner nature of sleep has been learned through the introduction of the electro-encephalograph. This is an instrument which, by means of electrodes attached to the skull, records the electrical activity of the brain. The tracings thus produced show a wave-pattern which varies with the level of consciousness and cerebral activity. It has been demonstrated that dreams occur during light sleep when the subject is still unconscious of the outside world but yet sufficiently aware to appreciate and remember temporarily his dreaming impressions. A person wakened from light sleep will often be able to recall his dream; suddenly roused from deep sleep he will usually have nothing to report.

All the experimental evidence suggests that everyone has dreams but that not everyone can recall them. Moreover it is a matter of common experience how quickly a dream is forgotten unless special steps are taken to preserve it, either by rehearsing it in full consciousness or by writing it down.

Significance of dreams. Sigmund Freud (1856-1939) said that 'the interpretation of dreams is the royal road to a knowledge of the unconscious activities of the mind', and he elaborated this thesis in his very important work, *The Interpretation of Dreams,* which he published in 1900. Freud was a positivist, committed to the belief that everything must have a cause, and he therefore maintained that dreams could not be as irrational as they often seemed. Instead he regarded them as symbolic of personal matters arousing strong emotion; lesser symbols which the mind substituted for inner conflicts which would otherwise disturb and interfere with sleep.

In his work as a psychoanalyst he used the analysis of dreams as a tool to explore the emotional life of his patients. His pre-occupation with sexuality as the force motivating all abnormal psychological activity was such that he would tolerate no dissent. As a result the birth of psychoanalysis and acceptance of its tenets and techniques was marred by his quarrels with his associates, Adler and Jung, who regarded dreams as an unconscious attempt to achieve a success and perfection which real life denied.

Nevertheless, despite these basic divergencies of view, the study of dreams remains as a useful and important part of psychoanalytic practice.

dropsy. The accumulation of fluid in the tissue spaces and body cavities. Dropsy is not a disease but a symptom of a variety of serious conditions affecting the heart, kidneys or liver.

The fluid is serum from the blood stream and its effusion into the skin and superficial tissues produces a swollen appearance.

The swelling from heart disease tends to occur in dependent parts; in kidney disease its distribution is determined more by relative tissue laxity. The affected areas 'pit on pressure'; i.e., pressure by an examining finger leaves a depression which disappears only slowly. Accumulation of fluid in the abdomen cavity is ascites; in the chest cavity it is known as hydrothorax.

Dropsy in heart disease is due to failing circulation; in kidney disease to diminished elimination of fluid associated with salt retention and protein depletion; in the liver disease, which produces ascites rather than tissue oedema, there is usually obstruction to venous blood-flow in the portal circulation resulting from cirrhosis of the liver or malignant disease.

Treatment. The first essential is accurate diagnosis to determine the cause of the dropsy.

Drugs to increase the flow of urine will assist in the elimination of surplus tissue fluid and a salt-free diet is usually prescribed. Fluid in the chest and abdomen may be removed by suction.

Otherwise treatment requires to be directed to underlying causes, but dropsy is always of serious significance and any measure may give only temporary relief from the symptom.

drowning. Drowning is asphyxia caused by the mouth and nose being submerged in fluid and the consequent exclusion of air from the lungs. For emergency treatment see ARTIFICIAL RESPIRATION.

Although most drowning accidents occur through falls into deep water, it is not essential that a person should be 'out of his depth', because toddlers get into shallow streams and inebriates stumble into ditches with equally disastrous results.

Moreover, individuals tend to panic in shallow water. They scream and struggle using up the air in their lungs, and with gasping inspirations inhale water as well as air. In a potentially dangerous situation a victim should try to remain calm, keep his mouth shut, breathe through his nose and endeavour to keep his head above water by treading water or doing a 'dog-paddle'.

These measures will at least improve the chances of successful rescue but every child should be taught to swim and have confidence in water from an early age.

drowsiness. A state of failing or impaired consciousness in which a person readily tends to fall asleep.

Drowsiness may be the normal preliminary stage of ordinary sleep, particularly likely to occur after excessive fatigue.

It may also be a symptom of any disease which impairs the circulation of adequately-oxygenated blood to the brain or causes deficient elimination of toxins as in heart disease or kidney disease with uraemia.

Many drugs produce drowsiness. Hypnotic drugs are given to induce sleep and the production of drowsiness is the first stage towards achieving the desired result. Tranquillizers on the other hand are given to reduce cerebral activity and anxiety while preserving normal awareness, and drowsiness is an unwanted side-effect. Attempts to overcome this dilemma have resulted in the great variety of formulations now being marketed.

There is, however, less obvious risk of drowsiness with many modern drugs given for quite different purposes; medicines given for heart disease, high blood pressure, troublesome cough, thyroid over-activity, diabetes, epilepsy, migraine, motion sickness and hay-fever are examples. Care is required when patients taking them have to drive road vehicles or work at tasks requiring care and alertness.

drug addiction. See ADDICTION.

drug rashes. Skin eruptions of diverse type produced by the toxic effects of drugs on the skin.

In most cases drug rashes are not precisely typical of any particular drug and may take any form, such as red patches, small haemorrhages in the skin or itchy weals. They can easily be confused with various infectious diseases but consideration of the history, the anomalous distribution, their variability, and the occurrence of weals should avoid mistakes. Rashes of these types occur with a wide variety of common drugs – aspirin, salicylates, barbiturates, sulphonamides, belladonna, coumarin, phenothiazine, penicillin and other antibiotics – to name only a few.

Some drugs on the other hand produce specific rashes with characteristics which can be recognized. Bromides, iodides, antipyrine, and phenolphthalein are the most common of these.

A third group of substances produce skin effects in a rather different way. Protein-containing substances such as vaccines and sera may produce an allergic skin reaction usually in the form of itchy swellings.

The treatment of drug rashes is to stop the drug and allay skin irritation with some suitable soothing lotion.

drugs. Any substances used in medicine for the treatment of disease or the alleviation of symptoms.

The study of drugs and their action upon living cells and tissues is known as pharmacology, a branch of knowledge which only began to achieve its present stature as a science during the present century.

The advent of the organic chemist and

developments in medicine and related sciences have resulted not only in the availability of an enormous range of completely new specific remedies but in the facilities to determine their mode of action and their effectiveness as therapeutic agents.

Vitamins, hormones, biological products creating immunity, sulphonamides, antibiotics and interferons are examples of drugs developed in modern times.

Hazards of drugs. The very potency and wide distribution of many new and powerful drugs has produced accompanying risks. Many may produce undesirable and dangerous side-effects or lead to ADDICTION. The well known thalidomide tragedy illustrates the completely unexpected effects which can result unless new products are exhaustively tested and controlled. Lastly, there is the danger of accidental or deliberate poisoning.

It is now more essential than ever that any drug should be taken in strict accordance with qualified instructions and that all medicines should be safeguarded from improper use or accidental ingestion.

drunkenness. A state of habitual intemperance in which the excessive consumption of ALCOHOL leads to chronic intoxication.

ductless glands. Glands which produce chemical substances to control various bodily processes but which have no secretory duct or tube. They are known also as ENDOCRINE GLANDS and the special substances or hormones which they produce pass directly into the blood stream.

ductus arteriosus. A blood vessel in unborn children joining the pulmonary artery to the aorta so that blood circulates without passing through the lungs, which are, of course, not yet functioning. The oxygen supply for the infant's blood is drawn from the mother's blood in the placenta.

After birth the ductus normally closes. An unclosed or patent ductus arteriosus is a fairly common variety of congenital heart disease but is easily treated by tying a ligature round the vessel.

dumbness. The state of being without the power of speech.

It is essential to differentiate between the child who has never spoken and the individual previously able to speak who has become dumb. In the latter the causes are either diseases affecting the speech centres in the brain – APHASIA – or disabilities affecting the mechanism of voice production – APHONIA.

The dumb child is a more complex problem. Speech is not an inborn ability; it is a skill which has to be learned by imitation, and if a child does not learn to speak by the usual time there is either failure to hear or inability of the centres in the brain to appreciate and reproduce what is heard. DEAFNESS is thus of two kinds: (1) where the fault lies in the ear or its connections with the brain; (2) where

the fault is in the brain centres. If the degree of hearing loss or brain-damage is considerable the child will be dumb or fail to acquire acceptable speech.

Dumbness in a child may therefore be due to (1) defects of the mechanism of hearing, (2) mental deficiency, and (3) aphasia due to brain damage. The speciality of audiology seeks to investigate the relative importance of these factors in the patient in order to make a decision about treatment and education.

duodenal ulcer. An ulcer of the small intestine, characterized by pain, sensation of fullness and tenderness in the pit of the stomach, the symptoms usually arising some two to four hours after a meal and being temporarily relieved by taking food. The immediate cause is excess quantity or undue acidity of secreted juices which in effect begin to digest the lining of the duodenum. Hence treatment involves alkaline drugs to combat excessive acidity, atropine or a similar drug to reduce activity and spasm of the stomach and duodenum, mild sedatives to improve physical and mental rest, avoidance of smoking or alcohol before meals (since these stimulate the flow of juices), and regular, well-chewed meals. Treatment generally starts with a very bland diet consisting mainly of milk, custard and junket, but progresses rapidly to a fairly normal diet with, however, permanent avoidance of highly indigestible foods. Surgical treatment is very seldom needed, and the very strict dietetic regime of the past is nowadays regarded as being needed for only a very few weeks.

Duodenal and gastric ulcer produce very similar symptoms and respond to much the same treatment, so clinical workers have tended to class them together; but they are widely different in respect of relative frequency in men and women and in rich and poor people, in probable causes and indeed in most of the features studied by epidemiologists.

Duodenal ulcer is four times commoner in men while gastric is about equally common in the two sexes; duodenal is more frequent in the more affluent social groups while gastric is rather commoner in the poor; and duodenal is on the increase whereas gastric is not. While both are similar to the extent that the mucous membrane is irritated and eroded by over-acid secreted juices, the underlying causes of duodenal ulcer appear to include an over-active, ambitious or worrying personality while gastric ulcer is associated more with nutritional factors.

While regular and well-chewed meals and avoidance of smoking before meals may contribute to the prevention of duodenal ulcer, the main preventive measure is clearly attention to personality development in the early formative years, including attempts to avoid excessive ambition without removing all desire for progress and attempts to create reasonable sense of security without inducing smugness and total incapacity for worry.

dura mater. The outermost of the three membranous layers which enclose the brain and spinal cord. It is tough and fibrous.

dust. Dust is any dry powdery material of a particle size small enough to remain suspended in (or be wafted by) the air.

Its importance in relation to medicine lies in the varieties of lung disease which it can produce when inhaled with air. Disease of this kind is known by the general name of pneumoconiosis of which there are many examples related to different trades and industrial processes.

Dusts may be either inorganic or organic and the distinction is of importance in relation to the type of disease which they produce.

Inorganic dusts. Of these the most damaging is undoubtedly silica in various forms. Typical industrial processes involving silica are sand-blasting, flint and pebble crushing, manufacture of refractory bricks and materials, pottery manufacture, grinding of metals, manufacture of scouring powders and abrasive soaps, quarrying, tunnelling and mining of all kinds.

It used to be thought that the disease condition silicosis was produced by damage from the sharp edged 'sandy' particles, but by some classic experiments it was eventually shown that silica (silicon dioxide) forms silicic acid in the tissues and that it is this that causes damage to the lung.

Another important factor is particle size; anything smaller than five-thousandths of a millimetre becomes increasingly hazardous.

Other common inorganic dust diseases are anthracosis of coal-miners, siderosis found in knife grinders and metal polishers and asbestosis affecting asbestos workers. Although each has some special features all are essentially due to silica in some form. Asbestosis carries a special risk of eventually inducing malignancy.

Organic dusts. A wide variety of trades produce organic dusts which although less harmful than silica may produce chronic respiratory disease of a bronchitic character. Byssinosis is related to the cotton industry and bagassosis to the conversion of spent sugar cane into insulating board.

Organic dusts also carry other hazards such as anthrax from wool-sorting and tetanus from jute processing. Mycosis of the lung may arise from malting or from the handling of mouldy straw.

Chemical dusts. Inhalation of these cause various types of poisoning. Compounds of chromium, lead, arsenic, zinc manganese, cadmium and nickel are the chief offenders.

House dust. In conclusion reference must be made to house dust which may cause illness in quite a different way. Compounded as it is of finely divided particles derived from textiles, feathers, hair and fur of pets, and even the dried and broken down tissues of the house mite, it contains allergens which may provoke attacks of asthma in susceptible subjects.

See also ASPERGILLOSIS.

dwarfism. A condition in which an individual animal or plant fails to grow to normal height having regard to its age and species.

The causation of human dwarfism is complex. Some races of mankind such as the pygmies are typically all very small although otherwise perfectly formed. Their stature is determined by their normal genetic inheritance and this is known as primordial dwarfism. Similarly small parents of all races tend to have small children.

Other varieties of dwarfism are due to disease or organic abnormality of some kind and these causes may be divided into (1) disorders of the endocrine glands, (2) various general diseases, and (3) genetic abnormalities.

Endocrine abnormality. Growth hormone is an internal secretion produced by the pituitary gland. Deficiency leads to the condition of infantilism, in which the individual is not deformed but is abnormally small for his age. The typical pituitary type dwarf is often not much more than 60 cm. (2 ft.) tall but is otherwise intelligent and well-formed. This is the Tom Thumb or circus-freak kind of dwarf, but another variety of pituitary abnormality can produce Fröhlich's syndrome or dystrophia adiposo-genitalis in which fatness and defective sexual development are the main features rather than extreme diminutiveness. Deficiency of thyroid secretion produces the thyroid dwarf or cretin who is mentally retarded, slow and apathetic, as well as being of small stature.

Other diseases. Retarded or deficient growth is seen in a variety of conditions which influence nutrition and development. Examples are rickets, coeliac disease, pancreatic disease and vitamin deficiency.

Genetic abnormalities. Best known of these is achondroplasia. In the achondroplasic dwarf the arms and legs are short in relation to the body ('human dachshund'). The condition is inherited as a Mendelian dominant, as is another rare disease, osteogenesis imperfecta, where there is both diminished stature and fragility of the bones.

In glycogen-storage disease which is inherited as a recessive characteristic there is excessive storage of glycogen and failure to bring it into the blood as required, so that the blood-sugar remains low and growth and development are retarded.

Treatment. For pituitary dwarfism, pituitary growth-hormone may be given by injection but the results are not particularly impressive. Cretins respond well to the administration of thyroxin although their mental retardation may not be improved. The treatment of vitamin deficiencies is straightforward. Little can be done to influence the other congenital and genetic conditions.

dysentery. Infection of the large intestine, characterized by severe diarrhoea, abdominal pain, painful desire to pass a motion and the presence of blood and mucus in motions.

1. Amoebic dysentery. This type is common in the tropics, caused by infection by a single-celled organism, *Entamoeba histolytica*, which usually reaches the victim from food or water contaminated from the excreta of a previous victim. Hence prevention is essentially a matter of proper sanitary facilities and personal hygiene especially by all food handlers. Typical symptoms are as indicated above, but some people have amoebic dysentery for long periods almost without symptoms. Emetine is still regarded as the drug of choice, though some of the newer antibiotics (e.g., paromomycin) are also claimed to be useful. The very fact that new drugs are being tried indicates that the existing treatments are not always fully effective.

2. Bacillary dysentery. Much commoner and occurring in all climates, the bacillary type is caused by infection by bacteria of the genus *Shigella*. The types most frequently seen are, in descending order of severity: the Shiga variety, common in the Far East, often associated with violent diarrhoea and dehydration, even to the extent of being confused with cholera; the milder Flexner variety which can nevertheless cause severe illness; and the relatively mild Sonne variety which usually results in two or three days of slight illness. Many other varieties exist. Transmission is normally by contaminated food or water, so prevention involves essentially the same measures as for prevention of amoebic dysentery. Soluble drugs which are absorbed from the gut to the blood stream (and so useful in many infections) are useless here. Treatment is by insoluble sulphonamides or insoluble antibiotics.

Bacillary dysentery, even of Sonne type, is serious in young babies. Diarrhoea occurring in a nursery or children's hospital should be regarded as dysentery until a definite diagnosis has been made.

dyslexia. An inability to read properly owing to a disorder of the brain causing letters to be confused (e.g., d and b) or the order of letters in a word to be altered (e.g., 'cat' read as 'tac'). Dyslexic children may be of normal intelligence, so that treatment, although difficult, is well worth attempting.

Until the last few years dyslexia usually remained undiagnosed and untreated, but diagnostic tests have now been developed and specially equipped teachers have had some success in treating the condition.

dysmenorrhoea. Pain during menstruation. Primary dysmenorrhoea is pain of this nature affecting girls from the start of their periods. The pain may be due to spasm of the uterus, congestion of the uterus, defective balance of hormones or emotional factors. In many cases the pain is relieved by drugs that relax spasm or by hormone treatment, including contraceptive pills. Secondary dysmenorrhoea is pain of this nature occurring in women who have previously had painless periods. It may be due to a number of gynaecological conditions and, if persisting, requires special investigation.

dyspareunia. Painful coitus. In males the common causes are inflammation and tightness of the foreskin, both easily treated. In women the condition may be due to a well-developed hymen, to inflammation of the vagina or to shrinkage of the vagina after the menopause, but in many cases it is the result of an involuntary contraction of the muscles immediately before coitus, i.e., an expression of unconscious aversion to sex. Medical examination should exclude or deal with physical causes. If none are found, a great deal of tact and patience is required to remove the underlying emotional causes which may be rooted in earlier unpleasant experiences.

dyspepsia. Discomfort after eating and difficulty in digesting food; see INDIGESTION.

dysphagia. Difficulty in swallowing. It may arise from any painful condition of the throat, such as tonsillitis or quinsy; from paralysis of the muscles of swallowing, in certain nervous diseases; from pressure of tumours in the vicinity of the throat; and occasionally from hysteria. Treatment depends on the cause.

dyspnoea. Undue BREATHLESSNESS and abnormal awareness of the effort of breathing.

E

ear. The organ of hearing and balance; it is divided into three parts.

1. The outer ear consists of the pinna (large and movable in many animals to help to collect and locate sounds) and the sound canal, or external auditory meatus, which passes inwards and forwards to end at the eardrum. Sound waves travel along the meatus and vibrate the eardrum.

2. The middle ear is a small cavity in the temporal bone, separated from the external meatus by the tympanic membrane or eardrum. The cavity is bridged by three tiny bones – malleus, incus and stapes (otherwise called the hammer, the anvil and the stirrup) – which pass vibrations from the drum to the inner ear. At the back the cavity has an incomplete wall, with the hole leading to the mastoid antrum, and in front of that there is a communication with the Eustachian tube leading to the back of the nose.

3. The inner ear consists of several cavities in the petrous part of the temporal bone. The cavities are collectively called the labyrinth and consist of (1) a central part called the vestibule with which all other parts communicate, (2) three semicircular canals all at right angles to each other, and (3) the cochlea, a spiral tube twisted on itself and resembling a snail-shell.

Movement of fluid within the three semicircular canals is responsible for the sense of balance. Inside the cochlea is the organ of Corti which is the true organ of hearing. The cochlea is filled with fluid and contains hair-bearing cells linked up with the auditory nerve, which carries impulses of hearing to the brain. Vibrations received by the eardrum are transmitted by the three bones in the middle ear, the last of which, the stapes, closes the small hole between the middle and inner ear. Thus the vibrations of these bones set up waves in the cochlear fluid and these stimulate the hair-cells. Here they are altered into electric currents which pass along nerve fibres to the brain.

Earache. Causes include:

1. Changes in atmospheric pressure (e.g., in an aeroplane) when a blockage of the Eustachian tube, as occurs in a head cold, makes it difficult to equalize the internal and external pressure on the eardrum.

2. Wax in the meatus (see below) especially in association with changes in atmospheric pressure.

3. A foreign body in the meatus. This is fairly rare in adults, though an insect has been known to fly in and be unable to get out, but not uncommon in children. A foreign body can often be floated out in a few drops of oil, a much less dangerous procedure than seeking to extract it with tweezers.

4. A boil in the meatus. An appropriate antibiotic may help, and warmth – e.g., application of a comfortably warm rubber hot-water bottle – may temporarily ease the pain.

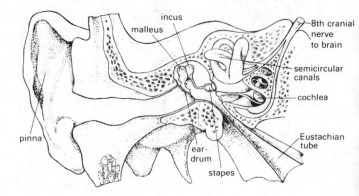

Anatomy of the ear

5. Inflammation or increased pressure in the middle ear known as otitis media; see below. This cause is very dangerous, since the infection may spread to the mastoid and thence to the meninges, causing meningitis. Hence, unless the cause of earache is obvious, a painful ear should warrant immediate medical attention.

Wax in the ears. Wax is a normal secretion of glands on the external ear canal. In some people wax accumulates and may obstruct the passage, causing temporary deafness, especially if water enters the ear during washing and makes the wax swell. The wax should be softened by introducing a few drops of slightly warmed olive or almond oil, and a day later very gently syringed out with warm water. Gentleness in syringing is essential, because excessive force may injure the eardrum. Various commercial preparations are said to be useful in breaking up wax or preventing its accumulation.

Otitis media or discharging ears. Children are particularly susceptible to inflammation of the middle ear (otitis media) occurring usually as a complication of upper respiratory tract infection or of specific diseases such as measles and scarlet fever. Enlarged and unhealthy adenoids are often present and infection reaches the middle ear by the Eustachian tube.

Usually there is pain, temperature and discharge of pus into the middle ear and on examination the eardrum (tympanic membrane) is reddened and may be distended. In pre-antibiotic days the pus accumulated until it escaped in one of three ways – by spontaneous perforation of the eardrum, by surgical puncture of the eardrum or by seeping inwards to cause inflammation of the mastoid bone and sometimes meningitis.

In chronic otitis the drum becomes perforated but, instead of the acute condition then clearing up, the discharge of pus continues for many months, and hearing usually becomes impaired.

The best treatment is an early administration of antibiotics to combat the infection, but in some cases it may be necessary to puncture the eardrum (paracentesis or myringotomy) to allow drainage of the pus. The ruptured eardrum with purulent discharge requires painstaking daily cleansing with cotton wool mops and the installation of antiseptic drops – spirit or hydrogen peroxide being commonly employed.

Other conditions. The middle ear is subject to abnormal deposit of bone cells (otosclerosis) and the inner ear may be the site of diseases both of balance and of hearing, e.g., Ménière's disease, causing HEAD NOISES, and DEAFNESS.

ecchymosis. The technical term for bleeding under the skin. A typical example is a bruise.

eclampsia. An acute but uncommon infection of the blood, occurring during pregnancy, labour, or the puerperium, and characterized by convulsions and coma. The cause is unknown.

Early symptoms include flashes of light, dizziness, headache and vomiting, and the urine has a high content of albumin. In the early stages rest, restriction of protein foods and the use of drinks to flush the kidneys are advocated. Where fits are actually occurring the patient should be given sedatives and placed in a quiet and darkened room under the care of a special nurse.

ECT. Electrical convulsive therapy. The treatment, which is essentially stimulation of a convulsion of about one minute's duration several times weekly by passing a current through two electrodes placed on the forehead, is beneficial in many cases of depressive illness (but not for corresponding cases of manic conditions) and has also some slight value in schizophrenia.

ectopic pregnancy. A pregnancy in which the embryo begins to develop elsewhere than in the uterus. Normally the ovum and sperm unite in one of the Fallopian tubes and the fertilized egg passes along to the uterus. In an ectopic pregnancy the fertilized egg becomes lodged in the tube or, much more rarely, in the ovary. Causes are normally grouped under two headings (1) those of congenital origin e.g., if the tube is unusually long or twisted or if there are indentations in the wall of the tube, and (2) acquired causes – damage to tube from previous disease.

The main symptoms are bleeding and pain, and differentiation from miscarriage is not easy. Since the condition is dangerous to the mother and since there is no chance of the embryo surviving, the normal treatment is removal of the tube and embryo by abdominal operation. Because the woman has a second tube, she can have further pregnancies.

eczema. See DERMATITIS.

effort syndrome. Also called disordered action of the heart (DAH) and soldier's heart. A neurotic state in which the individual complains of heart pains, palpitations and breathlessness, and has a loss of energy and an unwillingness to work; yet examination of the heart reveals no abnormality. Essentially the condition is an anxiety state and usually requires psychotherapy.

effusion. Leakage of fluid into one of the cavities of the body. The term is also sometimes used for the pouring out of fluid to the exterior.

ego. The conscious mind. Freud divided the mind into the super-ego (which has analogies to conscience), the ego (or personal consciousness) and the id (or primitive impulses).

ejaculatio praecox. Premature ejaculation of semen before coitus or early in coitus.

In some cases there is a lack of the normal control, so that in extreme cases the mere idea of a sexual situation can cause ejaculation. In other cases there is an extreme sensitivity of the urethra, and the ejaculation is not merely premature but sometimes painful instead of pleasurable.

The condition is a cause of a considerable amount of marital unhappiness but is seldom treated, because (1) the man generally feels shy and embarrassed and so hesitates to consult his doctor; (2) the wife who could often help by patience and reassurance is herself emotionally involved and distressed; and (3) the doctor, if consulted, is often perplexed since psychosexual problems are far removed from the illnesses that constitute the bulk of a general practitioner's work. A restoration of self-confidence is almost certainly the main necessity in treatment. To this end alcohol – by removing inhibitions and creating temporary confidence – often helps, but if neither counselling directed to restoring confidence nor the boosting of confidence by spirits helps, the advice of a psychiatrist may be required.

elbow. The hinged joint formed by the humerus (the bone of the upper arm), the ulna and the radius. The point of the elbow is the olecranon process of the ulna. The 'funny bone' is the point at which the ulnar nerve passes over the lower end of the humerus just under the skin.

There is a bursa, i.e., a small sac containing fluid, on the point of the elbow and this may become inflamed from constant pressure as from leaning on a table.

Injuries. The elbow joint is subject to sprains and dislocations, and the component bones may be fractured. Dislocations, the commonest serious injury, are usually backwards, while bending the elbow too far can tear ligaments and force a sprain. Frequent minor jarring of the joint produces the pain and stiffness described as tennis elbow, a condition involving either strain of the muscle on the outer side of the elbow joint or inflammation of the bursa lying beneath that muscle. Without treatment, other than some inevitable restriction of movement of the elbow, the symptoms disappear in about five or six months. Adequate rest of the muscle may shorten the duration appreciably, and an injection of hydrocortisone into the painful spot produces rapid alleviation of the pain.

X-ray examination is usually desirable to check whether sudden pain is caused by dislocation or fracture, so that the proper treatment can be undertaken. For other conditions the best treatment is rest.

Electra complex. Named by Freud after Electra's devotion to Agamemnon in the Greek legend, the Electra complex is excessive love by a daughter for her father, i.e., the female equivalent of the Oepidus complex.

To some extent the attraction of a child to the parent of the opposite sex is a natural phenomenon created by the equally natural phenomenon of the paren being more attracted to the child of the other sex. The expectant mother (more often than her husband) hopes that the baby will be a boy; the mother finds in the son whom she has reared the desirable qualities that originally attracted her to her husband; the daughter becomes the apple of her father's eye; and the chil naturally responds to the parent tha shows the greater interest and sympathy.

It is important that parents should try to show equal interest in – and sympathy with – children of both sexes. In extreme cases excessive attraction of a child to the parent of the opposite sex can not only make it difficult for that child to find a marriage partner but can also lead to repression and psychoneurosis.

electric shock. A person touching a 'live electric wire and receiving a shock may be unable to let go, or may fall to the groun unconscious and with breathing stopped. If the victim is still in contact, the rescuer should turn off the current if practicable or, failing that, should use insulating material, such as a dry stick or a piece o rubber, to remove the victim from the wire. If breathing has stopped, artificia respiration should be carried out.

electrocardiogram. A tracing (usually known as an ECG), made by an electrocardiograph, of the electrical changes in the heart muscles. The electrodes of the electrocardiograph which is essentially a sensitive galvanometer, are normally fastened on both arms and on a leg, with sometimes a fourth electrode placed over the heart They detect the impulses produced by the heart as it beats and they produce a record of these impulses as a tracing on paper The procedure in no way hurts the patient

Examination of the tracing reveals disturbances of rhythm, damage to heart muscle and imbalance between the two sides of the heart with remarkable precision.

The procedure is sometimes used in ordinary, thorough medical examination but is more often employed where there is a suspicion of some cardiac abnormality and is regularly used to check progress and recovery after a heart attack.

electroencephalogram. A record, made by an electroencephalograph (or EEG), o electrical changes in the brain. By placing the electrodes on different parts of the scalp the discharges from various portions of the brain can be studied.

Electroencephalograms are now used routinely for the diagnosis of mino varieties of epilepsy (which were formerly difficult to differentiate from othe conditions) and they are also valuable fo the recognition of certain other disorder of the brain. There is, however, some variation in the tracings obtained from normal individuals, with about one-eighth of ordinary persons having 'abnormal electroencephalograms. Hence an EEG, while a useful aid to diagnosis, cannot be used in isolation.

electrolysis. Chemical destruction of tissue by passage of electrical currents. The procedure is sometimes used to destroy birth marks, warts and the roots of superfluous hair.

elephantiasis. Gross enlargement of parts of the body (the legs below the knee being most often involved, with the scrotum, breasts and arms sometimes affected) due to obstruction of the lymphatic vessels by a parasitic worm, filaria. The embryos of the worms are conveyed to the body by the bite of an infected mosquito. Diethylcarbamazine is the only effective drug but sometimes causes allergic reactions which can be avoided or modified by the use of antihistamine preparations.

The term elephantiasis is also sometimes applied to an enlargement of the leg that may arise from inflammation and partial blockage of lymph glands after childbirth. See WHITELEG.

emaciation. Extreme loss of flesh and wasting of the body. Causes include: (1) various severe disorders, e.g., cancer, chronic nephritis and tuberculosis, (2) starvation, (3) dehydration, i.e., extrème loss of fluid, as in cholera, (4) terminal stages of a few rare organic diseases of the nervous system, and (5) anorexia nervosa and hysterical refusal of food. Progressive loss of weight is always an indication for medical investigation.

embolism. Blockage of an artery by an embolus, e.g., a fragment of a diseased heart valve, a fragment of a blood clot, a foreign body or an air-bubble. The effects of an embolism depend on the size and position of the vessel blocked. If the vessel is small and there is an alternative channel of circulation, the effects may be minimal. If the blockage is in an artery of the brain the embolism may cause paralysis of one side of the body (hemiplegia), if in the retinal artery it may cause blindness of one eye, and if in a coronary artery it may cause sudden death.

In some circumstances surgical removal of an embolus is practicable.

embrocations and liniments. Preparations that are rubbed into the skin for the treatment of muscle strains, joint sprains and injured ligaments, to encourage the dispersal of inflammatory nodules as in fibrositis. Soap liniment is a simple alcoholic solution of soap and camphor, suitable for most mild cases. Camphorated soap liniment is a stronger preparation containing a little ammonia as a stimulant. Camphorated oil is a much favoured application for the chest and back of children. Various other liniments are also in common use.

Most liniments are poisonous if taken internally. They should therefore be kept in a safe place, along with other poisons, and should not be applied to broken skin.

embryo. The unborn offspring from the time of union of the ovum and the sperm to the time, about two months later, when its form has become recognizably human. After that time the term 'foetus' is used.

The ovum is fertilized in the Fallopian tube and the resultant embryo is just large enough to be visible to the naked eye; it travels down the Fallopian tube to the uterus, implants itself in the uterine wall and divides and re-divides into a cluster of cells. The outer cells in due course form the placenta (from which the embryo draws nourishment from the mother) and the chorion, or outer membrane, enveloping the embryo. The inner cells form the amnion, or inner protective membrane, and the embryo proper.

Growth of the embryo proper occurs in three separate layers. The ectoderm or outer layer forms an outer wrapping and curls over to create an inner tube (the neural tube). The skin is later formed from the outer wrapping and the nervous system from the inner tube. The endoderm or inner growth layer later forms the digestive system and the lungs; and the mesoderm, or middle growth layer, forms the heart, muscles and bones.

As the embryo grows it essentially re-enacts human evolution. At about three weeks it has gill-slits, occurring in the same position as the gills of a fish; by a few weeks later it is definitely mammalian; and by eight or nine weeks it is identifiable as human in its structure.

By that age the embryo is about 4 cm. (1.5 in.) long, has a relatively enormous head of about 2 cm. (0.75 in.) and very rudimentary limbs. It has lost its tail and its heart has begun to pump blood through the system.

By about 16 weeks the foetus is roughly 10 cm. (4 in.) long and weighs approximately 100 g. (3.5 oz.), and by 24 weeks it has reached 20 cm. (8 in.) and 600 g. (21 oz.) and has some chance of survival if born prematurely.

emetic. A substance given to induce vomiting. This may be needed in cases of narcotic and irritant poisoning but should never be used in corrosive poisoning, i.e., in poisoning by strong acids and alkalis. An easily prepared emetic is a tablespoonful of mustard to half a tumblerful of water or two tablespoonfuls of salt to the same amount of water.

emission. See NOCTURNAL EMISSIONS.

emotion. The state of consciousness in which such sensations as joy, love, anger and hate are experienced.

The emotions give colour and vitality to life. They govern our behaviour to a greater extent than does reason and they enable us when strongly moved to perform feats of physical and mental endurance which would be impossible in the absence of emotion. The completely unemotional person tends to lack drive and to be unattracted to others.

Emotions, however, are considerably

modified by upbringing. We learn, for example, not to hit someone when we are angry, and a soldier learns not to run away when afraid. For the proper development of character, the emotions, which have free expression in a baby, must come increasingly under the general control of persisting sentiments. In a healthy mind there should be a reasonable balance between, on the one hand, expression of emotion and, on the other, conformity not only to the patterns imposed by training and associates but also to the sentiments created in the formative years. Full indulgence in such emotions as rage and lust with their characteristic actions can produce conflict with others and with the law, but to give free rein to the feeling without the action can harm the individual, e.g., the man who masks his barely controlled fury may have a dangerous rise in blood pressure or develop indigestion. On the other hand, excessive repression of emotions can contribute very materially to the production of PSYCHOSOMATIC DISEASE and also of NEUROSIS.

In the rearing of children the fostering of emotional health is particularly important, and there are four points to be especially noted.

1. For the child's emotional development he needs a sense of security, an awareness of continuing parental affection and a reasonably permissive atmosphere with only such rules and restrictions as are essential for his safety or for the well-being of the household.

2. Battles of wills should be avoided. Parental victory carries with it dangers of resentment and repression of feelings in the child and certainly does not help his emotional development; child victory is even more dangerous, leading to the 'spoiled' child who later has to learn with difficulty that a hard world will not conform to his wishes. It is better to distract the child, or ignore him, during an emotional crisis, and at an unemotional period to seek to discuss the situation in an attempt to work out a solution satisfactory to both parent and child.

3. The child (an imitator from infancy) should be made aware of his parents' love of fair-play, justice, beauty etc., and gradually brought to see that most human situations involve the feelings and desires of more than one person.

4. Complete supression of emotion should not be encouraged. The 'stiff upper lip' policy of the past can perhaps be correlated with the fact that one British adult in every nine receives treatment during his life for a disorder of emotional origin.

emphysema. A condition in which the fine air-cells of the lungs are distended and their dividing walls destroyed, so that less space remains available for the exchange of oxygen and carbon dioxide. Emphysema occurs as a result of the physical stress of frequent coughing, in chronic bronchitis and sometimes in asthma, or as a result of years of blowing wind musical instruments. It causes the chest to become enlarged and barrel-shaped, is associated with breathlessness, and may ultimately damage the heart.

Since lung tissues cannot be replaced, treatment consists essentially of dealing with the causal disease before the emphysema has developed. In existing emphysema residence in a warm, dry climate is often beneficial, breathing exercises may help and the patient should be given a portable oxygen inhaler to use at need.

empyema. A condition in which pus is present in the chest cavity, between the two layers of pleura. Before the era of antibiotics it was not uncommon as a complication of pneumonia, and it can also arise from wounds of the chest.

Symptoms are pain, breathlessness and swinging temperature. Treatment consists of removal of pus through a hollow needle inserted through the chest wall, followed by injection of penicillin solution. During convalescence breathing exercises are useful to promote expansion of the lung and to prevent adhesions.

encephalitis. Inflammation of the brain. It occurs (1) as a rare complication of almost all of the acute infectious diseases, (2) through virus infection, as in ENCEPHALITIS LETHARGICA, or rabies, (3) following wounds of the skull, (4) from spread of inflammation from the ear or nose, and (5) very infrequently as a complication of vaccination against some diseases.

Symptoms include headache, irritability, fever and vomiting, followed by convulsions and drowsiness. Sulphonamides and antibiotics are the drugs of choice.

encephalitis lethargica. An inflammation of the brain, caused by a virus, and characterized by headache, high temperature, double vision and disturbance of sleep rhythm – drowsiness by day and irritability at night. Complete recovery is unusual, the majority of victims being left with disturbance of muscular co-ordination (post-encephalitic parkinsonism).

There was a widespread outbreak in many countries from 1917 to 1923, but since then the disease has disappeared.

The condition is sometimes known as 'sleepy sickness' and should not be confused with SLEEPING SICKNESS, a tropical disease caused by a trypanosome transmitted by the bite of a tsetse fly.

endemic. Persistently present. The term is used to indicate diseases always present in a population, in contrast to epidemics: e.g., bronchitis is endemic in Britain, whereas at intervals there is an epidemic of influenza.

endocarditis. Inflammation of the lining of the HEART, particularly that of the valves. It can occur as a complication of rheumatic fever (rheumatic endocarditis) or from bacterial infection (bacterial endocarditis).

The heart valve becomes deformed, so that it does not close fully when the heart contracts. Apart from damage to the circulation there is a danger of a fragment of a deformed valve being carried in the blood-stream and producing an EMBOLISM.

Bacterial endocarditis responds well to antibiotics. Rheumatic endocarditis may largely subside after the rheumatic fever is cured, but in some cases the valves are so badly damaged as to warrant surgical repair.

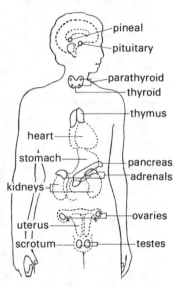

The endocrine glands

endocrine glands. The endocrine glands are ductless glands which pump the hormones or 'chemical messengers' of the body directly into the blood-stream. These messengers are as important as the brain and nervous system: for instance growth, menstruation and the changes that occur during pregnancy are in no way under the control of the brain, but are regulated by hormone secretion from the endocrine glands.

Study of these glands and the hormones they produce has widely affected scientific opinion about the functioning of mind and body, and has given increased understanding of human behaviour. Anomalies of development, idiosyncracies of personality and some mental disorders have been found to be related to variations in the activity of the glands.

Analysis of the exact functions of the various glands is difficult because (1)

several of the glands produce more than one hormone, e.g., the pituitary secretes at least eight; (2) several glands may be involved in a single function, e.g., growth depends largely on a hormone from the pituitary but partly on hormones from the thyroid and the sex glands; (3) there are complex relationships between the nervous and chemical functions of the body, e.g., the conscious emotion of rage stimulates the secretion of adrenaline by the suprarenal glands; and (4) the effect produced by a hormone depends not only on the amount of hormone secreted but also on the responsiveness of the organ or tissue, e.g., the same amount of secreted hormone may create excess, or normal amounts, or sparsity of facial hair.

The individual glands are; pituitary, thyroid, parathyroid, adrenal (or suprarenal), thymus, islets of Langerhans in the pancreas, male testes and female ovaries. These are described separately, but their interconnections should be remembered, e.g., a pituitary hormone stimulates the thyroid to produce more thyroxine and an excess of thyroxine lowers pituitary secretion.

Pituitary. The pituitary, a two-lobed gland about the size of a pea, lies at the base of the skull, beneath the central part of the brain and resting on a depression of the spenoid bone. Despite its small size the pituitary produces various hormones which in part control the other endocrine glands, so that it is often called 'the conductor of the endocrine orchestra'.

The front lobe of the pituitary secretes at least six hormones. These include a growth hormone which controls the growth of the skeleton, a thyroid-stimulating hormone, adrenocortico-trophin (ACTH), which controls the activity of the cortex of the adrenal glands, gonadotrophic hormones which regulate the activity of the ovaries and testes, and prolactin which is responsible for the secretion of milk in the nursing mother.

The rear lobe of the pituitary releases two hormones – vasopressin, which causes constriction of small arteries and also acts on the kidney, regulating water absorption and hence the amount of urine, and oxytocin, which stimulates the muscles of the uterus causing it to contract during labour.

The secretory activities of the pituitary itself are regulated partly by messages from the portion of the brain that appears to control emotions (hypothalamus) and partly by 'feed-back' from the hormones secreted by the other endocrine glands.

Thyroid. The thyroid gland in the front of the neck consists of two lobes (roughly 5 cm. long and 3 cm.) on each side of the windpipe and connected by a narrow isthmus. It manufactures two hormones, thyroxine and tri-iodothyronine. These secretions regulate the rate at which the body uses energy, e.g., speeding up the heart rate and the respiratory rate by extra secretion where necessary.

Parathyroid. These are four tiny glands (about 6 mm. by 2 mm.) lying behind the thyroid. Hormones secreted by these glands control the level of calcium and phosphorus in the blood by regulating the excretion of phosphates by the kidneys and by mobilizing calcium from its stores in the bones.

Adrenal or suprarenal. These are two bean-sized glands situated above the kidneys. The outer shell of each gland is called the cortex and produces several steroid hormones, one of which (aldosterone) regulates the levels of sodium and potassium in the blood and urine, while another (cortisol or hydrocortisone) permits the formation of glucose from protein – with excess leading to hyperglycaemia, and insufficiency causing hypoglycaemia. Other hormones from the cortex (androgens) are responsible for the development at adolescence of the scrotum, penis, prostate and larynx and for the growth of facial hair; and in both sexes they stimulate sexual activity.

The inner core or medulla of the suprarenals secretes two hormones, adrenaline and noradrenaline. Adrenaline combats the metabolic consequences of stress: that is to say, it raises the level of blood sugar by mobilizing glucose from stores in the liver, dilates the bronchioles to allow greater intake of oxygen and speeds up the heart rate. Noradrenaline constricts the peripheral blood vessels, reserving blood for the parts that are more important in fighting. In short, the suprarenal hormones prepare the body for 'fight or flight'.

Thymus. A two-lobed gland lying behind the breast bone and extending into the neck. It grows until puberty and thereafter shrinks away to practically nothing. The function of its secretion is imperfectly understood but it is concerned with the production of lymphocytes and of antibodies to infection and there is some evidence that it is also concerned with growth and development.

The islets of Langerhans. While the pancreas is a gland with a duct, carrying digestive juices to the small intestine, small portions of tissue embedded in the pancreas have entirely separate functions. They secrete insulin which is responsible for the level of blood sugar, for the utilization of sugar in the tissue and so for the production of energy.

The ovaries. Besides producing ova (eggs), the ovaries secrete various hormones including oestrogen and progesterone. These are responsible for the growth and development of the uterus and vagina at puberty, for the menstrual cycle and for the changes that take place in the uterus during pregnancy. Progesterone is thought to be the cause of fluid retention, weight gain and psychological change in pregnancy.

The testes. Besides producing spermatozoa, the testes secrete a hormone testosterone. It is responsible for the maturation of the spermatozoa and for the development and maintenance of masculine characteristics.

Additionally the stomach secretes hormones needed for digestion and the kidney produces a hormone which regulates the production of red blood corpuscles.

Diseases of endocrine glands. Only the main diseases can be mentioned here.

Tumour or syphilitic disease of the pituitary may result in either increased or decreased secretion, and may affect both lobes or only one. Increased secretion in a child causes giantism, resulting in a weakly giant of seven to eight feet tall and, in an adult, acromegaly. Decreased secretion causes stunting of skeletal development, depression of sexual function, mental retardation and increase of fat tissue. Diseases of under-activity go under various names, e.g., Simmond's disease, diabetes insipidus and Brissaud's disease, according to which symptoms predominate. Headaches and disturbances of vision, especially of colour vision, are common in diseases of the pituitary but have many other causes.

Thyroid over-activity without excessive secretion occurs from lack of iodine in food and water and creates simple goitre. Deficiency of thyroid secretion – from congenital causes, from tumours or from extreme lack of iodine – in childhood causes cretinism, and in adults myxoedema. Excessive activity of the thyroid causes hyperthyroidism or Graves' disease.

Over-activity of the parathyroids (most commonly caused by a benign tumour) leads either to renal calculus, from excess calcium in the blood and hence formation of a 'stone' in the kidney, or to signs of calcium excess in the blood, namely weight loss, lack of appetite, nausea, drowsiness and weakness. Tetany, still ascribed to parathyroid deficiency in some text-books, can actually be caused by such deficiency – which, however, practically never occurs except in rare circumstances of the parathyroids being damaged during an operation on the thyroid. It is far more often due to malabsorption of calcium or lack of vitamin D.

Over-active adrenals cause Cushing's syndrome, characterized by obesity, high blood pressure and absence of menstruation. Depending on the part of the gland most affected this can also cause masculinization of women, with increased facial hair and enlargement of the clitoris, and in males can lead to precocious puberty. Deficiency causes the progressive muscular weakness and skin pigmentation known as Addison's disease.

An enlarged thymus can cause pressure on the trachea which results in breathing difficulties; this is usually found in children who are fat, anaemic and lethargic (see STATUS LYMPHATICUS). Treatment is by irradiation of the thymus gland with x-rays.

Insufficiency of insulin production by the islets of Langerhans in the pancreas leads to the condition of diabetes mellitus.

Deficiency of the secretions of the ovary leads to absence of menstruation, lack of development of the female characteristics at puberty, and infertility. Decrease of ovarian activity in middle age is the main cause of menopause. Similarly, deficiency of testosterone from the testes may lead to failure to manufacture spermatozoa and hence to infertility or sterility, and also to failure of the development of the masculine characteristics at puberty.

endometritis. Inflammation of the mucus membrane lining the inside of the uterus. In the acute form the main features are abdominal pain, raised temperature and often a semi-purulent discharge from the uterus. The chronic form is characterized by pain both in the back and in the lower abdomen, and by a blood-stained discharge. The causes are numerous and treatment varies according to the cause. Hormones are often required, but some cases need operative treatment.

enema. Injection of liquid into the rectum to clear the bowel, to dispel persistent wind or, in some cases, to introduce fluid or nutrient (although a nutrient enema is usually called a rectal injection or RECTAL FEEDING). An enema is normally given before any major surgical operation.

A barium enema, containing a suspension of barium sulphate, is used in x-ray examination of the rectum and large intestine. Since the barium sulphate is opaque to x-rays, the bowel shows up clearly and any ulcers or tumours can be identified.

enteric. Literally, pertaining to the intestine. The term is used mainly for the group of infectious diseases including typhoid and paratyphoid fever.

enteric fever. A general name used to describe both TYPHOID FEVER and PARATYPHOID FEVER.

enteritis. Inflammation of the intestines, usually manifested by diarrhoea and abdominal pain. Causes include bacterial infection, virus infestation, chill, indigestible food, certain poisons, a grossly excessive meal and a heavy consumption of alcohol. If the condition is severe, bacteriological and biochemical examination of the motions is desirable. In mild cases an aperient should be given to remove any possible irritant, the patient should be rested in bed with only liquid diet for two or three days and an astringent such as chalk and catechu may be given.

enterostomy. A surgical operation by which an artificial opening is made in the intestine, usually to by-pass an obstruction created by a tumour or an ulcer. If the opening is made in the large intestine (colon) it is called a colostomy.

enuresis. See BED-WETTING.

enzyme. A highly specific catalyst produced by living cells within the body and promoting chemical changes, especially those in which complex substances are broken down into forms which the body can use. Examples are ptyalin (secreted by the salivary glands) which initiates the breakdown of starches to sugars; lactase (in gastric juice) which reduces lactose, the sugar in milk, to the simpler glucose; pepsin (also in gastric juice) which acts on protein; and tsypsin (secreted by the pancreas) which also acts on protein.

The enzymes – probably thousands in number – are in most cases essential to life. Certain poisons operate by inactivating enzymes, e.g., cyanides block the action of the particular enzyme that controls the release of oxygen from the red blood corpuscles.

Several hereditary diseases are due to enzyme deficiency, for example, phenylketonuria and cretinism.

Various enzymes are themselves activated by co-enzymes. For instance, the enzyme which causes blood to clot is at all times present in the blood but is activated only when a co-enzyme is liberated at the site of an injury.

In recent years the relationship between vitamins and enzymes has become appreciated. Most – and perhaps all – vitamins act as co-enzymes. Hence the underlying mechanism of most deficiency diseases is not simply the absence of the vitamin but the failure of an enzyme to act because of the absence of the appropriate co-enzyme.

eosinophil. A variety of white blood corpuscle containing large granules which are readily stained with the red acidic dye, eosin. Normally about 2 per cent of white blood corpuscles are eosinophils. An increase to above 4 per cent suggests the presence of – (1) certain intestinal parasites, or (2) some allergic conditions, especially asthma, or (3) various skin diseases, such as psoriasis, or (4) Hodgkins' disease or, very rarely, (5) a form of leukaemia.

ephedrine. An alkaloid drug with effects broadly resembling those of adrenalin and having the advantage that it can be taken by mouth. In some cases of asthma it eases the breathing by widening the bronchial tubes and bronchioles. It is useful in hay fever, is often included in drops or sprays to relieve nasal congestion, and is sometimes employed in eye-drops to dilate the pupil before eye examinations.

epidemic. An outbreak of disease simultaneously affecting large numbers of people. The term 'epidemic' (abnormal prevalence) was often used in contrast to 'endemic' (persistent prevalence). However 'epidemic' has in recent years come to mean simply 'widely prevalent', with the old distinction from 'endemic' lost. Likewise, the use of the term 'epidemic' is no longer restricted to infectious diseases. Thus we nowadays speak of bronchitis, coronary thrombosis, rheumatism, cancer and home and road accidents as the modern epidemics.

epidemiology. The science that studies the prevalence of a disease in the community, the groups affected and the groups spared, the methods of spread, and the effects.

Essentially while the clinician is concerned with the treatment of sick persons, the epidemiologist is concerned with disease and absence of disease in the community. Indeed the persons who escape are just as important to the epidemiologist as are those who develop the disease.

Clearly epidemiology can contribute enormously to ascertainment of the causes, and therefore of the means of prevention, of many diseases, and to working out the particular age, sex and occupation groups to which preventive techniques for particular conditions can most usefully be directed. Clearly, too, epidemiologists, clinicians and backroom laboratory workers should work together to elucidate the causes, methods of spread and means of prevention of diseases.

Yet unless the epidemiologist, the health education officer and the health visitor can collaborate, many of the findings of epidemiology will fail to improve the health of the community. To take two simple examples, epidemiological studies have proved beyond a shadow of doubt that the risks of damage from whooping cough vaccination are less than one-thousandth part the risks from whooping cough and can be further reduced by excluding the tiny proportion of children unsuitable for vaccination, and epidemiological investigations over a quarter of a century have established beyond a shadow of doubt that removal of fluoride deficiency where it exists in drinking water can enormously reduce dental disease without creating any disease whatsoever; but – because the epidemiological findings have not been suitably communicated to the public – a goodly number of parents still hesitate to have their children protected against whooping cough and many communities still resist the addition of fluoride to water deficient in it.

epidermis. The outer layer of the SKIN.

epididymis. A curved structure attached to the testicle, consisting of a twisted tube leading to the duct which conveys the sperms from the testicle.

epiglottis. A yellowish, leaf-shaped flap of fibro-cartilage situated at the back of the throat, behind the root of the tongue. During the act of swallowing the epiglottis is pressed against the opening to the larynx thus closing it, with the result that food enters the oesophagus. The not uncommon experience of choking during swallowing is a result of the epiglottis acting imperfectly or belatedly, so that particles of food enter the larynx and trachea.

The epiglottis

epilepsy. An ill-defined but common group of disorders characterized by recurrent convulsive seizures and affecting about one in every two hundred of the population.

Epileptic fits are a symptom of brain damage. Causes include hereditary defect, foetal injuries and disturbances of development, birth injuries, cerebral infections and head injuries, but in many cases no cause can be identified. In most cases the first seizures occur in childhood or adolescence, the condition is not progressive, and the person has a normal span of life.

In the severest form (grand mal) the fit is often preceded by an aura or warning such as flashes of light or ringing in the ears. This warning is usually the same for any one patient and may enable him to lie down in a safe place. With or without the aura the patient loses consciousness, becomes rigid with muscles contracted and teeth clenched for some seconds, and thereafter has violent jerkings of the limbs and facial muscles, passing in a minute or so to a comatose stage. The immediate treatment of a fit is to turn the patient on his side (lest he vomits and blocks his respiratory passages) and to place a soft object in his mouth (to prevent the tongue from being bitten).

A milder form (petit mal) is characterized by momentary loss of consciousness without convulsions; and a third form (psycho-motor seizures) is marked by restlessness and confused movements.

Various drugs (e.g., phenobarbitone and primidone) are useful for controlling fits, and an epileptic can lead a reasonably normal life. The only barriers to his physical and intellectual activity are those in which a fit would harm himself or other people.

See also CATAPLEXY.

epiphysis. Bone formed from a secondary centre of calcification. Most bones are originally formed of cartilage and later calcified. The part in which the process of calcification – technically termed ossification – first starts is called the primary centre (e.g., in the shaft of a long bone) and the portion calcified from that centre is known as the diaphysis. Ossification starts later at secondary centres (e.g., in the head of a long bone) and the portion calcified from a secondary centre is called the epiphysis.

Ultimately the epiphysis and diaphysis join and (because cartilage can grow but bone normally cannot) the growth of the bone ceases. The age of a child at death can sometimes be determined by examination of the diaphysis and epiphysis of several bones, since for any one bone the junction of the two tends to occur at a fairly constant age.

epistaxis. See NOSE BLEEDING.

epithelioma. CANCER of the surface cells (epithelium) of the skin or a mucous membrane. An epithelioma may appear as a wart, fissure or nodule. It grows fairly slowly but presently ulcerates, forming an ulcer irregular in shape and with hard floor and margins.

epulis. A benign (non-malignant) tumour on the gum, usually near a tooth socket. A minor operation suffices for its removal.

erection. The rigid state of the penis when filled with blood. Under physical or emotional stimulation (which affects the parasympathetic nerves) the muscles round the veins contract and prevent blood from leaving, so that, as more blood arrives from the arteries the organ becomes engorged, elongates and grows hard and erect.

Inability to have an erection (impotence) is usually a result of psychological difficulties and does not imply sterility. Conversely a man who is sterile, e.g., after vasectomy, can still have erections. Painful and involuntary erection is called priapism.

ergot. A drug, originally made from a fungus which grows on rye, which stimulates contraction of the uterus and is therefore used at the end of labour. Excess, as from eating infected rye bread over a period, causes poisoning, starting with itching and inflammation of the skin and going on to loss of sensation in the fingers and toes

and, in severe cases, to gangrene; this is known as St. Anthony's Fire.

The drug contains several different alkaloids and these are now generally used in pure form. Thus ergometrine is employed to stimulate uterine contractions, and ergotamine is used to relieve migraine. The alkaloids of ergot are compounds of lysergic acid and are therefore related to the hallucinogen LSD.

erogenous zones. Those parts of the body particularly sensitive to sexual stimulation, e.g. the lips, genitals and breasts.

eructation. See BELCHING.

erysipelas. A painful infection of the skin caused by streptococci, the same bacteria as cause scarlet fever.

The disease occurs most frequently on the face. The affected patch of skin is hot, dark red, painful, tender, rather shiny and with a definite raised edge. The disease spreads by extension of the edge, while blebs sometimes appear in the older portion. General symptoms include rise of temperature, headache and vomiting. Until the advent of sulphonamides and antibiotics erysipelas was considered a very dangerous disease, but it is nowadays easily controlled. The condition, however, is highly contagious, so that care is required in nursing.

In mediaeval times the disease was known as St. Anthony's Fire, and was confused with a different disease caused by ergot poisoning.

erythema. Abnormal reddening of the skin. Generalized reddening with raised temperature may indicate the beginning of an acute fever, e.g., scarlet fever or measles, while localized erythema with raised temperature suggests either early erysipelas or inflammation of a cut or wound. Erythema without rise in temperature is most commonly the result of an ALLERGY but is sometimes of toxic origin. A small irritable patch on the skin follows the bite of a midge or the sting of a nettle. A hot bath may produce a temporary generalized erythema, a blow may cause a localized erythema, and a blush is an erythema of emotional origin.

Pending investigation of the cause calamine lotion or a dusting powder may help.

erythrocyte. A red blood corpuscle. The colour is due to haemoglobin which carries oxygen from the lungs to the tissues.

erythrocyte sedimentation rate. The rate at which red blood corpuscles in a tube containing citrated blood fall out of suspension and settle at the bottom of the tube. A rapid sedimentation rate suggests the presence of active infection. However, the rate is also increased during pregnancy and in some forms of cancer.

The test (often known by its initials as the ESR) is useful to determine the presence of early infection or of late infection that has not yet cleared.

ethmoid. A light spongy bone situated at the roof of the nose, and wedged between the sockets for the eyes. The thin perpendicular central plate of the ethmoid forms the upper part of the nasal septum. The name ethmoid, meaning 'like a sieve', refers to the large number of holes in the bone; through these holes pass branches of the olfactory nerves, carrying sensations of smell to the brain.

eugenics. The science of the improvement of the human race by selective breeding. Essentially attempts to improve the mental and physical qualities of future generations fall into two groups – positive eugenics, or encouragement of the reproduction of desirable stock, and negative eugenics, or limitation of the reproduction of persons of undesirable stock.

Scientific positive eugenics is impracticable unless a community can select the qualities it deems most desirable (e.g., intelligence, beauty, physical strength or compassion). As regards negative eugenics we have to realize several points: (1) Increased knowledge of genetics enables us to forecast with reasonable accuracy the degree of probability of any two parents producing a child suffering from serious hereditary defect (e.g., spina bifida, Huntington's chorea, deaf-mutism and schizophrenia). (2) Improved antenatal and child health services greatly increase the likelihood of survival of children with such defects. (3) Oral contraceptives, male vasectomy and female tying of tubes make it possible for those who should not reproduce to enjoy normal sex lives. (4) Increased educational and occupational opportunities make it increasingly likely that the more intelligent citizens will be literate and will be members of occupational groups in which family limitation is normally practised. That is to say that unless there is widespread health education about family planning there is a real danger of a decreasing number of children of intelligent parents but no corresponding decrease in the number of children of less intelligent parents. (5) Genetic counselling, facilities for family spacing and, where necessary, family avoidance (coupled with health education on both) could drastically reduce the numbers of children born with serious hereditary defects.

Few informed workers would advocate obligatory sterilization of those who are likely to produce children with serious genetic defects; but an increasing number would suggest that the undesirability of procreation should be made known to such people and that facilities for contraception and sterilization should be made freely available.

euphoria. Abnormal elation. A feeling of well-being unrelated to actual circumstances. Alcohol and certain anti-depressant drugs produce this sensation of comfort which is undoubtedly useful in certain abnormal circumstances but is at most times dangerous in that it divorces

people from problems requiring to be solved. In this connection it should be remembered that alcohol and drugs are not the only creators of euphoria: Karl Marx called religion 'the opiate of the masses'; a declaration of war can produce a remarkable enthusiasm; and, at individual level, a young man whose proposal of marriage has just been accepted may well be in a state of euphoria.

Eustachian tubes. The two narrow passages between the cavity behind the eardrums and the back of the nose.

euthanasia. The securing of painless death, especially to a person suffering from incurable disease.

Advocates of euthanasia point out that we put incurably diseased animals to death and claim that human beings have at least an equal right to be spared suffering. Such advocates say that a temporary decision by a patient under emotional stress could be prevented by a legal requirement for him to request euthanasia twice at a specified distance of time, and that a requirement for two doctors to be involved would safeguard the patient against the persuasion of inheriting relatives.

Organized religion is opposed to euthanasia on essentially the same grounds as its opposition to suicide; and most doctors have so far taken the view that, while they should relieve pain and suffering, their function is to preserve life, not to end it.

excretion. The elimination of waste matter from the body. The working of the human machine depends on the maintenance of its energy supply and this requires the intake of sufficient fuel, i.e., food. The digestive system breaks down the raw fuel into sources of energy and waste products. Solid waste materials are excreted through the bowel, and liquid waste is excreted partly through the kidneys and partly in perspiration. Carbon dioxide and some water vapour are also excreted in the breath.

Efficient excretion is as essential to the body as is good ventilation to a house. Many minor and some major maladies are results of impaired excretion.

exercise. Physical exercise is essential for the growth and muscular development of children, and in adults is necessary for the proper functioning of the digestive, respiratory and excretory organs. Adequate regular exercise develops the muscles and maintains muscle tone, improves posture, deepens breathing and stimulates the circulation. Additionally it produces a sensation of well-being and appears to improve mental activity.

The type and amount of exercise needed varies with the individual's age, state of health, diet and other factors. In general exercise should not aim at the development of abnormal strength and endurance: big muscles have to be fed, and extra work is therefore thrown on the

Three different exercises

time spent on sport should bear in mind the Roman aim, 'a healthy mind in a healthy body'.

For those of sedentary occupation there are perhaps two points at which exercise is in special danger of being sharply reduced. The first is at the change from a learner (in school, college or university) with normal participation in organized games to an earner who has to find his own recreations and leisure activities. The second is at the period, which often coincides with promotion and increased preoccupation with work, when the middle-aged person begins to feel unfit for the strenuous pastimes of his youth. With a little care both risks can be avoided.

In middle and later life walking and golf are excellent forms of exercise, as is cycling and, in moderation, swimming. Considerable additional exercise can be secured by fairly minor changes of habits, e.g., walking to the second nearest bus stop (instead of the nearest) and in the office using stairs rather than the lift. Exercise should be regular, not spasmodic. Persons who have long discontinued strenuous activities should think of moderate ones and should be hesitant about re-starting violent activities: while somebody who has played tennis for many years may well continue at 60, to take up tennis again at that age, after having discontinued all vigorous activity at 46, is merely to put a heavy and unanticipated strain on the heart and indeed on the whole body.

Men and women who are becoming over-weight often try to counteract a sagging waist-line by increased exercise. The exercise, if reasonably moderate and regular, may be good for them in other ways but it tends to stimulate the appetite, and one has to walk many miles to use up the energy provided by a single additional slice of bread. Exercise is not a cure for obesity, a recipe for longevity or a means of preventing the ailments of old age; but regular, moderate exercise is usually beneficial.

Exercise, suited to a person's age and very gradually increased in persons of previously sedentary life, tends to be pleasant and therefore easily continued. By contrast, specific exercises – again adapted to age and physical condition – tend to be dull and to require much personal discipline for continuation. A person who considers himself in need of special exercises is perhaps as well to consult an expert about his needs, but it is a little difficult to suggest what expert to consult.

For example, in the U.K. (1) a health visitor can sometimes give very useful advice but in other cases may be preoccupied with the emotional and physical health of children and the health and well-being of the elderly; (2) a physiotherapist can sometimes give excellent guidance but in other cases has concentrated for years on the

digestive system and the heart.

Babies not yet walking should be given special daily periods for free kicking, unencumbered by clothing, but usually young children after babyhood provide their own exercise, although attention may be needed for those children who are prevented by physical disability from indulging in vigorous games. In older children and adolescents physical training and organized games are important, and those of academic disposition who grudge rehabilitation of persons recovering from serious diseases or injuries; (3) a general medical practitioner can sometimes be extremely helpful but in other cases is concerned almost exclusively with the diagnosis and treatment of illness; and (4) a gymnast can sometimes give very useful guidance but in other cases is preoccupied with the advanced training of athletes.

Three simple examples are given here:

1. To strengthen the muscles of the arms and shoulders, stretch the arms sharply to the sides and then swing them in an arc up above the head and down again.

2. To strengthen the leg and thigh muscles, start from a standing position and first rise onto the toes; from there bend the knees until the buttocks almost touch the heels and then slowly resume the standing position.

3.To strengthen the abdominal muscles, crouch with the weight on the hands which are placed rather more than the shoulder-width apart palms down on the ground; from there shoot the legs backwards till the body and legs are straight.

See also KEEPING FIT.

exophthalmic goitre. A condition in which the eyeballs protrude, giving a staring appearance, and the person is nervous and over-excitable. The cause is over-activity of the thyroid gland. See GOITRE.

expectorant. Any drug which aids the expulsion of phlegm or sputum (spit) from the bronchial tubes. Essentially expectorants – of which ipecacuanha, squills and senega are examples – increase the flow of mucus and so make the expulsion of phlegm easier, and they also stimulate the cough centre in the brain.

expiration. Breathing out.

exposure to cold. Prolonged exposure to cold, insufficient to cause frost bite, results in HYPOTHERMIA which may end in death. Less severe cold (with which a healthy person's body's temperature regulating mechanism can normally cope) can cause local effects. For instance, elderly people with little fat in their skin may develop an itchy rash on legs or arms; this is most marked on exposure to sharp changes of temperature, such as undressing in a cold bedroom or sitting close to a fire after enduring a cold external temperature. In susceptible persons cold causes the bluish-red, itchy swellings known as chilblains. Another example is where the feet have been long immersed in cold water: the numbness and cramp known as trench foot may develop.

In all cases gradual warming is the most important feature in treatment. Prevention includes adequate wrapping up before going outside in cold weather, reasonable heating of bedrooms and bathrooms and avoidance of alcohol for an hour or so before exposure to cold, because alcohol dilates the blood vessels of the skin and increases heat loss.

extension. The movement of straightening a joint or of treating a damaged arm or leg

by a steady pull to prevent the muscles from contracting.

extrovert. A person primarily interested in things outside himself, fond of company, sociable and out-going. The term contrasts with the isolated, inward-looking, self-centred INTROVERT.

It is probably incorrect to classify any person simply as an extrovert or an introvert. A person may, for example, be lively and outgoing at home and the 'life of the party' on social occasions, but quiet and self-centred at work. Another may be an active, forceful leader at work but quiet and subdued on social occasions. Yet another may be sociable and lively at most times but apparently introverted this month because of some domestic worry or personal illness while yet another may be shy with strangers but out-going with established friends.

Cross-section of the eye

eye. The eye may be regarded as a camera in which the light rays from an object are concentrated by a contractable diaphragm (the iris), focused by the lens, and received as an inverted image on the retina.

The spherical eyeball is protected by the eyelids and moved by six muscles – the superior, inferior, internal and external rectus muscles and the superior and inferior oblique muscles; these six are supplied by the third, fourth and sixth cranial nerves.

The eyeball has three coverings. (1) The sclera, or tough outer coat, forms the white of the eye and is continuous in front with a transparent, window-like membrane, the cornea. (2) The choroid, or middle coat, is a pigmented membrane which in front becomes the iris, the coloured diaphragm in front of the lens. The central opening in the iris is called the pupil. (3) The retina, or inner coat, contains the terminations of the optic nerve which are light-sensitive. There are two types of cells – the 'cones', with which we see in bright light, and the 'rods' which are used in dim light.

From front to back the eyeball therefore has: (1) the transparent cornea; (2) an anterior chamber between cornea and iris; (3) the coloured iris with a central hole, the pupil; (4) a posterior chamber between iris and lens; (5) the lens; and (6) a large rear portion extending from lens to retina and filled with a jelly-like fluid, the vitreous body.

The cornea acts as a transparent window, protecting the structures behind it. The iris controls the amount of light entering the eye. The lens focuses rays of light to produce a clear image on the retina in the function known as accommodation. When an individual is trying to view a distant object, the lens is only slightly convex and rays of light coming from the object are focused on the retina. To allow a nearer object to be seen clearly the lens is pulled into a more globular shape by the small ciliary muscle: in other words it 'accommodates' by becoming a lens of higher power, so that the diverging rays from the object are still brought to a focus on the retina. As people grow older the lens gradually loses its elasticity, so that from the age of about 40 or 45 years a person may need the aid of glasses for reading, sewing, or fine work. This natural loss of accommodation is called presbyopia. Defects of EYESIGHT can usually be corrected with glasses. Lastly the retina receives the images and transmits them along the optic nerve to the visual area of the brain.

Since the eyes are a short distance apart, the images which they receive must differ from each other. However, the difference is so slight that the two images can be 'fused' into one by the visual centre of the brain, and this blending of the two images received in binocular vision gives rise to the three-dimensional aspect of sight known as stereopsis.

Eyestrain. Prevention of eyestrain should begin in childhood. The child's bed should not face the window, the sun should not shine directly into the baby's eyes, and toys should be reasonably large. If there is any suspicion of short-sight the child's eyes should be examined and appropriate glasses regularly worn. Ideally, since children are liable to falls and other accidents, the lenses should be plastic, not glass.

In early school life teachers, health visitors and parents should be on the lookout for signs of eyestrain, such as rubbing of the eyes, frequent blinking and reddened eyelids; and attention should be paid to natural and artificial lighting in school and at home, with testing of the child's vision undertaken as a routine every year.

Eyestrain can also occur during years of prolonged study and at various later periods. Good lighting is an essential preventive measure, as is occasional testing of vision and the prescription of glasses where required.

Diseases. Short-sight (myopia), long-sight (hypermetropia) and uneven curvature (astigmatism) are considered under EYESIGHT. Other disorders of the eye include CONJUNCTIVITIS, CATARACT, GLAUCOMA, and SQUINT.

Watering eye. Persistent overflow of tears on to the face implies either over-secretion of tears or, more usually, blockage of the tear-ducts which would normally convey the secreted moisture to the nose. The condition is annoying and unsightly. Treatment varies with the cause, e.g., an astringent lotion may help to reduce excessive tear-secretion, a foreign body in the duct may be removed, and gentle syringing may help where the lachrymal sac is distended with mucus and pus.

Injuries. The commonest injuries affecting the eye are black eye and presence of a foreign body.

A black eye is simply a condition of bruising, caused by violence, and is best treated by immediate application of a cold, damp cloth.

A foreign body in the eye may be removed by repeated blinking or by pulling one eyelid over the other. If these measures are unsuccessful the upper lid may be rolled upwards, or the lower lid rolled downwards, over a pencil or knitting-needle, and the foreign object gently removed by application of the moistened corner of a clean handkerchief.

Injuries other than an obvious black eye and a removable foreign body call for medical aid. Such a condition might be a corneal abrasion, when the surface layer of cells is irritated or damaged; this will heal over rapidly (in about a day) with no scarring if it is not infected. However, if the substance of the cornea beneath the surface layer is damaged healing may take many months because the blood supply to the cornea is minimal. Such damage is found in corneal ulceration which may occur as a result of infection following injury, or infection by itself, as can happen with shingles of the face. If the damage is severe, scarring of the cornea will occur with consequent impairment of vision. Such a scarred cornea can be removed and replaced with a graft from a donor.

eyelids, diseases of. Common diseases of the eyelids include the following.

1. Cyst. A hard swelling of the gland of an eyelash, usually of the lower lid. It is painless but disfiguring. It usually requires removal.

2. Drooping eyelid (ptosis). This result of weakness of the muscle that raises the upper lid may be congenital, may arise after disease damaging the nerve which controls it (e.g., shingles) or may occur as a senile condition. Treatment often involves a small operation to enlist the aid of another muscle.

3. Ectropion. A condition in which the margin of the lower lid is turned outwards, so that the eye cannot be fully closed. Ectropion arises from contraction of scars (e.g., from ulcers or burns) or as a senile condition. A slight operation is often necessary for remedy.

4. Entropion. A turning inwards of the margin of a lid. The causes are similar to those of ectropion. A common treatment is to increase the normal 'pull' of the skin by removing a small piece of skin.

5. Ingrowing eyelash. A lid margin is displaced inwards and the lash irritates the conjunctiva causing pain and watering of the eye. The offending eyelashes can be removed with special forceps.

6. Stye. Suppurative inflammation of one of the glands at the margin of a lid. In very early stages an antibiotic may abort the stye. Where a hard, painful swelling has developed, hot antiseptic compresses may help to bring about pus formation, after which the abscess either bursts or can be opened by incision with a small knife.

7. Blepharitis. A crusty scaling of the lid margins fairly common in children; it may be associated with dandruff of the scalp and is often found in situations of poor general health.

Whether driving a car or reading a book, the lens of the normal eye can adjust the focus to see clearly.

eyesight. The optical principle to be kept in mind in considering eyesight is that rays of light entering a denser medium are bent out of their course. Thus light passing from air into the eye is first deflected by the cornea and again by the lens; the more curved the lens of the eyes, the greater is the bending that takes place.

As indicated under EYE, the eye is like a small camera with a shutter, a lens and a screen.

A normal or emmetropic eye is in perfect focus for objects at a distance of more than one metre. Rays from such objects reach the retina without any additional curving of the lens. Nearer objects are brought into focus by an appropriate degree of bulging of the lens, achieved without conscious effort, known as accommodation. An object very close to the eye cannot be brought into focus because the capacity of the lens to increase its curvature is limited.

The common departures from normal vision – excluding diseases of the eye – are hypermetropia (or long-sight), myopia (or short-sight), astigmatism (or uneven curvature), which are all errors of refraction, and presbyopia.

The long-sighted person requires a convex spectacle lens to help bring the light from a near object to a focus point on the retina.

Hypermetropia. The hypermetropic eye is either shorter from front to back than the normal eye or has a lens with less than the normal curvature. Either of these deviations from normality implies that, if no bending of the lens occurred, rays from a distant object would be brought to a focus not on the retina but on an imaginary point beyond it, so that the image produced on the retina would be blurred. Actually in the hypermetropic eye the lens fattens sufficiently to bring distant objects to a correct focus, so that the long-sighted person can see distant objects clearly. For nearer objects (for which a normal eye would need bulging of the lens) the hypermetropic eye needs greater accommodation so that for objects fairly near the eye there is a blurring because the lens is already bulging to capacity. Hence a long-sighted person can see distant objects (and can, for example, drive a car without spectacles) but cannot bring near objects to a focus (e.g., read a book). Correction of long-sightedness is by convex glasses which bend rays inwards and in effect do some of the work of the lens.

Myopia. The myopic eye is abnormally long from front to back or has a lens with more curvature than normal before any accommodation takes place. Hence rays from a distance come to a focus at a point in front of the retina and then spread out, producing blurring. Nearer objects can be brought to focus on the retina with less bulging of the lens than in the normal eye. Hence the short-sighted eye can clearly see near objects (e.g., a book held at average distance) but to focus distant objects requires the help of concave glasses which in effect balance the excessive curvature of the lens.

Presbyopia. From the age of 40 years

The short-sighted person needs a concave lens to help bring the light from distant objects to a focus.

presbyopia begins to develop, that is to say, the elasticity of the lens begins to decrease. Hence the normal eye begins to require a convex glass for near objects, 'reading glasses', and another glass which is only mildy convex as 'distant glasses'. Such persons can usefully obtain bifocal lenses, in which the upper segment corrects distant vision and the lower segment corrects near vision. Bifocal glasses save the person from having to switch from one pair of spectacles to another, e.g., a teacher who desires repeatedly to transfer his gaze from book to class and back again. Some such people find bifocal glasses a great advantage, but others find it very difficult to become accustomed to wearing glasses with the upper and lower parts of completely different focusing power. To lessen the sharp change from an upper segment for distant vision and a lower segment for near vision, attempts have been made in recent years to introduce an intermediate zone: tri-focal glasses.

The myopic eye, which previously needed a concave glass to counteract excessive curvature of the lens, requires a progressively weaker glass as presbyopia develops, then perhaps no glass for a period, and finally, when the ageing process has more than balanced the short-sightedness, a mildly convex glass.

Astigmatism. In the astigmatic eye the cornea at the front is not curved uniformly. Hence, unless the abnormality is balanced by a glass appropriately curved, the whole of an image cannot simultaneously come into focus. In regular astigmatism, the directions of greatest and least curvature are at right angles and a suitable cylindrical lens will readily correct the difference in refraction in the two axes. In irregular astigmatism, usually due to previous corneal ulceration, refractive power varies irregularly and is usually impossible to correct effectively with traditional spectacles, although if there is no scarring of the corneal surface, contact lenses can be very successful. Astigmatism can, of course, exist simultaneously with myopia or hypermetropia.

Finally, it should be mentioned that not all defects of vision can be cured by suitable glasses. Glasses can ensure that appropriate images are focused on the retina; but if the retina is detached or if the optic nerve is damaged, glasses will not restore vision.

F

facial nerve. The seventh cranial nerve carries impulses to the muscles of facial expression. It emerges from the base of the brain and passes through a small hole in the mastoid bone to emerge just below the opening of the ear. The nerve is liable to be damaged in inflammatory conditions of the ear and in mastoid operations.

facial paralysis. Paralysis or weakness of one side of the face due to damage of the FACIAL NERVE on that side. The paralysis does not affect sensation but creates a lop-sided appearance with the mouth drawn towards the unaffected side. It may arise following any damage to the nerve, as in head injury, infection (particularly in the ear, close to which the nerve passes on its course to the face) or exposure to intense cold. The condition often recovers quite spontaneously.

facial spasm. A disturbance of the facial nerve causing twitching of the muscles of one side of the face. Mild cases are best left untreated, although tranquillizers and sedatives sometimes help. In serious cases cutting of some branches of the facial nerve can be considered but the operation produces a permanent facial paralysis and should therefore not be lightly undertaken.

faeces. The technical name used for the motions or STOOLS discharged from the bowel.

failure. The dictionary definition of failure is 'a falling-short or cessation', and in a medical context the word may be used in either sense. Thus death may result from cardiac failure, but a diagnosis of 'heart failure' or 'kidney failure' (perhaps prefixed by 'chronic'), is often merely a convenient way of saying that the particular organ at a particular moment is inadequate to meet the demands made upon it.

It may, or may not, be possible to restore the failing action of an organ, either by reducing the demands made upon it (as, for instance, by rest and dietary measures), or by more active therapeutic procedures designed to improve function.

fainting. Temporary loss of consciousness through deficient blood supply to the brain.

Some persons faint easily from such causes as strong emotion, an over-heated atmosphere or the sight of blood. Other causes of fainting include a blow on the abdomen or on the head, acute pain, sudden change of posture (e.g., getting very quickly out of bed), and abnormal exertion.

If warning symptoms – such as dizziness and dimming of vision – appear, the faint can sometimes be prevented by getting the person to improve the blood supply to the brain by lowering his head; this is best done by bending forward with head between knees. Where fainting has occurred, clothing round the neck should be loosened, the head kept low and smelling salts, if available, held to the nostrils.

Sal volatile may be given in the preliminary dizzy stage and after the return of consciousness, but not during the unconscious phase.

While prolonged unconsciousness (over three minutes) or repeated fainting requires medical investigation, most occurrences of fainting are followed by immediate recovery even without treatment. After regaining consciousness, whether after treatment or spontaneously, the person should lie or sit quietly for about a quarter of an hour.

falling sickness. An old term for EPILEPSY.

Fallopian tube. The oviduct or tube which leads from each of the two ovaries to the uterus, and through which the unfertilized ova travel. Occasionally a fertilized ovum travels back into the tube and begins to develop there (ectopic pregnancy).

When a woman has had the number of children that she desires, she may elect to have the small operation of tying the Fallopian tubes. This operation, by stopping ova from reaching the uterus, renders her permanently infertile. Other methods of BIRTH CONTROL are not permanent.

family planning. Deliberate restriction of children born to the number desired and to the times at which their births are desired. See BIRTH CONTROL.

Faradism. Use of an interrupted electrical current to cause contraction of a muscle when the current is passing (as contrasted with Galvanism where contraction occurs only when a current is made and broken). Faradism is used to treat various forms of paralysis and muscle weakness.

fascia. A sheet of fibrous tissue. Fasciae are found in all parts of the body and vary in thickness and strength from the loose open-work structure of superficial fascia to well-defined anatomical entities which are dense, tough, and tendinous (deep fascia).

Fasciae connect the skin to the underlying structures, provide capsules for muscles, organs, blood-vessels and nerves, and subdivide muscle-groups. Some fascial sheets are themselves under muscular control so that they can tense or relax to conform with adjacent muscle-movements.

They are also of importance in suppuration and haemorrhage since pus or effused blood may flow along fascial planes to emerge at points remote from the actual lesion.

fasting. Deliberate abstention from food. A fasting person generally does take water as he would otherwise die in about three days. Assuming that he has water, he lives essentially on his own tissues. The glycogen, (sugar) stored in the liver is first utilized, and thereafter fat and protein are mobilized from the tissues.

In a healthy and well-nourished person a fast of two or three days may be harmless, and in certain diseases it is even beneficial, although it is accompanied by hunger-pangs and a feeling of weakness. In prolonged fasting the hunger-pangs disappear but the fasting becomes dangerous. A fasting person would die of starvation in about a month but might well develop deficiency diseases or infection (through lowered resistance) in less than a month. After prolonged fasting the return to food should be gradual, with no heavy meal during the first thirty-six hours.

Intermittent fasting, e.g., complete abstention for one day each week, or partial fasting for a few weeks, is on the whole commendable for well-nourished adults.

fat. A type of FOOD, and one of the essential constituents of the DIET but digested only in the presence of carbohydrates. For equal weights fats supply more than twice the energy of proteins and carbohydrates. In addition to providing sources of energy in concentrated form, animal fats (e.g., butter, which is about 80 per cent fat, cheese, cream and the fat of meat) carry the fat-soluble vitamins A and D, but certain vegetable oils differ from animal fats in not containing fat-soluble vitamins, unless these are artificially added.

Fats are derived from both animal and vegetable sources and are combinations of fatty acids and glycerin. At ordinary temperatures they may be either solid like lard, or fluid, like olive oil. They differ also in their molecular structure. If their carbon atoms are uniformly linked by single bonds they are said to be 'saturated fats'; if there are one or more double bonds they are 'unsaturated' or 'polyunsaturated fats'. Saturated fats are derived from animal sources and the other kinds are of vegetable origin. In recent years it has been suggested that too much animal fat (e.g., from butter, cheese and meat fat) raises the blood cholesterol level and may predispose the individual to coronary thrombosis, and that about half of the total intake of fat should be obtained from vegetable oils.

It is difficult to envisage a state which is solely fat deficiency although low fat diet has the disadvantage that it would result in a diminished intake of fat-soluble vitamins. In addition to being an energy source, fatty compounds are integral components of the structure of the cell.

fatigue. Weariness, normally occurring after prolonged physical or mental effort, and acting as a signal that the person suffering from it needs rest, change of activity, or medical treatment.

While fatigue is usually a sign of working too hard or too long or at unusual tasks or under bad working conditions, with the remedy obvious, abnormal fatigue without any of these causes may indicate that the person is suffering from an undiagnosed illness, such as diabetes or anaemia; or that he is under sustained emotional stress either at work or domestically; or that he has become bored and dissatisfied and requires a change of occupation, a good holiday or an interesting hobby.

Fatigue is usually easy to diagnose. Its manifestations include quickened pulse and respiration, perspiration and lowered body temperature, frequent yawning, impaired muscular co-ordination as revealed for example in handwriting, a feeling of tiredness, a reduced power of concentration and span of attention, weakened memory, impaired judgment, irritability, and increased liability to accidents.

Unless the cause is obvious, medical examination for possible undetected disease is desirable, and, if that is negative, attention to the emotional state including both manifest and hidden worries and conflicts.

In general a fatigued person needs REST and change of activity; and the persons hardest to treat are those in posts of responsibility who, while making errors of judgment because of exhaustion, often genuinely believe that the business or department would collapse if they took a fortnight off. Tonics and 'pick-me-ups' though advertised, are not of much value. Where immediate continuation of the activity is essential, as with a tired soldier during a battle, benzidrene will postpone fatigue for many hours. So to a lesser extent will strong coffee. Both of these, however, merely delay the onset of fatigue, and the subsequent physical and emotional exhaustion is all the greater. In fatigue of emotional origin tranquillizers may help, although generally the background condition requires treatment.

Where abnormal fatigue is found in children one should think of over-pressure either in school or at home, unsatisfactory environmental conditions again either in school or at home, anaemia, nutrition insufficient for rapid growth, insufficient recreation and unidentified defects of vision or hearing.

fattening. A deliberate attempt to gain weight. The young girl whose face begins to look 'pinched' and whose body loses its natural curves and the older woman with haggard appearance, dry and sallow skin and folds of loose skin on face and neck, often set out to eat more food in an attempt to gain weight. In many cases a good nourishing diet and a moderately restful life – including mental as well as physical rest – will produce the desired result.

Three sets of conditions should however be noted. (1) Excessive thinness, often coupled with excessive physical and mental activity, may be the result of an over-active thyroid gland, and a good diet will not correct that over-activity. (2) Loss of weight may be the first symptom of various diseases, such as tuberculosis and cancer. (3) Increasing or persistent thinness may be the result of worry, either in consequence of abnormal emotional or stress factors or as a result of the person having a worrying personality.

In general, therefore, a person who is steadily losing weight should consult a doctor. Treatment – sometimes surgical – is clearly needed in glandular upset, and may be life-saving in cases of undetected serious disease; in abnormal emotional stress tranquillizers may help, although what is really needed is modification of the factors involved; and the person of worrying personality, with its causes rooted in childhood, may need considerable psychological help.

Where fattening is attempted without medical aid a few points are worth noting. Physical and mental REST are important and since the person's appetite has probably been small, the increase in food should be fairly gradual, because otherwise there is danger of nausea and indigestion, especially if the new diet contains large amounts of fat. Carbohydrate foods are particularly valuable for weight gain, e.g., plenty of sugar in tea and coffee, and abundance of cakes and scones. Milk should not be forgotten as an easily digested source of extra calories.

fatty degeneration. Cellular damage accompanied by the appearance of fat-droplets within the cells. In most organs the fat has come from the affected tissue, but in the liver, which has a specific role in fat-metabolism, the visible fat which overfills the cells has been transported from elsewhere and accumulates because the liver-cells have become unable to deal with it.

There are various causes of fatty degeneration. It occurs as a result of deficient oxidation, as in anaemia, or from actual interference with local blood-supply, for instance to the heart muscle; from cell-poisons such as phosphorus, chloroform, and bacterial toxins; and from nerve injuries which tend to produce degeneration in the fatty myelin envelope of nerve-fibres on the far side of the injury and in the associated muscle-fibres.

fauces. The fairly narrow opening between the mouth and the throat, with the soft palate above and the root of the tongue below. On each side there are two folds, the pillars of the fauces, in which the tonsils are imbedded. When the tonsils are swollen the fauces may be narrowed to such an extent that swallowing becomes difficult.

favus. A skin disease, caused by a fungus, mainly affecting the scalp and sometimes the nails. Yellow cup-like crusts form and adhere together. When they drop off the portion of scalp is hairless and scarred. Infection is by direct contact with a person or a cat suffering from the condition. Treatment consists of removing the crusts and applying an appropriate antiseptic ointment. Where this does not suffice, exposure to x-rays may be necessary.

fear. Fear of things or situations that are known by experience to be dangerous is a normal human reaction, leading to the person taking special care, or avoiding the danger, or preparing to fight. Fear of the unknown is also in considerable part normal, although it is in some measure created or exaggerated by parental over-protection of children.

Both of these types of fear can to some extent be reduced in various ways. Calm consideration of the reasonably worst expectation can be helpful: it frequently appears that the worst that can be expected to happen is far less than the person in mental apprehension had vaguely anticipated. Another possibility is to discuss the fear with a trusted friend who can bring a rational and unemotional outlook to bear on the situation. Yet another is to steel oneself to tackle the source of fear, as in deliberately setting out to drive a car shortly after a terrifying skid.

In many cases, however, fear is a projection of hidden emotional conflict and cannot be fully dispelled until the conflict is resolved. Pathological fears and PHOBIAS are forms of NEUROSIS.

There appears to be little relationship between physical and moral fear. The man who will unhesitatingly tackle an unknown intruder may be afraid to express an unpopular opinion, and vice versa. Moreover, physical cowards who succeed in temporarily repressing their fears sometimes perform remarkable acts of bravery.

Fear of pain and fear of disease affect patients or prospective patients in two opposite ways. In some cases these fears cause a person to seek medical examination, but in many cases it is these very fears that make a person hesitate to seek expert advice.

Practitioners of health education are virtually unanimous in holding that an appeal to fear, e.g., by showing pictures of diseased lungs in a drive against cigarette smoking, does not achieve much long-term success.

febrile. Having a raised temperature.

fecundity. See FERTILITY.

femoral vessels. The main artery and vein of the thigh. The femoral artery passes from the abdomen in the middle of the groin where it can be felt pulsating and, if the thigh is moved slightly outwards, can be compressed against the head of the femur to stop bleeding. The artery passes down the inner side of the thigh and in the lower third passes behind to become the popliteal artery at the back of the knee. The femoral vein corresponds with the artery and drains blood from the leg. One of its tributaries is the long saphenous vein which is often varicose and liable to phlebitis.

head,
which
with the
acetabulum
forms
the
hip joint

neck

The femur

femur. The thigh bone, the longest and strongest bone in the body. Its head articulates with a cavity in the hip bone called the acetabulum, forming the hip joint; below the head is a narrowed part, the neck, and where the neck joins the shaft there is a protuberance, the great trochanter. The lower end consists of two bulges or condyles which articulate with the tibia and the patella in the formation of the knee joint. Fractures of the femur are not uncommon: displacement, pain and inability to move the limb are general features but beyond these the signs vary according to the part of the bone fractured.

Fracture of the neck of the femur is commonest in elderly people, especially elderly women. It used to be regarded as always being the result of indirect violence, e.g., landing heavily on the foot after missing a step on the stair. Increasingly however experts are beginning to question that explanation (though it is certainly true in some cases). If the hormone changes after the

menopause are followed by a diet poor in calcium the bone may become thin, especially at the neck, and incapable of supporting the weight of the body, which is often increasing about this time. So in at least some cases the situation is not that a woman falls and breaks her leg but that the leg breaks and causes the fall.

fenestration. An operation, for relief of deafness due to hardening of the bones of the ear, involving the making of an artificial opening into the inner ear. The operation is being increasingly superseded by newer operations that claim better results.

fertility. The ability to procreate children.

While fertility in women begins to decrease about the age of thirty and disappears at the menopause, and while fertility in men also decreases although much more slowly, most couples can produce as many children as they desire; and indeed the modern stress on family planning and birth control is testimony to the fact that most couples need assistance to keep them from having more children than they desire.

About one-tenth of marriages, however, are infertile although the partners desire to produce a family. Some of the causes of such infertility are:

1. Ignorance of sexual techniques, e.g., premature ejaculation by the man, or inadvertent avoidance by the couple of the days midway between the menstrual periods when the woman is most likely to conceive.

2. Physical ill-health, temporarily reducing the fertility of one of the couple.

3. Male infertility, which should not be confused with impotence. One not uncommon cause is orchitis occurring as a complication of mumps. Examination of the number and motility of the sperms in the seminal fluid will determine whether the man is the infertile partner, but male infertility is on the whole more difficult to treat than female infertility.

4. Female infertility due to a deficiency of hormones (which can often be remedied) or to various gynaecological conditions (for which there is often treatment) or to neurosis (which can usually be cured).

5. Sexual incompatibility, where both partners are fertile but, for reasons not yet fully understood, there appears to exist an antagonism between the sperms and ova of the particular partners.

Investigation of both partners at a sub-fertility clinic is desirable where a couple are more than two years without a wanted child. In many cases the condition can be cured, although it must be appreciated that some are as yet incurable, and in these cases alternatives have to be considered, e.g., artificial insemination of the woman with the husband's semen, or adoption.

In view of the age-old and still prevalent belief that in a childless marriage it is always the woman who is barren, it is perhaps desirable to state that in over one-third of investigated childless marriages the infertility is in the male.

Fecundity, i.e., abnormal fertility with a tendency to multiple births, is largely an inherited trait: twins occur about once in every eighty births and triplets about once in every seven thousand births, but the chances are appreciably higher in families with a history of multiple births in grandparents, parents or brothers and sisters. Apart from the hereditary element, it should be noted that some synthetic drugs employed to treat infertility occasionally lead to multiple births, even including quadruplets and quintuplets.

fester. To generate pus. The term is not much employed in medicine but is in popular use for any inflammation with formation of pus, as in an abscess, boil or ulcer.

fetishism. A fetish is an inanimate object which is regarded with awe or reverence, or creates sexual satisfaction on the part of a person who handles, destroys or steals it. Fetishism is the belief in or use of fetishes, and is thus a form of sexual PERVERSION.

In religious fetishism the object, e.g., the idol, the alleged fragment of Christ's cross or the bone of a saint, becomes gradually invested with the miracle-working or divine attributes of what it represents, until at last the idol-worshipper is not praying to his deity but concentrating all his hopes and fears on the idol.

In erotic fetishism certain articles of attire or objects used by the beloved person – or even by any member of the opposite sex – come to arouse the emotions of sexual pleasure, even sometimes to the point of orgasm, and attraction to the article or object is often to the exclusion of normal sexuality. Fetishism often starts with a part of the body, such as the hair, hand, foot or leg, and is transferred by association of ideas to the hat, gloves, shoes or petticoat.

Fetishism is predominately a male sexual deviation, and some psychiatrists claim that it does not occur in women.

Where fetishism is confined to secreting a handkerchief or a lock of hair and using it as a love-object, it probably does little harm, although it may prevent normal sexual intercourse and procreation of children; but where it involves the stealing or destruction of articles of attire, such as women's underwear hanging on a clothes line, it clearly requires psychiatric treatment.

fever. Otherwise known as pyrexia, this is any condition in which the bodily temperature is increased materially above the normal. High temperature may occur after exposure to great heat, after swallowing various drugs, and in severe nervous shock. •Normally, however, the term is reserved for a number of specific infectious diseases which produce pyrexia as one of their main characteristics.

Symptoms. The start of a fever is often marked by rigor or shivering, pallor, or in children convulsions, accompanied by a general feeling of illness, headache, backache and often sickness. After the chilly stage, which lasts for minutes or hours, the temperature rises rapidly, the skin feels hot and dry (although in a few fevers such as rheumatic fever and malaria profuse perspiration is a feature), characteristic rashes may appear, the tongue becomes furred and dry, appetite is poor, thirst is considerable, the pulse is rapid (although there are some exceptions), respiration is accelerated, urine is diminished and highly coloured, and headache, sleeplessness and delirium are common.

Classification. Continued fever is the term used when the high temperature persists until it falls, usually suddenly 'by crisis' as in lobar pneumonia, scarlet fever, measles and typhoid. Remittent fever is the name employed when the temperature varies, being high at one part of the day and normal or subnormal at another, as in bronchopneumonia and pulmonary tuberculosis. In intermittent fever, as in malaria, the high temperature occurs regularly only once a day, or once every two days, or once every three days.

Specific fevers. This term is sometimes used to differentiate from other causes of high temperature the particular fevers that are (1) caused by specific micro-organisms, and (2) infectious, i.e., transmissible from person to person. Other characteristics are that they run a fairly defined course and that an attack tends to confer an immunity which may be long-lasting (as after smallpox) or of short duration (as after influenza).

Most specific fevers have fairly consistent incubation periods during which the invading organisms multiply until numerous enough to produce symptoms. For instance, the incubation periods of both scarlet fever and diphtheria are one to four days, that of measles is ten to fourteen days and that of rubella is twelve to twenty-one days. A very few fevers have variable incubation periods: e.g., while the incubation period of typhoid is normally around fourteen days, it can be as short as seven or as long as thirty days, depending on the quantity of organisms swallowed and on various other factors.

Many fevers have a characteristic rash, such as minute red spots on a flushed background in scarlet fever, the slightly coarser spots of rubella and the more blotchy rash of measles; but in some, such as whooping cough and mumps, there is no rash, and in some others (such as typhoid and cerebrospinal meningitis) the rash is not always seen.

Treatment. Ascertainment of the exact cause and its treatment is highly important. Apart from such therapy skilled nursing plays the major role. In particular rest is essential (including, for example, in diphtheria not allowing the patient to subject his heart to the strain of raising his head from the pillow); warm baths stimulate the skin and excretory organs and so facilitate heat loss; tepid sponging is useful when the temperature passes above 104 °F., and should aim at reducing it to 100 to 101 °F. but not lower; frequent changes of clothes may be necessary if there is much sweating; dehydration must be avoided by drinking quantities of fluids; regular turning of the patient decreases the chance of lung involvement; the mouth and teeth should be carefully cleaned periodically; bed-sores should be prevented by scrupulous cleanliness and thorough drying, and in long fevers by hardening the pressure areas of skin with methylated spirits; and the nurse must constantly bear in mind that in most fevers the patient is infectious and his discharges and bed-linen are infectious.

Prevention. Measures include: health education to encourage routine immunization against many formerly common fevers (e.g., diphtheria, poliomyelitis, whooping cough, measles and rubella), and to encourage immunization in special circumstances against various other fevers (e.g., cholera, typhoid and typhus); hygienic measures to prevent diseases spread by faulty hygiene (e.g., typhoid and cholera); destruction of insects and their breeding grounds in areas liable to insect-borne infections (e.g., malaria and yellow fever); and, where infection occurs, strict isolation of patients, exclusion of visitors, recording names and addresses of all contacts (including members of the medical, nursing, paramedical and domestic staff), surveillance or quarantine of all contacts and investigation of the source of the outbreak, together with many other measures as appropriate, such as boiling of all water where a water-borne outbreak is suspected.

The reduction of food-borne specific fevers by personal and environmental hygiene, and the virtual eradication of many droplet-borne specific fevers by immunization and vaccination, together with education of the public about these measures, have been among the greatest triumphs of preventive medicine or indeed of all medical science.

fibrillation. The involuntary, uncoordinated action of individual muscle fibres, which alternately contract and relax in a rapid irregular fashion so that tremors occur and the normal muscular movements are impaired and weakened. It particularly affects heart-muscle (ventricular or AURICULAR FIBRILLATION).

Fibrillary twitching of muscles normally under voluntary control is a sign of several degenerative nervous diseases, such as Parkinson's disease. Effects are usually first seen in the smaller muscles of hands, forearm, and face.

Transient episodes of muscular twitching sometimes occur in the eyelids and around the orbits. This is generally unimportant and is related to fatigue or debility.

fibrositis. Alternatively called muscular rheumatism, this is a condition, probably rheumatic, but affecting not joints but soft tissues, characterized by pain and tenderness at localized 'trigger-points' and by muscular stiffness. Muscular strain, mental stress, chill and even dietetic errors are suggested as causes, with American experts particularly emphasizing the mental factors and calling the condition psychogenic rheumatism. Yet against the psychological factor is the fact that the condition occurs twice as frequently in outdoor as in indoor workers. According to the part of the body affected the disease may be called lumbago, sciatica, intercostal neuralgia or rheumatic headache.

Treatment involves rest, analgesics to relieve the pain, and application of heat until the muscular spasm is relieved. Thereafter normal activity can be resumed.

fibula. The long slender bone on the outer side of the leg. It is attached to the broader and thicker tibia at both ends, enters into the structure of the ankle joint at the lower end but takes no part in the formation of the knee joint.

Fractures of the fibula alone are not uncommon, usually caused by direct violence. Because the tibia acts as a splint they generally produce no displacement, although pain is produced by pressing the bone below or above the fracture. Fractures of both tibia and fibula are also not uncommon and may be due either to direct violence, such as a blow on the leg, or to indirect violence, which would fracture the fibula by, for instance, jumping from a height and landing heavily on the heels.

filariasis. Infection with certain tiny worms (filaria) transmitted from the blood of an infected person to another person by several species of mosquito. The incubation period is remarkably long, usually eight to twelve months. After developing, the worms block lymphatic vessels, causing painful and tender swellings, and subsequently the enormous swellings known as elephantiasis.

Diethylcarbamizine is the most effective drug so far, but it sometimes causes acute allergic reactions and it does not always secure a complete cure. Prevention includes anti-mosquito measures in endemic areas.

fingers. The five separate members forming the extremities of the hand. In man, apes and monkeys the fingers have the unusual characteristic that the thumb and the other fingers can be brought together for grasping. From the thumb inwards the others are named the index, the middle, the ring and the little finger, and each has three small bones (the phalanges). The knuckle joints are formed by the first phalanges and the metacarpal bones.

Fingers have great range of movement and are very richly supplied with nerves and nerve-endings; at their tips the sense of touch is particularly acute.

The fingers are subject to all the diseases of skin and bone, but are particularly liable to abscess, especially at the root of the nail, and to injury and septic inflammation. Chilblains are among the commonest affections of the fingers, and spasm of the fingers may arise in tetany and in writer's cramp. Scabies commonly makes its first appearance on the skin between the fingers.

first aid. See first aid section at the end of the book.

fistula. An abnormal channel or passage connecting two hollow organs (e.g., recto-vaginal fistula) or connecting a hollow organ with the body surface (e.g., anal fistula). In most cases a fistula develops from an abscess, fissure or operational wound, but occasionally fistulas arise from deep-seated disease of the bones or joints, and some fistulas are congenital. A fistula is easily infected and is often extremely painful. Treatment varies with the situation and the cause, but often involves surgery.

normal   flat

Flat foot

flat foot. A condition in which the arch of the instep is lower than normal so that in standing or walking the whole of the sole rests on the ground. Some of the main causes are (1) hereditary weakness of the tendon running from the back of the heel up the leg; (2) excessive weight, especially if coupled with standing for long periods; (3) badly fitting shoes; (4) certain acute and debilitating illnesses; (5) occasionally pregnancy; and (6) very occasionally accidental injury as in jumping from a height.

Prevention by well-fitting shoes and the adoption and maintenance of good posture is important, and in the early stages of the condition exercises and manipulation can help greatly.

In advanced stages it is necessary to differentiate between flexible flat foot in which the bones can be brought back into their normal position and rigid flat foot in which return to normal position is no longer possible. In the former case, which is often characterized by pain, manipulation, arch supports and special shoes are often valuable. In the case of rigid flat foot where changes have occurred in the bones and joints, there is deformity but seldom pain, and arch supports merely cause discomfort; it is best to leave the condition untreated.

flatulence. Uncomfortable accumulation of gas in the stomach or intestine, relieved by the passage of the gas through the mouth or anus. In some cases flatulence is caused by the swallowing of air during the gulping of food or drink, and in others it is essentially due to anxiety and the air is swallowed during unsuccessful attempts to belch.

In another group of cases the flatulence is a result of excessive fermentation of food in the stomach, either because the digestive juices of the particular person are poor in ferments or because the muscular wall of the stomach is flabby so that the food is not firmly held. In the gas production type the patient may learn by observation that certain foods produce flatulence and so learn to avoid them. The foods vary slightly from person to person, but cabbage, cucumbers, melons and nuts are common causes. Flatulence is also sometimes an indication of the presence of gallstones.

As a rule half a teaspoonful of bicarbonate of soda in a cup of warm water will relieve the immediate symptoms.

fleas. Wingless, blood-sucking insects that live as parasites on man and other animals. They have powerful back legs which enable them to jump several feet to a new host, carrying disease from the infected person or animal previously bitten to the one on whom they next alight.

There are several hundred varieties of fleas. The common man-inhabiting flea, *Pulex irritans*, causes unpleasant and itching bites but has seldom been

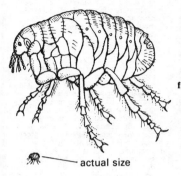

— actual size

Flea

incriminated in the spread of serious diseases although the possibility must be recognized. The rat flea, *Xenopsylla cheopis,* can feed on man as well as on rats and is the means of transmission of the bacterium of plague from rat to rat, from rat to man and from man to man.

A partially developed flea can lie dormant in dust for several months.

Measures of control include strict cleanliness in the home, the use of DDT and other insecticides in infested houses, suppression of rats and vermin by known methods of destruction, special attention to destruction of rats on ships arriving from infected ports and rat-proofing of ships so that rats cannot board them. In any area deemed to be at risk from plague, examination of the corpses of dead rats is useful, because plague in rats tends to occur before plague in human beings.

flexion. The movement of bending a joint.

flies. This is a general term for two-winged insects with jaws adapted for piercing and sucking. Some well known varieties are the house-fly (*Musca domestica*), the tsetse fly (transmitter of sleeping sickness), mosquitoes (some of which transmit malaria and yellow fever), gnats, etc. In Britain, although gnats are abundant and some forms of mosquito exist, the insect usually implied by the term is *Musca domestica* which, unlike the majority of flies, is capable only of sucking, not piercing.

Despite its lack of biting capacity the house-fly is a dangerous pest, because it can pick up from the excrement and sputum of persons and animals the bacilli of typhoid, dysentery, poliomyelitis, cholera and possibly tuberculosis. It carries the organisms on its hairy legs and abdomen and in its alimentary canal and infects food on which it lands or on which it feeds.

Flies breed in all forms of refuse and

excreta so long as they are warm and moist. Measures for fly control include the treating of manure heaps with suitable disinfectants such as strong solutions of borax, the keeping of all refuse in closely covered bins, the killing of adult flies with DDT (although DDT-resistant flies are now appearing), the use of other insecticides, and the covering of all food – especially food that will not subsequently be cooked – to prevent contamination.

floating kidney. A condition, sometimes related to rapid loss of abdominal fat, in which (as in MOVEABLE KIDNEY) there is an abnormal amount of mobility of the kidney. Usually there are no symptoms and the condition is discovered by accident, but if the mobility is such as to cause kinking of the duct connecting the kidney and the bladder (the ureter) there may be bouts of severe pain. Apart from that possibility, the condition is often blamed for vague abdominal discomfort and persistent indigestion. Abdominal massage and the wearing of a suitable belt may help.

floating ribs. The ribs are long curved bones springing from the spine and sweeping round to be attached to the breast bone, or sternum, in front. However, the two lowest ribs on each side are not attached to the sternum and are therefore sometimes described as 'floating'.

flooding. Excessive bleeding during menstruation. The technical term is menorrhagia. Since the blood loss varies appreciably from woman to woman, flooding is best defined as appreciably greater loss than the particular woman normally has. Common causes include anaemia, raised blood pressure, ovarian cysts or tumours, hormonal disorders and severe anxiety. Flooding also sometimes occurs in the periods immediately before the menopause. Treatment varies according to the cause but in general serious flooding warrants medical investigation. See also METRORRHAGIA.

fluke worm. Flat, bilaterally symmetrical worms with a very complicated developmental history. The schistosomes are mentioned elsewhere: see BILHARZIASIS. Another parasitic variety, the liver fluke, is here briefly described. It is a leaf-shaped worm, about 2.5 cm. (1 in.) long and roughly half as wide. The fluke lives in the bile ducts of a sheep and causes the serious and usually fatal disease of liver rot. The eggs, passed out with the excreta of the sheep, develop in damp spots into free-swimming, conical-shaped miracidia. If these reach an available water snail they enter its tissues and develop there, ultimately becoming cercariae which leave the snail, settle on blades of grass, and may be eaten by a sheep or occasionally by man. The clinical features of infection in the human are rather vague – high temperature, impaired appetite, abdominal pain and loss of weight. Diagnosis can be confirmed by a blood test. Many drugs are tried, but emetine hydrochloride probably gives the best results.

fluoridation of water. Artificial addition of fluoride to water supplies which show a deficiency of this mineral.

The fluoride content of water varies from about 0.1 parts per million to over 6 p.p.m. Prolonged studies of communities drinking water naturally high or low in fluoride (including 903 separate high fluoride communities in the U.S.A. alone) have shown several features.

1. The incidence of tooth decay decreases steadily as the fluoride level rises up to about 1 part per million; broadly the amount of dental decay in persons normally drinking water of 1 p.p.m. or above is only a shade over half of the amount in persons drinking water with less than 0.6 p.p.m.

2. There is no further decrease in tooth decay where the fluoride content is above 1 p.p.m.

3. Concentrations of above 5 p.p.m. produce harmless mottling of the enamel of teeth – dental fluorosis.

4. No toxic effects (e.g., on bones or arteries) have been demonstrated where the fluoride level is below 5 p.p.m. In particular analysis of deaths and diseases in communities drinking water of high and low fluoride content provides no shadow of evidence that consumption of water of high fluoride content (i.e., 1 to 5 p.p.m.) improves health except dental health and no shadow of evidence that consumption of water of low fluoride content has any effect except on dental health.

Virtually all dentists, doctors, health visitors, nurses and other health workers agree that a concentration of up to 1 p.p.m. is beneficial to dental health, that higher concentrations confer no proved benefit, and that the kidney can deal adequately with concentrations up to at least 5 p.p.m.

For over thirty years artificial rectification of fluoride deficiency has been a controversial and emotive subject. Fluoride up to the desired limit, usually 1 p.p.m., can be added very simply and with absolute guarantees against over-dosage. Advocates of artificial fluoridation point out (1) that the taste of the water is so little altered that few if any people can tell whether they are drinking rectified or deficient water; (2) that the cost of rectification is trivial by comparison with the saving on dental treatment; (3) that fluoridation reduces the emotional and physical trauma of toothache and of dental treatment; (4) that artificial fluoridation has been adopted in many communities (e.g., in more than two-thirds of the major cities of the U.S.A.), with absolutely no evidence of any harmful effects on the health of the people; (5) that claims that fluoridation is dangerous or harmful have been supported neither by scientific evidence nor by courts of law; (6) that opponents of fluoridation frequently shift their ground, arguing today that it causes one effect and tomorrow that it causes a completely different effect; and (7) that the professions with expertise in health matters are overwhelmingly in favour of fluoridation.

Opponents of fluoridation have perhaps lost the part of their battle relating to danger: it is difficult to maintain that fluoridation is dangerous when, without evidence of damage of health, many communities have drunk water naturally high in fluoride for centuries and other communities have consumed artificially fluoridated water for three decades. The opponents contend, with more effect, that artificial addition of fluoride is mass medication and a dangerous precedent which might be followed by the addition of other drugs, that it is wrong that adults with dentures or already damaged teeth should be forced to consume a substance that will do them no good, and that there are other methods – fluoride rinses, fluoride tablets and fluoride toothpastes – available for those who would benefit from extra fluoride.

In general topical applications, fluoride tablets, etc., are much less effective, although undoubtedly of some value, and very much more costly. Perhaps we have to come back to a basic question: are pre-school children, school pupils, adolescents and young adults who live in an area with water deficient in fluoride to endure the pain and discomfort of preventable tooth decay, and is the community to pay directly or indirectly for much treatment that would otherwise have been needless, or are the middle-aged and elderly to submit to drinking water to which there has been added a substance that will in no way benefit them?

There is, however, another point which may influence that question. In recent years there has been growing evidence of the association between soft water and high incidence of certain diseases of the heart. There is no suggestion that deficiency of fluoride is a factor, but if in due course we have to add perhaps calcium or magnesium to soft water for the benefit of the middle-aged and elderly, it will become increasingly difficult to resist the addition of fluoride for the benefit of the young.

fluorine. A chemical with many properties resembling those of chlorine, required in the human body as an ingredient of bones and teeth, present in many substances (e.g. fish, tea and beer) in small quantities and present to a varying extent in all natural water supplies. It occurs mostly in the form of its sodium and potassium salts (fluorides), and, like many other substances essential in small quantities for life, it is toxic if taken in large doses.

flushing. See BLUSHING.

foetus. The term is sometimes used non-specifically for the unborn offspring of mammals while in the mother's uterus, i.e., from conception to birth. Many writers, however, try to differentiate the embryo and the foetus. Where such distinction is made, the embryo is the early developing mass of cells, from the union of ovum and sperm up to the stage where the developing creature is recognizably human in form; and the foetus is the unborn child from the age of about 8 weeks.

At 8 weeks the human foetus is about 4 cm. long, the head is proportionately very large, the limbs are perceptible and the heart is pumping blood through the body and out to the placenta. Growth is fairly slow at first. By 16 weeks the foetus is about 10 cm. long and weighs 100 g. By 24 weeks it is about 20 cm., weighs around 650 g. and has a faint chance of survival if then born. At 28 weeks it is considered viable under English law, although a child born at this stage is dangerously premature and can survive only with very expert nursing. Most of the intra-uterine increase in weight occurs during the last ten weeks of pregnancy.

folic acid. A VITAMIN of the B group, found in liver, milk, spinach, yeast and various other foodstuffs. Deficiency causes the formerly fatal disease of PERNICIOUS ANAEMIA.

folie à deux. A curious condition in which a person, usually suffering from paranoid delusions of persecution or injustice, persuades a wife, sister or other closely associated person of the justice of the complaints, so that the second person comes to have the same delusions. If the two persons can be separated for any appreciable time, the person who has been 'infected' usually recovers completely.

fomentations. See POULTICES.

fomites. A term used to designate articles of clothing, bedding, toys, food utensils and so forth which have been in contact with a person suffering from an infectious disease and are therefore liable to spread the disease. See DISINFECTION.

fontanelles. Soft areas on a baby's head where the skull bones have not yet fused. In the new-born baby there are normally six fontanelles. Of these the largest, the anterior fontanelle, is a diamond-shaped aperture on the top of the head, about 2.5 cm. in diameter, and normally remaining unclosed until about 15 to 20 months. The second largest, the posterior fontanelle, nearer the back of the head, normally closes before 12 months, as do the others which are situated at the temples and behind the ears.

The presence of these soft areas makes obvious the importance of protecting a baby's head from injury.

Continued presence of an unclosed fontanelle after the age of 24 months is suggestive either of rickets or of some other state of defective development.

food. The term is sometimes used for solid nourishment as differentiated from drink, but is normally employed for anything -

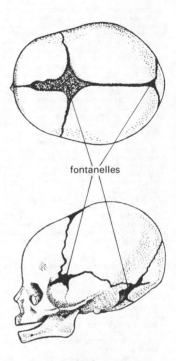

fontanelles

The fontanelles

solid or liquid - of nutritional value and passing into the digestive system.

Food is essential for various reasons. Firstly, the average adult at complete rest requires about 1,000 Calories a day for basal metabolism, i.e., to balance the energy used by the body in maintaining warmth, keeping the heart beating and lungs breathing, and so on. Secondly, additional food is needed to balance the energy used in all forms of activity - the amount of such energy varying from about 40 Calories per hour when relaxing about the house to as much as 600 an hour when engaged in very strenuous athletic activity. Thirdly, food, and in particular protein, is needed for growth and for repair of worn tissues: hence a growing child needs proportionately more food than an adult and an adolescent requires more Calories than an adult of the same size and sex engaged in the same activities.

The energy requirement is measured in Calories, one Calorie being the amount of heat needed to raise 1,000 g. of water through 1 °C. A gramme of protein or carbohydrate when completely absorbed and digested yields 4.1 Calories and a gramme of fat yields 9.3 Calories. Taking average sizes, a child of 2 years needs 1,300 Calories daily, a child of 5 years requires 1,700, a boy of 15 years needs about 2,800 and a girl of 15 about 2,300, a man of sedentary occupation requires about 2,500 and a woman of sedentary occupation about 2,100, while a man doing heavy manual work requires well over 3,000. Roughly, an adolescent needs 300 Calories a day more than an adult doing similar work, a pregnant woman needs an additional 200 and a woman breast-feeding her baby requires an additional 500.

The foods required by the body may be of animal or VEGETABLE origin; they are PROTEINS, FATS, CARBOHYDRATES, MINERAL SALTS and VITAMINS, together with WATER and ROUGHAGE. General insufficiency of food (MALNUTRITION), finally resulting in death from starvation, is rare in developed countries, although common enough in underdeveloped countries.

Proteins. The only foods containing absorbable nitrogen and sulphur, proteins are essential for replacement of worn out cells and tissues and in children for growth.

Fats. These are the most concentrated sources of energy and so are required in considerable amounts for very strenuous work and in very cold climates.

Carbohydrates. Sugars and starches are the most readily available sources of energy and therefore essential for children and others who use energy quickly. They are the body's main source of energy, they are required for the complete digestion of fat, and they are in general the cheapest forms of food.

Mineral salts. The body requires small but calculable amounts of various minerals, e.g., calcium, phosphorus, sodium, potassium, chlorine, sulphur and magnesium, and even smaller amounts of such minerals as iron, iodine, copper, cobalt, fluorine, manganese, selenium and zinc.

Vitamins. These are the 'trace substances' essential for growth and health.

Water. Water is essential for the functioning of the body. About two-thirds of the body weight is water, and there is constant loss by respiration, perspiration and excretion. About two or three litres are required daily, the amount varying mainly with the external temperature.

Roughage. If the bowel is to excrete waste products it needs sufficient material on which to function. Most of the unabsorbed and apparently valueless food material, which is nevertheless essential for bowel action, comes from the cellulose of vegetables.

Food may be adequate enough when purchased but may be damaged by cooking: in particular the water-soluble vitamins may be removed or destroyed by

cooking in water. The food, still adequate in Calories and in individual constituents, may be so cooked or so served as to be unattractive to the nose or the eye, so that, even if it is completely eaten, digestion is slowed down and the food is not fully utilized. Not least, food properly cooked and attractively served may be inadequate if there are factors interfering with chewing (e.g., lack of teeth) or interfering with the ingestion of the food (e.g., peptic ulcer or gastro-enteritis) or interfering with its absorption (e.g., diseases of the gall-bladder, liver or pancreas).

Fortification of food is the addition of necessary minerals and vitamins that have been removed by processing, or, in the case of synthetic foodstuffs, that are found in the naturally occurring substance for which the synthetic is a substitute. The major products so treated are flour (to which are added B vitamins, iron and calcium) and margarine (which is fortified by the addition of vitamins A and D).

The reverse process to fortification is adulteration of food in which the nutritive content of food products is diminished by their dilution, as can occur with milk, or the addition of cheaper, bulk-increasing substances, as can occur with flour.

In developed countries protein deficiency and vitamin deficiencies are rare and mineral deficiencies even rarer; the commonest error, particularly in the affluent sections of the population, is carbohydrate excess, i.e., the creation of obesity from over-eating sugars and starches. See also DIET.

food poisoning. An acute illness characterized by vomiting, diarrhoea or both, and by pain in the abdomen; it is usually caused by eating food contaminated by bacteria.

The disease is notifiable but is probably much commoner than is indicated by notifications. Many mild cases clear up without the victim having consulted a doctor, and in some cases that come to medical notice the infecting organism cannot be found and the disease cannot be differentiated from other conditions causing diarrhoea and abdominal upset.

Food poisoning should always be suspected if several people who have eaten the same food develop abdominal symptoms roughly simultaneously. In the most frequent type, poisoning by bacteria of the salmonella group, symptoms begin between twelve and thirty-six hours after eating the contaminated food, the time period varying with the number of organisms swallowed, the general health of the person and several other factors. In poisoning by staphylococci the symptoms begin between one and six hours later, and in the rare but serious botulism they appear in twelve to twenty-four hours.

Treatment includes rest in bed, abundant water or fruit juice to drink (to prevent dehydration) and in severe cases an appropriate antibiotic. If any of the

Milk bottles rendered inaccessible to birds and not left standing in sun

Food kept cool, wiremesh window

Wash hands after visit to lavatory but not in kitchen sink

Fruit and vegetables thoroughly washed, especially if eaten raw

Wash hands after using handkerchief preferably a disposable one

Dustbins to be kept in good repair and away from kitchens Wash hands after using same

Spoons used for tasting should not be put back in mixture

Always use the handle of cutlery when setting the table

Avoid fingering the nose whilst preparing food

Plates scraped, rinsed and stacked tidily. Cutlery stood in vessels of hot soapy water

All cuts covered with waterproof dressing

Tea towels should be clean daily

Prevention of food poisoning in the home

suspected food remains available portions of it should be sent to a bacteriological laboratory to try to establish the source and to save other people from becoming infected.

Bacterial food poisoning occurs in three main ways. (1) The bacteria or their toxins may be present in the animals or fowls which are subsequently served as meat or poultry products. (2) Cooked food may be contaminated by bacteria on the hands, cloths or utensils. (3) If food is kept warm for a long time after cooking, a few bacteria that have survived cooking or that have reached the food subsequently have time to multiply.

The hygiene of livestock, poultry and abattoirs is beyond the scope of this book, but much food poisoning could be prevented by scrupulous personal hygiene by all food handlers (e.g., thorough hand-washing after using the lavatory or blowing the nose), cooking food thoroughly (remembering that the temperature should be high enough to kill organisms in the middle of the joint or bird – frozen chickens should always be thawed out for twenty-four hours before cooking) and storing uneaten cooked food under conditions both of coolness and cleanness.

Non-bacterial food poisoning can occur from the eating of poisonous fruits or berries, or from the eating of unwashed fruit recently sprayed with poisonous pesticides.

foot. The portion of the lower limb situated below the ankle-joint. The foot consists of twenty-six bones forming a series of arches and some thirty-three joints, bound together by many strong ligaments. From back to the front of the foot the bones can be considered in three groups: (1) the seven tarsal bones, strong and compact, and so jointed that the foot can be rotated in any direction; (2) the five metatarsals, long bones running between the tarsals and the phalanges or toe-bones; and (3) the fourteen phalanges, two for the great toe and three for each of the other toes.

The foot is arched longwise so that in standing only the outer edge touches the ground, and in walking the weight is normally taken partly by this weight-bearing arch and partly by the ball of the great toe. There is also a second arch running crosswise at the ball of the foot.

Strain of the foot with pain and ultimate deformity may arise from badly fitting shoes with insufficent room for the toes or with inability for the foot to alter shape as the weight of the body shifts. Other causes include overweight and persistently bad posture.

Since the foot bears the entire weight of the body and of any additional burden carried, e.g., twenty stone in the case of a twelve-stone man carrying a sack with a hundredweight of coal, diseases and disabilities are not uncommon. See CLAWFOOT, CLUBFOOT, CORNS, FLAT FOOT, GOUT.

footwear. A general term for boots, shoes, sandals, slippers, etc.

In Britain fully 50 per cent of persons over middle age have foot trouble, traceable in the main to badly fitting footwear, and backache and other disturbances can also frequently be a result of foot trouble. All too often shoes are bought as articles of fashion without any consideration of their ultimate effect on the user's feet.

Firstly, new shoes should feel comfortable: if uncomfortable at the beginning they are likely to become more uncomfortable as time passes. Secondly, since there is much free movement from the ball of the foot forwards, the front part of the shoe should not only allow each toe to lie perfectly straight without side pressure but should permit some movement of the toes. Thirdly, since there is little movement behind the ball of the foot, there should be a reasonably close fit in this part. Fourthly, there should be a cut-in at the back to fix the shoe in position. Fifthly, high heels create an excessive incline from the heel to the ball and so force the toes forwards, restricting their movement; they also may cause weakening (through disuse) of the muscles at the back of the leg, and are, therefore, to be avoided.

Feet vary greatly and footwear – especially for children – should be chosen with care and with adequate time for trial of different types. Sufficient attention to boots and shoes in the first thirty years of life can save much discomfort and disability in middle and old age.

foreign body. Any substance which penetrates an individual's body, either through an opening such as the mouth, or through the skin. A particle of dust in the eye is a foreign body and so is mud in a cut. There is usually a defensive process put into action to counteract the presence of a foreign body – in the two examples given the eye 'weeps' to wash out the dust, and the white blood cells gather to engulf the bacteria in the mud.

forensic medicine. The branch of medicine concerned with the law, the proper application of justice and medico-legal problems.

Where the clinical expert looks at a wound, fracture, injury or case of poisoning and asks himself, 'How best can I treat it?', and where the community physician asks himself 'How can I aim to reduce the likelihood of a similar occurrence?', the forensic expert asks himself exactly how and when it occurred and whether it was the result of accident, self-inflicted injury or external violence.

Inevitably much of forensic medicine is unspectacular – involving, for example, knowledge of the laws relating to the granting of death certificates and of the laws regulating the sale of poisons.

However, problems of identification, post-mortem changes, the examination of blood and hair, differentiation of accident and suicide and murder, identification of types of wound, and medico-legal aspects of insanity are also all subjects that fall within the scope of forensic medicine.

foreskin. The prepuce, a fold of skin covering the head of the penis. It can normally be retracted. Tightness of the foreskin (phimosis) is a not uncommon inherited condition, leading in extreme cases to difficulty in passing urine, and sometimes to bed-wetting and to inflammation of the skin lining the head of the penis. Slight degrees of phimosis often respond to artificial retraction and in due course disappear, but failure to respond should be followed by the very trivial operation of CIRCUMCISION. This operation is sometimes performed for religious – quite apart from medical – reasons.

forgetfulness. Although often used as a synonym for AMNESIA, forgetfulness normally implies difficulty in recalling a few inter-related associations whereas amnesia implies the blocking off of a large number of these associations. Returning from a wedding I find that I cannot describe the bride's dress while my wife cannot remember a joke made at the reception: these are examples of normal forgetfulness. On the way home I sustain a head injury and cannot recall the entire wedding: that is amnesia, in this particular case retrograde amnesia.

Some forgetfulness of past events and experiences is essential if memory of the past is to serve as a guide in the present. We must be able to select important or relevant happenings for recall without being cluttered by unimportant and irrelevant details: we must be able to remember that a no. 24 bus will take us to our friend's new house without also recollecting that the number of the bus ticket was A 41258.

In the elderly it is common to have an impaired memory for recent events, as compared with clearer recollection of significant earlier events; this is probably explicable by the events being less vigorously noted – because of thickened arteries or cerebral anaemia or simply because as life experience extends fewer current events seem important.

Forgetfulness is in considerable part a defence mechanism: we forget the disagreeable appointment scheduled for today or we repress from our conscious memory the unpleasant experience of last month. Freud considered that most forgetfulness is the result of such unconscious repression, and pointed out that repressed memories reach consciousness in distorted forms, e.g., in dreams and in slips of the tongue. Some forgetfulness, however, is explicable simply in terms of lack of interest: in the example in the first paragraph I would probably have remembered the bride's dress if I had expected to be asked about it, but my mind dismissed it as being of no

long-term interest to me. A child, fired by his teacher's enthusiasm, remembers the causes of a historical event; his neighbour, bored and uninterested, forgets them in an hour.

A good or bad memory is in large part innate. To some extent, however, forgetfulness can be decreased in several ways. (1) By conscious or subconscious realization that a particular experience is important to us: a lawyer will develop a remarkable ability to recall legal precedents while remaining unable to recollect the names of the flowers in his garden. (2) By forming connecting links with information already in the mind: because Mendel's genetic experiments were ignored until long after his death I had difficulty in 'placing' him chronologically until I appreciated – by chance – that he was born in the same year as Pasteur (1822). (3) By mechanical methods: e.g., tying a knot in a handkerchief as a reminder of an engagement or deliberately repeating a name several times to impress it on the memory. (4) As a very temporary measure, by the use of artificial linkages, such as mnemonics – useful where the information is required for only a few weeks but of little use for the permanent retention of information.

Diagram of (a) a simple fracture, and (b) a compound fracture of the leg

fracture. A break in a bone. Fractures may be caused by direct violence, as when the skull is fractured by a blow on the head; by indirect violence, as when a fall on the outstretched hand causes a fracture of the wrist; and occasionally by muscular action, as when sudden spasm of the thigh muscles causes fracture of the patella. In old people a spontaneous fracture may very occasionally occur without injury: in such a case the person does not 'fall and break his leg' but rather 'breaks his leg and therefore falls'.

A simple fracture has no external wound communicating with the surface. A compound fracture has such a wound. A simple or compound fracture may be complete (dividing the bone into two parts) or incomplete, common in children (where the break does not extend right across the bone); and it may be comminuted, where the bone is broken into several pieces, or impacted, where one end of a broken bone is driven into the other.

There is pain and tenderness near the site of the fracture, loss of movement in the limb or unnatural mobility, deformity (i.e., alteration of the shape and outline of the fractured bone), shortening of the affected limb, and crepitus (i.e., a grating sound when the broken parts rub together).

Whatever the type of fracture it is likely to require an x-ray to determine the exact nature of the break and amount of displacement, careful manipulation by a doctor to place the broken bones in complete alignment, and splinting in the position of best alignment.

Where a fracture is suspected or diagnosed the immediate aims should be to prevent further damage, to reduce pain, to guard against shock and to secure prompt medical attention. In general the victim should not be moved unless he is in a position of danger, and if he has to be moved a splint – e.g., an umbrella, walking stick or board covered with any available soft material – should be placed from above the joint above to below the joint below the fracture and tied with bandages or slings to reduce movement.

freckles. Localized deposits of brownish colouring matter in the superficial layers of the skin, arising after exposure to the sun's rays. Freckles are peculiar to northern races and found particularly in persons with fair or red hair. They can be regarded as nature's attempt to provide a sunshade for the tissues underneath.

Freckles are harmless and in general not unattractive, but where prevention is desired it involves the wearing of broad-brimmed hats and the use of sun-screening creams. Where existing freckles are deemed disfiguring they can be very slowly modified by the use of various soothing lotions and by avoidance of exposure to the sun. Attempts to remove freckles by peeling agents are dangerous.

fresh air. See VENTILATION.

Freud. Sigmund Freud (1856-1939) was the founder of psycho-analysis and is perhaps the most outstanding figure in the entire history of psychology and psychiatry.

He is often described as the discoverer of the unconscious, but he made no such claim; Schopenhauer and Hartmann had suggested the existence of unconscious mental activity about the time Freud was born. What Freud did was essentially to explore the hitherto unknown territory of the unconscious, to indicate the strength and complexity of unconscious motivation to devise methods of investigating the unconscious, and to cure neurotic and some other disorders by bringing their causes to the surface.

A physician and a distinguished neurologist before he became interested in psychology, Freud started with cases of neuroses, and found that – first under hypnosis and later by using techniques of free association – patients could be gradually led to bring to consciousness long forgotten experiences which were responsible for their present illnesses. The method worked. It rendered the psychoneuroses curable.

Even more importantly, it led Freud to a concept of unconscious motivation. Essentially he divided the mind into the superego (which has analogies with conscience), the ego (or conscious mind including things of which we are at present conscious and things that can easily be brought to consciousness), and the id (the vast unconscious portion in which lie many forgotten experiences and repressed desires which motivate many of our actions). A mechanism which he termed the censor prevents the appearance in the ego of ideas and desires incompatible with a person's general ethical and other code of what is acceptable; but the ideas and desires emerge in distorted or hidden form – as symbols or substitutes, as trivial accidents or 'slips of the tongue' and in dreams – and they constitute the motivation for many of a person's actions.

Because Freud used 'sex' in a very wide sense, including virtually the whole of our desires for pleasure and affection, and regarded it as the mainspring of human behaviour, his views throughout most of his life were regarded as highly controversial. Himself a highly moral man, he was accused of being a destroyer of moral values and of being obsessed with sex, and his ideas, such as those of a male child's love for his mother and jealousy of his father, were easily distorted by his adversaries.

Time, however, has been on Freud's side. His discoveries of unconscious motivation and of methods of exploring the unconscious rank among the greatest of human achievements; and his work has rendered possible the successful treatment of psychoneurotic and psychosomatic diseases and also of the psychological element in many organic diseases. While no pioneer can hope to be completely accurate in the exploring and mapping of a vast and previously unknown territory most modern psychiatrists accept something like 90 per cent of Freud's teaching as beyond dispute.

Friedreich's ataxia. A hereditary disease transmitted through either sex and characterized by progressive loss of co-ordinated movement as a result of degeneration of the nerve columns in the spine and cerebellum.

Awkwardness of gait and a tendency to stumble are early signs and often appear before the age of 6 years. As the disease progresses the gait becomes more irregular and clumsy, the patient walks with feet wide apart, and he begins to reel from side to side when walking. Later similar lack of co-ordination appears in arm movements. The disease, while progressive, does not appreciably shorten life. There is as yet no specific treatment.

frigidity. Inability to derive pleasure from sexual intercourse, commoner in women than in men. It may arise through both partners being ignorant of sexual matters, as where the husband reaches his climax too hurriedly and with insufficient preliminary sex-play, leaving the wife unsatisfied and coming to regard intercourse with distaste. Perhaps more often it has its origin in conscious or unconscious faulty attitudes to sex: because of inadequate or erroneous sex education intercourse is associated with ideas of sins, dirtiness or fear. Again, it may be due to a physical cause which renders intercourse painful, or to sheer fatigue.

In general there is a difference between the attitudes of the sexes: the woman is more affected by 'atmosphere' in sex relations and needs to be brought gradually to the stage where she desires intercourse; whereas the man has a more physical and more rapid desire. Given mutual love and respect, and a willingness to learn sex manners, many couples can themselves overcome frigidity. If they fail, they should first seek medical help lest there is any physical cause, and in the absence of a physical cause should seek the aid of a psychotherapist. Psychotherapy is usually needed if the woman has a persisting view of sex as sinful or dirty.

A marriage in which one partner has normal sexual desires and the other is frigid is unlikely to be successful. So it is important that a couple in these circumstances should study sex manners and should, if necessary, seek medical and psychiatric aid.

fringe medicine. Systems of treatment that fall outside the scope of orthodox medicine. Examples are ACUPUNCTURE, chiropraxis, HOMEOPATHY, naturopathy and OSTEOPATHY.

Acupuncture is discussed in a separate article. Chiropraxis, or manipulation of bones, has considerable prestige in the U.S.A. where there are 25,000 practising chiropractors, but is almost unknown in Britain. Homeopathy, treatment by minute doses of drugs, appears to be in a phase of decline in most countries. Naturopathy, or treatment by diet, seems to vary enormously with individual practitioners – from a vegetarian diet to the use only of foods grown without the aid of fertilizers. Osteopathy, treatment – like chiropraxis –

by manipulation of bones, is the most popular form of fringe medicine in Britain (there is a school for osteopaths in London, although only a fraction of all practising osteopaths have attended that school), and osteopaths appear to have abandoned the idea that they can treat all diseases and have begun to concentrate on diseases and disorders of bones, joints and muscles.

It is unlikely that any system of treatment for which thousands of persons are willing to pay has absolutely no merits. The marked hostility of the medical profession to the various forms of fringe medicine is based on three main points:

1. Very few homeopaths, naturopaths, etc. have had any long, rigorous training with periodical examinations, practical and theoretical. A qualified doctor can use any form of treatment, including fringe methods, but doctors – after lengthy study of anatomy, physiology and pathology – object to diagnosis and treatment being undertaken by people who have had much less training or no training at all.

2. Orthodox practitioners maintain that the causes of diseases are numerous and that no one form of treatment (e.g., exercises, diet, drugs or surgical operation) will suffice for a mass of entirely different diseases. They allege that practitioners of fringe medicine seem willing to treat almost any disease by the one method.

3. Orthodox doctors claim that the results of new treatments attempted by them are subjected to rigorous scientific testing, including, for example, the 'double-blind' method. In this system patients matched for age and sex are respectively given the old or the new drug, while the doctor responsible for assessing the patients' progress is left unaware of which drug was given to any one patient; treatments by practitioners of fringe medicine, they say, are not subjected to any such rigorous testing.

On the other hand, persons who have not been cured by orthodox medicine often visit chiropractors, homeopaths or osteopaths, and some of them are cured or improved. Fringe practitioners would claim that they are getting the 'difficult' cases, the 'simple' one having been cured by orthodox doctors. Traditional physicians while not denying that fringe practitioners tend to get their own failures suggest that a good proportion of illnesses are psychological in origin, and that the cure or alleviation depends more on the confidence inspired by the fringe practitioner than on the method of treatment employed. In response, the unorthodox worker would doubtless ask why – if the inspiring of confidence is all that is needed – it should be regarded as their monopoly: why should the orthodox doctor, presumably no less capable of inspiring confidence, attribute his cures to method (not confidence) but attribute the cures of some of his failures to confidence (not method)?

frontal sinuses. Two air cavities in the frontal bone of the skull, situated above the eyes and connected with the nose. They may become infected from the nose, causing headache and a feeling of fullness. Occasionally pus may form in them, sometimes necessitating an operation for its removal.

frostbite. Injury to the skin and underlying tissues through exposure to intense cold and consequent constriction of peripheral blood vessels.

Frostbite arises most commonly in the toes, fingers, ears and nose. The affected part becomes 'dead', white and hard. On recovery it can become painfully inflamed, with blisters which rupture, producing ulcers and sometimes even gangrene.

Prevention is largely by taking adequate precautions, including the wearing of sufficient warm, suitable clothing (loose enough to allow free circulation of blood) and avoidance of exposure to cold in persons with poor circulation. It is important to remember in connection with prevention that frostbite is not related to the temperature (32 °F. or 0 °C.) at which water freezes; the colder the atmosphere the greater the risk of frostbite, but cases have occurred considerably above 32 °F.

Treatment involves very gentle warmth – in a comfortable room but not close to a fire or stove, and bathing of the affected parts with cold water. The old remedy of massaging with snow is now discredited: the rubbing is more likely to harm the tissues than to benefit them.

frozen shoulder. Pain and stiffness due to inflammation of the BURSA in the shoulder joint. Spontaneous recovery tends to occur in three or four months but can sometimes be hastened by injection of procaine (a local anaesthetic allied to cocaine) either alone or mixed with a hydrocortisone (a cortocosteroid).

fugue. A disturbance or restriction of consciousness, predominantly occurring in hysterical illness.

The patient continues to act in a purposeful manner but retains no conscious remembrance of having done so,

and may disclaim any knowledge of his identity or whereabouts. A hysterical fugue with such amnesia, or loss of memory, represents a subconscious attempt to escape from some predicament.

See also AUTOMATISM and DOUBLE PERSONALITY.

fundus. The bottom of a structure. The term refers to the rounded part of a hollow organ furthest from its opening and it is most commonly used in relation to the uterus, bladder, and the upper portion of the stomach. The spherical rear part of the eyeball to which the retina is attached is known as the fundus oculi.

fungus. A low form of vegetable life, of the botanical class thallophytes, distinguished mainly by absence of chlorophyll. Fungi are parasitic on living plants or animals. Yeast, moulds, mushrooms and toadstools are fungus growths. Acthinomycosis, ringworm, favus and asperillosis are fungus diseases affecting man.

Fungi are medically important in at least four ways: (1) certain toadstools are highly poisonous; (2) some moulds cause infection, just as bacteria do; (3) some fungi cause allergic reactions; (4) some are highly important for the obtaining of drugs, e.g., yeast (essential for production of alcohol) is an excellent source of the B vitamins, and moulds are the source of pencillin and other antibiotics.

'funny bone'. In its path from the armpit to the wrist the ulnar nerve at the elbow lies close to the skin and also just over the swollen end of the humerus. So a very minor injury can temporarily compress the nerve between an external hard object and the bone, producing a tingling sensation popularly known as 'striking the funny bone'.

furred tongue. A condition in which the tongue is covered by a whitish-brown layer consisting of cast-off surface cells, food debris and bacteria. Causes include constipation, digestive disorders and some fevers. The condition itself is of little significance.

furunculosis. The technical term for 'suffering from BOILS'.

G

gait. The way a person walks often gives a clue to his psychological make-up or current emotional state, e.g., depressed people tend to walk slowly with bowed head and bent shoulders, and elated people with vigorous and springing step. Yet many trivial causes, such as a blister on the heel or the need to hurry for a bus can temporarily alter the gait.

In infants congenital dislocation of the hip, if missed earlier, may be suspected from a waddling gait. In children faulty gait may indicate bad posture, which can be corrected by suitable exercises, or early disease of the hip joint; and a jerky gait is observed in chorea. In adults a reeling gait suggests over-indulgence in alcohol or disease of the cerebellum; a 'broad base' gait with feet well apart is found in locomotor ataxia; a high-stepping gait is common in neuritis of the legs; and a shuffling gait occurs in paralysis agitans and after a stroke.

It should of course be remembered that an unusual gait may simply be a mannerism.

gall. Another name for BILE.

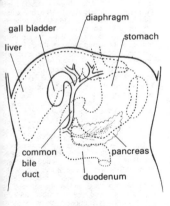

The gall-bladder

gall-bladder. A pear-shaped muscular bag situated on the under-surface of the liver. It acts as a receptacle for BILE. From the gall-bladder bile travels along the cystic and common bile ducts to the duodenum.

For inflammation of the gall-bladder, see CHOLECYSTITIS.

gallstones. Solid, pebble-like masses formed in the gall-bladder. There are three main varieties – multiple faceted stones composed of calcium and bile pigment, single stones of cholesterol, and pure granules of bile pigment.

The commonest cause is chronic inflammation of the gall-bladder (causing albumen to be added to the bile, with precipitation of calcium, and formation either of a stone of calcium and bile pigment or of a nucleus round which cholesterol crystallizes). Other probable causes include excess of cholesterol in the diet and stagnation of bile.

Gallstones occur mostly between the ages of 30 and 60 years, are found in 20 per cent of women and 7 per cent of men, and are particularly associated with child-bearing, sedentary occupation and obesity.

Stones may exist for years and cause no trouble, or cause only occasional mild discomfort, heart-burn and flatulence. If a stone passes down the cystic and common bile ducts, which lead from the gall-bladder to the duodenum, and becomes lodged, there is intense pain (often tranferred to the right shoulder), collapse, vomiting, high fever and rigor, with – through blockage of the duct – jaundice appearing in due course. The condition is at first liable to be mistaken for a perforated peptic ulcer or acute appendicitis.

Prevention is largely by early recognition and treatment of CHOLECYSTITIS, and by attention to diet. During an attack the pain may be controlled by injection of morphia and atropine, and various drugs may be used to aid the passing or the dissolving of the stone. If the stone is duly passed, it has to be considered whether it was an isolated event or is likely to be repeated, and x-ray examination may provide useful information on this point. If stones are numerous and attempts to dissolve them unsuccessful, surgical treatment will be required – the gall-bladder being either opened and drained or else removed.

Galvanism. Use of a constant electrical current which causes muscular contraction only when it is made and broken (unlike FARADISM which uses alternating current), Galvanism is employed in the diagnosis of muscle and nerve injuries, and also in the treatment of neuritis, arthritis and synovitis.

gammaglobulin. The plasma or fluid part of the blood is a sticky solution composed mainly of two types of protein, albumin and globulin. The globulin component, produced by the lymphatic system, can be separated by chemical means and further fractionated. When this is done it is found that antibodies to infection are particularly associated with the so-called 'gamma' fraction (IG). Gamma-globulin or human immuno-globulin is now prepared from 'pooled' human sera and is available for the prevention and treatment of certain infections. By using sera from persons known to have natural or induced immunity to specific diseases it is also possible to produce hyper-immuno-globulin, as for instance, vaccinial immuno-globulin. Certain persons have a genetically determined deficiency of gammaglobulin and suffer from hypo-gammaglobulinaemia.

ganglion. A swelling or cyst containing a jelly-like substance and developing as a round, hard mass on a tendon sheath or joint capsule. The back of the wrist is the commonest site. A ganglion is painless and harmless but, if unsightly, can easily be removed surgically.

The term is also used for a 'junction' in the nervous system, where nerve fibres connect with each other.

gangrene. Mortification; death of the tissue in one part of the body.

Dry gangrene is essentially due to loss of blood supply to the part affected. For instance, old people with hardened and thickened arteries may develop gangrene of the toes and this may spread to the foot. Causes include any interference with the blood supply, e.g., blockage of an artery, injury to an artery, or extreme spasm of an artery in severe cases of Raynaud's disease. Diabetes and chronic nephritis favour the development of gangrene which may also occur following frost-bite, burns, crushing injuries and ergot poisoning.

The dead part becomes hard, dry, wrinkled and (from diffusion of disintegrated haemoglobin) dark brown in colour, with a sharp line of demarcation from adjacent living tissue. Attempts to preserve the circulation and close attention to the feet and hands of those at risk may prevent gangrene. Where it occurs surgical removal of the dead tissue is usually necessary.

Gas gangrene is a complication of severe wounds in which tissue is crushed. Bacteria, mostly *Clostridia welshii*, breed in the damaged tissue which first becomes reddish, then greenish-yellow and finally black, while bubbles of gas appear between the muscle fibres. Apart from pain, swelling and discoloration, the symptoms are those of acute toxaemia. Antibiotics and drainage of the wound help, especially if used early, but in many cases amputation is necessary to preserve life.

gargle. The process of applying a cleansing or antiseptic solution to the back of the throat. It consists of taking a very small mouthful of the liquid, throwing back the head and making the liquid bubble in the throat without swallowing it. Gargles are quite useful in cases of tonsillitis and pharyngitis. Two simple gargles are: (1) crystals of potassium permanganate in

warm water in sufficient amount to turn the water faintly pink (not red which would be so strong that it would damage the tissues); and (2) salt (half a teaspoonful to a tumbler) in warm water.

Although gargles are of some use, their value has been overrated in the past. In general, throat infections need treatment with appropriate antibiotics or sulphonamides; and for a mildly inflamed throat rest from speaking and smoking is far more important than the use of a gargle.

gas poisoning. See CARBON MONOXIDE.

gastric ulcer. An ulcer is an eroded open sore on the surface of the skin or a mucous membrane. A gastric ulcer is such a sore occurring in the wall of the stomach.

The stomach contains highly acid gastric juice which digests the protein of food but does not normally affect the living tissue of the stomach wall, because that wall is protected by gastric mucus. However, about 20 per cent of people have a short and over-active stomach, a higher than normal concentration of acid gastric juice, and a deficient secretion of the protective mucus. In such persons any minor injury of the stomach wall (e.g., from a sharp swallowed substance or even from hard and insufficiently chewed food) is likely to be extended by the action of gastric juice on the damaged area, so causing an ulcer.

The main symptom is pain in the region of the lower end of the breast bone, recurring regularly about half to one-and-a-half hours after food, and usually relieved by an alkaline drink or tablet. Other features are tenderness over the pit of the stomach and sometimes vomiting of blood-stained stomach contents. For accurate diagnosis a TEST-MEAL is often required (to determine the chemical characteristics of the gastric secretion) and an x-ray after a barium meal (to render the stomach temporarily opaque to the rays).

Treatment is based on rest, an easily digested diet, and the giving of antacids to neutralize excess acid and of other drugs to diminish secretion of acid and to reduce the movements of the stomach.

Gastric and DUODENAL ULCER are very similar clinically and sometimes classed together as peptic ulcer, though there are some differences in symptoms, e.g., while the pain of a gastric ulcer comes on fairly soon after a meal and is not relieved by eating more food, the pain of a duodenal ulcer comes on about two hours after eating and is temporarily relieved by further eating. There are, however, considerable differences in the groups of people who suffer from each type and in the underlying causes: gastric ulcer is a disease of the poor more than of the rich; emotional stress and worry, while playing some part in the production of gastric ulcer, play a far more important part in duodenal ulcer; and faulty dietetic habits – e.g., meals at very irregular intervals – are very important in causing gastric ulcer but relatively unimportant in the other condition.

gastritis. Acute gastritis usually follows ingestion of unsuitable or grossly excessive food or large amounts of alcohol. An intense form occurs after the swallowing of some poisons. Symptoms include headache, discomfort in the upper abdomen, nausea and sometimes vomiting. Initially the diagnosis is difficult: typhoid often has a similar onset; cancer of the stomach is also similar although there is more pain and a wasted appearance; and gastric ulcer is not dissimilar although the pain has more relation to meals. After diagnosis has been made treatment consists of giving a laxative, withholding food for a day or so and giving a mild alkali.

Chronic gastritis occurs as a sequel to repeated acute gastritis; following prolonged excess of alcohol, condiments, tea or tobacco; or in association with various severe diseases, such as chronic nephritis and diabetes. Symptoms include poor appetite, diffused pain after food, bouts of headache and vomiting, especially in the morning. After serious diseases have been excluded, treatment is on the same lines as for GASTRIC ULCER.

gastro-enteritis. Inflammation both of the stomach and of the intestines. The condition is characterized by diarrhoea and vomiting, high temperature, and signs of dehydration. In severe cases and especially in young children treatment of the dehydration is essential, so frequent drinks should be taken.

There are four groups of causes: (1) infections such as cholera and dysentery; (2) defects of metabolism or absorption e.g., indigestion following excess starches, diarrhoea following too much protein, and various conditions (such as coeliac disease) resulting from inability to digest fat; (3) emotional and nervous conditions, e.g., nervous diarrhoea; (4) various other causes, such as allergies or tumours of the colon.

Severe cases and outbreaks affecting more than one person are best regarded as due to infection until the contrary is proved. Pending diagnosis the patient should be given no solid food for a day or so but encouraged to drink sufficient water. Antibiotics and other drugs should not be given until the cause has been established, because they may mask the cause.

general paralysis of the insane (GPI). A chronic progressive disease of the brain occurring ten to fifteen years after the contraction of syphilis that has been inadequately treated or left untreated. See SYPHILIS.

general practitioner. A doctor who undertakes diagnosis and treatment without limitation of the age or sex of his patients and without restriction of the types of illness handled. The general

practitioner seeks to provide primary medical care for all individuals who have accepted him as their personal physician.

The term 'family doctor', sometimes used as a synonym, expresses the broad meaning but is less accurate because (1) persons working far from their families may need a general practitioner but can hardly be said to have a family doctor, (2) members of a family may elect to enroll with different practitioners, and (3) in the group practice that is becoming increasingly common – and is necessary to enable doctors to have freedom from emergency calls when not on duty – a family, even if enrolled with one practice, may in three successive episodes of illness be treated by three different members of the practice.

Although the general practitioner cannot claim the clinical expertise of the specialist or the preventive and epidemiological expertise of the community physician, he should not therefore be considered of lesser importance. He has chosen to exercise his skills over a wider range and in less detail, and he is in many ways the key medical figure who calls in appropriate clinical or community specialists at need.

Nearly half the doctors in Britain are general practitioners. They are paid a fee calculated on the number of patients on their list, with the fee increased for elderly persons (because of greater liability to illness) and with additional payments permitted for some services (e.g., supervision during pregnancy and childbirth). A person is free to choose his own practitioner and to change that practitioner at any time; and a practitioner can refuse to have a patient on his list, either because the list is full or because he considers the particular patient unreasonable.

Some private practice still exists in Britain. A patient who thinks he will get better service by paying for it directly may consult any practitioner privately, with the single exception that a practitioner cannot accept as a private patient somebody for whom he is already receiving a fee from the National Health Service.

The current tendency in Britain is very much towards group practice, where perhaps six doctors, five health visitors, four district nurses and a receptionist accept responsibility for a 'panel' of 14,000 patients or prospective patients. There are advantages to the professionals, for instance a doctor can know that he is liable for night calls on only one night out of six. Also there are advantages to the patients such as the better equipment that a multiple practice can provide, and the knowledge that the doctor who attends in an emergency is not exhausted because of his previous night's sleep having been disturbed by another emergency call.

genes. Minute particles inside the cells which pass on all the physical and mental characteristics that a person inherits, e.g., blood group, colour of eyes, colour of hair, mathematical ability, linguistic ability, etc. Large numbers of genes, far too small to be visible under a high-powered microscope, are located in a line down each of the chromosomes. See GENETICS.

genetic guidance. Counselling of married couples, or preferably of persons contemplating matrimony, as to their degree of risk of producing a child seriously handicapped by hereditary disease. Essentially such guidance is based on two factors: detailed study of pedigree and microscopic examination of the chromosomes of body cells.

Where a family has a history of hereditary disease inherited as a dominant gene (see GENETICS), as in Huntington's chorea or congenital dwarfism, the ascertainment of risk is easy: the son or daughter of a sufferer has a 50 per cent chance of inheriting and transmitting the disease, but the nephew or niece of a sufferer, provided the parents were unaffected, will not transmit the disease. Where there is a family history of disease inherited as a recessive gene, as in cystic fibrosis or deaf mutism, the ascertainment of risk is more difficult, because the disease may miss a generation or a couple of generations and then reappear. Where several genes are involved, as in spina bifida and schizophrenia, the full skills of a geneticist are needed to estimate the risk of producing a damaged child.

Most of the highly developed countries have genetic clinics to which persons of suspicious family history or couples who have produced a handicapped child can be referred. Essentially these clinics perform three functions: (1) they reassure many couples who wrongly think themselves at risk because of the illness of a relative of one of them; (2) in cases of bad heredity they can advise married couples or couples contemplating marriage of their degree of risk of producing a seriously damaged child; and (3) in the case of a pregnant woman they can sometimes determine whether the foetus is seriously damaged, although in this case the investigation is pointless unless the woman is prepared to have the pregnancy terminated if necessary.

Since improvement in maternal and child health services enables a higher proportion of handicapped children to survive, and since in some hereditary diseases (e.g., Huntington's chorea and schizophrenia) even a direct transmitter may reach child-bearing age before showing any signs of the disease, genetic clinics are clearly very important, but it should be appreciated that they cannot stand on their own. For their success there also has to be a well-developed service (such as health visitors in the U.K.) to reassure many people who falsely suspect that they may be transmitters of hereditary disease (and who might

otherwise swamp the clinics) and to persuade others who may be at risk that it is desirable for them to attend genetic clinics.

Assessment at a clinic is not the end of the story. The geneticist's job is essentially to say, 'If you produce a child there is a 10 per cent chance that it will suffer from a particular disease'. Thereafter there must be people – health visitors, general practitioners, social workers – prepared to discuss with the couple the seriousness or otherwise of the possible disease, the degree of risk in relation to that seriousness, the means of having a full sex life without producing children (contraceptives, tying of female tubes, male vasectomy) and the methods of compensating for natural desire to have children (e.g., adoption).

genetics. The study of the factors which determine the transmission of inherited characteristics from parents to offspring. An individual's total make-up is not entirely determined by genetic factors, since heredity and environment go together to mould the human being.

The narrower field of medical genetics is concerned primarily with the transmission of hereditary diseases. These are becoming of greater relative importance both because many non-genetic conditions can now be successfully prevented or treated and because facilities for effective treatment result in many more children with congenital defects surviving to adult life.

Biological inheritance. The old name for this was Mendelism because the broad principles of heredity were originally worked out by an Austrian monk, Gregor Mendel, about 1850, and later verified in 1900 by independent workers.

Mendel experimented with ordinary pea-plants and identified paired characteristics in which they varied. As an example he found that if he interbred plants with red flowers all the offspring had red flowers too. If he bred red-flowered plants with white-flowered plants all the hybrid offspring had red flowers and he concluded that redness was a dominant characteristic, and that whiteness was recessive. If he then interbred the red/white hybrids he obtained both red flowers and white flowers in the proportion of three to one, but of the three reds one was a pure red which would continue to breed true and the other two were red/white hybrids. This became known as the Mendelian ratio and on the basis of this he formulated two laws. These were the law of segregation (that paired characteristics were inherited one from each parent) and the law of independence (that paired characteristics were inherited independently). The second is now known not to be wholly true because 'linkage' can occur unless the separate characteristics are carried on separate chromosomes.

Chromosomes and genes. The next step came with the growing elucidation of cell-structure.

The cell-nucleus contains chromatin, made up from protein, ribonucleic acid (RNA) and deoxyribonucleic acid (DNA). In the resting phase chromatin appears as a network of nuclear material but when the cell is about to divide the chromatin becomes defined into rod-shaped bodies called chromosomes. In man there are forty-six of these, arranged in twenty-three sets of similar pairs (diploid chromosomes), one member of each pair having been derived from father and mother respectively. As cell and nuclear division proceed each chromosome splits longitudinally and separates (mitosis) to form a new but identical chromosome. Collectively these are again reconstituted as two sets of twenty-three and shared between the two daughter cells.

An important exception to this general rule occurs in the ovum and sperm (gametes). Since these unite to form the zygote the union would produce twice the proper number of chromosomes, so during maturation they undergo a process called meiosis and their individual chromosomes are reduced to twenty-three. Twenty-two of these are autosomes and similar in both sexes but the remaining chromosome is known as the sex-chromosome and occurs in two forms, x and y. All female gametes contain an x-chromosome; male gametes have either an x or a y. Accordingly when they join to form an embryo or zygote the sex-chromosome pair resulting may be either xx in which case the child will be female, or xy resulting in a male. See also CHROMOSOME.

The DNA appears in the chromosome as a long complex molecule like a double thread or tiny twisted rope-ladder with its steps made up of the bases adenine, thymine, cytosine and guanine. The order in which these bases occur along the ladder forms the genetic code. If the DNA becomes disarranged as by chemical agents or radiation a mutation results. Most mutations are harmful but natural selection tends to retain favourable ones and reject the unfavourable.

The genes are the units of inheritance, also bi-parental in origin, and they occupy corresponding positions on the chromosomes. As already mentioned a gene occasionally alters by spontaneous or induced mutation and it can then be present in two or more forms known as alleles. If an individual inherits from each parent the same allelic form of a particular gene he is said to be homozygous for that gene position; if different alleles are present he is heterozygous. When a particular allele gives rise to an obvious physical characteristic in a heterozygote it is said to be dominant but if the characteristic only appears in the homozygote it is recessive. In addition to their function in determining

sex the sex-chromosomes carry other genes affecting other characteristics and hence the inheritance of such genes is sex-linked but, since the human y-chromosome is much smaller than the x-chromosome, linkage is mainly to x.

It can now be explained how the foregoing considerations work out in practice.

Dominant inheritance. While the y-chromosome of a father can pass only to his sons and his x-chromosome only to his daughters all the other autosomes of both parents pass equally to sons and daughters. When two unequal genes (alleles) meet in a pair the stronger prevails and is said to be dominant. Pigmentation for instance is dominant to albinism which is an undesirable trait. In general, dominant genes are related to normal or beneficial characteristics, but the rule is by no means invariable; achondroplasia, short, webbed or additional fingers and toes, Huntington's chorea, diabetes insipidus and some eye defects, all relatively common, are due to dominant inheritance and will appear in heterozygotes. On the average, affected persons married to normals will have affected and normal children in equal proportions. Normal children of the union marrying normals will have only normal offspring.

Recessive inheritance. The effects of a recessive gene are seen only in homozygotes, where both parents carry the gene and contribute an affected chromosome to the offspring. Albinism is recessive to pigmentation and so two apparently normal persons may marry but if each is a heterozygous carrier of albinism there is a one in four chance of an albino offspring (Mendelian ratio). There are many recessively inherited diseases but most of them are individually uncommon. The chances of marrying someone with the same harmful gene are low but marriage with a close relative obviously increases the risk and similarly the effects of modern treatment in securing the survival to adult life of patients with such conditions as cystic fibrosis and phenylketonuria also have implications for the future. Amongst other recessive conditions are amaurotic familial idiocy, Friedrich's ataxia, Ménière's disease, deaf mutism and osteosclerosis.

Because these conditions continue to be carried by apparently normal heterozygotes they may reappear after missing a generation or two.

Sex-linked inheritance. The classic example is HAEMOPHILIA in which the male victim carries the gene in his one x-chromosome. So far all sex-linked diseases have proved to be x-linked and nearly all are recessive. Thus in haemophilia an affected male cannot transmit the disease to his sons, whose x-chromosome must have come from the mother, but his daughters will be heterozygous (one x from mother and another x with the weak gene from the father) and they will be able to transmit the condition to the next generation. Muscular dystrophy (Duchenne type) is inherited similarly.

Mixed inheritance. Some conditions do not quite follow these rules precisely, probably because of segmental interchange between chromosomes and hence may occur either as dominant, recessive, or sex-linked types. This is true of congenital deafness, other types of muscular dystrophy, and retinitis pigmentosa. Pyloric stenosis, spina bifida, hare-lip and cleft palate, congenital dislocation of the hip, congenital heart disease, diabetes, schizophrenia, manic-depressive psychosis and spondylitis also show evidence of a partial or complex inheritance.

Chromosome abnormalities. The abnormality may be of number or of structure where chromosomal breaks have led to loss or rearrangement of chromosomal material. The best known condition is mongolism or Down's syndrome where there is an extra no. 21 chromosome making a total of forty-seven in all. Hence the name 'trisomy 21'.

Genetic counselling. Persons with a family history of inherited disease or who have already had an abnormal child are naturally concerned to know what are the risks of the condition arising or recurring in their family. Genetic Advisory Centres are now available in most main hospital centres, and the family doctor if he cannot resolve the problem himself can make arrangements for consultation in order that appropriate advice may be given. See GENETIC GUIDANCE.

genitals. Those parts of the REPRODUCTIVE SYSTEM which are on the body surface.

genu valgum. See KNOCK KNEE.

geriatrics. The branch of medicine concerned with the health and diseases of those who are AGEING.

Old people differ from younger adults in many respects. For instance their recovery from any illness tends to be slower but, because of risk of joint stiffening, are often have to be got out of bed at an earlier stage of the illness. Again, while younger adults, when ill, generally have a single disease, old people may well suffer from a number of simultaneous diseases and disabilities. To take another example, if a young adult has normal appetite and an adequate and well-balanced diet, we can usually forget about deficiency diseases; but in respect of the nutrition of an old person we have to consider such points as: (1) the food available (having regard to the relative poverty of many old persons), (2) the foods actually used (having regard to likes and dislikes acquired over many years and also to possible chewing difficulties), and (3) digestive and absorptive capacities (which may make it desirable that a pensioner with an apparently well-balanced diet

should nevertheless receive vitamin supplements).

germ. A germ or micro-organism is a minute living creature which cannot usually be seen without a microscope. The term is mostly reserved for micro-organisms which cause disease (pathogens) but can be used also for harmless micro-organisms and for micro-organisms that are actively useful, such as the mould from which we derive penicillin or the yeast used in baking. Germs include BACTERIA, VIRUSES and RICKETTSIA. Bacteria can be seen through an ordinary microscope; examples are organisms that cause typhoid, bacillary dysentery and diphtheria. Viruses are much smaller and can be seen only by using an electron microscope; examples are those that cause chicken pox and influenza. Rickettsia are to some extent intermediate. An example is the organism that causes typhus.

Yeasts and moulds are included under the term 'germs', and so usually are somewhat larger single-celled organisms, PROTOZOA, such as the germ which causes amoebic dysentery.

Germs enter the body in three main ways: by inhalation of air particles carrying them, by swallowing of food containing them, or by penetration of the skin or access through an open wound.

In many cases bacterial and rickettsial diseases can now be prevented by immunization, or treated by antibiotics. Both prevention and treatment of virus infections is more difficult: vaccines have been devised for only a minority of these infections, and many virus diseases are resistant to antibiotics.

German measles. Otherwise known as rubella, this is a mild, infectious, feverish disease, caused by a virus. There is a rash which is less coarse than that of measles, mild catarrhal symptoms and enlargement of the glands behind the ears. The incubation period is about eighteen days and the duration of illness is about three days. One attack results in permanent immunity.

Although a trifling illness, rubella is of considerable importance if it occurs during early pregnancy because of the risk of viral damage to the developing foetus. Rubella during the first three months of pregnancy may cause congenital cataracts, deafness, mental deficiency and congenital heart disease, and may sometimes produce miscarriage.

In order to prevent this situation arising some countries are attempting to eradicate rubella completely by immunizing all children (of both sexes) while other countries, including Britain, are trying to prevent the occurrence of the disease during pregnancy by offering immunization to all girls aged about 13 years, and in some cases by also offering immunization to young women, not yet pregnant, who have neither had rubella earlier nor been immunized against it.

If, despite the availability of immunization, a woman develops rubella during the first three months of pregnancy, the question of abortion should be considered. It should be noted that rubella later in pregnancy causes no risk to the child, and that rubella in early pregnancy – whether followed by a therapeutic abortion or by the birth of a deformed or a healthy child – carries no risk to subsequent children.

gestation. The period during which the unborn child develops within the uterus, i.e., from conception (the union of the ovum and the sperm after intercourse) to birth. In the human female it averages 266 days, although 6 days longer and 6 days shorter are both considered to fall within the limits of normality.

giardiasis. Infestation of the bowel by a pear-shaped microscopic parasite, *Giardia lamblia*. Infection, just as in typhoid and paratyphoid, comes from consuming food or drink contaminated by the excreta of sufferers, so the condition could be eliminated by proper sewerage and good personal hygiene.

In highly developed countries the disease is rare but by no means unknown, but in some countries infestation is so common in apparently healthy children that some experts question whether the parasite really does any harm. In at least a proportion of cases, however, it causes diarrhoea and abdominal discomfort with the passing of motions containing excessive fat, perhaps because the parasites line the mucous membrane of the intestine and hinder the proper absorption of fat. Tablets of mepacrine hydrochloride (100 mg. daily for a week) usually effect a complete cure.

giddiness. See DIZZINESS.

gigantism. See ACROMEGALY AND GIGANTISM.

gingivitis. See GUMS.

glanders. A dangerous infectious disease, caused by a bacillus, occurring mainly in horses but occasionally communicated to persons in close contact with horses. In man the condition usually starts with spots on the nose, semipurulent nasal discharge, and symptoms of pneumonia and general fever follow. If untreated the disease is fatal in about 90 per cent of cases.

For treatment a combination of streptomycin and a sulphonamide is usually advised.

glands. Organs which manufacture and release substances necessary for the working of the body. There are two broad types, those with ducts which carry their secretions, and those that pass their secretions directly into the bloodstream.

Examples of glands with ducts include the various salivary glands required for digestion, and the sweat glands needed for release of perspiration. Glands without ducts secrete hormones or chemical messengers; these are the ENDOCRINE GLANDS, such as the pituitary and the thyroid.

Additionally, the term 'glands' is used for lymph glands or nodes which are interposed in the course of lymphatic vessels and through which the lymph is filtered. Apart from arresting inert or harmful substances (including bacteria) lymph glands manufacture lymphocytes which are important for the destruction of bacteria.

Inflammation of glands has, consequently, two separate meanings. Firstly, it applies to swelling of organs of secretion: e.g., in tonsillitis and scarlet fever the neck glands are enlarged, and swelling of glands behind the ears is an indication of a rash being that of German measles. Secondly, the term applies to the lymph nodes, as when infection of the gland spreads up the lymphatic vessels to produce reddening of small glands near the elbow and swelling of glands in the armpit.

glandular fever. An acute infection characterized by fever, sore throat, swelling of cervical and other lymph glands, and enlargement of the spleen. The symptoms last for about a month, and diagnosis – formerly rather difficult – can nowadays be made by blood-test.

The cause and mode of transmission are not yet understood, although it is thought that the spread is from the nose and throat of infected persons. The normal treatment consists simply of rest and light diet, and spontaneous recovery occurs in four or five weeks. Many drugs have been tried but none have been shown to shorten the disease, although antibiotics are useful if complications occur, such as tonsillitis.

Probably many cases have remained undiagnosed in the past. Now that we have an accurate means of identifying suspected cases we may hope to learn more about the cause and method of spread. So far, however, we are largely working in ignorance: for instance, authorities in the U.S.A. regard the disease as too common to justify isolation, whereas in Britain isolation is recommended.

glans penis. See PENIS.

glaucoma. A disease of the eye caused by increased pressure of fluid within the eyeball. If untreated the increasing pressure damages the optic nerve and retina, and causes blindness. The cause is obstruction in the drainage of fluid from the eyeball. Very occasionally the condition occurs in infants through a developmental abnormality, but usually the disease appears only above the age of 50 years.

Acute glaucoma may start with severe pain in the eye, disturbance or blurring of vision, and sickness. Chronic glaucoma comes on gradually, with little pain but steady deterioration of vision; there are attacks of 'mist before the eyes' and the seeing of rainbow rings round a distant light.

Early diagnosis is important because of the danger to sight in untreated cases.

Indeed the risk of glaucoma is one reason why it is advised that persons over 50 should have their eyes examined every two years. Pressure can be estimated by the specialist's finger or by an instrument called a tonometer.

In early cases treatment with suitable drugs is often effective. Where drugs fail, a small operation may create an outflow canal for the excessive fluid. Once the retina and optic nerve have been damaged, treatment may prevent a worsening of the condition but cannot undo the damage already done.

glioma. A tumour of the tissue connecting and enfolding the substance of the brain (neuroglia). The commonest intracranial tumour of adults, glioma may occur in the cerebrum or less often in the cerebellum or pons. While symptoms vary with the site, frequent ones are headache, mental changes such as stupor and dullness (especially in tumours of the frontal lobes), vomiting (especially in tumours of the cerebellum and pons), visual disturbances and vertigo. Unlike a cancer a glioma does not spread by secondaries to other parts of the body; but because of its situation it may be dangerous. Whether it can be removed depends on its size and position.

glossitis. Inflammation of the TONGUE.

glottis. The entrance to the main air-way from the throat (pharynx) to the voice-box (larynx). It alters in width according to the movement of the vocal cords, opening for breathing but narrowing for speaking or singing.

Oedema of the glottis – usually the result of an allergy that causes swelling and inflammation – is a serious condition requiring urgent medical attention.

glucose. A simple form of sugar found in ripe fruits and in honey, and tasting less sweet than cane-sugar (sucrose).

While starches have to be converted to sugars by intestinal juices before being absorbed, and while even sucrose requires chemical action in the intestine, glucose can be immediately absorbed and so can provide a very quick source of energy. The energy is created during the combustion of glucose and oxygen to water and carbon dioxide.

Where nourishment is needed very quickly glucose has an advantage over all other foods, and where a patient has to be fed through a vein a solution of glucose is essential; but apart from these circumstances glucose has no special advantages.

If sugar is excreted from the body in the urine, the condition is known as GLYCOSURIA.

glycosuria. The presence of sugar in the urine. This is normally an indication of the existence of DIABETES MELLITUS. However, glycosuria also occurs in certain other circumstances. (1) A few people have a lowered kidney threshold for the transfer of sugar to the urine. (2) Many people temporarily have sugar in the urine after a very large, carbohydrate meal. (3) Temporary glycosuria can occur after severe emotional shock. (4) It is also found in some diseases of the nervous system.

Glycosuria should therefore not be regarded as establishing that a person has diabetes, but merely as justifying the use of a glucose tolerance test. In this test the patient eats a specified and known amount of glucose and his blood and urine are examined at half-hourly intervals to ascertain how the body is dealing with the glucose.

gnat. A general term employed to describe all forms of small, biting flies, such as midges and MOSQUITOES.

goitre. A persisting enlargement of the thyroid gland. If not associated with general symptoms of disturbed thyroid function it is a simple goitre commonly seen in adolescent girls and young women.

The thyroid is an endocrine gland producing the hormone thyroxin, a complex organic compound containing iodine. In the tissues this acts as a catalyst to increase the rate of oxidation and so influences metabolism.

The symptoms of the various types of goitre depend on whether the gland produces excess thyroxin (hyperthyroidism), or too little (hypothyroidism).

Endemic goitre. Certain parts of the world have been notorious for a high incidence of very large goitres. 'Derbyshire neck' was well-known and some parts of Switzerland had a similar reputation. This proved to be due to a deficiency of iodine in water and soil. The use of iodized table salt (1 part sodium iodide to 100,000 parts sodium chloride) has now virtually eliminated endemic goitre.

Hypothyroidism. Under-production of thyroxin leads either to cretinism or myxoedema. In cretinism thyroxin deficiency begins during foetal life and unless treated early a child so affected is dwarfish, apathetic, somnolent, and usually mentally deficient. In the adult, thyroid deficiency causes myxoedema, a condition marked by a lowered basal metabolism with resultant intolerance of cold, and by mental slowness, loss of hair, and thickening of the skin and subcutaneous tissues.

Hyperthyroidism. This condition is commoner in women than in men, usually occurs between the ages of 15 and 50 years, and tends to have a hereditary element. Precipitating factors include sudden severe fright or shock, prolonged worry and overwork, and tumours of the gland.

Symptoms include tiredness, nervousness, tenseness, anxiety, tremors of the hands, rapid pulse, excessive perspiration, and in some severe cases emaciation and protrusion of the eyes. The last named symptom accounts for the alternative name, exophthalmic goitre.

There are essentially three possibilities

for treatment. (1) Rest in bed, absence of excitement, a good diet, elimination of any septic foci and use of antithyroid drugs. This is certainly the method of first choice for younger patients. (2) The use of radio-iodine to lessen the activity of the gland. (3) Thyroidectomy – surgical removal of part of the gland.

General. Apart from metabolic effects, goitres may cause other symptoms merely from their presence. Large goitres may extend behind the breast bone (retro-sternal goitre) to compress the trachea and cause difficulty with breathing and secondary effects such as bronchitis and emphysema. The laryngeal nerves in the neck may be affected causing hoarseness and loss of speech.

The thyroid gland may also be the seat of local tumour growth either cancerous or nonmalignant.

old treatment. Preparations of gold are sometimes used for the treatment of rheumatoid arthritis. The usual preparation is sodium aurothiomalate (Myocrisin) given by injection either as a watery or oily solution. It probably acts by providing a general stimulus to the body's immunity mechanisms.

Although opinion has been somewhat divided about the efficacy of gold therapy, the results of recent controlled trials by the Arthritis and Rheumatism Council have been in its favour. What is certain, however, is that gold salts are very toxic, and readily cause severe damage to the liver, kidney and the blood-forming elements in the bone marrow. Gold therapy requires very careful control and should be discontinued on the appearance of skin rashes, albuminuria, jaundice, or on any reduction in the white blood-cell count (leucopaenia).

onadotropic hormones. Internal secretions affecting the gonads or sex-glands. Two such hormones are produced by the front lobe of the pituitary gland.

In the female they are responsible for the initiation of sexual development and the subsequent control of the production and maturation of the egg-cells, with their enclosing follicles, which in turn produce the sex-hormones oestrin and progestin. These are related respectively to sexual activity and to the changes in the uterus which lead either to menstruation or to preparation for pregnancy should a ripe ovum become fertilized.

Similarly, in the male they initiate the sexual development which occurs at puberty and continue to stimulate the formation of sperms and the production of male sex-hormone.

onads. The reproductive glands of the body comprising the ovaries in women and the testes (or testicles) in men.

onorrhoea. The commonest of the venereal diseases, caused by infection of the urethra and genital tract by the gonoccus (*Neisseria gonorrhoea*).

The disease is almost always acquired by sexual intercourse with an infected person. Two other possible sources of infection are (1) the eyes of babies during passage through the birth canals of infected mothers (ophthalmia neonatorum), and (2) of female children through contamination with infected material, e.g., a lavatory used only minutes before by an infected person.

Symptoms appear between two and ten days after infection. In the male there is slight tingling of the urethra, followed in a day or two by a little pain on passing urine and by a purulent discharge from the urethra; but apart from these mild symptoms the patient usually does not feel ill. In the female the same symptoms occur but are often even milder and are completely absent in about one-third of cases. There is thus a faint possibility in a man and quite a chance in a woman that the disease will remain unrecognized in its early stages.

Apart from the fact that the person with unrecognized gonorrhoea can unknowingly infect a sexual partner, untreated gonorrhoea can produce serious results. In the male the condition may become chronic and cause stricture of the urethra, inflammation of the prostate gland, or infection spreading to other parts of the genito-urinary system. Similarly, in the female upward spread may involve the cervix, uterus, Fallopian tubes and ovaries with a risk of permanent sterility.

In both sexes the blood stream may spread the organism more widely to cause arthritis or heart complications.

Since the introduction of penicillin the treatment of acute gonorrhoea has become both rapid and effective. In all developed countries venereal disease clinics are accessible and well-publicized in all areas, and immediate advice should be sought when suspicious symptoms arise.

For preventive and social aspects see VENEREAL DISEASES.

gout. A disease in which there is an increase of uric acid in the blood. This results from a failure of the body-chemistry to deal with purines, which are substances produced during the digestion of protein, and which also occur naturally in certain foodstuffs. Examples are xanthine, caffein and theobromine found in tea and coffee; malt, as in beer, is also a source of xanthine.

In gout, deposits of sodium urate occur in the body tissues and especially in the cartilage of joints, to cause symptoms of acute or chronic arthritis. The cartilage of the ear is another common site, and urinary stones also occur. The deposits of sodium urate are sometimes visible as nodules.

Gout tends to be hereditary and is traditionally associated with over-indulgence in rich foods and wines, but can occur in the absence of such excesses.

Acute gout responds to treatment with colchicine, an alkaloid derived from the autumn crocus (*Colchicum autumnale*);

Grafting: skin from the abdomen taken via the wrist to a site on the cheek

and anti-inflammatory drugs such as phenylbutazone, with or without steroids, are often used as well.

For long term treatment the aim is to prevent recurrence by lowering the uric acid blood level either by increasing the rate of uric acid excretion (cinchopen group of drugs) or diminishing its production (allopurinols). Cinchophen is toxic and its administration requires care and supervision. The diet should be adjusted to be as simple as possible with ample fluid, and purine-containing items should be restricted.

grafting. The surgical implantation of portions of skin or bone to repair defects resulting from injury.

Skin-grafting is mainly required after extensive burns and there are several procedures. In the commonest method a strip of epidermis (the outer layer of the skin) is shaved off the thigh or upper arm and transferred to the new situation. This is relatively easy if the dermis beneath the skin graft duly grows, but if the regrowing dermis contracts, an unsightly scar may be produced.

Alternatively, a flap of skin (including dermis as well as epidermis) may be detached at one end from its original part of the body, placed in the cleaned gap, but left with the other end of the flap attached to the original part until there is a firm growth in the new situation. This method gives better cosmetic results, but for a face wound it may necessitate an arm being bound near the face for an appreciable time.

Bone-grafting is used in repair of fractures or for joint fixation. Suitable strips of bone are cut, usually from the tibia in the lower leg, and implanted to provide a scaffolding for new bone growth.

Modern organ TRANSPLANT is also a form of grafting but it is essentially the grafting of tissues or organs from one individual to another. The difficulties are of an entirely different scale of magnitude and the procedure is complicated by the body reaction to tissues which are not its own.

granulation tissue. In a clean cut where the skin edges can be brought together, the separated tissues soon re-establish their continuity and this is known as 'healing by first intention'. If tissue is missing, as in lacerated wounds or ulcers, a vascular mass of soft tissue gradually grows from the base of the wound to fill up the deficiency and ultimately develops the epithelial form of the outer skin layer or is covered by skin. This is granulation tissue bright red in colour and bleeding readily when touched. It contains many fibrous tissue cells (fibroblasts), and wounds thus healing by 'granulation' or by 'second intention' produce scarring, puckering and sometimes contractures as the fibrous tissue retracts.

granuloma inguinale. A venereal disease not uncommon in some tropical countries characterized by ulcers in the genital region; it is in general curable by an appropriate antibiotic.

gravel. Small concretions composed of mineral salts originating in the kidney or bladder and usually causing some pain and bleeding when intermittently passed with the urine. Gravel differs from stone or CALCULUS in the urinary tract only in the size of the concretions.

greenstick fracture. A fracture occurring in the long bones of children generally under the age of 12. Since the 'bone' is still cartilaginous and only partially ossified breaks incompletely in the manner of a green twig. The bending stresses produce a fracture of the convex side of the bend and a longitudinal split of the shaft.

griping. A common term for abdominal COLIC -an intermittent type of spasmodic pain produced by excessive intestinal contractions. It is mostly used in relation infants in whom such symptoms may reflect an unsuitable diet or an unskilful nursing technique which encourages flatulence.

Abdominal colic also occurs in more serious conditions such as enteritis, intussusception or volvulus. If it persists or recurs, or if the infant appears to be seriously affected, advice should be sought without delay.

groin. The junction of the lower abdomen and thigh on each side is marked by an oblique fold, which, with the immediately adjacent and underlying parts, is known as the groin or inguinal region.

Near the surface, the area contains lymph glands and it overlies the upper attachments of the thigh muscles on the front of the leg which swing the leg inwards. Within it runs the inguinal canal traversed in the male by the spermatic cord and by the round ligament of the uterus in the female. The large blood vessels of the leg lie below the canal.

Conditions affecting the groin are related to these structures. Local sepsis may cause enlargement and inflammation of glands; inguinal or femoral HERNIA may occur; in boys an undescended testis may remain in the canal. It is a common site for fungoid skin disease, favoured, especially in the obese, by moist skin surfaces rubbing together.

Pain may be a symptom of strain of the muscles, and penetrating wounds give concern because of the proximity of large blood vessels and the peritoneal cavity containing the abdominal organs.

group psychotherapy. A method of treating neurotic illnesses by assembling a small group of patients under the leadership of a psychotherapist or psychiatrist who guides and encourages them in free and frank general discussion about their individual and common problems. The members of the group become more aware of the deeper causes of their neurotic behaviour, and are helped to conquer their emotional difficulties by a clearer understanding of how these are caused and by mutual support.

Group psychotherapy may be used both as an adjunct to individual psychoanalysis, or, in the view of some psychiatrists, as a more effective substitute.

The underlying principles of group psychotherapy are also employed (not necessarily with professional supervision and leadership) in the support of people with a variety of personality problems, such as alcoholism, gambling, smoking and drug taking. Associations, such as Alcoholics Anonymous, exist to encourage such activities and undoubtedly achieve good results.

Since the success of group psychotherapy depends on the participants being able to talk freely and make confident personal relationships amongst themselves, it is important that groups should not be too large. Five to ten persons is regarded as the optimal size.

growing pains. Limb and joint pains in young children were formerly regarded as an almost normal accompaniment of growth but rheumatic infection in childhood is often an insidious disease which may ultimately cause serious damage, especially to the heart. So such pains should not be ignored, especially if there are other suggestive symptoms such as recurrent sore throat, pallor, fatigue, loss of appetite, failure to develop healthily, or jerky movements.

'Growing pains' should be investigated. This will usually entail electrocardiographs and blood tests. One simple test is to note the pulse-rate when asleep; it may not show the normal slowing-down. If suspicions of rheumatic infection are confirmed, long-term penicillin may be advised as a preventive measure.

Other causes of pain in childhood are often related to some orthopaedic defect – flat feet or weak ankles – especially if the pain occurs towards the end of the day or after over-fatigue, or during rapid growth.

These conditions need appropriate treatment with attention to footwear. Muscular tone can be improved by exercises, massage and improved general nutrition.

growth. The word has several meanings. In phrases like 'growth in the breast' it is used as an alternative to tumour; in phrases like 'the child's mental and physical growth' it means development; but when we speak of 'biological growth' we are talking principally of increase in size. The present article concerns the latter meaning.

In many organisms the increase in size from conception to adult status is of astronomical proportions. For instance, a full-grown man is thousands of millions times larger than the fertilized ovum from which he originated. Even so, the adult body is not complete and permanent, except in form, because there is a constant interchange as cells waste away and are replaced. Similarly, with a part of the body such as the skull, it is clear that it cannot grow in a simple way of just adding cell to cell. It must increase in size by additions on the exterior and removals on the interior in order to maintain its shape.

Even as simple increase in size biological growth must be considered as two processes. One of these is the formation of inert matter to produce an end-product, an accretion, or a crop. Obvious examples are the hair, the nails and the outer layers of the skin; less obvious are accumulations of fat and glycogen; still less obvious are the blood cells, both red and white corpuscles, which are manufactured from cells in the bone-marrow and cast out into the blood-stream. In health the cells that manufacture corpuscles are never found in the blood; they stay in the bone-marrow and maintain their numbers by cell-division.

Cell-division is the other type of

biological growth. It is multiplicative and always associated with the activity of nucleo-protein whereby two strands of nucleic acid replace a single ancestor in continuous succession. Outside the body, as in tissue culture, cells grow like this indefinitely if food is provided and waste-matter removed. What is still not certain is whether this is their normal behaviour or whether their unnatural environment has caused some change in their metabolism. Whatever the reason there must be some difference to account for their behaviour, because land animals do not grow indefinitely and something must determine this. It may in fact be only the geometry of size in relation to design. Weight-bearing capabilities impose an effective limit on size and undoubtedly contributed to the evolutionary disappearance of the very large animals of prehistoric times. Aquatic animals, because they are supported in water, are not subject to the same limitations and so we have whales ten times as heavy as the largest elephant (10 tons) and many fish which continue to grow throughout their life. Another interesting point is that growth is not necessarily irreversible; the absence of a skeleton allows some simple animals to reduce in size when food is short.

Biological growth is best studied by graphs plotting size against age. Broadly the curve starts off slowly as cells adapt to their environment, then accelerates rapidly but at diminishing rate and finally levels off. In other words, the rate of multiplication of cells falls progressively, as if living matter steadily lost its ability to maintain its early reproductive rate.

growth in childhood. Amongst mammals the state of development of their offspring at birth varies very widely. At one end of the scale we have young animals like colts, calves or lambs who can stand up and move independently as soon as they are born and at the other end helpless blind kittens and still-foetal marsupials, like young kangaroos, who require to be sheltered in a maternal pouch.

The human infant is something of a compromise between the advantages of being born in a state of developmental advancement and the disadvantage of the birth-hazards imposed by his relatively large brain and head. At birth he is uncommonly helpless and dependent but his sensory system is well-developed and he is well-equipped to demand the attention which his senses tell him that he needs.

On average the new-born infant weighs about 3.4 kg. (7.5 lb.) and a relatively large proportion of this is fat. During the first nine months weight growth is rapid – a useful rule-of-thumb is that birth weight should double in six months and treble in a year. Most of this weight gain is skeletal growth and fat, but at about a year old there is a shift in emphasis from fat to muscle as the child learns to move

independently and begins to walk, and this happens again at about 5 years as activity increases.

After one year of age the rate of growth is much less: although birth weight trebled in the first year it does not treble again until the child is 9; however, from 10 onwards children begin to enter into the period of puberty, a new phase of accelerated growth with increased metabolic activity, increased food uptake, and a corresponding increase of tissue-mass. The weight gain in the six years from the age of 10 to 16 is approximately the same as in the nine years from 1 to 10.

Although children at birth weigh on average about 3.4 kg. and are about 50 cm. (20 in.) long there are wide variations even allowing for the fact that girls tend to be slightly smaller. Basically, size and weight depend on two factors – the size of the parents and the length of the development in the uterus before birth.

Growth after birth depends very much on nutrition. If this is good, departures from the average are likely to be due to inherited characteristics, but malnourished, sick, or debilitated children show major delays in both growth and development. In underdeveloped countries where there is total calorie and protein deprivation, a child of 6 may only be as large as one of 4 from countries where nutrition is adequate. Over-nutrition and under-exercise however produce opposite effects and there is some evidence that growth rate is related inversely to length of life.

Since at least the year 1800 people have been growing bigger and maturing earlier. This has been due to improved nutrition with adequate calories, protein and vitamins on the one hand, and on the other, reduced energy expenditure from warmer homes, better clothing and no child-labour. The energy thus saved is available for growth. Another testimony to better early nutrition is the lowering of the age of onset of menstruation, which has fallen from 15 to 12.

Although many factors can effect growth there have been attempts to arrive at some formula by which ultimate stature can be predicted. As a general rule it can be said that the length of male infants at birth is about 27 per cent of their adult stature. The corresponding figure for females is 30 per cent. Girls reach 90 per cent of their final height by 12 and boys by 14. Another way of estimating is to determine 'skeletal age' as opposed to chronological age. This can be done by x raying the hand to examine the stage of ossification – that is, the change from cartilage to bone; the pattern of ossification is very regular in relation to stages of development.

Over-nutrition is perhaps the chief danger of the present generation in developed countries. Fat children tend to grow up to be fat adults with reduced life expectancy, and children over-large and over-mature for their age by comparison with their contemporaries tend to develop psychological difficulties.

gullet. See OESOPHAGUS.

gumboil. An abscess occurring within the expanded margins of the upper and lower jaws containing the teeth and covered by the gums.

The abscess is usually associated with the fang of a decayed tooth and infection makes its way down the pulp-canal and through the opening at the end of the root to infect the tooth-socket. Suppuration ensues with swelling and pain, and pus ultimately tracks through the bony socket and overlying gum or between the tooth and the wall of the socket.

Treatment is by hot mouth-washes to hasten suppuration and evacuation of pus, and by the administration of analgesics and an antibiotic. Surgical incision may be required when the abscess shows signs of 'pointing' (i.e., coming to the point at which the surface breaks) but sometimes the associated tooth will have to be extracted. Dental treatment is needed in any event. With proper care of the teeth and regular visits to the dentist, gumboils should seldom if ever occur.

gumma. A painless inflammatory swelling occurring in the tertiary or late stages of SYPHILIS.

gums. The layer of tissue (gingiva) which covers the tooth-bearing margins of the jaws. Gum-tissue consists of a dense fibrous layer connected to the underlying bone and covered on its surface by vascular membranes. Extensions of the gums, known as papillae, occupy the spaces between the necks of the teeth and prevent lodgement of food-debris.

Diseases. Inflammation of the gums is known as gingivitis; the gums become congested and often bleed, either when food is being chewed or when the teeth are being brushed. There is also some tenderness, so that solid food tends to be swallowed without chewing, creating risk of indigestion. At a late stage the gum margins may shrink away from the teeth, leaving the necks of the teeth exposed.

Apart from occurring in certain serious diseases (e.g., scurvy) and certain acute poisonings (e.g., by mercury) gingivitis starts gradually through defects of dental hygiene, allowing food debris to collect and to form breeding grounds for bacteria. Care of the gums, by regular brushing, massage and the removal of debris before it destroys gum-tissue by pressure can help to prevent gingivitis. Treatment involves removal of all debris (usually by a dentist), mouth-washes and daily massage of the gums with the finger.

Advancing age may cause the gums to recede, allowing infection to reach the sockets and loosen the teeth.

gynaecology. The branch of medicine which deals with diseases peculiar to women and in particular those involving the genito-urinary tract and the hormonal control of the reproductive system. Doctors practising gynaecology are known as gynaecologists but the speciality is nearly always combined with obstetrics which deals with pregnancy and childbirth.

Gynaecologists also concern themselves with problems of contraception and the investigation and treatment of sub-fertility and sterility.

H

habit. A fixed or constant routine practice established by constant repetition.

Most habits are physical actions of one kind or another forming a response acquired by deliberate or unconscious learning, but mental reactions and the formation of thoughts and ideas may be similarly conditioned. Once established, habits are remarkably stable; they tend to become automatic or easily elicited, and they are difficult to break.

The effect of habit is to simplify the movements required to achieve a desired result, to make them more accurate, and to minimize fatigue; indeed a purpose of all education is to make useful actions automatic and habitual. The acquisition of a new habit or the breaking of an old one requires motivation, repetition and resolution to persist. After the age of 30 it becomes increasingly difficult to alter a person's character and behaviour.

'You cannot teach an old dog new tricks'. The same principles hold good in the inculcation of new ideas, and the psychological techniques of influencing the young by the constant repetition of exhortations (usually under conditions where members of a group reinforce each other) are the methods of the more unscrupulous political leaders.

Health education. In any developed country elaborate measures are now taken to protect people from most hazards in their environment. There remain malign influences which only individuals themselves can overcome – obesity, alcoholism, smoking, uncleanliness, carelessness and disregard for others, to name only a few.

The task of those undertaking HEALTH EDUCATION is to apply to the community at large the principles of habit formation and habit alteration in relation to patterns of conduct which will best serve the purposes of better health for all.

haematemesis. Vomiting of blood. The bleeding usually comes from a chronic ulcer of the stomach or duodenum and may be very considerable. Other causes are cancer of the stomach and varicose veins at the lower end of the oesophagus (usually associated with liver disease). Susceptible persons may develop gastric bleeding after taking aspirin, and rarer causes include a form of anaemia and a form of purpura.

In contrast with blood from the respiratory tract (haemoptysis), vomited blood is usually brownish rather than red owing to alteration by the gastric juice; it is acid in reaction because it is mixed with stomach contents; and it is vomited rather than coughed up.

The treatment is complete rest and sedation with transfusions of saline, plasma, or whole blood if necessary. Fluid by mouth is avoided for two or three days followed by gradual return to a suitable light diet. Cases of recurrent haematemesis may require an operation.

haematoma. An accumulation of blood which has leaked into the tissues usually resulting from violence without an external wound, as in blows from a blunt instrument or falls on a hard surface. Milder injuries, which have broken the blood vessels but caused less damage to the tissues, result in BRUISES, when the blood is diffused and does not accumulate.

Head injuries may be seriously complicated by a haematoma within the skull.

A haematoma sometimes occurs after surgical operations when failure to secure complete stoppage of bleeding allows further bleeding within the operation site.

The area over a haematoma is swollen, tender, discoloured and fluctuant to touch. Small haematomatas generally absorb spontaneously; if large they will require to be drained.

haematuria. The presence of blood in the urine due to haemorrhage in the urinary tract. The appearance of the urine may range from deep red to faint pink depending on the amount of bleeding, or red cells may only be detectable microscopically.

Although haematuria may occur in a variety of general medical conditions, it is usually due to some local abnormality affecting the urinary tract. Stones in kidney or bladder, infections, malignant growths and prostatic enlargement are the commonest causes. In 'essential haematuria' no obvious cause can be found and the bleeding probably proceeds from some congenital weakness in the kidney.

Haematuria always calls for investigation, and treatment will be for the condition causing the bleeding.

haemoglobin. The oxygen-carrying pigment of the red blood corpuscles. It is a complex organic compound composed of a protein globin combined with haematin, which is a compound of iron and porphyrin.

Haemoglobin forms a loose compound with oxygen – oxyhaemoglobin – which readily gives up oxygen on tissue demand to become reduced haemoglobin.

Aerated blood from the lungs, passing along the arteries, contains oxyhaemoglobin and is bright red. It returns from the body by the veins, stripped of its oxygen, and then has the bluish-red colour of reduced haemoglobin.

Assessment of anaemia measures the amount of haemoglobin in blood. The normal figure is 14.8 grammes per 100 ml. of blood.

Some hereditary abnormalities in the haemoglobin molecule are related to certain rare blood diseases such as sickle-cell anaemia and thalassaemia.

haemolysis. A breakdown of the membranes of red blood corpuscles so that their contained haemoglobin is liberated into the plasma. It is caused by osmosis when the pressure of the corpuscles and the plasma is unbalanced, so that plasma diffuses into the corpuscles which swell and ultimately rupture.

Haemolysis occurs in certain hereditary and acquired types of anaemia (hereditary acholuric jaundice being perhaps the best known), in destruction of red blood cells by parasites (as in malaria), and in some allergic conditions.

haemophilia. A disease in which blood clotting is abnormally delayed. It is a sex-linked inherited condition which affects only males (see GENETICS). However, the genetic defect is carried on the mother's x-chromosome so that an affected male cannot pass the defect to his sons with the result that the occurrence of cases in a family always skips a generation.

Haemophiliacs bleed excessively from trivial wounds and may bleed internally into muscles and joints with resultant disability. Care should be taken to avoid any injury.

Blood clotting is a complex process primarily initiated by the ferment thromboplastin liberated from damaged areas, from the plasma, and from the plasma platelets which adhere to injured tissues. In haemophilia there is absence of this 'clotting-factor' or anti-haemophilic factor (AHF).

Certain hospitals are designated as haemophilia centres and sufferers should register locally because minor injuries and operations require special measures such as plasma transfusion and administration of concentrated AHF.

haemoptysis. The spitting of blood from structures below the larynx, especially the lungs. The blood is bright, frothy and alkaline, whereas in haematemesis (vomiting of blood from the stomach) the blood is brown and acid. Causes of haemoptysis include pulmonary tuberculosis, cancer of the lung or bronchus, chronic venous congestion as in mitral stenosis, bronchiectasis, various parasitic diseases, scurvy, and occasionally measles. Treatment varies with the cause.

haemorrhage. The formal term for bleeding, defined as any escape of blood from the blood-vessels. For immediate treatment see First Aid section at end of book.

Bleeding from various sites is given special names: (1) from the lungs and air-passage, haemoptysis; (2) from stomach or duodenum via mouth, haematemesis; (3) from bowel, melaena; (4) from urinary tract, haematuria; (5) from the nose, epistaxis; (6) abnormal uterine bleeding, metorrhagia.

Primary haemorrhage is the immediate result of injury to a blood vessel and its characteristics vary according to the type of vessel: (1) arterial, which is bright red and pulsating; (2) venous, which is dark-blue or purple and in a steady stream, and (3) capillary, which is a steady reddish ooze from cut tissues where no large vessel is involved.

Reactionary haemorrhage is the recurrence of bleeding from a wound within twenty-four hours of initial stopping. It may be due to slipping of an insecure ligature or to the restoration of normal blood pressure which displaces the clots.

Secondary haemorrhage is recurrence of bleeding after a period of twenty-four hours without bleeding. This happens when infection in the wound weakens the walls of blood vessels, which give way under pressure. It usually occurs eight to ten days after injury.

If blood escapes through a wound in the skin it is said to be external haemorrhage, but if it escapes into the tissues under undamaged skin it is said to be extravasated and the result is a bruise or a haematoma. If blood escapes from damaged vessels into the body cavities, the result is a concealed or internal haemorrhage; this may be difficult to diagnose except by the general signs of haemorrhage.

Features. The local signs of external haemorrhage are obvious. In cases of internal haemorrhage, pain, tenderness and dullness on percussion over body cavities may provide the doctor with an indication of the site of any haemorrhage when general symptoms arouse suspicion of its occurrence.

The general signs of severe haemorrhage are those of shock and collapse owing to diminished blood volume so that less blood reaches the brain. The patient is restless, feels faint and looks pale; the skin is blanched, cold, and clammy; the respiration is in rapid gasps and distressed; there is apprehension and complaint of thirst, and the pulse is rapid, weak and easily compressible. If the haemorrhage is not controlled unconsciousness and death soon supervene.

Children and old persons bear loss of blood badly but while the former rapidly recover from the effects, recuperation is slow in the aged.

The body's reactions to haemorrhage are clotting of the blood, contraction and retraction of the walls of cut vessels and the fall of blood pressure which occurs after severe haemorrhage.

Treatment. The active treatment of haemorrhage is by immediate arrest of the

Haemorrhage: the skeleton, principal arteries and pressure points

The general symptoms of haemorrhage should be treated by warmth, fluids, elevation of the foot of the bed, cardiac stimulants and in severe cases transfusion of plasma or blood.

haemorrhoid. See PILE.

hair. A single hair is a filamentous outgrowth on the surface of the body derived from the cells forming the skin; hair, collectively, is an aggregation of such filaments covering the scalp and some other parts of the body.

Hairs are found on nearly every part of the body-surface except the palms and soles but they vary very much in length, thickness and colour. A hair consists of a root implanted in the skin and a shaft or projecting part. The root is lodged in a skin depression called a hair-follicle and at its base it is expanded as the hair-bulb which contains the hair-papilla or growing point supplied with blood vessels and nerve fibres. This is continuous with the cells of the dermis.

Opening into the follicle, near its outer end, are the ducts of one or more sebaceous glands to provide an oily dressing for the hair so as to maintain its lustre and waterproof qualities. Straight hairs are round or oval in cross section and grow from straight follicles. They are generally stronger than curly hairs which are flattened and owe their curliness to a curve in the follicle.

Care. If it is kept clean, untangled and not deprived of its natural oils hair will remain glistening and mobile and give an appearance of healthy vitality.

The routine of normal care for the hair is simple. It should include a weekly shampoo and thorough combing and brushing every day. The natural oily dressing of the hair is provided by the sebaceous glands around the hair-follicles and brushing stimulates the scalp and glandular activity and helps to disperse the secretion along the hair. Harsh soaps should be avoided since they dissolve the sebaceous material and leave the hair dull and lustreless. Proprietary shampoos are less apt to do this and if the hair is exceptionally 'dry' application of olive oil, lanolin, vaseline, or special dressings which mimic the natural secretion will ensure an attractive sheen.

Permanent waving is carried out by forming the hair round rollers and applying heat or chemicals so that it retains the required curvatures. The chemicals may affect sensitive skins and the risk of this should be ascertained beforehand by testing a small area. Hair dyes require similar precautions.

In certain circumstances hair requires more particular attention. The scalp may harbour the head-louse *(Pediculus capitis)*, a well-known parasite. The female lays eggs called nits which adhere to the hairs at their roots. This infestation (pediculosis) is particularly likely to be found in school children or even in adults

bleeding at the point of severance of the vessel. In venous and capillary bleeding local pressure usually suffices. In arterial bleeding pressure should be applied to a 'pressure point' between the wound and the heart. These are points at which the arteries are close to a bone so that the pressure is more effective in reducing blood-flow. Alternatively the wound may require to be explored and the cut ends secured by ligature. Application of a tourniquet is a temporary expedient only: it will cause gangrene of a limb if left on too long.

Styptics, applications which contract the blood vessels or hasten clotting time, are sometimes useful for capillary bleeding, and elevation of a limb combined with local pressure will stop venous bleeding.

especially if they have elaborate coiffures which they are reluctant to disturb unduly. A search of the scalp will disclose nits and the hair should then be treated with an insecticidal shampoo and thoroughly fine-tooth combed to get rid of nits.

Dandruff is an accumulation of fine flakes of the dead superficial layers of the skin of the scalp. It may be caused by deficiency or excess of normal sweat secretion or there may be a low-grade superficial infection of the sweat glands (seborrhoea). The scalp should be washed several times a week using a detergent shampoo. Preparations containing 1 per cent cetrimide are available and are of service in true seborrhoea because of their anti-infective properties.

Superfluous hair. Hair grows on most parts of the body. If it is so profuse, long, or dark at any site as not to conform with fashion or conventional appearance it is known as superfluous hair. Women in particular are distressed by the growth of obvious facial hair, by hairy legs, or by the occurrence of isolated long hairs on the face or neck.

Various methods are employed to eradicate superfluous hair or to minimize its anti-cosmetic effect. Bleaching with hydrogen peroxide will make it less obvious, commercially produced depila-tories will remove it temporarily, or some areas can be shaved. Isolated single hairs can be pulled out by tweezers and because of resultant damage to the hair-papilla take longer to grow again than if cut. Electrolysis will destroy unwanted hair permanently but is impracticable except for limited use.

halibut oil. A liquid fat obtained from the liver of the halibut. It contains vitamin A and vitamin D and is a much richer source of both than cod-liver oil. Since fish-oils are not very palatable it is advantageous to be able to give the required dosage of vitamins in a smaller bulk of oil.

Commercial preparations are available in vials with a dropping-pipette or as three minim capsules which are the equivalent of four teaspoonfuls of cod-liver oil. The recommended daily dosage is for infants eight to ten drops, and for adults one or two capsules.

halitosis. See BREATH, OFFENSIVE.

hallucination. Something perceived or appreciated by the senses which has no basis in reality. Hallucinations may thus be sensations of seeing, hearing, smelling or touching and they are most commonly experienced by patients with mental disease or persons under the influence of drugs. They may also be provoked by extreme fatigue or by emotional stress.

A peculiar example is the so-called 'phantom limb', a condition in which a patient who has lost a limb experiences sensations which persuade him that the amputated member is still there.

Hallucination must be distiguished from DELUSION in which there is a false belief rather than a false sensation.

hallucinogen. A drug which alters mental and emotional processes, producing visual or auditory hallucinations. The commonest are (1) cannabis (marihuana or hashish), a mild and probably non-addictive hallucinogen with a long history of ritual use in certain religious cults; (2) mescalin, which produces stronger dreams or ecstatic states; and (3) LSD, which produces a state of mental disorientation thought to resemble that of schizophrenia.

None of the hallucinogens has much medical application and the unauthorized possession of any of them is illegal in Britain; but while at the one extreme LSD is generally recognized as highly dangerous, at the other extreme cannabis is judged by many experts to do no more harm than tobacco or alcohol.

hallux valgus. See TOE.

hammer toe. See TOE.

hamstring muscles. A group of muscles at the back of the thigh which are attached by tendons to the bones of the lower leg. These muscles by contracting bend the knee, and they also take part in straightening the hip.

hand. Apart from his superior brain capacity man owes his success in evolutionary terms largely to the design of his hand which provides a thumb which is capable of reaching across to the fingers, so that grasping is strengthened and precise manipulation is made possible. This ability is common to the higher mammals, known as primates, which include man and the apes, monkeys and lemurs.

The skeleton of the hand consists of the wrist (or carpus), made up of eight small bones articulating with each other and with the bones of the forearm; the palm (or metacarpus), consisting of five elongated bones known as metacarpals; and the five fingers or digits, which each contain three phalanges – except in the thumb, which has only two.

The movements of the hand and fingers are produced mainly by muscles situated in the forearm whose power is transmitted by long tendons running in tendon-sheaths to their points of attachment. There are also palm muscles concerned with movements of the thumb and little finger and with the spreading of the other digits.

On the palmar surface the skin of the hand is thick and dense and firmly attached to the underlying tissues. It shows characteristic markings especially over the tips of the fingers where the highly individual patterns provide the basis for the science of identification by fingerprints. The extremities of the fingers are protected by the nails which have evolved from claws originally intended as weapons, tools or grasping equipment.

Inspection of the nails can be a useful diagnostic procedure since they may show 'clubbing' in severe respiratory or cardiac disease or other abnormalities of shape, colour, or texture. Examination of the hand as a whole may often be equally informative. Its general position, the condition of the skin, the presence of rheumatic nodules, twitching of small muscles, and general tremor, can all provide clues for the acute observer.

Diseases. As a universal tool, the hand is particularly exposed to injury – burns, cuts, penetrating wounds, impact, crushing, dislocation and peculiar damage such as having skin stripped off by machinery.

Burns and cuts present no special features and are treated on routine principles. Bleeding from cuts is generally profuse, and they should be carefully sutured especially on the palm, where an irregular painful scar may cause later disability. Special attention should be given to antisepsis since deep infections can be troublesome. In the palm infection can spread in the tissue spaces and into tendon-sheaths to cause a painful abscess and later disability if the tendons become fixed by scar-tissue.

A whitlow is an acute septic inflammation of the deep tissues in a finger, often developing at the side of the base of a nail. The cause is infection by bacteria, usually through a prick with a dirty pin or other sharp object. The main symptoms are throbbing pain, swelling and redness; and if the condition remains untreated there is danger of the infection spreading over the hand and extending up the arm. In cases treated early hot fomentations or kaolin poultices often suffice. In more severe cases an appropriate antibiotic or sulphonamide may be required, and sometimes an incision is needed to allow pus to escape.

Fractures are common in crush and impact injuries. Any of the palm or finger bones may be broken and are best healed in plaster of Paris with traction if necessary to secure good position. Bennett's fracture is a fracture of the base of the thumb – a common injury in boxing. It is difficult to reduce satisfactorily, and may cause arthritis later. 'Mallet-finger' results from cutting the tendon on the top of a finger, so that the finger cannot be straightened at the last joint. If not recognized at the time of injury and appropriately treated, an operation may be required.

Dupuytren's contracture is a permanent bending towards the palm of the little finger and sometimes also of the ring and middle fingers. This is due to contraction of the tissues of the palm often caused by repeated irritation as from continued pressure of tools on the palm.

handicapped persons. People with appreciable and lasting physical or mental disability. Although the general meaning is clear enough the exact definition varies from country to country. There are at least three reasons for this variation.

1. There is no universal acceptance of what degree of disability is appreciable enough to be designated a handicap. For instance, in the U.K. there are about five million persons who have some pain and limitation of movement from osteoarthritis or rheumatoid arthritis: are all of them handicapped, or only the 150,000 who are housebound, or does the boundary lie somewhere between minor pain and stiffness and inability to go beyond the house? Again, a blind person clearly has a serious handicap but may be perfectly capable of earning a living; a person with full vision in one eye and blind in the other is incapacitated from certain jobs but is obviously not a handicapped person, but at exactly what point in partial sightedness is the term applicable?

2. There is no general agreement as to how lasting a condition must be before the person is graded as handicapped. Probably in all countries a person with a serious inherited disability, e.g., spina bifida or phenylketonuria, would be deemed handicapped, although in some cases of spina bifida surgical operations can remove the handicap and in most cases of phenylketonuria early dietetic treatment can convert the person to a normal individual. In most of the advanced countries a person with a paralysed limb following a stroke would not be classified as handicapped until after treatment and rehabilitation had failed to restore the limb to functioning capacity: but experts differ as to how long these measures should be continued before being regarded as having failed.

3. Handicapped persons are often divided into handicapped children and handicapped adults, but exact meanings differ. In the U.K. a handicapped child is between the age of birth and 16 years, and there are fairly specific criteria for the borders of the various types – blind, partially sighted, deaf, partially deaf, educationally subnormal, maladjusted, physically handicapped, and so on; but neither the age range nor the criteria are identical with those in other countries; and in Britain itself large regional differences in the proportions of children with handicaps of different types (e.g., a variation in educationally subnormal children from under five per thousand children in the south-east to over nine per thousand in Wales) suggest that standards of assessment are far from uniform. For handicapped adults criteria are usually much less clearly defined and the term is sometimes used to cover all handicapped persons other than children, and at other times employed merely for handicapped persons of working age. Clearly for estimating things like the amount of need for help it is desirable to include all adults, but for considering the need for sheltered workshops or special training only persons below pensionable age need be counted.

Because of such differences, international comparisons are not of much value, but as a rough indication of prevalence it may be mentioned that in the U.K.

about a million people (almost 2 per cent of the population) are on disability registers, and the numbers are growing slightly each year – partly because of the greater survival of handicapped infants and partly because of general prolongation of life and the frequency of handicap in the very old.

Services for handicapped children, e.g., open-air day or residential schools for delicate children, are not further considered in this article.

For handicapped adults most of the advanced countries have some residential provisions, such as hostels for the infirm elderly, occupation centres for the mentally handicapped and special centres for some varieties of physically handicapped persons. The latter may be long-term centres or short-term resettlement centres which seek to help the individual (e.g., after a long illness in hospital) to become able to cope with a domestic environment or to resume some form of remunerative employment.

By reason of sheer numbers, however, the vast majority of handicapped adults must live in their own homes. Where the handicap is severe and they are living alone they are often struggling desperately to keep going and to maintain their independence against progressively disabling disease, and in great need of help which may range from assistance with the heavier aspects of housework to personal help over such things as dressing and washing. Where the handicapped person lives with a relative he may have more physical help and more companionship but if there is no external aid the strain on the relative is enormous.

Available services vary from country to country but those of the U.K. may be outlined as illustrative. Britain, apart from Northern Ireland, has separated its health services and social services, and there are really four components.

1. Ascertainment of handicap and of changes from time to time needed in the nature and amount of help is inevitably done mainly by health workers, in particular health visitors, home nurses and general medical practitioners. The health visitors also give guidance on many problems of physical and emotional health; the home nurses undertake any skilled nursing required; and the doctors are concerned both with medical treatment at home and with questions of temporary or permanent admission to a geriatric hospital.

2. Financial aid is provided from national funds at specified rates, and from national funds also come certain expensive items of equipment.

3. Personal services, other than preventive and remedial medical and nursing treatment, are the reponsibility of the social work department of the local authority. These services may include practical assistance with housework (e.g.,

the supplying of a part-time home help), a mobile meals service, provision of social centres and appropriate recreational facilities (and transport to them), provision of library and wireless facilities, assistance with adaptations to the house (e.g., a widened door to the toilet to permit access of a wheel chair), provision of suitable appliances, assistance with home employment and with the marketing of goods produced, provision of subsidized or free holidays, and admission to old people's homes or appropriate centres.

4. Voluntary bodies play important roles supplying visitors to reduce the loneliness of the handicapped and producing many appropriate gadgets for their use, and in some cases providing residential homes or special centres. However, since the registered handicapped are equivalent to about 3 per cent of the total population of working age, and since there are an even greater number of elderly persons who need some help but are not registered as handicapped, the services are necessarily thinly spread. This applies whether we think of geriatric hospitals (with shortage of nurses), of old people's homes and special centres (with difficulty of providing enough staff without excessive burden on the ratepayers), of health visitors (in short supply and with important duties to the young in addition to ascertainment, advice and guidance for the handicapped and the elderly), of home nurses, of social workers, of home helps or of any other workers.

There is no easy solution to the vast problem of catering for the needs of the steadily increasing number of handicapped persons. Clearly in the health field there is a spectrum of health and disease services — fostering of good health, prevention of disease, diagnosis of illness or defect, treatment, rehabilitation, and supportive care of the physically or mentally handicapped. If decisions are left mainly to health workers they may feel that public money is more usefully devoted to the prevention of handicaps (e.g., reducing diseases of hereditary origin, removing the main causes of stroke and coronary thrombosis, vaccinating against diseases like poliomyelitis and preventing the known causes of osteoarthritis) or to the treatment and rehabilitation of such persons as can be restored to full working capacity than to helping those who are incurable. In other words, they may seek to concentrate scarce resources on the provision of more health education officers and health visitors, or more hospital nurses and physiotherapists. Yet in common humanity we cannot let the handicapped drag out the remainder of their lives with minimum subsistence and minimal help. On the other hand, where social services and health services are separated they compete for scarce funds (and if social services get the bulk on humanitarian grounds there is an unending increase in the numbers of handicapped persons).

There is also constant argument between health workers and social workers about whether a person who can no longer manage at home is more suitable for a short-staffed geriatric hospital or for a short-staffed old people's home; social workers are dependent on health workers both for diagnosis of the original handicap and its extent and for information about changes in the medical condition perhaps necessitating more help; and health visitors and other health workers, after recommending perhaps an additional home help session per week for a deteriorating client or a bath grip for a person who has difficulty in getting out of a bath, feel frustrated when their recommendation is 'checked' by a social worker of short training and with very little health knowledge, and even more frustrated when the duly corroborated recommendation fails to produce prompt action.

Whether health services and social services are better combined or separate is arguable, but it is clear that, as the number of handicapped persons increases, the solution is threefold: such increase as the national economy can stand in health workers concerned with the prevention of handicap; such increase as the economy can stand in paid workers for support of the handicapped (e.g., home helps); and extensive use of voluntary workers, particularly persons in the first decade of retirement, themselves still physically and mentally fit and prepared to act as part-time unskilled assistants both to health workers and to social workers.

hand-washing and food sanitation. Bacterial food poisoning and infections such as dysentery are due to micro-organisms derived from the intestinal tracts of persons who may or may not show signs of disease. Some are also of direct animal origin and appear in raw foodstuffs, particularly meat and poultry.

Such organisms can easily be spread to other persons by food-handlers who do not thoroughly wash their hands after visiting the toilet, or who handle raw meat and then proceed to prepare other food. Staphylococcal food poisoning may also be passed on by hands contaminated by discharges from skin diseases, superficial injuries, boils or infections of the nose, throat and ear.

All toilets should therefore be equipped with wash-hand basins and with hot water, soap, nail-brush and individual arrangements for hand-drying – paper towels or hot air. Food-handlers should be impressed with the need to use these facilities, and the advice is equally applicable in the home.

Steps should also be taken to minimize opportunities for hand contamination – no smoking; do not touch mouth, nose, hair, etc. at work; wash hands after using handkerchief; handle food with fork, tongs, etc.

hangover. A colloquial term for the unpleasant after-effects of over-indulgence in alcohol (or more rarely in food). The symptoms include a dull headache and sensation of dazedness, a general feeling of discomfort and sometimes dizziness. Many remedies have been advocated, e.g., strong black coffee to improve alertness, various bitters and sauces to stimulate gastric juice and biliary secretions, and – on doubtful physiological grounds – a further small quantity of alcohol ('a hair of the dog that bit you').

In general a hangover is an indication that a person has exceeded his limits of toleration and should in future keep within these limits. Many points, however, are still unexplained. For example, a whisky drinker who knows his normal capacity may develop a hangover after consuming a quantity of sherry containing considerably less alcohol than he can normally take in whisky. Again some workers have claimed that a person who takes alcohol to about his limit of toleration is more likely to have a hangover if he smokes heavily while drinking than if he does not smoke in that period.

hare-lip and cleft palate. Hare-lip may appear only as a slight notching of the red margin of the upper lip on one or both sides or may be present as a complete fissure running into one or both nostrils. In cleft palate there is a gap along the mid-line of the roof of the mouth and this too may vary from a split in the uvula and soft palate at the back of the mouth to a complete division of the hard palate so that there is a passage between mouth and nose. Both defects are congenital malformations and are usually inherited.

In severe cases a child is unable to suck. There is risk of choking and infection through fluid getting into the air-passages, and feeds need to be carefully given by pipette or tube.

Repair of the mouth and lip requires plastic surgery. Hare-lip can be dealt with in the first few months but cleft palate treatment is usually postponed until about 1½ years of age. A series of operations and the co-operation of a dental surgeon may be required, and the results of treatment are generally excellent. Later on, even after successful repair, speech difficulties may need help from a speech therapist.

Harvey, William. An English physician, William Harvey (1578-1657) was the discoverer of the CIRCULATION OF THE BLOOD.

hashish. An Arabian name for preparations of CANNABIS made from the plant Indian hemp *(Cannabis indica)*. The dried leaves and stalks are smoked or made into beverages or confections and taken as a drug for their intoxicating effect.

hay fever. An acute attack of nasal catarrh resembling a common cold. There is usually profuse watery nasal discharge, sneezing and conjunctivitis and there may also be asthmatic symptoms. It is an allergic response, primarily to pollen, but other allergens cause similar symptoms. True hay fever recurs every summer when pollens are in the air. The Meteorological Office provides information about pollen counts, and risk increases when the index rises over thirty.

Treatment. In an acute attack antihistamines and ephedrine are usually prescribed. Sodium cromoglycate is also useful.

Persons who suffer repeatedly may be skin-tested with various allergens in an attempt to identify the one responsible for their recurrent attacks. Once this is ascertained a course of desensitizing injections may prove helpful.

In the pollen season sufferers should avoid districts where the pollen count is high.

headaches. Headache is a symptom of many conditions ranging from serious organic disease of the brain to the less well-defined type of pain which accompanies conditions of worry, anxiety and strain, and which is to be regarded as of psychosomatic origin.

It is convenient to consider first headaches which originate from causes outside the skull. Very often these headaches are localized and arise from fibrositis affecting either the related nerves carrying sensations or from the muscles of the scalp and neck. Massage and local treatment may prove helpful. In the same category are headaches caused by inflammatory conditions affecting the teeth, the nose and its sinuses, the eye or the ear, in all of which treatment must be directed to the primary cause. Eye-strain caused by a need for spectacles also requires consideration, especially in young persons.

Within the skull, the brain itself is insensitive to pain but the sheaths surrounding it are supplied by sensitive nerves.

General disorders, including indigestion, constipation, nephritis, uraemia, and jaundice can give rise to headaches and they also occur as an almost inevitable symptom of fever.

Diseases within the brain will of course tend to cause headaches – these include meningitis, encephalitis, brain abscess, cerebral syphilis and such conditions as tumours or haemorrhage, which press on the brain.

In the same way disturbances of the blood supply to the brain due to blood pressure problems, anaemia or decompression disease will also result in headaches.

Alcohol is perhaps the commonest drug causing headaches but overdoses of many potentially poisonous substances, and some particular drugs which interfere with the function of haemoglobin, may also be responsible.

'Tension' headaches are a common complaint in nervous individuals under strain. Since migraine, a particular type of very sudden headache, is now generally regarded as being due to spasm of blood vessels supplying the brain, it is likely that nervous or tension headaches are produced in a somewhat similar fashion.

With such diverse causes it is clear that no single line of treatment can be recommended for headaches. In most cases the traditional analgesic based on a combination of aspirin, phenacetin and caffein will produce some relief of symptoms but more basic causes must be sought for and eliminated or relieved so far as proves possible.

head injuries. These arise from either direct violence, such as a blow on the head, or indirect violence, as in a fall on the feet or a blow on the chin, which cause jarring to the head.

Scalp lacerations bleed profusely and generally heal well after cleaning-up and careful suturing.

Blows to the head may cause concussion in which there is no gross damage but brain-function is temporarily disturbed by pressure effects producing symptoms of shock; there may be unconsciousness, nausea, giddiness and mental confusion. Any case with concussion demands careful subsequent observation to ensure that there is not also contusion of the brain with haemorrhage or an actual skull fracture.

Fractures vary in type. A direct blow may produce a depressed fracture with a portion of the skull driven inwards to compress the brain. Blows with a blunt instrument, or indirect violence from falls on the feet or a blow on the chin, tend to produce linear fractures. The danger of these, especially when involving the base of the skull, is damage to blood-vessels which results in intra-cranial haemorrhage. Depressed fractures and intra-cranial pressure from haemorrhage require surgical treatment.

In general, head injures need expert assessment and even the less serious benefit from prolonged rest. Even with the best care there may be troublesome after-effects from severe injuries such as epileptic seizures and psychological disturbance.

Most head injuries occur in industrial and traffic accidents. Risks can be reduced by safety precautions - re-inforced headgear, seat belts and crash helmets.

head noises. Persistent recurring noises in the head, also known as tinnitus. The term does not include impressions of such sounds as voices, bells or musical sequences. These are hallucinations, often accompanying mental disease, and a patient with tinnitus, which is much more a 'ringing in the ears', should be reassured that it has no psychiatric significance.

Many people over 65 with tinnitus also have presbyacusis or senile deafness. Noisy occupations, arteriosclerosis, and various diseases affecting the ear, or the nerve carrying the sensations of hearing, or even the brain itself, may make the patient experience continuous high-pitched noise.

Ménière's disease is characterized by fluctuating deafness, tinnitus and vertigo. Although its primary cause is unknown, abnormalities in the ear (particularly of the cochlear and vestibular lymph-spaces) have been demonstrated. The disease occurs usually after 50, more often in women, and sounds heard may be distorted as well as lessened. High tones are sharpened and low tones flattened giving a 'Punch-and-Judy' quality to voices.

In presbyacusis noises are generally continuous and high-pitched; in Ménière's disease they tend to be intermittent and to be heard as low-pitched humming, roaring or banging.

Some other conditions also produce head noises — wax in the ear, otitis media, tic of eardrum muscle, intra-cranial aneurysm, high and low blood pressure and also certain drugs such as salicylates and quinine.

Tinnitus is difficult to treat effectively but patients usually learn to adapt to it.

health

absence of health

disease
without symptoms

symptoms following
organic change

There is no clear boundary between health and disease

health. A state of physical, emotional, mental and social well-being, in which the body is functioning harmoniously and efficiently and the person is reasonably in tune with his environment and with most of his associates. Health is more than absence of disease: many people who are persistently tired, dull, apathetic and incapable of enjoying life are nevertheless not suffering from any diagnosable illness.

Health (or absence of health) depends essentially on three sets of factors.

1. Heredity. Apart from various serious defects being inherited (e.g., spina bifida, cleft palate, schizophrenia) HEREDITY can create an increased or a decreased liability to many diseases. Again, much of one's intelligence is a matter of inherited potential, although no intelligence can develop to its full inherited capacity in the absence of appropriate stimuli, such as suitable toys, books, associates and, not least, encouragement. Similarly, stature is basically inherited but requires adequate food, fresh air and exercise.

2. Effects of early years. A young child malnourished to the extent of developing rickets will carry the bony deformity for life, and a person undernourished in the formative years will never develop to his full anatomical and physiological potential. Similarly, the youngster reared in a house that lacks books and magazines and in a family that despises book-learning is unlikely to become a keen reader. The under-exercised sedentary child is later liable to the diseases associated with lack of exercise. The youth who has been deprived of parental love may have difficulty in ever forming bonds of affection.

3. Current or recent aspects. While predisposition or resistance to certain diseases is largely a matter of nature (heredity) or nurture (earlier conditions and influences) current or recent conditions commonly trigger off disease. Thus the elderly man develops a heart attack by frequently sprinting for a bus, the lonely and introverted widow acquires senile delusions from lack of companionship (and perhaps also from inadequate diet), the person who gourmandizes at Christmas has a bilious attack, and the adolescent who slims vigorously to get rid of 'puppy fat' has an increased liability to tuberculosis.

Improvement of health. This can also be discussed under three main headings: cure or palliation of disease, prevention of disease and promotion of health.

1. Treatment of disease or injury. This is clearly very important. Yet it has obvious limitations. In the first place it is useless where the lack of health first shows itself in sudden death, e.g., where the man who has for years eaten too much animal fat, smoked forty cigarettes a day, taken little exercise and worried constantly about his work or about marital problems, but has never been so ill as to consult a doctor, dies from a coronary thrombosis. In the second place, treatment is inevitably often far less than complete restoration of function, e.g., where an undiagnosed diabetic develops diabetic gangrene necessitating amputation of the foot. Thirdly, treatment is often slow, e.g., it may take many months of skilled medical and nursing care to restore to health the person who has a (preventable) traffic or domestic accident or the person who develops poliomyelitis. And fourthly, because of the amount of medical, nursing and paramedical time involved, treatment

is very costly, whether the cost falls on the state or on the individual.

2. Prevention of illness and injury. The importance of prevention is becoming increasingly recognized. It had a massive triumph in decreasing deaths of children in the first few decades of this century: following the creation of maternity services and child welfare clinics, the establishment of a profession of health visitors and general improvements in sanitation and hygiene, the infant death rate in England and Wales fell from 129 per thousand births in 1911 to 59 per thousand births by 1934, years before the improvements in treatment created by the introduction of antibiotics and sulphonamides. An equally massive advance in the middle years of the century was the virtual elimination of many serious infections (e.g., diphtheria and poliomyelitis) by immunization and education of the public about its desirability.

Yet prevention of serious hereditary conditions (by discouraging persons likely to convey them from producing families) is still in its infancy, and attention is only beginning to be devoted to the prevention of diseases of later life (such as coronary thrombosis and stroke) and of diseases due to emotional and social factors.

3. Promotion of health. The fostering of good health has an overlap with the prevention of disease. The beneficial effects can be seen in respect of the improved health of children since the creation of home visiting by health visitors, the setting up of child health clinics and the provision of welfare foods: children are taller and heavier and suffer from fewer diseases than in the past. On the emotional side, counselling of parents on child management (including, for example, the need to give the child an assured base of security and love from which to start exploring his 'world', and the dangers of over-strictness, over-indulgence and inconsistency) has already begun to improve the mental health of the young and to promote the development of personalities fit to cope with the normal stresses of life.

Yet, apart from health promotion for pre-school children, most of the vast field of promotion of health remains as a future task for health workers. In respect of family spacing and family limitation little time has been devoted to advising the woman (not a carrier of hereditary disease) about the dangers – to her children as well as herself – of having so many children in rapid succession that she cannot give them adequate personal attention. The School Health Service has been more concerned with the important task of finding and remedying defects than with the even more important job of improving emotional and physical health. Often children leave school without having been taught even the elements of human relations. Adolescents and adults have in the main been left without counselling on the maintenance and improvement of health; and the young elderly (persons nearing retirement age) who could remain in good health for many years have in general been neglected until their health deteriorated to the stage of illness.

Perhaps the most hopeful sign for the future in the U.K. is the expressed intention of the Government, despite financial stringency, to train and appoint more health education officers and more health visitors. After all, a 1 per cent reduction in treatment services could give us at the same cost something like a 25 per cent increase in preventive and promotive staff, with enormous benefit to the health of the people.

health education. Education aiming at improving or maintaining the physical and mental health of persons and of the community, preventing or reducing disease, decreasing the likelihood of relapses or recurrences, and promoting the efficient use of the health services.

Health education has four overlapping branches: individual counselling, e.g., by health visitors in the home; group discussion, e.g., with parents of young children or pre-retirement groups; teaching of larger groups, e.g., school classes; and use of mass media, e.g., books, exhibitions and television programmes.

This education has played a major role in the reduction of maternal and infant mortality, the removal of the so-called 'dirt diseases' (like impetigo and ringworm), the elimination of many infections by public acceptance of immunization, the reduction of home and traffic accidents, and the general acceptance of the need for family-spacing.

Over the years, however, the concept of health education has changed – from the old idea of an articulate expert instructing willing listeners, to the modern idea of creating changes of attitude and behaviour by discussion in which the learner both talks and formulates his decisions, while the 'instructor' needs, in addition to articulacy and health knowledge, insight into the social pressures, prejudices and beliefs of the persons taught.

The main professional sources of health education include the following: (1) Health visitors, whose post-nursing education (in health teaching, psychology and elements of sociology) and whose unrivalled tradition of access to homes without the presence of emotionally disturbing factors such as illness or social emergency, place them in an ideal position for one-to-one teaching and for the formation and counselling of small groups. (2) General medical practitioners who, although primarily concerned with diagnosis and treatment, can make a large contribution. (3) Midwives, whose contact with their patient, though brief, is intimate. (4) Other health professionals, such as physiotherapists, home nurses, hospital nurses, community physicians, hospital doctors, etc. (5) Environmental health officers (formerly called sanitary inspectors) especially on prevention of food-borne diseases. (6) Social workers, although their primary skill and main function is in a different sphere. (7) School teachers, especially in respect of younger children, although for the health education of older children teachers have the limitation already indicated for social workers. (8) Writers and other publicists, although to some extent they – like teachers and social workers – can only act as relayers of information initially provided by health professionals. (9) Health education officers who act as co-ordinators of health education and advisers on audio-visual aids and resource material.

health screening. The aim of health screening is the systematic examination of sections of the population to detect hidden defects and initiate appropriate measures to correct them or to lessen their effect. In relation to the infant, toddler and schoolchild the problem is simple because there are already organized arrangements for the supervision of all children up to school-leaving age. Great progress has therefore been made in the early detection of abnormalities such as congenital dislocation of the hip, phenylketonuria, and defects of sight and hearing, and also in carrying out general developmental assessment as a guide to educational placement and general supervision during the formative years.

With the adult population the problem is more difficult. There exists a vast amount of hidden disease which has not progressed to the point at which the patient goes to the doctor. It is logical that steps should be taken to examine populations systematically to detect abnormalities and to institute appropriate treatment.

Screening procedures for the adult population vary considerably. They may be offered to the public at large or within defined age-limits; they may be applied to selected groups of a particular practice or clinic; or they may be a project for the better care of a specific group' of employees. Screening may be aimed at a single disease (e.g., diabetes) or it may be a 'blunderbuss' procedure covering many different diseases. Most screening campaigns search for a variety of pathological conditions. Even 'Well-Women Clinics', primarily established to look for early signs of cancer in the cervix, normally extend their work to include other gynaecological conditions, breast disease and the checking of urine samples.

Multiple screening. There is as yet no agreement as to what tests are most profitable to include.

The usual programme includes a selection of the following: (1) Height, weight, and skin-fold thickness, indicative of general nutrition and obesity. (2) Chest radiology, revealing abnormalities of heart and lungs. (3) Blood samples, for the detection of anaemia and of any abnormalities in the chemical content of the blood. (4) Urine samples, for indications of diabetes or nephritis. (5) Heart and lung function such as electrocardiographs, blood pressure estimations, and respiratory capacity. (6) Special senses, that is tests of vision, colour blindness, ocular tension (for glaucoma), and hearing. (7) Personal and family history, by questionnaire. (8) Personality assessment, by questionnaire, designed to elicit indications of mental instability. (9) Uterus, with cervical cytology, testing for cancer. (10) Breasts, giving instruction in the technique of self-examination for early detection of cancer.

Screening of older persons. It is probably wise not to include pensioners in general screening surveys. Older persons have their particular problems and need a more personal approach. An individual and sympathetic but none the less systematic scheme provides an opportunity for assessing and explaining any abnormalities and also for exploring the more practical difficulties which affect the health of the elderly, e.g., household composition, problems of retirement or bereavement, domestic and social help, meals, special diet and medication, ability to shop, cook and housekeep, financial problems, and worries from mental or physical difficulties.

Industrial health checks. Many firms now realize that facilities for health supervision are a matter of common prudence and help towards good staff relations. They are applied both to executives and to work-people. It is equally important that the sales director should not have a coronary infarct in the middle of an export drive, and that those on the shop floor should not be prematurely incapacitated by industrial disease.

General. Screening programmes are gaining in popular support, and they can already claim substantial successes especially when directed against a single disease where the problem is well-defined and the prospects of successful intervention are good.

However, a very large question mark still hangs over the large-scale multiple procedures. The difficulty is not in organizing and carrying out such a programme but in interpreting the results and being able to act upon them effectively. It may even be a disservice to a patient to uncover signs of departure from normal which one cannot influence beneficially.

health services. These vary vastly from country to country. In some developing countries there is about one doctor for every hundred thousand people, and there are hardly any qualified nurses; in some advanced countries there is more than one doctor for every thousand people, and nurses have years of full-time training and sometimes university degrees. In some countries disease prevention and health maintenance are priorities, while in others little is attempted except treatment of such sick people as can afford to pay or can secure charitable services. The degree of state funding also varies from none at all in some countries to fully nationalized health services in others.

In Britain three stages may be considered.

1. *Before 1948.* Such services as existed for disease prevention and health promotion (e.g., antenatal clinics, domiciliary midwifery, maternity hospitals, visiting of mothers and children at home by health visitors, child health clinics, school health services, and supervision of the purity of water and food) were administered by local authorities and coordinated by a salaried doctor called the medical officer of health. For treatment services at home, the upper and middle classes employed general medical practitioners on a fee-for-services basis, and the less affluent, unless covered by insurance, had either to find the fee or find a doctor generous enough to treat the poor without charge. Over two-thirds of hospitals were run by local authorities, with patients paying according to their means, and the remainder were 'voluntary hospitals', financed by charitable donations and state grants.

2. *In 1948* the services were reorganized as the now world-famous National Health Service, with the cost falling partly on a newly constituted national health insurance scheme, partly on ordinary revenue, and to a small extent on local authority rates. Services for promotion of health and prevention of disease continued to be administered by local authorities and headed by medical officers of health, with the functions of health visitors considerably extended and with home nurses coming under the jurisdiction of local authorities.

The general practitioner service became a service under which the patient was entitled to treatment without direct charge (although some exceptions like prescription charges were introduced later) and the GP received a sum for each person on his list, but was free to treat on a fee-for-service basis persons not on his list.

All hospitals, whether previously voluntary or local authority, were placed under the control of nominated hospital boards. Hospital staff other than senior doctors and senior dentists were salaried, including junior doctors so that aspiring consultants no longer had to endure years of poverty. Consultant doctors and dentists could opt to be either full-time and salaried (as about half of them were) or paid for a number of theoretically calculated sessions and entitled to undertake private work.

In general the health of the people, as measured for instance by average age at death or by infant mortality rates, improved enormously. Defects, however, became apparent. To take an example: there was no co-ordinated planning, e.g., a heart transplant operation might occupy the full time of five doctors and seventeen nurses on a single patient, but it was no concern of the hospital boards that prevention of the births of children born with severe handicaps through maternal rubella or prevention of coronary thrombosis in the middle-aged was being thwarted by sheer shortage of health visitors. Again, as the health visitor's post-qualification training improved and as the general practitioner's income ceased to depend on the amount of illness, it became increasingly obvious that two experts could collaborate and reinforce each other, but the GP was in a separate service.

Yet again nursing began to rise to full professional status with its own expertise and priorities, but both in hospitals and in local authority services there was tremendous medical domination; there was, for instance, a reluctance to accept that health visitors (with at least four and a half years of professional education) might undertake developmental screening of infants just as capably as general practitioners, an unwillingness to believe that dietitians could function without being 'supervised' by a doctor, a contentment with a situation in which all the highly paid posts in a department were filled by doctors and perhaps a single dentist, while the administrative and teaching heads of health visiting, midwifery, nursing and other large services were paid less than a trainee consultant.

Perhaps the biggest defect of all was that more than 60 per cent of the available money was spent on curative and palliative services in hospital and most of the remainder on curative, palliative and supportive domiciliary services, with very little expended on promotion of mental and physical health, health education and prevention of disease.

3. *The National Health Service of 1974.* Various tentative experiments took place; for instance, in Oxford (with many other towns following) general practitioners and health visitors, although still paid by executive councils and local authorities respectively, began to work in close association; in Aberdeen the medical officer of health gave up his dictatorial powers and formed an administrative group (including the chief nursing officer and the chief health education officer) to advise the local authority on matters of policy; various hospitals employed general practitioners on a part-time basis; liaison health visitors appeared in many hospitals; and in some cases joint appointments were made of doctors or nurses working partly in hospital and partly in the local authority services.

Finally, the social work services having already been separated off and left with local authorities, in 1974 the strictly environmental services (i.e., those of the former sanitary inspectors) were left with local authorities and all other health services – whether hospital or otherwise, and whether curative, palliative, educative, preventive or supportive – were placed under nominated health boards, with each board having an executive group of chief officers: a medical officer, a nursing officer, a secretary or administrator, and a finance officer, with the chief dental officer and the chief pharmacist attending when their services were under discussion.

Many difficulties remain. The tradition of spending nearly all the available money on treatment and palliation will not easily disappear. The variation in methods of payment remains, with about half the clinical consultants spending part of their time on private work, with general practitioners remunerated by annual fee for each person on their list (including a larger fee for each elderly person) and also fees for certain items of service (such as vaccinating a child), with some workers, e.g., general dental practitioners, paid entirely on items of service and with most members of the various health professions salaried. This variation could have unfortunate results, e.g., some dental officers might resent the efforts of health education officers and health visitors as tending to reduce the amount of dental treatment needed, and some general medical practitioners might prefer that they themselves should immunize 50 per cent of children and provide family planning services for 30 per cent of women (with due payments for items of service) rather than that clinic services with salaried staff should raise the immunization level to 90 per cent and the family planning figure to 60 per cent.

Not least, the rigid separation of health needs and social needs may make for difficulties, with the health visitors – selected nurses with subsequent full-time training both in health teaching and in social science – uneasily poised between the Health Board and the Social Work Department, employed by the former but often knowing more about the social needs and problems of their clients than do the less numerous and in most cases less highly trained workers of the Social Work Department. This difficulty may arise too in the case of home nurses who in the past recommended appliances for the handicapped (such as wheel chairs and walking aids) but now find that the issue of such appliances is controlled by the Social Work Department.

Yet, despite these and other difficulties, the integration of curative and preventive health services should substantially assist forward planning.

health visitor. A qualified nurse, with additional training in psychology, sociology and health teaching, whose primary functions are the health education and medico-social counselling of individuals, families and small groups. She (or he) works either from clinics or in collaboration with general practitioners, but always acts as an independent expert with separate priorities.

The health visitor is an essential and indispensable member of the team providing a health advisory service to families and individuals, and his or her main functions have been thus summarized by the Council for the Education and Training of Health Visitors:

1. Prevention of mental, physical and emotional ill-health, and alleviation of the consequences of such ill-health.

2. Early detection of ill-health and surveillance of high risk groups.

3. Recognition and identification of need, and mobilization of appropriate resources.

4. Health teaching.

5. Provision of care – including support during periods of stress, and advice and guidance in case of illness as well as in the care and management of children.

Health visitors are still in short supply, although numbers are increasing. A recent official circular advocates one per 3,000 population (a figure already achieved by a few districts that recognized early the importance of improving health and reducing preventable disease), but many areas have less than one per 4,500, or less than two-thirds of the number really needed. Yet if a serious attempt is to be made to reduce disease by the education and unobtrusive counselling of the people in matters pertaining to emotional, physical and mental health, the health visitor is from her background, her training and her tradition of access to the homes of the people, almost certainly the key to success.

hearing aids. For the elderly, unsophisticated, and non-mobile patient the old-fashioned ear-trumpet is still very good. It is simple to use, costs nothing to run, and is free from background noise.

However, the ordinary person with irreversible hearing loss seeks an aid which will be inconspicuous in use but will still make sound louder and speech more intelligible. Modern aids are electromagnetic devices consisting basically of microphone, amplifier, and receiver. Miniaturization of electrical components and the replacement of valves by transistors has enabled smaller and smaller aids to be developed with increased flexibility to match different needs.

The heart of a hearing aid is the amplifier. Its degree of amplification is known as gain, usually of the order of 60 decibels at a frequency (pitch) of 1,000 Hertz. With an input of 65 dB, which is the average strength of ordinary conversation, an output of 125 dB will result. Since the maximum the receiver can handle is only a little more than this it does not help to shout: only distortion will result. Amplifiers can be designed to be more efficient on certain frequencies. All aids have a control for volume which may operate automatically and some have also a tone-control. Microphones do not pick up sound uniformly over the whole possible range of pitch: the smaller they are the more restricted their range, but fortunately high tones are least likely to be lost.

Selection. Before choosing a hearing aid the type of DEAFNESS should be investigated. It is important to discover the amount of hearing conveyed in the normal way by air-conduction through the outer ear to stimulate the normal process of hearing, compared with the amount of hearing being conveyed by bone-conduction. A tuning-fork vibrated first while not quite touching the head and then while touching the skull will show the difference. According to the result the patient will benefit most either from a hearing aid which is inserted into the ear to amplify air-conducted sound, or from an aid placed behind the ear to help bone-conduction. In nerve deafness neither may be effective.

Types. There is a range of styles of aid, each designed for specific uses.

1. Body-worn – microphone and amplifier worn on the body. There is a cord to the ear-mould with a single cord to both ears. National Health Service 'Medresco' aids are of this type, and there are various models – adult, child, and 'special' with more gain but limited frequency. Commercial aids are legion.

2. Post-aural aids – contained in a case which fits behind the ear. A National Health Service model is becoming available.

3. Spectacle aids – components housed in an enlarged side-piece of a spectacle frame and sound conveyed by a tube or vibrator.

4. In-the-ear aids – generally have poor gain and limited frequency and are subject to 'squeal' (acoustic feed-back) because of the proximity of the receiver to the microphone.

5. Non-wearable aids – used in schools and for speech training. There is an amplifier and headphones, either single, or multiple for groups of children. The perimeter of the classroom is wired and individual hearing aids have a pick-up coil so that children can move about freely in the classroom. A variation of this is the use of a VHF radio-transmitter by the teacher.

heart. A hollow muscular organ designed as a pump whose purpose is to circulate blood to all parts of the body. In shape it is conical with base uppermost and apex pointing downwards. It is situated centrally in the chest, behind the breast-bone and close to the lungs, with one-third of its bulk to the right, and two-thirds to the left of the mid-line. It is enclosed within a fibrous sac known as the pericardium and weighs

about 480 to 560 g. (17 to 20 oz.) in males and rather less in females.

Internally it is divided by muscular partitions into four chambers – the right and left atria (or auricles) above, and the right and left ventricles below; the right and left halves of the heart are completely separated and not in communication. However, the atria and ventricles of each side are connected through openings, each guarded by a non-return valve. The right valve is the tricuspid valve; on the left side is the bicuspid or mitral valve.

Heart: anatomy

The heart is composed of a special type of muscle, the myocardium, a term which also differentiates it from its delicate lining membrane, the endocardium (which also covers the valves), and its external sheath, the pericardium. The muscular walls of the atria are relatively thin compared with those of the ventricles and the left ventricle wall is about twice as thick as that of the right, since its work in propelling blood through the whole body is much greater than the work of the right ventricle, which is merely circulating blood through the lungs.

The blood supply to the heart itself comes from the right and left coronary arteries, branches of the aorta. Narrowing or blockage of these arteries reduces blood to the heart-muscle and causes myocardial ischaemia – the so-called 'heart-attack'.

Cardiac action is as follows: venous or deoxygenated blood returns from the body by the superior and inferior venae cavae to the right atrium, passes to the right ventricle and is pumped through the pulmonary arteries to the lungs. After oxygenation there it returns to the left atrium by the pulmonary veins, passes to the left ventricle and is propelled through

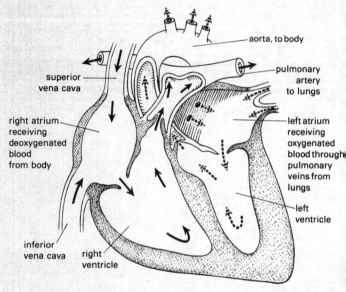

Heart: blood flow

the aorta and so to the rest of the arterial system, supplying oxygenated blood to the whole body.

Rate and force of cardiac contraction are controlled by the 'pacemaker', an area of specialized tissue at the base of the heart which is sensitive to chemical and nervous stimuli. Impulses arising in the pacemaker are propagated by a band of specialized muscle-fibre (the bundle of His) to the atria and ventricles so that their contractions are regulated and co-ordinated.

The blood output of the heart is about 3 to 5 litres per minute but can rise to ten times as much during violent exercise.

Diseases. More than one-third of all deaths occur from various types of heart disease, which are the result of pathological processes affecting either the heart-muscle (myocardium), its lining membrane (endocardium), or its outer covering and enclosing sac (pericardium). Before describing these in detail, mention must be made of congenital heart disease which is an important cause of disability in infants and children.

1.   Congenital   heart   disease. Embryologically the primitive heart is a single continuous tube consisting of an atrial part, a ventricular part, and the aortic bulb. In the course of development

each of these divides and eventually forms the right atrium, ventricle, and pulmonary artery and the left atrium, ventricle, and aorta.

If this process goes wrong congenital abnormalities result, such as defects in the wall dividing the right and the left sides of the heart, narrowing of either the pulmonary artery or the aorta, or persistence of certain structures which are needed in foetal life to draw oxygen from the mother's blood, because the unborn child cannot use its own lungs. The defects may be due to adverse influences during intra-uterine life, notably the occurrence of German measles (rubella) in the mother. Rubella vaccination of adolescent girls is therefore a very important preventive measure; and advances in heart-surgery have been conspicuously successful in dealing with many such abnormalities and restoring normal life-expectancy.

2. Diseases affecting the myocardium. Acute myocarditis occurs mainly from (1) a complication of specific fevers such as diphtheria and typhoid fever, (2) rheumatic fever, (3) blood disorders such as uraemia and acidosis, and (4) sudden interruption of the blood supply to the heart-muscle as by thrombosis or embolism.

Chronic myocarditis on the other hand is predominantly the result of vascular disease resulting from raised blood pressure causing arteriosclerosis, from degeneration of vessel walls as in arteriosclerosis and syphilis, and from the general atrophy which accompanies old age. Angina is essentially severe pain due to shortage of blood to the heart muscle.

3. Diseases affecting the endocardium. Acute endocarditis occurs from invasion by bacteria, e.g., during rheumatic fever. The heart valves are particularly affected, becoming either narrowed (stenosis) so that the blood flow through them is diminished, or unable to close fully (incompetence) so that some of the blood flows backwards when the valve is supposedly closed. Both stenosis and incompetence lessen the efficiency of the heart as a pump. Chronic endocarditis occurs following acute endocarditis, or as a sequel to very prolonged physical strain, syphilis and some other diseases. Both in acute and in chronic endocarditis the commonest conditions are mitral incompetence, mitral stenosis and aortic incompetence. Many cases of these can now be treated successfully by heart surgery.

4. Hypertensive heart disease. High blood pressure occurs either as an isolated condition – 'essential hypertension' – or as a secondary effect in other diseases. Death-rates were rising rapidly until about 1950; since essential hypertension is regarded as a stress disease this may have been due to the increased strains of modern life. From 1950 the rates have shown a modest decline and this period coincides with the introduction of hypotensive drugs. As a preventive measure it seems reasonable to advocate systematic search for cases of seriously elevated blood pressure so that affected individuals may be treated and helped to live less stressful lives.

5. Arteriosclerotic heart disease. This is the main cause of the blood supply to the heart muscles being insufficient and accounts for most cardiac deaths in men of middle age and beyond. The recorded rates continue to rise steeply. There is no known single cause: rather there is a 'web of causation' which includes many risk factors. It has been demonstrated that if a man's age, blood pressure, serum cholesterol level, body bulk, physical activity, and smoking habits are all known, the risk of his having a coronary attack can be predicted with considerable accuracy.

Obesity, inertia, and raised fat levels in the blood, are all related to over-eating and are susceptible to dietary restriction and the substitution of unsaturated fats for those of animal origin. Machinery has lessened the need for activity at work and leisure pursuits are becoming more sedentary - spectator sports and television. The statistical association incriminating cigarette smoking is impressive; its effects are probably due to action on the sympathetic nervous system.

Coronary artery disease thus provides great opportunities for health education: avoid stress, eat less, reduce animal fats, stop smoking, and take more exercise – things easy to advocate but difficult to advocate successfully to a man who does not yet feel ill, thinks himself only mildly overweight and smokes heavily because of stresses beyond his control.

6. Diseases affecting the pericardium. Inflammation of the pericardium most usually accompanies the conditions producing endocarditis but it occasionally occurs in pneumonia, in tuberculosis, in terminal illness generally, and as a complication of trauma to the chest. Its importance lies in its disabling effect on cardiac action.

7. Disorders of cardiac rhythm. These affect the functional efficiency of the heart and result from damage to the 'pacemaker' and conducting mechanism brought about by almost any of the diseases described above.

8. Heart-block. This occurs when disease or degeneration of the 'pacemaker' causes partial or complete arrest of the impulses governing the heart beat. The ventricles then contract more or less independently and pulse-rate may fall to 20 or 30 beats per minute. Severe cases may have fainting or convulsive attacks from cerebral anoxia, a condition in which insufficient oxygen reaches the brain.

Some patients are now treated by the implantation of an 'artificial pacemaker', which is electrical. See also HEART, DISORDERED ACTION, HEART FAILURE and HEART SURGERY.

heartburn. A peculiar burning sensation felt behind the lower part of the breast-bone, and often accompanied by flatulence and belching. It is common in chronic indigestion and is presumed to be due to irritation of the lower end of the oesophagus by the stomach contents. Antacids usually afford relief but heartburn is not specifically due to the action of gastric hydrochloric acid since it may occur in achlorhydria.

heart, disordered action. Another name for EFFORT SYNDROME.

heart failure. A very general term, indicating inability of the heart to maintain an efficient circulation, so that the person gradually finds that he cannot undertake customary physical exertion without symptoms of distress.

Basically failure develops from heart-muscle (myocardial) insufficiency or from some interference with the stimuli which cause its rhythmical contraction (see HEART). Lessened contraction or slowing rate of contraction causes less blood to be pushed through. Heart-muscle may be weakened by toxaemia or by interference with its blood supply, but insufficiency may also develop when the heart is called on for more work than it is capable of performing. This happens when there is excessive resistance in either the pulmonary or systemic circulation or when narrowed or leaking valves impair the heart's mechanical efficiency as a pump. For a time these difficulties are met by compensatory changes, the heart increasing in size and muscularity to pump more forcibly, but eventually compensation fails.

Slower or irregular contractions of heart muscle occur in toxaemia, in poisoning by certain drugs, in endocrine disorders, particularly thyrotoxicosis, and in myocarditis and myocardial degeneration. Clinically cardiac failure is regarded either as acute or chronic.

Acute heart failure. The most common cause is coronary artery thrombosis, leading to cardiac infarction. The symptoms are severe pain in the cardiac area, often radiating down the left arm, with palpitation, severe breathlessness and collapse, leading in extreme instances to unconsciousness and death. Although the onset may be unexpected it is likely that gradual diminution of cardiac reserve will have been noted before the actual attack. Other causes of sudden failure are toxaemia from infections, notably diphtheria, sudden changes in rhythm as in fibrillation or heart-block, and less usual incidents such as pulmonary artery embolism.

Cases of acute heart failure need complete rest and expert care, and most general hospitals now deal with such patients in intensive-care units where the cardiac action can be monitored and immediate steps taken to institute appropriate treatment.

Chronic cardiac failure. The main causes of more gradual failure of the heart are (1) myocardial insufficiency from disease of the blood vessels, (2) disturbances of rhythm, (3) increased pressure in pulmonary circulation due to chronic bronchitis, emphysema and pulmonary fibrosis, (4) increased pressure in systemic circulation due mainly to arteriosclerosis or chronic nephritis, and (5) mechanical effects such as adherent pericardium or the presence of mediastinal tumours. The salient features are increasing breathlessness on exertion, palpitation, and oedema of dependent parts, especially legs and ankles. Waterlogging of tissues may develop and with right-sided heart failure there is often a troublesome cough and profuse, watery sputum. Impaired circulation also affects other systems to produce indigestion, sleeplessness, restlessness, impaired memory, diminished urinary output, and albuminuria.

Treatment is based on rest, light diet, cardiac tonics such as digitalis, the administration of diuretics, and sedation as indicated.

heart murmur. An abnormal sound heard on listening to the heart with a stethoscope.

Since many children have in the past been needlessly debarred from taking part in athletic activities because a general practitioner heard a murmur, it is important to stress that murmurs of no significance are much commoner than murmurs of significance.

Soft murmurs while the heart contracts (systolic murmurs) can be heard in many apparently healthy hearts. Observation over many decades of persons with such murmurs has revealed no evidence of heart disease, and post mortem examination of such persons after their death from unrelated causes has shown healthy hearts. Again, a soft, blowing murmur is common in anaemia, in several fevers and in various other illnesses, and tends to disappear when the condition is cured.

However, certain murmurs occurring at the various valves of the heart indicate disease of the particular valve. Broadly these are of two types: stenosis (narrowing or shrinkage) where the valve is unable to resist the pressure of blood in a contracting chamber of the heart; and incompetence (leaking) where the valve cannot efficiently close and so permits a back-flow of blood during the phase of relaxation.

heart surgery. Despite the increasing competence of general surgery, the difficulties of cardiac surgery still loomed large as late as 1930 and the prospects of progress seemed dim. The operative problems facing the would-be heart surgeon were much more daunting than those of his colleagues in other fields because a functioning circulation was essential to life and the heart could not just be shut-off, stopped, and emptied of blood while the operator repaired its defects.

The earliest operations were therefore those which could be done entirely from outside the heart or at least by some rapid procedure which, although allowing limited access to its interior, would interrupt its action for only a brief period. Such operations rectifying minor congenital abnormalities or enlarging a narrowed valve in mitral disease, were undertaken with encouraging success.

Since those early beginnings there have been great advances. The surgeon's need was for more time and this was met by the development of heart-lung machines which could maintain the circulation while the heart was stopped and bypassed. Some use was also made of the principle of hypothermia: lowering body-temperature reduces tissue-demand for oxygen and gives the surgeon perhaps eight minutes to work instead of four.

Although reliable heart-lung machines were the key to progress this has not been achieved without help from other specialities, and especially in the fields of anaesthetics, blood-transfusion and pharmacology (for anticoagulant drugs). Above all, the ability to undertake cardiac operations on a more or less routine basis meant that it was necessary to know exactly what defect was present in order to plan procedures and give some sort of assessment of the likely results of treatment. Thus diagnostic tests had to be developed to a greater degree; and it has turned out that the use of x-ray diagnosis has supplied the answer.

A wide range of operations is now undertaken. Commonest are repairs of congenital defects, repair or replacement of valves, and procedures to replace narrowed or diseased sections of the blood vessels supplying the heart muscle.

Even more dramatic have been recent developments in heart TRANSPLANT using healthy hearts from cases of sudden accidental death. The surgical problems of transplant operations have been overcome, but the factors still preventing reliable results are those of tissue-rejection. The most satisfying successes of cardiac surgery have been in dealing with congenital heart disease. Perhaps 75 per cent of 'blue babies' (i.e., those with a hole in the central wall of the heart that allows the blood to mix between the two sides) can now be saved; and older children with lesser defects can in most cases be assured of growing up to lead a normal life. Valve operations on well-chosen adult cases also give encouraging results.

heat. The effect of heat on matter is to increase the activity of molecules and hence their energy; thus energy and heat are interchangeable.

Body temperature is maintained at a constant figure of 37 °C. (98.4 °F.) by a temperature-regulating centre in the mid-brain. Heat production results from the metabolism of food and from muscular activity, and heat-loss occurs mainly from the body surface by radiation and convection and particularly by the evaporation of sweat.

If heat-loss exceeds heat-production the body attempts to correct this by shivering in order to produce more heat from additional muscular activity. If this fails the condition of hypothermia will ensue. In a climate with high temperatures and high humidity heat-loss is insufficient and the body temperature will rise to produce hyperpyrexia. This may result in heat-exhaustion, HEATSTROKE, or muscular cramps due to excessive loss of salt in perspiration.

In medicine heat is also used therapeutically. Poultices or heating-pads induce increased blood flow and relax muscle spasm. This increases cell activity, stimulates repair and healing, and relieves pain and tension. General application (by an electric-blanket or hot-air cage) is used to counteract shock. If continued it will cause increased perspiration and is sometimes used to assist in the elimination of waste-products as in kidney disease.

heatstroke. A state of general collapse brought about by exposure to excessive heat. It is synonymous with sunstroke but exposure to the sun is not essential.

The condition mainly occurs in tropical climates when the shade temperature reaches about 43 °C. (110 °F.). Exercise and high atmospheric humidity increase the risk. Symptoms are usually sudden in onset with malaise, headache, restlessness, nausea and vomiting. The body temperature may rise to 43.3 °C. (110 °F.) or more with mental excitement, delirium, convulsions and, sometimes, coma and death.

Prompt and adequate treatment is required, with cold sponging and ice-packs to lower body temperature, and the replacement of fluid and salt. Recovery may be followed by signs of heart strain and mental disturbance. Later re-exposure to heat may induce further attacks more readily than before.

height and weight. Variation occurs in all biological phenomena and in any population it is a matter of everyday observation that individuals differ widely in bulk and stature. Considerable variation in height and weight is quite compatible with normality. There are many reasons why this is so: no population is homogeneous; it is made up of a variety of racial types, and individuals are also affected by their personal heredity. Apart from these genetic considerations bodily development is influenced by nutrition, exercise and disease during the period of growth. In adult life fluctuations of weight should be investigated.

Tables which purport to show ideal heights and weights have to be employed with these considerations in mind but they are sufficiently representative to indicate whether a person is seriously under-or over-weight. Those given on the following pages relate to adults; for children's tables, see DEVELOPMENT.

For adults, three weights are given for each height related to small, medium or large build. All weights given are for unclothed persons. The weights shown for age 30 should ideally be maintained throughout life although some authorities are prepared to accept a further rise of roughly 0.5 kg. (1 lb.) per year until the age of 45 as still being within acceptable limits.

Attempts have been made to devise formulae as a substitute for tables. Two useful rules of this kind for adults are (1) ideal weight in kg. = height in cm. minus 100 or, alternatively, (2) ideal weight in kg. = height in cm. multiplied by chest measurement in cm. divided by 240.

heliotherapy. See SUNLIGHT TREATMENT.

hemiplegia. Paralysis affecting one side of the body. Nerve-fibres controlling voluntary movements of arm and leg originate from either side of the cerebral cortex of the brain, and cross over to the opposite side in the brain-stem, before continuing on their way to the muscles.

MEN

Height in cm. (in.)	Weight in kg. (lb.) at ages shown		
	20 YEARS	25 YEARS	30 YEARS
149 (59)	45.7 - 50.7 - 57.0 (101 - 112 - 126)	47.5 - 53.0 - 59.3 (105 - 117 - 131)	49.3 - 54.8 - 61.6 (109 - 121 - 136)
152 (60)	46.6 - 51.6 - 58.0 (103 - 114 - 128)	48.4 - 53.9 - 60.7 (107 - 119 - 134)	50.2 - 55.7 - 62.5 (111 - 123 - 138)
154 (61)	47.5 - 53.0 - 59.3 (105 - 117 - 131)	49.3 - 54.8 - 61.6 (109 - 121 - 136)	51.1 - 56.6 - 63.4 (113 - 125 - 140)
157 (62)	48.9 - 54.3 - 61.6 (108 - 120 - 135)	50.7 - 56.1 - 62.9 (112 - 124 - 139)	52.1 - 58.0 - 65.2 (115 - 128 - 144)
160 (63)	50.2 - 55.7 - 62.5 (111 - 123 - 138)	52.1 - 58.0 - 65.2 (115 - 128 - 144)	53.4 - 59.3 - 66.6 (118 - 131 - 147)
162 (64)	51.6 - 57.5 - 64.8 (114 - 127 - 143)	53.9 - 59.8 - 67.0 (119 - 132 - 148)	55.2 - 61.1 - 68.8 (122 - 135 - 152)
165 (65)	53.4 - 59.3 - 66.6 (118 - 131 - 147)	55.7 - 61.6 - 69.3 (123 - 136 - 153)	56.6 - 62.9 - 70.7 (125 - 139 - 156)
167 (66)	55.2 - 61.1 - 68.8 (122 - 135 - 152)	57.0 - 63.4 - 71.1 (126 - 140 - 157)	58.4 - 64.8 - 72.9 (129 - 143 - 161)
170 (67)	56.6 - 62.9 - 70.7 (125 - 139 - 156)	58.9 - 65.2 - 73.4 (130 - 144 - 162)	59.8 - 66.6 - 74.7 (132 - 147 - 165)
172 (68)	58.4 - 64.8 - 72.9 (129 - 143 - 161)	60.2 - 67.0 - 75.2 (133 - 148 - 166)	61.6 - 68.4 - 77.0 (136 - 151 - 170)
175 (69)	59.8 - 66.6 - 74.7 (132 - 147 - 165)	62.0 - 68.8 - 77.5 (137 - 152 - 171)	63.8 - 70.7 - 79.3 (141 - 156 - 175)
177 (70)	61.6 - 68.4 - 77.0 (136 - 151 - 170)	63.8 - 71.1 - 79.7 (141 - 157 - 176)	65.7 - 72.9 - 82.0 (145 - 161 - 181)
180 (71)	63.8 - 70.7 - 79.3 (141 - 156 - 175)	66.1 - 73.4 - 82.4 (146 - 162 - 182)	67.9 - 75.6 - 85.2 (150 - 167 - 188)
182 (72)	65.7 - 72.9 - 82.0 (145 - 161 - 181)	68.4 - 76.1 - 85.6 (151 - 168 - 189)	70.7 - 78.4 - 87.9 (156 - 173 - 194)
185 (73)	67.9 - 75.2 - 84.3 (150 - 166 - 186)	71.1 - 78.8 - 88.3 (157 - 174 - 195)	72.9 - 81.1 - 91.1 (161 - 179 - 201)
187 (74)	69.7 - 77.5 - 87.0 (154 - 171 - 192)	72.9 - 81.1 - 91.1 (161 - 179 - 201)	75.6 - 83.8 - 94.3 (167 - 185 - 208)

Table of ideal weights at various heights and ages; three weights are given in each instance, and refer to small, medium and large builds. All weights given are for unclothed persons.

WOMEN

Height in cm. (in.)	Weight in kg. (lb.) at ages shown		
	20 YEARS	25 YEARS	30 YEARS
142 (56)	43.0 - 47.5 - 53.0 (95 - 105 - 117)	43.9 - 48.9 - 55.2 (97 - 108 - 122)	45.3 - 50.2 - 56.6 (100 - 111 - 125)
144 (57)	43.5 - 48.4 - 53.9 (96 - 107 - 119)	44.9 - 49.8 - 56.1 (99 - 110 - 124)	46.2 - 51.1 - 57.5 (102 - 113 - 127)
147 (58)	44.4 - 49.3 - 55.7 (98 - 109 - 123)	45.7 - 50.7 - 57.0 (101 - 112 - 126)	47.1 - 52.1 - 58.4 (104 - 115 - 129)
149 (59)	45.3 - 50.2 - 56.6 (100 - 111 - 125)	46.4 - 51.2 - 58.0 (103 - 114 - 128)	47.5 - 53.0 - 59.8 (105 - 117 - 132)
152 (60)	46.6 - 51.6 - 58.0 (103 - 114 - 128)	47.1 - 52.5 - 59.3 (104 - 116 - 131)	48.4 - 53.9 - 60.7 (107 - 119 - 134)
154 (61)	47.5 - 53.0 - 59.8 (105 - 117 - 132)	48.4 - 53.9 - 60.7 (107 - 119 - 134)	49.8 - 55.2 - 62.0 (110 - 122 - 137)
157 (62)	48.9 - 54.3 - 61.1 (108 - 120 - 135)	50.2 - 55.7 - 62.5 (111 - 123 - 138)	51.1 - 56.6 - 63.8 (113 - 125 - 141)
160 (63)	50.2 - 55.7 - 62.5 (111 - 123 - 138)	51.1 - 57.0 - 64.3 (113 - 126 - 142)	52.5 - 58.4 - 65.7 (116 - 129 - 145)
162 (64)	51.1 - 57.0 - 64.3 (113 - 126 - 142)	52.5 - 58.4 - 65.7 (116 - 129 - 145)	53.9 - 59.8 - 67.5 (119 - 132 - 149)
165 (65)	53.0 - 58.9 - 66.1 (117 - 130 - 146)	54.3 - 60.2 - 67.5 (120 - 133 - 149)	55.7 - 61.6 - 69.3 (123 - 136 - 153)
167 (66)	54.8 - 60.7 - 68.4 (121 - 134 - 151)	55.7 - 62.0 - 69.7 (123 - 136 - 154)	57.0 - 63.4 - 71.6 (126 - 140 - 158)
170 (67)	56.1 - 62.5 - 70.2 (124 - 138 - 155)	57.5 - 63.8 - 71.6 (127 - 141 - 158)	58.9 - 65.2 - 73.4 (130 - 144 - 162)
172 (68)	57.5 - 63.8 - 72.0 (127 - 141 - 159)	59.3 - 65.7 - 73.8 (131 - 145 - 163)	60.2 - 67.0 - 75.6 (133 - 148 - 167)
175 (69)	59.3 - 65.7 - 73.8 (131 - 145 - 163)	60.7 - 67.5 - 75.6 (134 - 149 - 167)	61.6 - 68.4 - 77.0 (136 - 151 - 170)
177 (70)	60.7 - 67.5 - 76.1 (134 - 149 - 168)	62.0 - 68.8 - 77.5 (137 - 152 - 171)	63.4 - 70.2 - 78.8 (140 - 155 - 174)
180 (71)	62.9 - 69.7 - 78.4 (139 - 154 - 173)	63.4 - 70.7 - 79.7 (140 - 156 - 176)	64.8 - 72.0 - 81.1 (143 - 159 - 179)

Table of ideal weights at various heights and ages; three weights are given in each instance, and refer to small, medium and large builds. All weights given are for unclothed persons.

Any disease, such as haemorrhage, thrombosis, embolism or tumour, which results in damage to only one side of the brain, causes paralysis of varying extent on the opposite side of the body.

Because speech centres are situated in the left of the brain, loss of speech facility (aphasia) is associated only with right hemiplegia but impaired muscular action may cause speech difficulties (dysphasia) irrespective of the side involved.

hemp. See CANNABIS.

heparin. A complex organic substance, secreted by connective tissue cells, which acts as an anticoagulant of the blood (i.e., it reduces blood-clotting). This it achieves mainly by inhibiting the conversion of pro-thrombin to thrombin. It is prepared commercially from cattle lung and is injected into the vein in conditions where it is desirable to reduce the tendency of the blood to clot, such as in cases of thrombosis. The effect of a single dose lasts for about two hours but a 'sustained-release' preparation is also available.

hepatitis. Inflammation of the liver. Although this may be a complication of various infections or result from poisoning by certain drugs, the most common cause is a virus infection and two distinct types are recognized.

1. Acute infective hepatitis tends to occur in local outbreaks and is probably a food-borne infection. An attack usually starts with the appearance of jaundice and bile-coloured urine, followed by symptoms of toxaemia – loss of appetite, headache and fever. The jaundice may take some weeks to clear up and convalescence may be prolonged.

2. Serum hepatitis is due to a specific virus known as SH or 'Australia' antigen. Cases result from contact with infected blood. The disease may be serious and is a hazard in blood transfusion, in renal dialysis, and in transplant surgery, and since it may also be communicated by improperly sterilized syringes and other instruments it often affects drug addicts and may occur after tattooing.

Gammaglobulin is used both for the prevention and treatment of infective hepatitis. It is particularly important that cases of hepatitis should avoid alcohol for at least a year after an attack because of its toxic effect on liver cells already weakened by the disease.

heredity and environment. Heredity is the organic relationship between parents and offspring which leads to the transmission of characteristics and diseases from earlier ancestors. The study of the factors which determine this transmission is known as GENETICS. Human inheritance is bi-parental (derived partly from the father and partly from the mother), and it is a matter of common knowledge that obvious traits of parents, such as skin and eye colour, curly hair, and shape of nose, reappear in their children.

These are examples of biological inheritance the content of which is determined at the time of conception when an egg-cell and sperm-cell unite to produce a fertilized ovum or zygote. At early stages of development the human embryo looks exactly like that of any other mammal but it contains within itself a biological code of instructions which determines its future conformation and characteristics.

Heredity is only partly responsible for an individual's total make-up because development after birth is influenced by every conceivable environmental factor – and even before birth, as witness the thalidomide disaster.

No two persons are exactly alike. Identical twins arise from a single ovum and share a common biological inheritance but although they may look alike they may develop quite differently in different environments. This is the fundamental difference between inherited and acquired characteristics. A parent with six toes (quite a common deformity) has a good chance of producing a child with six toes too, but a parent who accidentally loses a toe will never have a four-toed child.

The inheritance of mental traits is no different from the inheritance of physical characteristics. The capacity to learn is inborn just as is ability for music, or mathematics, or any special skill. Exploitation of such capacities depends on environmental opportunities.

In relation to disease the same situation is found. Many diseases are now known to be due to abnormalities present in the biological inheritance – haemophilia and colour-blindness are familiar examples – and similarly there may be inborn characteristics which only become manifest after interaction with the environment, as an increased susceptibility to develop specific diseases.

Although heredity is a complex subject the basic laws are now well understood and they have practical applications in the production of improved breeds of plants and animals and also in GENETIC GUIDANCE.

hermaphroditism. The combination of essential male and female structures and functions in one individual. Although this is normal in flowering plants and in lower animals of such types as worms, molluscs, snails and polyps, it is a very rare abnormality in mammals, and in man very few examples of true hermaphroditism have ever been recorded.

In the cases of 'sex change' which are occasionally seen the condition is really pseudo-hermaphroditism. Either ovaries or testes are present as usual but malformation or imperfect development of the external sexual organs leads to a child being regarded as of the opposite sex to its real hormone condition. Difficulties then arise at puberty or in later life when the error becomes apparent. However, it is now possible to determine genetic sex positively by chromosome examination and specialist advice should be sought immediately.

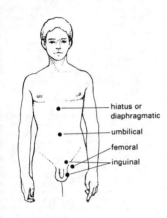

- hiatus or diaphragmatic
- umbilical
- femoral
- inguinal

skin

cavity — lining membrane

abdominal organ

Hernia

hernia. The protrusion of some organ or part of an organ through a weak spot in the wall of its containing cavity, the protrusion remaining covered by the lining membrane of the cavity and by the overlying soft tissues and skin.

Hernia is most frequently seen in the lower abdomen (where it is popularly called 'rupture') and appears as a swelling in the groin. In inguinal hernia a portion of bowel passes down the inguinal canal in the pelvis and in men may reach the scrotum. Femoral hernia occupies the femoral canal alongside the main blood vessels to the leg. Both these types may be controlled by the wearing of a TRUSS. Other abdominal hernias include umbilical hernia (through the umbilicus), incisional or ventral hernia (through a weak abdominal scar) and hiatus or diaphragmatic hernia in which congenital or acquired weakness of the diaphragm allows abdominal contents to bulge into the chest cavity.

So long as a hernia can be returned to the abdomen by external manipulation it is 'reducible' and can generally be controlled by a truss. If adhesions form it becomes irreducible, and is then more likely to become a potential danger as the section of the intestine concerned may become obstructed or strangulated by the wall through which it has protruded. Both of these situations will necessitate an emergency operation.

Trusses are rather unsatisfactory because although they have relieved the situation, they have not corrected it; most hernias can be satisfactorily repaired by a relatively simple and effective operation at negligible risk.

heroin. Di-acetyl morphine, a powerful alkaloid derived from opium. Although less depressant of the respiratory centre than morphine it is perhaps the most dangerous drug of ADDICTION. Its use is now restricted and may be prescribed for addicts only in special centres. In underworld jargon it goes by various names such as 'boy', 'horse', 'jack', 'schmee' and 'schmeck' or 'smack'.

herpes. A superficial skin infection due to the virus *Herpes simplex* and not to be confused with herpes zoster, more commonly known as SHINGLES. A crop of small watery blisters usually occurs on the face around the margins of the nose and mouth; these dry up and form crusts which separate in about a week. It is frequently seen in association with the common cold or with more serious infective illnesses such as pneumonia. No treatment is really required. The lesions may be dabbed with spirit and kept dry.

herpes zoster. See SHINGLES.

hiccough (hiccup). A troublesome symptom produced by repeated sudden spasms of the diaphragm with simultaneous closure of the glottis.

Usually transitory and unimportant, it is often produced by taking food or drink too rapidly with sudden distension of the stomach. Expedients such as holding the breath, sucking an ice-cube, or holding a hot-water bottle over the stomach soon bring relief.

In a more prolonged form it occurs as a symptom of serious disease of stomach or bowel (because of irritation to the diaphragm), and it may complicate the after-treatment of operations on the upper abdomen. It is also common in uraemia and cirrhosis of the liver, and occurs in encephalitis lethargica. Hiccough from such causes exhausts the patient and is very difficult to treat without resorting to powerful sedation.

high blood pressure. See BLOOD PRESSURE.

hip. The joint between the pelvis and the upper end of each femur, or thigh bone. The rounded head of the femur fits into a cup-shaped cavity (acetabulum) on the pelvis and this ball-and-socket design ensures that it is both freely movable and strong enough to withstand the stresses imposed by weight-bearing, walking, running, and jumping. It is further supported by ligaments and the overlying thigh muscles.

Injuries. Dislocation of the joint may occur as may fracture of the narrow neck of bone between the rounded head and the shaft of the femur.

Diseases. (1) Tuberculous arthritis, formerly common in children, is now less often seen since milk became largely free from bovine tuberculosis; (2) Perthes' disease, an obscure degenerative process, affects the femoral head during growth; (3) osteo-arthritis, a degenerative joint disease, is found in older persons.

Congenital dislocation. It has been recognized since the time of Hippocrates that some new-born infants have hip-joints which are either dislocated or easily dislocatable because the socket is too shallow to retain the head of the femur.

The cause is unknown. The incidence is about 1.25 cases per 1,000 births and females are three times more commonly affected than males. The condition can be recognized in new-born infants within their first week of life by a manipulative test. If it is not recognized and treated promptly the patient develops a characteristic 'dipping' gait and is liable to osteo-arthritic changes and further crippling.

Treatment is simple: the hips are placed in full abduction, the legs splayed at 90 ° from the line of the body. Splints or plaster may be used but in many cases the application of specially bulky 'nappies' will suffice to maintain the required position. With prompt diagnosis, splinting is seldom needed for longer than twelve weeks and follow-up of cases has shown uniform success. If the diagnosis is missed subsequent treatment is much more difficult and prolonged, and not always so effective.

The virtual eradication of this condition is one of the unappreciated triumphs of preventive medicine and testing for the condition should be a routine of every doctor, health visitor or nurse with responsibility for the care of a new-born infant.

Hippocrates. Hippocrates of Cos (about 460-370 B.C.) is traditionally regarded as the 'father of medicine'. He emphasized the scientific basis of medicine, distinguishing it from philosophy and religion.

Hippocratic oath. The oath, attributed to Hippocrates but in all probability of earlier origin, traditionally taken by doctors when they qualify. The oath makes seven pledges: (1) that the doctor will hold those who taught him as dear to him as his own parents; (2) that he will impart knowledge of medicine only to his own sons, his teachers' sons and recognized students; (3) that he will treat patients to the best of his ability and judgment; (4) that he will not perform surgical operations but will leave them to persons specializing in that line; (5) that he will not have sexual relations with patients or members of their households; (6) that he will not give poison

and will not give a woman a pessary to cause abortion; and (7) that he will keep to himself all information obtained.

histamine. A substance produced in all body tissues by the breakdown of the amino-acid, histidine. Its main action is to enlarge small blood vessels and so increase the blood supply to the tissues. Abnormally large quantities of histamine, or of closely related substances, are produced in conditions of allergy, in shock, and in certain injuries. Excess histamine is the principal cause both of inflammation and of allergic symptoms. Drugs which reduce the action of histamine are called ANTIHISTAMINES.

histology. The study of bodily tissues under the microscope. This investigation of the structure of the cells in tissues and organs has contributed enormously to our knowledge of physiology and pathology.

histoplasmosis. A disease of the lungs caused by infection with *Histoplasma capsulatum*, a fungus found in the dried excreta of bats and various birds. The disease has an acute form with symptoms resembling those of influenza, and a more severe chronic form which resembles tuberculosis of the lungs and spleen. The condition is almost unknown in Britain but is not uncommon in the U.S.A.

Prevention would seem to lie mainly in avoidance of air-borne spores in caves, old silos, etc. Most cases recover without special treatment, but where this is not so, antifungal antibiotics are worth trying.

hives. An allergic reaction to foods (especially strawberries, shellfish, eggs and chocolate) or less commonly to antibiotics or to pollen, causing reddish, itching, circular weals. Prevention is difficult and involves identifying the cause so that the patient may try to avoid it. Calamine lotion or a paste of bicarbonate of soda applied to the itchy skin may help, but in severe cases antihistamine drugs are desirable.

hoarseness. A rough, grating or 'husky' tone of voice. When air is forced through the larynx and between the vocal cords a sound is produced which is then modified by movements of the palate, tongue, mouth and lips to form intelligible speech. The pitch and tonal quality of the basic sound is determined by the tension and position of the vocal cords.

Inflammatory conditions and tumours affecting the larynx and vocal cords interfere with this mechanism and the vocal cords themselves may become paralysed from damage to their nerve supply. Any of these conditions may affect the character of the voice.

Persistent hoarseness calls for examination of the larynx to determine the precise cause.

Hodgkin's disease. A condition, also known as lymphadenoma, in which there is a painless progressive enlargement of lymph glands near the body surface, and ultimately of lymphoid tissue throughout the body. It can occur at any age but most commonly in males under 40.

The initial stages are followed by the development of general symptoms of anaemia, lassitude, breathlessness, and loss of weight, and the occurrence of a characteristic fluctuating fever. There is often itching and the skin may become sallow or pigmented.

The disease was formerly always fatal, few cases surviving for more than five years, but modern treatment either by radiotherapy alone or combined with courses of cytotoxic drugs (i.e., drugs which prevent cells from reproducing, so that the enlargement of the lymphoid tissue is halted) has considerably improved the prospects of securing some remission for considerable periods.

holly berries. The fruit of the holly tree (genus *Ilex*) occurring as clusters of bright red or scarlet berries. Children should not be allowed to eat the attractive berries. They are mildly poisonous and will cause abdominal pain, headache, vomiting and purging.

If vomiting does not occur spontaneously, an emetic (e.g., a tablespoon of mustard in a glass of water) should be given to induce it, followed later by a laxative. The berries are so bitter to taste and are usually rejected so promptly, that it is unlikely that any serious harm will result.

home nursing. The term is used in two senses.

1. Visiting of patients in their homes by home nurses (formerly called district nurses), who are qualified nurses with a short training. Since many patients are not ill enough to need the continuous skilled nursing care provided in hospital but nevertheless require some skilled nursing, e.g., injections and changing of dressings, a home nursing service is an essential element in any comprehensive system of health care, and the visits of the nurse are also very reassuring to the relatives undertaking the general care of the patient.

2. Caring at home for a sick or ailing relative. Everyone likely to be faced with the task of caring for a sick or ailing relative at home should endeavour to acquire some basic knowledge of the skills needed to provide for a patient's comfort and happiness. Many simple manuals are readily available and in many areas the British Red Cross Society and other organizations provide classes of instruction.

Practical comments and advice on home nursing are given in the article on NURSING. Special precautions are necessary in relation to cases of infectious illness. These are dealt with in the article on DISINFECTION.

homeopathy. A system of medical treatment based on the proposition, '*similia similibus curentur*' (let likes be treated by likes).

The system was introduced by Samuel Hahnemann about 1812.

Ordinary medical treatment concerns itself with diet, physical measures, and pharmaceutical remedies. It was in relation to the last that allopathy and homeopathy parted company. The allopaths advocated strong medicines to relieve symptoms: the homeopaths attached less importance to suppression of symptoms than to the support of natural healing by minute doses of drugs directly affecting diseased cells and organs. Their procedure was to test a drug on a healthy body; to equate the symptoms produced with similar symptoms occurring in disease; and to give the selected drug in such small doses that it could produce no injurious effect. For example, arsenic causes watery diarrhoea and so was recommended for cholera.

The homeopaths maintained that curative doses must be minute (one part in ten thousand to one part in a million, or even greater dilutions) so that the amount of drug actually received was so infinitesimal that it was difficult to believe that it could be of much effect. Nevertheless, homeopathy continued to attract adherents and by 1870 or so had won a measure of grudging acceptance. Homeopathic hospitals and practitioners became established in many centres, especially in America where by 1900 one-quarter of the practitioners were said to be homeopaths.

Although homeopathy is still practised, it is in decline. In its time it exercised a powerful influence on medical practice by reviving interest in the rational use of drugs. The methods suggested by Hahnemann for study of their actions laid the foundations of pharmacology. The huge doses of the allopaths are no more. They have gradually been eliminated from orthodox medical practice and been replaced by newer drugs whose use is based on a scientific approach to their development and use. For this at least some credit must be accorded to Hahnemann.

homicidal mania. Mental disease which leads to the killing or attempted killing of another individual.

In manic-depressive psychosis the patient alternates between extremes of depression and excitement. In the manic phase he may become quarrelsome, aggressive and intolerant of restraint and may strike those who seek to restrain him.

In schizophrenia and paranoia any homicidal act may be of a more deliberate and calculated character. Such a patient may suffer from delusions of persecution, with the result that he may attempt to kill people whom he falsely imagines to be seeking to injure him.

homosexuality. A sexual attraction between persons of the same sex either with or without sexual activity of a physical nature. Homosexuality between women is known as lesbianism and the prostitution or seduction of boys by adult males is pederasty.

Homosexuality can sometimes be a problem in boarding schools but this is no more than an adolescent exploratory phase of development which has been termed 'puppy pruriency'. It occurs also under circumstances where the sexes are segregated under abnormal conditions as in prisons, reformatories, at sea, or in the armed forces.

These examples, however, do not represent true homosexuality, because there is no real change in personality and homosexual attitudes and activities are outgrown or abandoned when opportunities with the other sex become available. Nevertheless in such segregated communities, when discipline is poor and standards low, the opportunities for the seduction of young people by older confirmed homosexuals are obvious and call for vigilance on the part of those who are responsible for the conduct of such schools and institutions.

Various theories have been advanced as to the cause of homosexuality. It clearly cannot be regarded as a form of degeneracy, since many homosexuals are gifted and artistic. It has not been proved to be due to genetic or endocrine causes, although recent work suggests that these may account for some cases.

Psychological influences are probably more important: Freud contended that it arose from over-attachment to the mother, especially in circumstances where the father had proved an unsatisfactory parent or had died, with the result that the child's personality tended to become excessively feminine. The fact that some homosexuals have responded to treatment by psychological methods lends weight to this view.

Homosexuals vary in type. Some may be exclusively so motivated; some may be bisexual and seek heterosexual relationships as well; some are transvestists who take pleasure in dressing as women; and some are trans-sexualists, playing either an active or passive role with another male.

The attitude of society to homosexuality is variable and undecided. Lesbianism has always been ignored by the law. In male homosexuality importuning and especially seduction of youth is generally condemned. On the other hand the law in the U.K. has been changed so that homosexual acts in private between consenting males over 21 are no longer crimes. Whether this is right or wrong is a matter for argument. No enlightened person would deny that the homosexual temperament should receive understanding and sympathy. Though changing social attitudes now encourage much more open discussion of the social and moral issues involved, and though more people can accept homosexual relationships as 'different' rather than 'perverted', homosexuality is still regarded by many with fear and intolerance.

hookworm disease. Anaemia arising from infection with hookworms, which are of two main types: *Ankylostoma*, prevalent in Egypt and the Middle East, and *Necator* (slightly smaller), common in Central and South America. An alternative name for the disease is ankylostomiasis.

The hookworm's eggs, passed with the faeces of a victim, hatch in warm, damp earth. The hatched embryo penetrates the skin of feet or legs in contact with the contaminated soil, and travels by the blood stream to the lungs and ultimately to the intestine, where the now adult worm 'hooks' itself in and sucks blood.

The symptoms are simply those of severe anaemia, and diagnosis is made by examination of the faeces, in which eggs can be seen under a microscope.

Treatment is with drugs which dislodge the hookworm and the anaemia also requires attention.

hormones. The 'chemical messengers' produced by the ENDOCRINE GLANDS such as the pituitary and the thyroid. Hormones play a vital part in many of the activities of the body.

hospitals. Hospitals were little more than shelters until Florence Nightingale's sustained campaign both for nursing training and for better accommodation and equipment. Thereafter hospitals became respectable, nursing became a profession, death rates fell dramatically and cures became more frequent. Yet hospitals still carried the stigma of pauperism: the senior physicians and surgeons gave their services free and few patients who could afford to be treated at home or in a nursing home entered a hospital ward.

In the middle of the twentieth century all this changed. Medical and surgical advances at unprecedented pace made the treatment of serious disorders impracticable at home or in a small nursing home: radiological, biochemical, bacteriological and other facilities could normally be made available only in a large unit. So hospitals became the normal places for the treatment of serious illness.

housemaid's knee. A form of bursitis in which the bursa in front of the knee-cap becomes inflamed as a result of pressure from frequent kneeling, so that the part becomes hot, swollen, tender and red. Prevention is by using a thick, soft mat when kneeling. Treatment involves rest, firm bandaging and in some cases removal of fluid by a needle and syringe.

humerus. The bone of the upper arm. It forms, with the glenoid cavity of the scapula, a ball and socket JOINT which is capable of a wide range of movement but easily dislocated. At the lower end it forms a hinge joint with the ulna.

hunger. The sensation of desire for food. It arises strongly in the early stages of fasting or starvation but is lost in later stages. Hunger pains, which disappear after eating, occur when a meal is delayed beyond its normal time and are also a symptom of gastric ulcer.

untington's chorea. A hereditary disease characterized by disordered and involuntary muscular movements and by progressive mental deterioration. There is as yet no cure, though sedatives and tranquillizers help to relieve the symptoms.

The disease usually appears at 35 to 50 years, by which time the individual will probably have completed his family; by the Mendelian laws of GENETICS about half of his children are likely to carry the gene and to transmit it to their offspring who will in turn have their children before they show signs of the disease. The disease could be eliminated by successful GENETIC GUIDANCE.

ydatid disease. A disease due to a tapeworm (*Taenia echinococcus*) conveyed to people and sheep from infected dogs. The eggs are passed in the faeces of the dogs and are eaten by sheep in which hydatid cysts form. Humans become infected by handling the dogs or eating food contaminated by their excreta. The embryo worms develop in the stomach and pass by blood-vessels to the liver (or occasionally the kidney or brain) where they form cysts which produce symptoms by pressure. Treatment is by surgical removal.

ydrocele. A collection of fluid in a sac-like cavity, most commonly the scrotum. The condition, which sometimes follows an injury and is sometimes congenital, usually appears gradually in middle-aged men as a smooth, uniform, pear-shaped, painless swelling which may cause a dragging sensation from the weight of the fluid. The inherited form also occurs in children. The usual treatment is periodical 'tapping', i.e. drawing off the fluid through the outer layer of tissue.

ydrocephalus. The term means 'water on the brain'. The condition is characterized by abnormal enlargement of the head through accumulation of cerebrospinal fluid in the cavities of the brain. The accumulation results either from excessive secretion of cerebrospinal fluid or from blocking of the opening through which it normally escapes from the brain cavities into the sub-arachnoid space surrounding the brain and spinal cord. In most cases intelligence is defective, and convulsions may occur.

The condition is mostly seen in association with SPINA BIFIDA, but occasionally occurs as a complication of meningitis or brain tumour.

Mild cases may clear spontaneously. More severe cases can be treated by an operation in which a tube is introduced behind the ear and into a vein in the neck, so that the excess fluid is carried by the tube from the brain to the blood stream. In a severe untreated case there is progressive destruction of brain tissue with consequent deterioration of cerebral functioning.

hydrochloric acid. A strong corrosive acid which in dilute form is a normal constituent of gastric juice and is used in the process of digestion. Excessive hydrochloric acid in the stomach – technically known as hyperchlorhydria – is an important factor in causing gastric ulcers.

In a case of hydrochloric acid poisoning an alkali, such as baking soda or milk of magnesia, should be given as soon as possible, followed by milk or white of egg. Emetics to induce vomiting must not be used. See First Aid section at end of book.

hydrocyanic acid. See PRUSSIC ACID.

hydrophobia. An alternative name for RABIES.

hydrotherapy. Treatment of disease by means of water.

In the past there was extensive use in medical practice of hot, tepid and cold baths for various conditions, and also of sulphur baths, effervescing or carbonic acid baths, alkaline baths, peat or mud baths, and even paraffin wax baths. Most of these are nowadays regarded sceptically.

Hydrotherapy today is virtually restricted to the use of swimming baths in the rehabilitation of patients suffering from partial paralysis or severe arthritis; because the water partially supports the weight of the body, movement is easier than in air.

hydrothorax. Accumulation of watery fluid in the pleural cavity between the layers of pleura, the tissue which surrounds the lungs. Inflammatory causes of active pleural effusion include tuberculosis and occasionally pneumonia and lung abscess. Passive accumulation of fluid from the blood also occurs as a late symptom in cardiac failure, some varieties of nephritis and certain forms of cancer. The fluid is removed by the simple operation of 'tapping', but in the active forms treatment of the underlying cause is also essential.

hygiene. Hygiene is essentially the science of maintaining or, improving health, although the term is sometimes restricted (wrongly) to purely physical aspects of health.

Environmental hygiene, or the creation and maintenance of an environment compatible with good health, includes such matters as establishing water supplies and safeguarding their purity, setting up proper systems of sewage disposal and preventing the contamination of water or food by sewage, ensuring that infectious persons are segregated in isolation hospitals, building and maintaining fit houses, ensuring that at each stage from the grower or manufacturer to the householder food is clean and not contaminated by germs, protecting the public from noxious vapours, maintaining the purity of the air and providing reasonable protection against excessive noise.

Personal hygiene includes such items as ensuring that persons in each age-group have adequate amounts not just of total calories but of proteins, mineral salts and vitamins; ensuring that each person drinks sufficient fluid, both for temperature regulation and for removal of waste products; prevention of obesity, not just in the middle-aged and elderly (in whom the results appear) but also in children and adolescents; provision of facilities for exercise and encouragement of people to take exercise appropriate to their age and state of health. It also means inducing people to wear clothing that will protect against heat loss but will also allow free movement; making people aware of the need for adequate rest and sleep – with sleep needs varying from the infant's 14 hours to the old person's 6 or 7 hours; and encouraging the development of leisure interests and recreations.

The aspect of personal hygiene usually implied in the popular usage of the word means making people aware of the importance of washing their hands after using the lavatory and before handling food; encouraging people to have regular baths for the removal of the solid constituents of sweat and of oily sebum, with cleansing of the genitalia, toes and arm-pits particularly important. Personal hygiene is a matter of persuasion and education, not legal enforcement. Health teaching in school is clearly important, but some habits and attitudes are best inculcated before school entry, and some aspects are perhaps best taught after leaving school.

Mental hygiene includes at its lowest level the development of affection and of consideration for others and the instillation of codes of behaviour that respect the desires and needs of other people. At a higher level it involves knowledge of elementary psychology, in order, for example, to avoid entering into argument with somebody who is clearly in a temper; awareness of the customs and traditions of persons of different background, race or religion; insight into the long-term and short-term effects of habits and behaviour on mental and physical health; and some awareness of many factors of importance in modern life – of which genetics, contraceptive facilities, economic stresses, problems of bereavement and social services are examples.

hymen. The membrane that partially closes the entrance to the vagina in women. Although it is normally ruptured on the first occasion of intercourse, its intact presence is not absolute evidence of virginity and its rupture is not evidence of absence of virginity. It can occasionally be ruptured during violent exercise and can – very occasionally – remain intact after intercourse.

hyperaemia. The congestion of blood which occurs in any part of the body that ha[s] become inflamed, and which causes th[e] reddening and heat of inflammation.

hyperaesthesia. Excessive sensitiveness [of] any of the senses but especially of the ski[n] so that, for example, a tap may be felt as [a] sharp blow. Hyperaesthesia is common [in] hysteria, occurs in some diseases of th[e] spinal cord and is sometimes noted [in] women during their menstrual periods [or] at the menopause.

hyperemesis gravidarum. Excessiv[e] vomiting in pregnancy, usually beginnin[g] as an exaggeration of morning sicknes[s]. There are two overlapping types: (1) th[e] neurotic variety – with retching an[d] vomiting at all hours and a risk [of] dehydration; and (2) the toxic variety where, in addition, the patient looks tox[ic] (with muddy skin and sunken eyes) and th[e] scanty urine contains albumin. Diagnos[is] cannot be certain until investigations hav[e] confirmed that such conditions as gastri[c] ulcer and strangulated hernia are n[ot] present. The cause is not yet full[y] understood. Treatment involves rest an[d] quiet, good nursing, and in some case[s] antihistamine drugs and tranquillizers. [In] the toxic variety the pregnancy may hav[e] to be artificially terminated.

hyperglycaemia. A condition characterize[d] by excess sugar (glucose) in the bloo[d] usually occurring because the pancreas [is] not producing an adequate amount [of] insulin. Hyperglycaemia is the basi[c] feature of DIABETES MELLITUS.

hyperidrosis. Excessive sweating, ofte[n] accompanied by an unpleasant odou[r]. Generalized excessive perspiration occur[s] from heat, exertion, fear, feverish an[d] toxic states, and also in hyperthyroidis[m] and some diseases of the central nervou[s] system. Fat people are liable to it i[n] conditions of heat or exertion, and it [is] more a condition of adolescents and youn[g] adults than of older persons. The localize[d] forms are common in nervous or highl[y] emotional people, in sufferers fro[m] exophthalmic goitre and in heavy drinker[s]; these tend to affect the feet, hands, arm[-] pits, genital region or face.

Frequent washing is essential an[d] application of a dusting powder of zinc an[d] salicylic acid is useful, but it is als[o] necessary to investigate the cause an[d] treat it, and to relieve any associate[d] anxiety or feeling of guilt.

hypermetropia. A defect of EYESIGHT commonly known as 'long sight' wit[h] which there is usually difficulty in readin[g] or sewing.

hyperpiesis. High BLOOD PRESSURE.

hyperpyrexia. Bodily temperature sub[-] stantially above the normal 37 °C. (98.[4] °F.). The condition occurs in many sever[e] fevers and also in sunstroke. Apart fro[m] the rise in temperature, the skin become[s] hot and dry, and the patient's condition [is] one of apathy followed by stupor an[d] coma. Hyperpyrexia is most likely to occu[r] in persons with defects of the sweat gland[s] or after the administration of sweat-inhibiting drugs such as atropine. Treatment includes spraying the body with cold water.

ypertension. High BLOOD PRESSURE.

yperthyroidism. See GOITRE.

ypertrophy. Increased growth of tissue mainly by multiplication of its cells. It may occur (1) from hormone stimulation, as in the growth of the breasts and uterus during pregnancy; (2) from frequent exercise, as in the muscles of athletes; or (3) as a compensatory mechanism, as when the heart enlarges to pump blood more vigorously into narrowed arteries.

Hypertrophy should be differentiated from TUMOUR (neoplasm). In hypertrophy the cells are increased in number but are completely normal.

ypnosis. A special form of sleep or trance induced by an operator who suggests the idea of sleep in various ways, e.g., by getting the patient to look at a bright object and by monotonously repeating a phrase. Hypnosis is not effective unless two conditions are satisfied: (1) that the patient is willing to co-operate, and (2) that the operator can hold the patient's complete attention. With a skilled operator about 80 per cent of willing persons can be hypnotized.

Hypnosis can be used to enable a patient to recover long-forgotten memories which, long repressed into the unconscious, may nevertheless be the causes of diseases, such as psychoneurosis. Hypnosis is therefore of considerable value in establishing the cause of neurotic diseases, thus permitting rational treatment.

A hypnotized person can also be given instructions which, after awakening, he will follow - provided they are compatible with his general codes of behaviour - without realizing that they have been implanted in his mind. For instance, hypnosis can be used to help a person who desires to stop smoking but lacks the will-power to do so. Again, in the absence of anaesthetics, operations have been painlessly performed under hypnosis: but with anaesthetics virtually 100 per cent effective no surgeon would willingly rely on a procedure with a failure rate of one in five.

Although very valuable for reviving repressed memories and for giving curative suggestions, hypnosis might be abused. A generous person might be induced to give money on awakening to an apparently desirable cause, and an unmarried girl already thinking about sexual relations with her lover might be persuaded to lose her virginity. Hence patients should consult only hypnotists of known integrity and should preferably be accompanied by reliable friends. Moreover, in unskilled hands hypnotism can do considerable emotional damage; and, while it can cure a particular symptom - e.g., a stammer - it does not treat the underlying cause of the symptom.

Despite the suggestion by many writers of fiction, there is absolutely no evidence that hypnotic subjects will, after hypnosis, obey instructions which are repugnant to them, e.g., that a person of normal standards could be hypnotically persuaded to commit a serious crime.

hypnotic. A drug which promotes sleep but does not relieve pain. Hypnotics should be differentiated from NARCOTICS (such as morphia) which relieve pain and induce sleep, ANODYNES (such as aspirin) which reduce pain without causing drowsiness and TRANQUILLIZERS, which relieve anxiety.

The barbiturates are by far the most commonly used hypnotics. Other sleep-stimulating drugs include chloral hydrate, paraldehyde, bromides and nitrazepam (Mogadon). Every known hypnotic has some potential unfortunate side-effect, e.g., the barbiturates are mildly habit-forming and are also thought to repress dreaming which some experts deem to be necessary for mental health.

hypochondria. Abnormal preoccupation with one's real or imaginary ailments. Concern with health is normal, especially in persons suffering from illness or disability, but the hypochondriac makes his ailments the absolute centre of his thoughts, and if a mild symptom which he regards as an indication of serious disease is satisfactorily explained, he promptly finds another symptom to worry about.

The condition should be differentiated from MALINGERING and HYSTERIA. The malingerer alleges illness that he does not have; the hysteric produces illness in himself; the hypochondriac generally goes to work, discusses his symptoms with anybody who will listen, consults a series of different doctors, studies medical textbooks and spends a relatively happy life considering new methods of investigation or of treatment. There is often a deep underlying cause of hypochondria, e.g., it may be a defence mechanism in work failure or marital failure or a self-punishment for imaginary guilt. So extreme cases need skilled psychological investigation.

hypodermic injection. A method of giving drugs in solution by injecting them under the skin, using a syringe and a hollow needle. The method is sometimes employed for quick action but is more often used for drugs which, if swallowed, would be destroyed in the digestive tract. The injection is normally made in a part of the body where the skin is loose and where blood-vessels can be avoided. The outer and upper part of the arm and the buttock are the usual sites.

hypoglycaemia. Deficiency of sugar in the blood (below the 0.09 to 0.12 per cent level in the blood of a normal person who has not eaten for some hours). Since all carbohydrate absorbed from the diet is converted into glucose, stored as glycogen in the liver and muscles, and immediately available for release to provide energy, deficiency of sugar in the blood is relatively rare. Essentially it occurs in three sets of circumstances: (1) where there is over-activity of the insulin forming tissue of the pancreas (an extreme rarity, in contrast to the frequent under-activity that causes the hyperglycaemia of diabetes); (2) in severe disease of the liver where that organ is unable to store glycogen (again an extreme rarity); and (3) in cases of excessive dosage of insulin to diabetic patients. The body's need for insulin varies from time to time with the amount secreted by a healthy pancreas adjusting to the need. In the diabetic the need similarly varies, so that what was a correct dose of insulin yesterday may be an excessive dose under the different bodily circumstances of today.

Early evidences of hypoglycaemia – nearly always due to insulin dosage disproportionate to the immediate circumstances – include general uneasiness, chilliness, hunger and perspiration; and if untreated the patient may lose consciousness and ultimately die. Treatment at the early stage consists of the immediate eating of sugar. All diabetic patients should be instructed to carry a lump of sugar at all times and to recognize the symptoms which should lead to the immediate eating of the sugar.

Where a diabetic patient develops coma the attending doctor has to make a swift decision. A diabetic (hyperglycaemic) coma may be caused by a missed insulin injection, the onset is usually slow, the skin is dry, the blood pressure is reduced, respiration is deep and slow, the breath may smell of acetone and the urine will contain ketones. Heavy dosage of insulin and replacement of water and salt deficiency are essential for the preservation of life. In hypoglycaemic coma there may have been a missed meal or unusual exertion, the onset is rapid, the skin is moist, the blood pressure is normal or raised, respiration is rapid and shallow, the breath has no smell of acetone and the urine has no ketones although it may contain sugar. An intravenous injection of a glucose solution may save life. Clearly a mistake, resulting in the giving of glucose to a patient in hyperglycaemic coma or in the giving of insulin to a patient in hypoglycaemic coma, is likely to cost a life.

hypothalamus. The part of the middle brain which regulates the sympathetic and para-sympathetic nervous systems, the body temperature, and to some extent the emotions. It also controls the pituitary gland, which in turn influences the other endocrine glands.

The enormous role of the hypothalamus is only in the process of becoming appreciated. While the cerebral hemispheres are pre-eminent for intellectual functions, it appears that the hypothalamus is the centre concerned with excitement, elation and depression, the link between the central nervous systems and the autonomic nervous system and the link between the nervous systems and the endocrine glands.

hypothermia. Chilling of the body technically after the temperature falls below 35 °C. (95 °F.); see COLD, EFFECTS OF. This is a common and serious condition in old people because (1) the body's heat regulating mechanism often becomes inefficient in the elderly; (2) many old people live in grossly underheated accommodation; and (3) many old people are relatively insensitive to cold and unaware of the need for more warmth or more clothing.

Hypothermia can lead, without symptoms of discomfort, to drowsiness, slumber and death. Apart from sometimes causing death directly it is probably a factor in the increased death rate of old people in winter from such diseases as pneumonia and bronchitis. Prevention is partly a matter of lessening poverty and partly of educating old people about the need for a proper DIET, clothing and household warmth.

For some operations on the brain or heart a measure of hypothermia is deliberately employed to lessen oxygen requirements; the patient is restored to normal bodily temperature as soon as the operation is over.

hypothyroidism. See CRETINISM.

hysterectomy. Surgical removal of the uterus. The operation is required in cases of fibroid tumours of the uterus and cancer of the uterus, and sometimes in cases of excessive menstruation not relieved by the simpler method of curettage, i.e., scraping the lining of the uterus.

If the vagina and ovaries are left in position, hysterectomy does not remove either sexual desire or ability to have intercourse, although of course it makes conception and childbirth impossible. A woman contemplating the operation should ascertain whether the surgeon proposes to remove only the uterus or also the ovaries. As normally undertaken the operation leaves a faint vertical or horizontal scar on the abdomen, and necessitates ten to fourteen days in hospital with avoidance of heavy work for a further six to eight weeks.

hysteria. A psychoneurosis, in which signs of physical and mental illness are produced by the unconscious action of the mind. Essentially the sufferer from hysteria is one whose personality has failed to meet the full responsibilities of life; a person who unconsciously produces his symptoms partly as an expression of frustration and helplessness (and in effect a cry for help), partly as a means of escape from an intolerable situation, and partly as a compromise between an unconscious wish and its conscious inhibition or repression.

Hysteria can take the form of almost any illness, producing for example blindness, dumbness, deafness, tremors or paralysis. By far the commonest variety consists of outbursts of uncontrolled emotion, occurring mostly in persons of a highly emotional temperament and persons with little self-control. While the typical hysteric is emotionally unstable and self-centred, hysteria can occur in very stable persons after prolonged strain and considerable suppression of emotion.

In simple hysterical outbursts three forms of treatment are advocated by different schools of thought, and all three often work. (1) Allow the emotion to expend itself without interruption: 'let her have a good cry'. (2) Allay the emotion by quiet reassurance and suggestion. (3) Remove the emotion by firm handling, e.g., a sharp slap. In persisting and recurring cases intensive psychotherapy may be needed, including a search for the unconscious strivings that have given rise to the disease.

I

ichthyosis. A hereditary condition in which the skin is abnormally dry and scaly. It varies greatly in severity but in general causes no itching and no impairment of general health. There is as yet no specific cure, but the condition may be helped by frequent warm bathing followed by application of ointment based on petroleum jelly or application of cold cream. The affected skin should also be protected from cold.

icterus. A technical name for JAUNDICE.

id. A term used by psychoanalysts for the most instinctive and deeply unconscious part of the human mind, the reservoir of many hidden and repressed impulses and wishes, and the unconscious source of much human behaviour. It contrasts with the ego, the conscious and rational part of the mind, and the superego, the censor or conscience that holds in check the self-gratificatory impulses of the id. See FREUD.

identical twins. See TWINS.

idiosyncrasy. Mental attitude or behaviour peculiar to a person, or peculiar reaction by a person to a particular substance. The term is often used in the sense of allergy to some drug or food.

ilium. The main bone of the pelvis which is formed by the union of three bones at the acetabulum, the cup-shaped cavity that receives the head of the femur in the formation of the hip joint. The three are the ilium (uppermost), the pubic bone (in front) and the ischium (behind).

The ilium is a flattish, curved bone. To its outer surface are attached the muscles of the buttock, while the iliacus muscle is attached to its concave inner surface. The bone has a crest at the top, to which are attached several abdominal muscles. The crest ends in front in a prominence (the anterior iliac spine) to which the inguinal ligament is attached; and at the back it articulates with the sacrum, while below that junction is a notch through which the sciatic nerve passes down to the thigh.

illusion. A false perception arising from genuine external stimulation, such as a shadow being mistaken for a man or a noise misinterpreted as a voice. Illusion should be differentiated from delusion, where a false belief persists in defiance of reason, and from hallucination, where the false sensation occurs in the absence of any external stimulation. Since our senses are imperfect, illusions are common in normal people, but are removed by investigation and reasoning. In some diseases illusions tend to persist.

imagination. The ability to create images independent of previous perception.

While remembering is essentially a selective reproduction of past perceptions, as in recollecting the appearance of a house we lived in or the sound of a relative's voice, imagination, although inevitably based largely on past experiences, is much wider and freer. We may, for example, imagine a known house but with fewer or additional rooms and placed in an entirely different setting, or envisage a combination of two objects, such as a horse that can fly, or convert a reporter's brief, factual story into a novel with realistic characters and specific motivation.

Some try to differentiate imagination, as an extension or manipulation of the real, from fancy or fantasy, which steps outside the bounds of reality or possibility. For instance *Alice in Wonderland* is glorious fantasy, whereas the best modern science fiction displays rich imagination.

Imagination is a necessary process of mental life, a means whereby we can reach forward into the future or back into the past, and a method whereby we can grasp – however dimly – possibilities that lie ahead. When a young child says, 'I saw a lion in the garden', he is not telling a lie but beginning to use imagination.

Many people have primarily a visual imagination, fewer an auditory imagination, and perhaps still fewer a spacial imagination. Clearly poets, artists and inventors possess imagination of unusual quality. At the other end of the scale are people almost without imagination.

immaturity. A state of being not completely formed or developed. Any child is therefore immature. The term is normally used, however, for adults whose judgment or behaviour is childlike or for children whose attitudes and conduct resemble those of considerably younger children.

Immaturity should be clearly differentiated from mental deficiency and backwardness. Mental deficiency means appreciable intellectual impairment and of course has, as one feature, an inability to make mature judgments. Backwardness implies either a milder degree of intellectual impairment or educational retardation such as may occur from long illness or very poor home conditions. An immature person may be of low intellect (combining immaturity and backwardness), of average intellect, or of high intellect (sometimes shown by obtaining degrees and higher degrees).

Immaturity is perhaps best explained by comparing an intelligent, mature man of 40 with the same person as a boy of 16. At 16 his intelligence is fully developed but we do not expect him to display fully balanced judgment, self-control, general competence, evaluation of priorities, ability to modify aggression and capacity to react normally to stresses; and we would tolerate minor abnormalities of conduct that would be intolerable in an adult. When a man frequently acts like a boy of 16 (or in more extreme cases like a child of 10) we call him immature.

Immaturity is essentially a failure of the personality to develop properly. Its causes are not yet fully understood but its prevention would seem to lie mainly in the provision throughout childhood of a healthy emotional climate – where the child knows he is loved and secure but is not mentally choked by excessive affection, where he is, in large measure, free to investigate and to learn from his own mistakes but is neither over-indulged nor dominated, and where he gradually learns self-control and self-evaluation by example and precept. In many cases an immature person is the son or daughter of an immature parent, but the explanation lies in the upbringing, not in heredity.

immunity. In ordinary speech immunity simply means the state of being protected or exempt, e.g., having once been tried and acquitted a man is immune from any other trial for that particular offence. In medicine, however, the term is applied specifically to power to resist invading germs or their toxins.

Natural immunity. The species, the race, the family or the person may have a natural immunity to a disease. Thus no human being suffers from hog cholera. Europeans are much more resistant to measles than are South Sea Islanders, and, if they develop the disease, have it in much milder form. Some families are notoriously susceptible to various infections while other families have a tradition of escaping them. Of two persons eating exactly the same infected food, one may develop the particular food-borne disease (e.g., typhoid) while the other remains healthy. While this natural immunity depends in part on general health and adequate body store of vitamin A, it appears that in each of the above examples the leucocytes (white blood corpuscles) of the particular species, race, family or person have a marked capacity to engulf or destroy invading bacteria of the relevant type and the antigens produced by the bacteria.

Again, people who have recovered from certain infections have an acquired natural immunity. Even in the era when smallpox was very common it was almost unknown for a person to have two attacks during his lifetime. The same holds with various other infections (e.g., rubella and poliomyelitis) while, for many other infections, illness is followed by a temporary immunity lasting for some years. The mechanism is perhaps best understood by thinking back to days when no specific treatments existed. The victim

of an infection in those days either died or else his body learned the art of manufacturing antibodies (to combat the invading antigens) or antitoxin (to neutralize the toxin produced by the bacteria); and today, although the body is assisted by the administration of antiserum, antitoxin or antibiotics, it still acquires during the illness the power to manufacture appropriate antibodies. This power remains – permanently or for an appreciable time – so that, if the body is again invaded by germs of the same type the antibodies promptly destroy the invaders. A fair comparison would be with the defence forces of a country: before the first attack there was no standing army, so a defence force had to be mobilized and trained with desperate urgency (although nowadays there is also foreign aid, e.g., antibiotics); if the attack has been successfully resisted, there is now a standing defence force which can deal effectively with future invaders, although it could still be overwhelmed by sudden onslaught by an invading army of quite abnormal size (as in a laboratory accident involving many millions of bacteria).

Active artificial immunity. This is the result of 'tricking' the body into producing the relevant antibodies or antitoxins. If we deliberately inject into the body very small, carefully measured doses of either (1) the original germ, weakened by many generations of growth under artificial conditions (as in immunization against tuberculosis) or (2) the organism or toxin after being inactivated by heat or an appropriate chemical (as in immunization against diphtheria), the body responds by beginning to manufacture antibodies or antitoxins, and, exactly as after recovery from the disease, retains this manufacturing power, so that invaders of the particular type will be efficiently destroyed.

In most developed countries active immunization is now offered against diphtheria, tetanus and whooping cough (usually simultaneously to reduce the total number of injections); poliomyelitis (usually by mouth); measles; rubella – GERMAN MEASLES – (either to older children in the hope of eliminating the disease or to girls of about 13 years to give them maximum protection against developing the disease in pregnancy to the danger of the unborn child); and tuberculosis where deemed necessary. Similar immunization is available when needed against typhoid, paratyphoid, plague, cholera, typhus, yellow fever and several other infections. Protection against diphtheria, tetanus, whooping cough, poliomyelitis and measles should be regarded as the birthright of every young child, while protection against rubella should be afforded to older girls.

Many forms of immunization have tiny disadvantages. Diphtheria-whooping cough immunization is remarkably free from reactions or side-effects, but needs a reinforcing dose about three years later. Protection against typhoid and paratyphoid can cause a sharp feverish illness and the protection lasts for only two years. Smallpox vaccination – which has eradicated the world's greatest killing infection – causes serious illness about once in a million times. Immunization against influenza is of variable efficacy because there are many strains of influenza virus: by the time an outbreak has swept through a few countries it is generally possible to produce a specific vaccine that gives high protection against that particular strain for six to nine months; but at the beginning of the next outbreak a vaccine produced against the strain that caused the previous epidemic gives a poorer – but by no means negligible – protection against the new strain.

Artificial immunization against any serious infection is really an intermediate stage: the ultimate aim is to eliminate the disease altogether. For such eradication a hundred per cent protection of the community is not essential: once the protected persons are so numerous as to make it unlikely that a case of the disease will come into contact with a susceptible person, the disease tends to die out.

Immunization procedures have eliminated smallpox, made poliomyelitis and diphtheria extreme rarities, and are in the process of greatly reducing many other formerly common diseases. Despite the glamour of heart transplants and artificial kidneys, immunization procedures stand as one of the three main life-saving discoveries of recent centuries, the other two being the discovery and isolation of vitamins and antibiotics. It is interesting, however, to note certain differences between the three: the effect of antibiotics depends simply on administration of the right antibiotics to the persons who are ill and therefore seeking treatment; the effect of the discovery of vitamins depends in small part on their administration to the persons who are ill but mainly on education of the not-ill community; and the effect of immunization depends entirely on health education of parents as to the need for protection of apparently healthy children, with – perhaps inevitably – considerable opposition from cranks.

Passive artificial immunity. It is possible to achieve temporary protection against infection by injecting serum from a protected person or animal into a person susceptible to the particular disease. For instance, if a debilitated child is in contact with measles and not previously immunized, active immunization is useless (because the disease would develop before the body had acquired the power to produce antibodies) but injection of a few millilitres of serum (concentrated from the blood of a person who has had measles or been immunized against measles) will provide circulating antibodies that can in the immediate future destroy the virus of measles. The protection lasts only three or four weeks, until the circulating antibodies in the bloodstream become worn out; it will tide the child over the immediate danger but does not stimulate active production of antibodies. It can be life-saving in protecting an exhausted child from immediate attack, but leaves the child at normal risk if he becomes a contact a month later. A refinement of this passive and temporary immunity procedure is to give the debilitated child a smaller or slightly delayed dose of serum from an immune person: this, deliberately insufficient or too late to prevent the disease by passive immunization, will produce a very mild attack, with subsequent active acquired immunity.

Broadly, natural immunity is a phenomenon interesting to doctors, passive artificial immunity is an infrequent but useful procedure, and artificial acquired immunity is one of the biggest advances of medical science.

immunization. The process of artificially producing IMMUNITY to an infectious disease by introducing appropriate substances into the body.

Inoculation, in the sense of arm-to-arm transmission of smallpox from a mild case to an uninfected person, was started by Chinese physicians, spread through Asia and was introduced to Britain by Lady Mary Wortley Montague in 1718. This method often created immunity, sometimes caused a mild attack and very rarely led to a severe or even fatal attack. Jenner in England, having noticed that milkmaids seemed resistant to smallpox, in 1796 started vaccination with lymph from cows that had suffered from cow-pox: although the full explanation was not discovered for about a century and a half, the virus was the same but modified by passage through generations of cows. Although some modifications were later made, e.g., sheep lymph for calf lymph, vaccination eliminated smallpox from country after country.

After Pasteur in France and Koch in Germany had shown how germs cause infections, methods of producing immunity by weakened or killed organisms were increasingly developed, and it seems likely that almost all infectious diseases will be eradicated before the end of this century. It has to be remembered, however, that such eradication depends either on legal enforcement of immunization or on active persuasion of the people by health education.

It was formerly customary to differentiate vaccination and immunization. Vaccination involved the use of live but weakened organisms, as in protection against smallpox and yellow fever, while immunization involved the use of killed organisms, as in the protection against typhoid or diphtheria. The distinction is becoming blurred, however. For instance, the Salk method of protecting against poliomyelitis by injection of a killed virus is strictly immunization and the Sabin method of protecting against the same disease by administering a weakened and harmless virus by mouth is technically vaccination, but it seems absurd to use different terms for the two processes.

impaction. A condition in which the broken ends of a fractured bone are driven together and firmly interlocked, so that – for healing without deformity and pain – the bone has to be reset before being allowed to knit together.

An impacted tooth is one that has grown out of line, has become firmly wedged in the gum and is unable to break fully through to the surface.

impetigo. A skin disease commonest in children, in conditions of poverty and poor hygiene. It is due to staphylococcal infection and usually shows as small blisters which become purulent and produce dirty, greenish-yellow crusts, with some inflammation of the surrounding skin. The disease appears most commonly on the face and hands, and is highly contagious (i.e., spread by direct physical contact).

Treatment consists of gently removing the crusts with lint or cotton wool soaked in soapy water, and then applying an ointment containing a suitable antibiotic. If the infection is spreading, injections of an antibiotic may also be needed. One of the triumphs of community health services – including education on personal hygiene and on nutrition – in recent decades has been a drastic reduction in impetigo and in other diseases (e.g., ringworm and scabies) associated with dirt and poverty.

impotence. Inability to perform or complete sexual intercourse. It occurs mostly in men, in whom the numerous causes include (1) congenital malformations, deformations or injuries of the penis, preventing erection and penetration; (2) disorders of the glands and nerves controlling the sex organs, including common after-effects of mumps in adolescents or young adults; (3) lessened desire and potency through old age, exhaustion, illness, drugs or alcohol; and (4) many emotional causes, as for example when a man is potent with a prostitute but not with his wife (sometimes because he is over-anxious). Impotence also occurs in women, where the causes include structural abnormalities, spasm of the muscles, revulsion created by faulty or absent sex education, or fear caused by an unhappy first experience of intercourse.

Treatment varies with the cause. Rest, reassurance and understanding from the partner, with pre-intercourse 'courting' and sex play, may suffice in cases due to exhaustion, worry, slight fear or temporary illness. Medical examination may be needed in some cases, and

sometimes psychological help is useful.

While alcohol in moderation may allay nervousness and decrease inhibitions, alcohol in large quantities tends to increase desire but diminish capacity for performance. Aphrodisiacs, though often used, are in general valueless.

Impotence should be differentiated from STERILITY. The impotent man may produce sperms and – by permanent or temporary cure of his impotence or by artificial insemination – become a father. The sterile person, on the other hand, may have normal sexual desires and be perfectly capable of having intercourse.

incontinence. Inability to control the reflex emptying of URINE from the bladder (urinary incontinence) or of the bladder and rectum (double incontinence). The commonest causes are: (1) loss of co-ordination in the nervous system, as in brain damage or senility, and (2) diseases of the bladder or rectum. Treatment varies with the cause, but if the patient is prepared to co-operate the condition is in large measure curable. Failing cure, incontinence pads and rubber sheeting are required.

incubation period. The interval between infection and the appearance of symptoms. In this period the invading germs multiply until they are numerous enough to overwhelm the defence mechanisms of the body and produce the disease.

The common cold and influenza have short incubation periods (one to three days normally), but most other virus diseases have long incubation periods (e.g., measles, ten to fourteen days). By contrast, most bacterial infections have short incubation periods (e.g., staphylococcal food poisoning, a few hours; or diphtheria, one to four days). In general the incubation period for any infection spread from nose to nose (by breathing infected droplets) is fairly well defined for any one disease; but for food-borne infections – e.g., typhoid – the period varies with the amount of infected food consumed, or rather with the quantity of germs in it.

For diseases caused by droplet spray the incubation period is still an excellent guide. For instance, a rash which might be a rather fine measles or might be a rather coarse rubella (German measles) is likely to be rubella if the incubation period has been nearer three weeks than two, and a rubella contact who does not develop the disease within twenty-three days can be regarded as having escaped. For diseases transmitted by eating infected food the advent of refrigerators (and deep freezes) has considerably altered the picture: infected food may be kept in a refrigerator (with the germs neither killed nor multiplying) for a week, so that the period from purchase to appearance of the disease is a week longer than would have been anticipated. See p. 204.

Indian hemp. An alternative name for CANNABIS or hashish, smoked as a mild

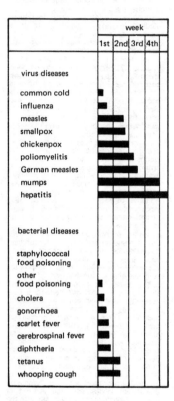

	week			
	1st	2nd	3rd	4th
virus diseases				
common cold				
influenza				
measles				
smallpox				
chickenpox				
poliomyelitis				
German measles				
mumps				
hepatitis				
bacterial diseases				
staphylococcal food poisoning				
other food poisoning				
cholera				
gonorrhoea				
scarlet fever				
cerebrospinal fever				
diphtheria				
tetanus				
whooping cough				

Average incubation periods

narcotic and sedative, producing pleasurable dreams.

indigestion. Normally the stomach carries on its work of digestion without its activity giving rise to any sensations or reasons for complaints, but some people do in fact experience discomfort related to the eating of food. This is loosely called indigestion or dyspepsia but it may arise from a variety of causes. The symptoms usually include one or more of the following: upper abdominal discomfort or pain; a feeling of fullness after eating; flatulence; nausea; heartburn; water-brash; hiccough; constipation, or diarrhoea. Another common manifestation is the skin condition known as rosacea in which there is chronic congestion of the small blood vessels of the nose and central part of the face.

Dyspepsia may be experienced in many abdominal conditions including chronic appendicitis, colitis, chronic gall-bladder disease, cirrhosis of the liver, and tumour and also in general diseases such as gout nephritis, anaemia and heart conditions but more commonly it is related to diseases specifically affecting the stomach itself.

Acute gastritis is usually due to dietary indiscretion. Over-eating, indigestible foods, hurried, imperfectly-chewed irregular meals, excessive fats, spices, and especially alcohol, can irritate the stomach lining and upset the digestive function Certain drugs such as aspirin are also liable to cause gastric upset. The condition usually responds quickly to simple treatment – a laxative, starvation, fluids and the giving of antacids.

Chronic gastritis may develop as a sequel to repeated attacks of acute gastritis but more often it will have been chronic from the beginning. Such cases call for fuller investigation with x-ray examination and test-meals to eliminate the presence of more serious conditions Prolonged treatment will probably be required with careful dietetic control and suitable drugs.

Peptic ulcers of the stomach or duodenum are a particularly common cause of indigestion. Usually they are accompanied by more definite pain usually of a characteristic pattern related to the intake of food. Suspicion of such conditions also calls for full investigation and a careful regime of subsequent treatment.

Nervous dyspepsia is a condition occurring in neurasthenic patients and accompanied as a rule by other signs of anxiety and stress such as headache backache, insomnia and loss of appetite. In these cases there is no abnormality of the stomach and treatment has to be directed towards the patient's general physical and mental health.

Intestinal carbohydrate dyspepsia is caused by a failure of starch digestion in the intestine and is characterized by excessive flatulence. Starch granules can be found microscopically in the stools Treatment is by restriction of starches and their replacement by sugar, with the giving of diastatic ferment, available in tablet form.

Antacids are much employed in the treatment of dyspepsia. They act by neutralizing the gastric hydrochloric acid The simplest and most readily available is sodium bicarbonate or baking-soda but its reaction rapidly evolves a large volume of carbon dioxide and may worsen the symptoms of flatulence. Calcium carbonate and magnesium carbonate neutralize hydrochloric acid more slowly over a longer period and are probably better, particularly as the latter is also a mild aperient. Aluminium hydroxide and magnesium trisilicate are also popular forms of treatment since they neutralize acid without gas formation.

Antacids of various proprietary brands are very extensively employed as self-treatment without medical advice. Their use in excess carries a risk of developing alkalosis with headache, nausea, vomiting and drowsiness – symptoms which resemble uraemia.

induction. Used in normal speech for 'introduction' or 'initiation', the term is applied in medicine to induction of labour, i.e., the artificial starting of childbirth, either (1) because of delay in the natural starting of labour (post-maturity), or (2) because the birth of a slightly premature child is desirable on account of danger to either mother or child. The old method of giving 300 mg. of quinine at four-hourly intervals for a day and then 30 ml. of castor oil is quite effective but nowadays it is usually replaced – or reinforced – by injections of pituitary hormone. In some cases rupture of the membranes is required.

industrial diseases. See OCCUPATIONAL DISEASES.

infancy, psychology of. The quality of parental care given to an infant is of vital importance for his future personality development and mental well-being. The evidence for this assertion comes from studies of children in institutions, of the early childhood of adolescents with psychological illness, and of the progress of children who have been deprived in infancy. It is of course not a new discovery because many writers from Aristotle onwards have regarded a child's mind as a blank slate on which only experience can write the elements which ultimately determine personality. There is however a growing appreciation that psychological development tends to proceed by steps related to experiences which are common to every child and that personality can be profoundly affected by the manner in which those successive steps and their individual problems are handled. It has been suggested that personality can be conceived as comprising three elements; the id or the deepest unconscious part of the mind influenced by pleasant or unpleasant experiences; the ego controlling conscious experience and interaction with the environment; and the super-ego, or conscience, concerned with moral and judicial attitudes.

The personality of the infant is determined by what happens to its id and ego, especially at periods of transition.

Birth provides the earliest of these transitions and although not remembered consciously it is obviously a traumatic experience. The foetus secure in its insulated environment is suddenly and forcibly squeezed through a dark passage and cast out into an unfriendly environment. To neutralize the damaging effects of this transition a great deal of mothering is required, with the child's senses stimulated by the feel and warmth of the parent and also by the sound of her voice. The effects of maternal neglect at this stage can often be seen in very young motherless babies whose failure to thrive requires to be treated by cuddling and by vigorous excitation of the sucking reflex. This highlights the emotional importance of breast feeding which provides solace and relief of tensions, but the infant will accept a substitute procedure without harm providing that the maternal cuddling and nursing which is an inevitable part of breast feeding is not also abandoned.

Weaning is the next stage. Since the infant's pleasures and satisfactions are centred around the act of nursing he is disturbed if this is suddenly withdrawn. The transition should be achieved gradually and there is advantage in starting the process by the fourth month. With longer delay it is more likely that the infant will become over-dependent on his mother and that he will retain immature character traits.

Toilet training is a further important step which can produce emotional anxiety and tension in both mother and infant. Excessive zeal at too early an age will result in the child associating the procedure with discomfort and compulsion, and he also soon learns to appreciate that this is a situation which can be used as a potent weapon to secure his mother's praise, discomfiture or attention. Conflict will result either in a performing or a non-performing reaction and according to the theorists these are associated in later life with personalities which are respectively careless, wasteful and extravagant or compulsive and fastidious. Before the age of 12 months the child can be given the opportunity to perform regularly, provided that no conflict element is introduced. By the end of the first year the child will be more ready to co-operate, and conflict is less likely to arise. As in any habit-training the basic principle is to avoid showing much disappointment at failure and to praise success so that a child gradually learns to conform to a pattern of desired behaviour.

See also CHILDHOOD, PSYCHOLOGY OF.

infant feeding. In its early months an infant depends exclusively on milk with the addition of appropriate vitamins. The natural source of this milk is its mother's breast and reference should be made to the article on BREAST FEEDING.

Where bottle feeding is necessary, expert advice on individual regimes should be obtained from the health visitor or other professional worker. An infant requires 35 ml. of milk per kg. (2.5 oz. per 1 lb.) of 'expected' body weight per day, usually divided into six feeds at three-hourly intervals until 3 months of age and five feeds at four-hourly intervals thereafter.

Weaning should be commenced at 3 to 4 months or when the child reaches 7 kg. (151 lb.) in weight, by the gradual introduction of mixed feeding – cereals, vegetables and protein supplements. Commercially prepared infant foods of this type are available and provide a safe and convenient method of extending the infant's diet.

infantile convulsions. See CONVULSIONS.

infantile diarrhoea. Diarrhoea is one of the commonest disorders of infancy and an important cause of death during the first year. It is significantly less frequent in breast-fed infants partly because of the greater risks of contamination of the bottle feeds and partly because of the difference in composition of human milk and other milk-feeds.

Outbreaks of infantile diarrhoea are common in children's wards and institutions. The infectivity is very high and since infants withstand fluid loss badly there is apt to be a considerable risk of death.

Minor attacks of diarrhoea may be treated by discontinuing the usual feeds and substituting a solution of sugar (1 tablespoonful) and salt (1 teaspoonful) in 1 litre (2 pints) of boiled water, but if the condition persists, or the baby appears generally ill, medical advice should be sought without delay.

infantile paralysis. See POLIOMYELITIS.

infantilism. The persistence of childhood characteristics into later life. There is impaired physical development, delayed sexual maturation and often mental retardation. Diminutive stature (DWARFISM) is not synonymous with infantilism. There are three groups of causes.

1. Endocrine causes. These include thyroid deficiency producing cretins; pituitary deficiency producing a condition called dystrophia adiposo-genitalis (Fröhlich's syndrome) and other similar conditions; and deficiencies of the sex glands (eunuchoidal infantilism). The rare condition of progeria where infantilism is associated with premature ageing also occurs.

2. Disease of other organs. Delayed development may result from coeliac disease; from congenital disease of the kidney (renal rickets); from pancreatic insufficiency; from congenital heart disease; or from forms of mental defect.

3. Constitutional and metabolic disease. Various chronic infections such as congenital syphilis and chronic tuberculosis may retard development. Malnutrition, vitamin deficiencies, rickets, diabetes and a glycogen-storage disease (in which there is inability to mobilize glycogen when it is needed) are other causes.

The management of cases of infantilism depends primarily on an accurate assessment of the cause followed by appropriate treatment.

infant mortality rate. The number of deaths of infants under one year of age per thousand live births in the particular year. In underdeveloped countries and in developed countries in the past it is – or has been – very high. For instance, in England and Wales it was 151 in 1901, i.e. rather more than one baby out of every seven died before reaching its first birthday; and as late as 1911 it was 129 representing more than one death in every eight babies.

The main causes of these deaths, in highly developed countries in the past and to a large extent in underdeveloped countries today, fell into four groups: (1) developmental conditions (including birth injury, prematurity, malformations, etc); (2) respiratory diseases; (3) infantile gastro-enteritis (infantile diarrhoea); and (4) acute infectious diseases (including measles, whooping cough and tuberculosis), with malnutrition and bad housing playing appreciable parts. With improved nutrition, better housing, provision of antenatal services, better obstetrics and provision of child health services, the infant mortality rate in highly developed countries has fallen dramatically, reaching figures as low as 11 per thousand births in Sweden and Finland; and it is sometimes said, with reason, that the reduction of baby deaths represents the biggest health advance of all time. As a concrete example, the rate for Scotland fell from 129 in 1900 to 18 in the 1970s.

Because young babies are the most vulnerable group in the community the infant mortality rate has for many decades been regarded as the best index of the health services and social circumstances of an area, tending to be high in places with bad housing, overcrowding, maternal ignorance and poor services.

Equally useful as an index is the perinatal mortality rate, which is the total of all stillbirths and deaths under the age of 1 week expressed as a rate per thousand of all births (live and still).

The factors influencing the perinatal mortality rate have been subjected to exhaustive and detailed examination in the U.K. in the British Perinatal Mortality Survey. A large number of interesting points have emerged. In particular the standard of prenatal care has proved of enormous importance: if there was no prenatal care at all the perinatal mortality rate was five times as high as the general average; or, in approximate figures, while about 2 per cent of all pregnancies ended in stillbirths or early infant deaths, 10 per cent of pregnancies with no prenatal care ended with these tragedies. Perhaps because unmarried women are more reluctant to seek prenatal help than married women, the perinatal death rate was almost twice as high for illegitimate pregnancies as for the pregnancies of married women.

Again there was an interesting relationship with the mother's age: stillbirths and early infant deaths were fewest when the mother was between 20 and 30 years, slightly more frequent if she was a little under 20 or a little above 30, and appreciably commoner if she was 40 or over. The mother's height also appeared to play a part, perhaps because a tall woman usually has a large pelvis. Another factor that emerged was that first babies had a higher than average risk, second babies had the lowest risk of all, third babies came close to first babies in risk, and fourth and subsequent babies had an appreciable and steadily rising risk.

The survey also confirmed that the amount of risk remained highest in the least affluent and least educated groups.

infant welfare. Organized and systematic arrangements for the protection and promotion of health in infancy. Infant welfare arrangements seek to ensure that every child is given the best possible chance of survival and healthy development, but equally important is the proper supervision of pregnancy because prenatal influences have a profound effect on subsequent progress.

A comprehensive scheme for welfare therefore has three components: adequate prenatal and childbirth services; an infant consultation clinic; and organized home supervision by HEALTH VISITORS or similar public health nurses with subsequent training in health maintenance. At all stages there must also be recognition of the importance of HEALTH EDUCATION for the mother as provided by mothercraft classes and individual tuition. To ensure that all these provisions are fully utilized the persistence and professional expertise of the qualified health visitor are indispensable.

Prenatal supervision aims at the detection and appropriate timely treatment of conditions likely to lessen the chances of infant survival. Amongst these are haemolytic disease of the new born (RHESUS incompatibility) and factors such as maternal conditions likely to cause premature birth. Skilled obstetrical management will reduce the possibility of injury or other problems at the time of birth.

A high proportion of infant deaths occur during the first four weeks of life. To reduce these the essentials are special facilities for premature babies, expertly controlled feeding, and strict measures to avoid infection. Routine tests are now employed to detect congenital dislocation of the hip and metabolic disorders such as phenylketonuria, but systematic examination by a doctor experienced in dealing with newly born babies is desirable to detect other indications of abnormalities.

In later months most infant deaths occur from infections of the respiratory or digestive systems. The influence of the child health clinic and of the health visitor are of paramount importance in educating the mother in general hygiene, feeding methods and commonsense precautions in order to minimize these and other risks. Steps are also taken to have infants immunized against various diseases in accordance with a routine schedule. Child welfare schemes are now increasingly providing for developmental assessment by systematic medical examination during the first year at 6 weeks, 6 months and 10 months of age in order to detect deviations from normal development, or defects such as deafness or poor sight which will prejudice progress.

The psycho-social aspects of child welfare and the enormous role of the HEALTH VISITOR therein are considered elsewhere.

infarct. A small portion of tissue that has died through loss of blood supply as a result of blockage of an artery by a blood clot (thrombus) or a foreign body (embolism). Infarction is rare in tissues that are supplied by a mass of small, inter-communicating arteries, because if one channel is closed the blood travels by other channels. It is relatively common in the heart (causing coronary thrombosis) and not uncommon in the brain, lungs, kidneys and intestines.

infection. The condition that arises when disease-producing micro-organisms successfully invade the body, establish themselves and multiply. The common sources of infection are discharges or excreta from the body of a person suffering from the disease or of a carrier, or, less frequently, the body of an infected animal. Droplet infection, which is spread in talking, laughing, coughing and sneezing is much the most frequent. The main paths of infection are:

1. Inhalation, in which the organism (e.g., the virus of measles or influenza) is breathed out by a patient and inhaled by the next victim, with the organisms settling on the mucous membrane of the nose, mouth or pharynx, and thereafter passing to any part of the body in which they can breed.

2. Ingestion, in which the food or water contaminated from the excreta of a case or carrier (as in typhoid and paratyphoid) is consumed, the organisms reach the digestive tract, and in due course pass to any portion of the body.

3. Inoculation, in which the organisms gain access through a wound in the skin or mucous membrane (as in tetanus) or enter through previously intact skin transmitted by the bite of an infected mosquito (as in malaria).

4. Very rarely transmission before birth, as in transmission of syphilis through the placenta or infection with gonorrhoea while the child is passing through the birth canal.

After the micro-organisms have obtained a habitation they breed, some germs doubling every half hour (so that one unopposed germ might become about 100 million in about fifteen hours) while the defence mechanisms of the body (e.g., white blood corpuscles) endeavour to kill them off. This is the INCUBATION PERIOD (fairly specific for any one disease) in which the organisms multiply before symptoms of the disease appear.

The symptoms of infection vary with the disease but often include: (1) nervous system: headache, malaise, insomnia, drowsiness, high temperature, rigor, shivering, delirium and convulsions; (2) circulatory system: rapid pulse, irregularities of heart beat, pallor, cyanosis and coldness of extremities; (3) alimentary system: dry mouth, furred tongue, loss of appetite, thirst, nausea, vomiting, diarrhoea or constipation; (4) respiratory system: rapid respiration and sometimes breathlessness; (5) excretory system: hot dry skin (or perspiration), scanty and highly coloured urine, and diarrhoea or constipation; and (6) muscular system: general weakness and prostration.

Until about a hundred years ago half the population of highly developed countries died as the result of infections. Developments which have enormously reduced the danger of infections include: (1) antisepsis and later asepsis which removed the likelihood of infection after surgical or gynaecological operations; (2) purity of water supplies, installation of sewerage systems and improved food hygiene, which together made food-borne and water-borne infections uncommon; (3) vaccination and immunization against an increasing number of diseases – incomparably the biggest medical development of modern times; and (4) the introduction first of sulphonamides and later of antibiotics which rendered possible the successful treatment of many infections.

infectious diseases. Diseases which result from the successful invasion of the body by living organisms. These organisms may be bacteria, viruses, rickettsia or protozoa. Invasion of the body by fungi is more usually called mycosis and the presence of more complex metazoan animals such as worms or flukes is parasitism or infestation rather than infection.

Infectious diseases are essentially preventable. The measures necessary are good hygiene, the protection of food and water supplies, the early identification, isolation and treatment of cases, the quarantining or surveillance of contacts, and the protection of individuals by specific immunological procedures where these are available. There are statutory powers for the notification and control of certain infections.

inferiority complex. A persistent feeling of guilt or unworthiness which dominates the thinking and actions of persons of inadequate or ill-balanced personality. It may occur in association with some physical disability either real or imagined or as an expression of some inner conflict with society. It may not always be obvious that a patient has feelings of inferiority as he may seek to conceal them by projecting his shortcomings on to other persons or by

rationalizing them in some way, and his conduct may be aggressive or boastful rather than self-deprecatory.

It seldom helps such patients merely to tell them that such feelings are unwarranted. Rather they should be assured that there is a logical reason for their symptoms and encouraged to devote patience and thought to uncovering and bringing into the open the half-forgotten secrets of events which in the past have engendered feelings of shame or guilt.

infertility. See FERTILITY.

inflammation. The changes which occur in living tissue when it is injured (provided that the injury is not of such severity as immediately to destroy its structure and kill it). The usual signs of inflammation are swelling, pain, redness, heat and impaired function.

Inflammation may be produced by bacteria and their toxins or by trauma, injurious chemicals and the effects of physical agencies such as heat, cold, electricity, ultra-violet light, x-rays and other forms of radiation. It should be regarded as a defensive reaction of the body to repair the damage. If this is successful, resolution is said to occur, but with more severe injury the inflammatory processes may progress to suppuration, ulceration or gangrene before healing ultimately becomes possible, or a state of chronic inflammation may ensue.

The treatment largely depends upon the cause. The principles are to remove or neutralize or destroy the cause, to encourage blood flow to the part (hyperaemia) by the application of warmth, and to secure rest for the affected part.

In medical terminology words which mean that inflammation has occurred end in '-itis', e.g., tonsillitis.

influenza. An acute infectious disease due to the influenza virus, occurring as world-wide (pandemic) or local epidemics or as sporadic outbreaks. It has a short incubation of one to three days and the onset is usually sudden with raised temperature, headache, pains in the back and limbs, upper respiratory symptoms resembling a common cold, and a tendency to more serious inflammatory complications in the respiratory system. Recovery from the acute phase is often followed by fatigue and depression which may last for some time. Five clinical varieties are recognized according to the incidence of main symptoms: (1) febrile, (2) respiratory, (3) malignant with severe general toxaemia, (4) gastro-intestinal, (5) nervous with headache and depression.

There are two main types of virus – influenza A and influenza B. The 'A' variety is usually found in the widespread winter epidemics which tend to recur every two or three years. Sporadic local outbreaks are more often the 'B' variety but its antigenic properties are variable and this makes it difficult to formulate a uniformly effective vaccine.

Vaccination is, however, a useful measure and should be offered to groups of persons at special risk, especially hospital staffs, community nurses, the elderly, and those with chronic cardiac or respiratory disease. It is also widely used in industry as a precaution against a high incidence of influenza during the winter which might disrupt work or production.

infra-red rays. Infra-red rays are given off by any body heated to just below redness and infra-red lamps for therapeutic purposes are basically very simple, consisting of a blackened electric bulb or a specially-shaped coil of resistance wire with a reflector. The cabinet type infra-red heat cage employs several such sources.

Infra-red rays occupy a position in the electro-magnetic spectrum just beyond the red end of the band of visible light and with waves of greater length in the range 7,700 to 4 million Angstrom units. (One AU = one ten-millionth of a millimetre.)

When absorbed by the skin infra-red rays liberate heat and cause the tissues in that area to rise in temperature, which has a sedative effect on sensory nerve-endings, produces dilatation of blood capillaries with improved circulation and induces perspiration. Heat relieves pain and muscle spasm, improved circulation helps resolution of inflammation, and perspiration aids elimination of waste-products. Because of these effects infra-red radiation is used in the treatment of neuritis, arthritis, neuralgia, fibrositis, traumatic inflammation and cellulitis and also in spastic paralysis before massage or manipulation, and in general diseases such as chronic nephritis where there is defective elimination of waste material by the kidneys.

ingrowing eyelash. See EYELIDS, DISEASES OF.

ingrowing toe-nail. See NAIL, INGROWING.

inguinal region. Another name for GROIN.

inhalation. Inhalation is synonymous with inspiration and is the act of drawing air or other vapour into the lungs. It is also a general descriptive term for any medicament intended to be breathed in as a vapour or powder.

This form of treatment is employed for various conditions affecting the respiratory tract. In nasal congestion, the common cold or tonsillitis, menthol, eucalyptus, or friar's balsam is added to boiling water in a jug surrounded by a towel so arranged as to form a funnel through which the patient breathes in the resultant medicated vapour. In bronchiectasis inhalation of vaporized creosote is a traditional remedy but probably only acts by inducing coughing and the expulsion of sputum.

In the treatment of asthma use is made of anti-spasmodic inhalations, usually prepared as pressurized aerosols or ultra-fine powders. Their constituents include adrenalin, ephedrine, isoprenaline,

salbutamol and sodium cromoglycate.

inheritance. See HEREDITY AND ENVIRONMENT.

inhibition. The blocking of any impulse or action. Inhibition occasionally has a physical basis, as when we desire to eat a food that disagrees with us but deliberately refrain because we know the consequences. More often, however, it is a result of social conditioning, e.g., we want to hit the person who has annoyed us but have learned from childhood that society disapproves of violence; or it may be a result of psychological conflict, e.g., the pupil wants to dispute the teacher's spelling of a word but refrains because of either respect or fear.

Inhibitions in moderation are conducive to the harmony of existence: a man wants to make violent love to a woman but is restrained because the place is unsuitable or because the woman is unwilling or because he is married and has feelings of guilt. In excess, however, inhibitions indicate a lack of self-confidence, a feeling of inferiority and an inadequate development of the personality.

One of the effects of alcohol is to reduce inhibitions. It can be useful in enabling a normally shy person to take his part in conversation; but the removal of inhibitions can lead to uncontrolled aggression.

Fatigue and exhaustion can increase inhibitions, so the first line of treatment of excessively inhibited persons is attention to general health. Many such persons, however, require prolonged psychological treatment.

injection. The procedure of using a syringe and needle to introduce into the body some fluid substance for therapeutic purposes.

Injections may be intradermal, i.e., given into the substance of the true skin or dermis; otherwise they may be given deep into the skin (subcutaneous), into the muscle (intra-muscular) or into the vein (intravenous), and these are variously employed in accordance with the needs of treatment or the characteristics of the material injected.

Injections may also be made into specific sites to ensure some desired local action. Examples are the induction of local anaesthesia, and the treatment of neuralgia and arthritis.

inoculation. The procedure of inducing active IMMUNITY against an infectious disease by introducing into the body a controlled dose of the causative organisms.

insanity. An imprecise term for MENTAL DISEASE. Its use has been largely abandoned by psychiatrists although the law still regards as insane a person who is incapable of forming moral judgements, who does not appreciate the nature and consequence of his acts, and who is incapable of managing his property and affairs.

insect bites. See BITES AND STINGS.

insomnia. Inability to fall asleep or achieve sleep that is adequate and restful. Almost everyone complains of sleeplessness from time to time, but it can be a distressing symptom of many disease conditions and measures to secure sleep for such patients are an important part of their treatment.

The treatment of insomnia in an individual who is otherwise well requires a careful consideration of all the relevant circumstances. Sleep only occurs if there is full physical and mental relaxation and there must be no extraneous conditions preventing this. Disturbing factors such as pain, cold, heat, light and so on, should be eliminated. In the elderly the prevalence and importance of cold feet should be appreciated. Many persons complain that their thoughts are more active in bed and this may be a pointer to worries and anxieties which should be identified and assuaged. Psycho-neurotics tend to compound the effects of worrying by worrying about the dangers of not sleeping and require to be reassured that this is not deadly. Many persons exaggerate the extent of their insomnia and it is important to investigate this aspect of the problem.

Various simple measures may help to re-establish a satisfactory sleep-pattern. In elderly persons digestive processes are slower and the last meal should be taken five hours before retiral. Tea and coffee act as stimulants and should be avoided at bedtime but a warm milky drink or a small dose of whisky is useful. No great volume of fluid should be given lest rest is disturbed by the need to pass urine. For the ordinary adult something light to read in bed, with the bedside-lamp within easy reach, is a good way to achieve relaxation.

Inability to sleep is very characteristic of any feverish illness particularly if accompanied by headache or the breathing problems of bronchitis or pneumonia. For these acute cases much can be done by nursing technique. Tepid sponging, bed re-making, a comfortable posture, bladder-emptying and a mild sedative are illustrative of the lines on which to proceed. In more chronic respiratory disease with a troublesome cough, the administration of a sedative cough mixture will often secure relief.

In chronic heart failure adequate rest may have quite remarkable effects in improving the efficiency of heart and circulation and sufficient sedation to secure this is generally justifiable. Similarly, sedation may be needed in uraemia, thyrotoxicosis, neurasthenia, delirium tremens, and mental disturbance.

The use of sedatives requires careful consideration. If given they should be employed in an attempt to re-establish the habit of sleep and then be gradually reduced and withdrawn. Fear of sleeplessness thereafter may be countered by having a single dose at hand to take if necessary, with the main supply held elsewhere to avoid risks of accidental overdosage. The type of sedative to be prescribed should be related to the sleep-pattern. If there is difficulty only in falling asleep a quickly-acting, quickly excreted hypnotic is best. For wakefulness later in the night a slow-acting drug is more suitable. Alcohol should not be recommended except for the elderly because of the risks of increasing dependence.

inspiration. Breathing in.

insulin. The hormone, produced by the islets of Langerhans in the pancreas, which controls the metabolism of sugar (glucose). Insufficient production of insulin is the cause of DIABETES MELLITUS which is essentially an accumulation of glucose in the blood. Excess of insulin, usually arising from overdosage of a diabetic patient, dangerously decreases the amount of glucose in the blood (hypoglycaemia).

intelligence. The faculty of reason or the total of a person's abilities to meet and to deal with various situations. When a person is faced with an unfamiliar set of circumstances he has to decide what to do. In making his decision he either has in mind the result which he wishes to achieve or, on the basis of past experience, attempts to foresee the result of any action and regulates what he actually does in accordance with his forecast. He is in short attempting to shape the present and the future by his knowledge and experience of the past and obviously his success in dealing with a particular situation will depend not only on his native intelligence but on the relevance of his cultural background to the immediate problem.

This illustrates the difficulties which surround any attempt to define intelligence in precise terms and to devise means of assessing it. It is now generally agreed that intelligence must be regarded as consisting of both general and special aptitudes. The standard INTELLIGENCE TESTS (as usually applied) primarily attempt to determine basic or general intelligence as shown by abilities of perception, memory and reason, and to neutralize the effects of special experience or knowledge.

intelligence tests. Everybody knows that the level of intelligence varies in different persons. We could choose from our acquaintances one whom we deem highly intelligent, one quite intelligent and one rather dull-witted. Yet our highly intelligent friend, who handles numbers so easily and spots the logical fallacy in an argument, may be a poor linguist and may lack the ability to undertake a simple household repair; and our dull-witted acquaintance may be the one who can best find his way in a strange town or who manages to improvise a tool for an unusual job. Clearly, even if we could devise a test independent of past experience, no one test could fully measure mental capacity.

In the eighteenth and nineteenth centuries many psychologists tried to evolve single 'scientific' tests of intelligence but inevitably failed. Then a French psychologist, Alfred Binet

(1857-1911) had the idea of creating a whole series of sub-tests for children of different ages. The group of tests for any one age-group would contain items designed to test comprehension of words, understanding of numbers, recognition of shapes, memory, capacity for finding analogies, and so on; and the battery of tests for, for instance, children of 7 years would contain items that less than half of 6-year-old children could manage successfully but that more than half of 8-year-old children could do.

After trying many such tests on large numbers of children and discarding some of the tests as unsatisfactory Binet and his co-worker Simon produced in 1905 their battery of tests for establishing a child's 'mental age'. For example, think of a child who is very good when dealing with numbers but less good when dealing with shapes and spaces. He manages all the tests for 7-year-olds, all except two of the tests for 8-year-olds (failing on two involving shapes) and only two of the tests for 9-year-olds (two involving numbers). Balancing his successes in the 9-year-old group against his failures in the 8-year-old group his mental age can be stated as exactly 8 years.

However, it is long-winded to have to say, 'This bright girl has a mental age of 10 years and a chronological age of 8 years'. So the refinement was introduced of expressing the mental age as a percentage of the chronological age and calling the result the intelligence quotient (often known simply as IQ). Thus the bright girl just mentioned would have an IQ of ten-eighths multiplied by a hundred, i.e., 125; and an exactly average person would have an IQ of 100.

The tests were basically simple and performed in a short time. For example, a 3-year-old was expected to be able to point to his nose, eyes and mouth, to repeat two digits, to name well-known objects in a picture, to give his family name and to repeat a sentence of six syllables. The original Binet-Simon scale was later revised and extended, and by 1921 further revisions – notably by two American psychologists, Terman and Merrill – were in world-wide use. The immediate international acceptance showed how great had been the need for a reasonably accurate measuring device.

Since this initial breakthrough, psychologists have produced further tests in bewildering variety. One difficulty with the Binet-Simon tests was that they used words and therefore placed illiterate children and children from homes in which there was little communication at a disadvantage. So an important step was to devise non-verbal methods of assessing illiterate children. The Collins, Drever and Wechsler Scales and the Penrose-Raven Progressive Matrices are examples of these.

Again, the tests were at first used largely

for backward or handicapped children, to determine whether a child could benefit from ordinary education – see BACKWARDNESS IN CHILDREN and MENTAL DEFICIENCY -but soon came equally into use for the identification of bright children, e.g., for admission to secondary schools or later to universities and other institutions of higher learning. Naturally psychologists began to extend their activities to the testing of adults.

If tests were to be useful in the selection of the most suitable person for admission to a particular advanced course or for a post as a senior civil servant, a high ranking army officer or a managerial post in industry, it was obvious that something more than a rough assessment of general intelligence was needed. The managing editor of a large newspaper, the head of a university, a general in the armed forces and a top civil servant all need good general intelligence but require also certain different qualities or aptitudes; and, while promotion to a top post might be on displayed ability in the particular field, it would be wasteful of talent to appoint persons to important junior posts in line for promotion simply on assessment of general intelligence. So, in addition to tests for general intelligence, tests were devised for specific aptitudes, personality, imagination, patience, stability, and so forth. Some of the better known tests used for assessing perseverance, personality, imagination, association fluency and other character traits include the Dewey-Will Temperament Test, the Attitude Scale, the Mosaics Tests and the Rorshach Ink-Blot Test.

The application of such procedures gained momentum after the success of the U.S. Army Alpha Test of the Second World War and the success in Britain of similar tests to select people for wartime posts demanding particular qualities. In older children such tests provide a sound basis for vocational guidance and, especially in America, many business firms now carry psychological assessment to what are perhaps excessive lengths, sometimes using for their prospective employees tests which are poorly conceived and inadequately standardized.

Nevertheless, intelligence tests can do much to prevent square pegs from occupying round holes, and they will be more and more used in the future.

intercourse, sexual. See COITUS.

intercurrent. An intercurrent disease is one that occurs during the course of another disease that is already present, e.g., a person suffering from a heart attack may develop intercurrent pneumonia. While the term is applicable to any second disease developing before complete recovery from the first, by far the commonest intercurrent diseases are infections, because a person who is seriously ill has a very low resistance to any infection.

interferon. In 1956 Isaacs and Lindenmann found that embryonic cells of a chicken treated with killed influenza virus produced a substance that interfered with the growth of influenza virus in other cells. This substance, a complex protein, was appropriately named interferon, or more correctly chick-interferon. Later it was discovered that human cells when stimulated by appropriate antigens including bacteria and viruses produce human-interferon (or to be more accurate a number of allied substances known as human-interferons), and that an interferon produced by one antigen (e.g., a particular bacterium) may interfere with the growth of several different viruses and bacteria.

For relatively large germs such as bacteria the discovery is probably not very important. Sulphonamides and antibiotics can be produced more easily and at much lower cost, and appropriate ones are much more effective in destroying bacteria. Viruses, however, are in general not susceptible to either sulphonamides or antibiotics. The use of antibiotics in viral diseases (e.g., measles) has been essentially to deal with complications, to kill off bacteria that invade tissues already weakened by the primary disease. Apart from the use of antibiotics for complications and the possibility of injecting serum obtained from the blood of a person convalescent from the particular disease or otherwise immune to it, and apart from good nursing and attention to symptoms, a viral disease has simply had to run its course.

The discovery of human interferons and of their range of action produces exciting possibilities for the treatment of diseases caused by viruses.

Additionally, just as human beings with a life-span of something like 70 to 120 years undergo alterations over thousands of years, viruses with a very brief life-span can undergo changes from year to year. So new viral diseases appear from time to time: Lassa fever and new varieties of influenza are examples. When a new disease appears it takes some months to produce a vaccine for its effective prevention, and treatment by use of serum obtained from the blood of immune persons does not become practicable until a sizeable number of people have developed immunity, either through recovering from the disease or through being immunized with a hastily prepared vaccine. In other words, until now neither treatment nor prevention has been available during the early months of an outbreak of a new viral disease. Although the obtaining of an interferon from a human donor and its purification for use on another person is at present a difficult and costly procedure, it seems likely that interferon may provide at least an emergency treatment for new viral diseases.

The long-term answer to any disease caused by a virus is to seek to eradicate it by developing a suitable vaccine and persuading susceptible people to accept vaccination: as has happened with smallpox and as is likely to happen with poliomyelitis, if enough people are rendered immune the virus cannot find human cells in which to breed and so disappears. By contrast, treatment, however effective, helps only the sufferer and does not reduce the amount of disease. Furthermore, while sulphonamides and antibiotics will actively kill bacteria, an appropriate interferon appears merely to reduce the multiplication and growth of viruses – to make it easier for the body's defences to cope with the invaders rather than to take part in the battle. Moreover, there is recent evidence that interferons are useful in at least some types of cancer (though further trials are needed), and there are possibilities of manufacturing interferons from cells cultivated in laboratories. The discovery of interferon may in course of time be ranked with the discovery of penicillin as a major contribution to man's war against disease.

intestine. The section of the DIGESTIVE SYSTEM which extends from the lower opening of the stomach to the anus. It comprises two distinct parts known as the small and large intestine.

Obstruction. Any condition which impedes the normal passage of intestinal contents through the small and large intestine. See BOWEL.

Tumours. Non-malignant tumours of the intestine are rare but overgrowths of fatty or muscular tissue occur occasionally, and slightly more common are polypi or pedunculated tumours arising from the mucous membrane and its related glands. Single polypi may reach a considerable size and become a cause of intussusception but they are more often small, multiple and widespread and may arise as a sequel to chronic inflammatory disease such as intestinal tuberculosis or long-standing dysentery.

Malignant tumours practically never effect the small intestine but cancer of the colon is the commonest growth in the large intestine. It generally arises at the flexures and at narrow parts such as the upper part of the rectum and the ileo-caecal valve. The symptoms are those of chronic intestinal obstruction and call for full investigation.

intoxication. In everyday usage, intoxication is taken to mean incapacity due to over-consumption of alcohol, but scientifically it is employed to describe functional impairment brought about by any poisonous substance or toxin.

Such toxins may arise from external (exogeneous) causes, particularly bacterial products or drugs, or they may be endogeneous, arising within the body from metabolic faults such as uraemia or acidosis.

intra-uterine device. An appliance inserted

into the cavity of the uterus to prevent conception. It was until recently thought that an IUD acted mainly by creating an obstruction, but to block the entrance to the uterus entirely is very difficult. More probably the main effect of an IUD is to irritate the muscles of the uterus so that it tends to expel any fertilized egg before it can attach itself to the uterine lining and to stimulate the uterus into producing a substance that kills the fertilized egg.

Though developed in the early years of this century, intra-uterine devices were little used between 1920 and 1950, but from mid-century onwards such appliances as the Zipper Ring, the Lippes Loop, the Margulies Spiral and the Birnberg Bow became popular. These are fairly small appliances which are placed in the uterus, usually by a doctor. In a small percentage of cases they are spontaneously expelled (and the woman may not know that she has lost her protective) or cause bleeding and have to be removed; but in about 96 to 97 per cent of cases they remain in position and prevent pregnancy.

In general an efficient IUD gives greater protection than vaginal methods - such as the Dutch cap and spermicidal jelly or cream - but has the limitation that it needs insertion by a doctor. To a great extent all these have been replaced by oral contraceptives, but the IUD is still useful for women (e.g., from multiproblem families) who cannot remember to take an oral contraceptive regularly.

intravenous feeding. An emergency method of giving a patient liquid nourishment - usually a saline solution with glucose added - by direct slow injection into a vein. A needle inserted into a vein is connected to an apparatus which drips in the liquid at the required rate, care being taken to ensure the absence of air which if present might block a blood vessel. The method is used if the patient is unconscious for a prolonged period, is too ill to eat or is unable to eat because of disease of the mouth, throat or stomach.

introvert. An inward-looking person concerned mainly with his own thoughts, valuing his own society, liking solitude and often enjoying reading or music. In the words of Jung, the inventor of the term, 'Introverts are taciturn, impenetrable, often shy natures who form a vivid contrast to the open, sociable or at least friendly and accessible characters (the extroverts) who are on good terms with all the world'. Morbid introversion occurs in schizophrenia and paranoia, with the personality withdrawn into itself and expended on fantasy formation.

Most people, however, are neither pure introverts nor complete extroverts but a mixture with perhaps one or the other normally predominating, as is more fully discussed in the article on EXTROVERTS.

intubation. The insertion of a tube. The term is used mainly in relation to intubation of the larynx in order to maintain a clear airway. The larynx may become obstructed in laryngeal diphtheria and other infections affecting the air-passages; in cellulitis of the neck and laryngeal cancer; by inflammation resulting from the inhalation of injurious vapours; and occasionally as an allergic phenomenon.

Intubation is also a necessary preliminary to specialized methods of anaesthesia.

intussusception. A condition in which a segment of bowel becomes telescoped into the part immediately below. It usually occurs in the small intestine or at the junction of the small intestine with the colon and it is the commonest cause of acute intestinal obstruction in children.

Cases usually occur between the age of 6 months and 2 years, most often in well-nourished and vigorous boys, and are probably due to disturbance of the normal digestive movements of the intestine by some irritation of the mucous membrane lining the intestine wall.

The symptoms are those of violent and persistent abdominal colic, often with the passage of blood-stained mucus, followed by signs of toxaemia and collapse. Vomiting is not usually marked until the later stages of complete obstruction.

Intussusception requires emergency surgical treatment.

iodine. A non-metallic element occurring as a greyish-black crystalline solid. In very small amounts, iodine is essential to the body because it is used by the thyroid gland in the manufacture of its hormone. Lack of iodine in childhood can produce physical and mental retardation (although cretinism is more commonly due to a defect of the thyroid gland itself) and deficiency in adult life produces simple goitre, with the thyroid enlarging through excessive activity in an attempt to produce enough hormone without sufficient iodine for its manufacture.

Iodine compounds are plentiful in the sea, but in some inland areas the soil contains practically no iodine and consequently food grown in these areas is deficient in iodine. Switzerland, the Tyrol, the Himalayas and Derbyshire are notorious for lack of iodine. Where such deficiency exists it can be easily remedied by addition of a very small quantity of iodine to table salt, and iodized salt is now in common use wherever iodine is scarce.

Iodine is only very slightly soluble in water but dissolves readily in alcohol. A solution of iodine in alcohol - tincture of iodine - is an excellent antiseptic for sterilizing intact skin but is too strong for use in wounds.

Radioactive iodine compounds are employed to treat an enlarged and overactive thyroid gland and sometimes to treat cancer of that gland.

iritis. The iris is a thin circular disc of tissue between the cornea and the lens of the eye, with a central circular aperture, the pupil.

Iritis is inflammation of the iris and may be acute or chronic. The eye appears reddened and the pupil is small and loses its natural lustre and colour. There is pain and sensitivity to light, and tears are formed. Most cases are due to bacterial or toxaemia. Syphilis, gonorrhoea, tuberculosis and rheumatism are the commonest causes.

The basic essentials of treatment are first to ensure dilation of the pupil with atropine in order to draw it away from the lens, which lies immediately behind it, and thus prevent any adhesions developing, and second to lessen inflammatory reaction by cortico-steroids. Appropriate measures are also required to treat whatever general condition caused the iritis.

iron. A familiar metallic element with magnetic properties. Iron is of importance in medicine because it is an essential constituent of haemoglobin, the oxygen carrying pigment of the blood. It is thus an indispensable MINERAL SALT in the diet, the daily requirement being 15 to 20 mg. The best sources are meat, liver, eggs, spinach, beans, peas, and whole wheat, but milk is poor. Additional supplies of iron are required in pregnancy and while breast feeding, and mothers should take iron tablets, usually containing ferrous sulphate. Infants may also suffer from nutritional anaemia but proprietary infant foods contain added iron.

Lack of iron in the diet results in anaemia, and for its treatment both tablet and injectable forms of iron are available. Iron preparations may cause gastro-intestinal irritation or more serious symptoms if taken in overdose.

Iron tablets should be kept secure from accidental swallowing by small children. Many cases of serious poisoning have occurred.

irradiation. The treatment of disease (e.g., cancer) by exposure of the diseased cells to x-rays, ultra-violet light or radioactive material; also the sterilization of food, medical instruments, etc. by similar methods. While irradiation is a useful weapon for certain serious conditions, it must also be remembered that it is a potentially dangerous weapon. For instance, while irradiation is useful in the treatment of certain cases of leukaemia, excessive irradiation can actually cause leukaemia – as shown in its increased incidence in survivors of the atomic bomb explosions in Japan and also in persons with anchylozing spondylitis treated by radiotherapy of the spine.

isolation. A control procedure adopted in relation to cases or carriers of highly infectious diseases who are segregated in an attempt to prevent them transmitting infection to other susceptible individuals. A limitation imposed on the movements of contacts who may be under suspicion of having contracted infection is known as QUARANTINE.

In the past most fever or isolation hospitals were constructed on the pavilion principle with large multi-bedded wards in which a number of patients with the same disease were segregated as a group. This type of construction is now obsolete and modern design is based on wards containing a number of single-bed units with complete structural separation by full-height partitions. These are usually called cubicle wards but the name is not a good one since 'cubicle' has a connotation of partitioning to less than full height.

Each chamber is separately ventilated and has its own toilet and washing facilities. They are constructed as a single row and served by an external or permanently ventilated internal corridor. In some designs mechanical ventilation or air-conditioning is also provided to minimize risks of cross infection.

Separate rooms of this kind are obviously important but do not obviate the need for separate nursing – an aseptic technique for fever nursing in which the patient and everything concerned with him is treated as infectious and the nurse wears a protective gown and mask left behind in each cubicle and carries out a 'surgical scrub' of her hands before proceeding to other patients. A similar routine carried out when cubicle isolation is not available is usually referred to as 'barrier nursing'.

Home isolation when patients are not admitted to hospital, should follow the same principles. The patient should be accommodated in a separate well-ventilated room preferably at the top of the house.

Aerial connection between sick room and the rest of the house can be restricted by a sheet over the door moistened with disinfectant and this has at least an admonitory value in reminding persons of the risks and the need for care. Separate utensils should be set aside and boiled or disinfected, and nothing should pass out of the room without disinfection. Attendants should carry out the rules of barrier nursing and visitors should be restricted or forbidden. Any who are allowed entry must adopt similar precautions of protective clothing and thorough hand-washing and disinfection.

isoniazid. A synthetic compound manufactured from isoniatinic acid and used for the treatment of tuberculosis. It is usually given by mouth in doses of 100 mg. twice daily. The drug acts specifically against the germ which causes tuberculosis but has little action against other bacteria.

isotope. Two atoms are said to be isotopes if they are of the same chemical element but have different masses, i.e., a different number of electrons moving round the same proton. An isotope may occur naturally or may be created by nuclear bombardment. Thus uranium has three naturally occurring isotopes and at least ten artificially manufactured isotopes.

Radio-active isotopes can be used in medicine for three purposes: for research, e.g., to trace the movement of chemical substances in the body; for diagnosis, e.g., to facilitate x-ray investigation of a suspected lesion; and for treatment, e.g., the use of radioactive iodine to treat cancer of the thyroid gland.

itching. The skin is particularly well-supplied with sensory nerve-endings susceptible to various irritants; chronic irritation insufficient to cause actual pain is experienced as itching or pruritus.

In many cases the cause is obvious: insect bites, infestation by parasites such as the scabies mite, fungoid skin infections, eczema or other chronic skin conditions, or local discharges or disorders of the blood's circulation (such as occur in chilblains or varicose veins).

In other cases there is general itching for no apparent local reason. This type of itching may occur in certain general diseases where there are circulating toxins, as in jaundice, diabetes, gout and nephritis; in certain blood diseases such as leukaemia and lymphadenoma; in old age where there is senile atrophy of the skin; from the use of certain drugs especially opium and heroin: or as a sympton in psycho-neurosis.

Treatment should be directed towards the precise cause. Alkaline baths and lotions may relieve general pruritus; calamine lotion, anti-histamine creams, or oily preparations containing 1 or 2 per cent phenol or camphor are useful as local applications.

Local pruritus most often affects the anus, scrotum or vulva, but may occur anywhere. Often itching starts from a transitory cause, leads to scratching and is then aggravated by the scratching. Threadworms are a common cause of anal itching, vaginal discharge may start itching of the vulva, and sweating, irritation of clothes and nervous factors are other causes. Removal of the cause is essential, extreme cleanliness of the part is useful, and the application of an alkaline lotion followed, when dry, by a fine zinc oxide dusting powder may do much to relieve the symptoms.

J

jaundice. Jaundice (icterus) is not a disease but is a yellowish appearance of a patient occurring in various conditions and due to the deposition of the bile-pigment (bilirubin) in the skin and mucous membranes. Early indications of jaundice may be detected by inspecting the 'white' of the eyes.

Bile is a clear yellow or orange fluid secreted by the liver cells and contains mainly bile-salts and the bile pigments bilirubin and biliverdin. It passes to the intestine via the gall bladder and the bile-duct. Bile-salts are required for the digestion of fats but the bile pigments are waste products from the haemoglobin in the blood.

Jaundice thus results from excess production of the bile pigment or a failure to eliminate it so that it accumulates in the blood-stream and stains the tissue. This occurs in three groups of conditions: (1) haemolytic anaemias where there is excessive destruction of red cells, (2) disease of the liver where the liver cells are unable to transfer bilirubin to the gall bladder, and (3) obstruction of the bile-duct, preventing bile passing from the liver to the intestine.

Jaundice therefore requires detailed investigation to determine its exact cause which may be a blood disease, liver conditions such as hepatitis, cirrhosis or toxic necrosis, or bile-duct obstruction due to chronic inflammatory conditions, gall stones or neoplasm.

A transient form of jaundice occurs in a large proportion of new-born infants – icterus neonatorum. This is due to the breakdown of foetal haemoglobin which is in excess of requirements once the child begins to breathe, and to the still immature liver function. It also occurs in haemolytic disease of the newborn which is caused by the blood abnormality known as RHESUS FACTOR. Investigation of Rh factors is now a routine procedure in all antenatal clinics; it has been found that exposure of the child to ultra-violet light helps the jaundice to clear and this form of treatment is now commonly employed in maternity hospitals.

jaw. The skeletal framework of the mouth in which the teeth are set, consisting of an upper-jaw, or maxilla, which is continuous with the skull, and a movable lower jaw, or mandible. The opposed margins are covered by the gums or gingiva and are expanded as the alveolar ridges or alveoli to provide the tooth sockets.

The mandible hinges with the skull at the temporo-mandibular joint, easily felt immediately in front of the ear, and often subject to derangement. It has cartilage rather like that in the knee-joint, and looseness of this may cause 'clicking-jaw', movements being accompanied by an audible snap. Also relatively common are unilateral or bilateral dislocations of the jaw which can usually be slipped back easily into place, even by patients themselves.

Jenner. Edward Jenner (1749–1823), medical practitioner in Gloucestershire, was the inventor of smallpox VACCINATION. See also IMMUNITY.

jogging. Trotting or running at a slow pace. With physical work being largely superseded by sedentary work many people have become aware that they are having too little exercise and so jogging has become increasingly popular. Its big advantage is that it occupies minimal time, but its main disadvantages are first that it provides no mental, aesthetic or emotional satisfaction – unlike, say, a quick game of tennis – but is solely a means of ensuring some exercise; and second that for accelerating the heart beat and deepening the breathing it is much less efficient than shorter but more violent exercise. See KEEPING FIT.

joints. The bones of the skeleton are connected to each other in accordance with functional requirements by joints or articulations. These may be (1) immovable as in the joints between the individual bones of the skull, (2) slightly movable as between the vertebrae or the individual bones of the pelvis, or (3) freely movable comprising mostly the joints of the limbs and extremities. In the slightly movable joints the opposed bony surfaces are united by intervening tough and elastic fibro-cartilage but in the freely movable joints the bony surfaces are completely separated from one another and are covered by smooth and dense hyaline cartilage. Such a joint is enclosed in an articular capsule lined with synovial membrane, lubricated by synovial fluid and strengthened externally by strong fibrous bands called ligaments.

The stability of a freely movable joint is maintained (1) by the shape of the joint surfaces, (2) sometimes by internal ligaments and shaped pieces of fibro-cartilage, (3) by the external ligaments, and (4) by the surrounding muscles and tendons. Freely movable joints may be of the ball-and-socket type, permitting movement in all directions (e.g., the hip or shoulder), or of the hinge type (e.g., the knee), or they may permit only pivot or gliding movements (e.g., the atlas vertebra).

Ball and socket joint

Hinged joint

The mechanics of joints

Joint diseases. Any inflammatory condition affecting a joint or joints is termed arthritis. Acute arthritis may develop as a result of bacterial infection from penetrating wounds or as a complication of other diseases such as rheumatic fever, gonorrhoea, pneumonia, typhoid fever, gout and dysentery. It may also be due to tuberculosis or syphilis. Haemorrhage into joints occurs in haemophilia, scurvy, other severe blood diseases and sometimes as a complication of the administration of serum. Certain diseases of the spinal cord produce degeneration of joints supplied by the affected nerves. Most of the foregoing are relatively rare but the familiar types of chronic arthritis are very common and cause widespread disability. Of these, rheumatoid arthritis occurs mainly in children or young adults, more often females, and it tends to affect the smaller peripheral joints many of which may be involved simultaneously or progressively. In juveniles the condition is called Still's disease.

Osteo-arthritis affects mainly the larger joints in older persons. Degenerative changes and over-stress damage the joint surfaces and produce pain and disability. Osteo-arthritis of the spine is known as spondylitis. A peculiar condition known as 'hysterical joint' is occasionally seen in neurotic subjects. A single joint, usually in a limb, appears to be fixed, very painful, and resistant to passive movement but no pathological process can be demonstrated. The disability disappears under anaesthesia and cases of this type often form the basis of so-called 'miracle cures'.

Joint injuries. Apart from penetrating wounds or contusions from direct violence these are either sprains due to tearing of the supporting ligaments or dislocations where there is displacement or separation of the bony surfaces. Both conditions are produced by forces compelling the joint to exceed its normal range of movement.

jugular vein. The right and left internal and external jugular veins are the four veins that convey blood from the head and neck to the chest.

Jung. Carl Gustav Jung (1875-1961) of Zürich became famous as the disciple and co-worker of FREUD but broke with him in 1913, not because of any difference on fundamentals but because they disagreed on certain additional concepts of Jung's. In particular, Freud had seen the libido (i.e. the individual's innate drive for pleasure and satisfaction) as primarily based on sex whereas Jung regarded it as also including other basic drives, e.g., that connected with hunger. The majority of Jung's views however, such as the idea that neurotic symptoms represent a retreat from life's difficulties or a retreat to the dependence of childhood, are essentially those of Freud and the psychoanalysts.

Jung's most controversial contribution to psychology is his theory of the collective racial unconscious: the idea that inherited racial experience creates part of our unconscious life, so that events outside our individual experience help to mould our actions, fantasies, dreams, symbols and mythologies. By no means all psychologists accept this idea.

He was also in large measure the co-developer (with Freud) of PSYCHOANALYSIS with its use of the association method.

His differentiation of people into EXTROVERTS and INTROVERTS has passed into everyday usage.

K

kala-azar. A tropical infection characterized by a very long incubation period (sometimes several months), irregular but repeated bouts of fever, progressive enlargement of the spleen and the liver, and sometimes diarrhoea and symptoms of bronchitis. The disease is caused by a tiny parasite, transmitted by the bite of the female sand-fly after it has become infected by sucking blood from an infected person or animal. Diagnosis depends on identification of the parasite in a blood specimen or in material drawn from the bone-marrow or the spleen. Antimony drugs, injected into a vein or a muscle, have become the standard treatment.

keeping fit. Since virtually all of us suffer from inherited weaknesses, faults in our upbringing or defects in our domestic or working environment, optimum physical, emotional and social health is probably beyond our fair expectations, although in the next century a majority of people may achieve it. Reasonably good health, however, should be within the grasp of most of us, and many diseases and disabilities are essentially self-induced.

Many articles in this book relate in whole or in part to the promotion of good health and the prevention or reduction of disease. All that can be done here in a single article is to bring together a few of the main points.

A fundamental difficulty about devising a regime designed to maintain or improve physical, emotional and social health is that we possess as yet very inadequate measures of health, as opposed to measures of disease. We have, for instance, no real justification for saying that an international footballer aged thirty is physically healthier than a non-athlete of the same age with no signs of present or impending disease, or that a man of seventy who still publishes articles on his particular subject is mentally healthier than a man of the same age who devotes his time to watching television and reading light novels.

However, most experts would probably agree that ten of the desirable conditions for fitness are (1) sufficient sleep; (2) adequate, well-balanced and not excessive diet; (3) reasonable but not excessive exercise; (4) either work activities or leisure activities that stimulate the brain without inducing strain; (5) interesting hobbies or recreations; (6) aims or beliefs that give some purpose to life; (7) short-term goals to provide interim satisfactions; (8) some congenial and trusted associates; (9) a satisfactory environment both at home and at work; and (10) facilities for the prompt treatment of disease or disability, and preferably for the recognition and rectification of these before they produce symptoms.

There are also desirable negative conditions of general applicability, e.g., avoidance of drugs, cigarettes and excessive quantities of alcohol; and many negative conditions that apply to persons who do not enjoy perfect health, e.g., restriction of carbohydrate intake by a diabetic and avoidance by a person with raised blood pressure of situations liable to increase the blood pressure further. The reasons for the negative conditions are fairly obvious but it may be useful to discuss the positive ones enumerated above.

Sleep. The need for adequate sleep is probably the most non-controversial of the ten selected points. The amount required varies with age, e.g., a month-old baby needs about twenty hours a day, a child of 7 years needs about thirteen hours and an adolescent of 15 needs about nine hours. While these are approximate averages there are also considerable individual variations, especially in adults: many require about eight hours a night but some remain healthy on much smaller amounts.

Insufficient sleep results in fatigue, irritability, inability to concentrate and impaired general health.

Where a person finds difficulty in getting to sleep (otherwise than through pain, worry or external noise) either a gentle walk or a warm (but not over-hot) bath before bedtime often helps.

The worst thing a sleepless person can do is to fret about his failure to fall asleep. By such fretting he will almost certainly ensure that he remains awake. Assuming that circumstances are compatible with slumber (e.g., reasonably warm bed, adequate fresh air without draughts, and quietness) he is better to rest quietly and to read an interesting but not too exciting book. Except under abnormal conditions (e.g., for some days after the death of a much loved relative) few people require sedatives and the immediate recourse of many non-sleepers to sedatives is a thing to be deprecated. On the other hand many middle-aged and elderly persons have used sedatives for many years without apparent harmful effect, and perhaps the opponents of sedatives have over-stated their case.

Diet. Of all the requirements for health, diet is the one that has been most extensively studied, and also the one on which the enquirer is confronted with the largest number of allegedly health-creating alternatives, e.g., lacto-vegetarian diet (including milk and eggs but no form of flesh), fully vegetarian diet, or even diet consisting of foods untouched by fire. Diet is also the thing on which there exists the largest number of religious taboos and dislikes.

The average requirement of first and second class protein, fat, carbohydrate, mineral salts and vitamins is reasonably worked out. (See articles on these various subjects.) There are, however, many variations. To mention three: (1) size: during the British rationing of the Second World War many a man of well over average stature was appreciably undernourished through having to exist on the same rations as a person of three-quarters of his weight; (2) stage in life: for instance a growing adolescent and an expectant mother both require slightly more food than an adult of the same size; and (3) individual variation: one person has a digestive system so efficient that he utilizes virtually every particle of food, is healthy on a minimum diet and gains weight if consuming appreciably more than the minimum, while another of identical size but with a digestive system of lower efficiency loses weight and decreases his resistance to disease when consuming a minimum diet and appears to be healthy when consuming perhaps 10 per cent more than that minimum.

For quantity a good index is provided by weight. If a person is gaining weight he is over-eating, unless he is thin and deliberately trying to increase his weight. If a person is losing weight, he is under-eating unless he is deliberately trying to reduce obesity.

As for quality, three points may be noted. A person who is substantially overweight is likely to be eating too much carbohydrate (e.g., sweets, cakes, bread, rice and potatoes) and possibly too much animal fat (e.g., butter). While dietary deficiencies often comprise several components of the diet together, the deficiency most commonly associated with poverty is that in first class protein: persons living near the bare subsistence level should therefore look for reasonably cheap forms of protein, e.g., in many parts of the world cheese and fish are appreciably cheaper than meat. Thirdly, in several northern countries, probably because of poor growth of many fruits and green vegetables, shortages of the water-soluble vitamins – c and the b group – are not uncommon.

Exercise. Exercise more violent than a particular person can stand is manifestly harmful: most of us have heard of an elderly man who had a coronary thrombosis after sprinting for a bus. Excessive exercise that creates exhaustion (as opposed to a pleasant feeling of tiredness) is also harmful. In reasonable amount, however, exercise keeps the muscles in trim, improves digestion by better burning up of foods, increases the rate and force of the heart beat and deepens breathing. Because highly developed nations have moved within three generations from a state of affairs in which the average person walked to his place of employment and then did manual work to a state in which he travels by bus or car and then does sedentary work, many people have far less exercise than their grandparents had.

Once we have passed beyond these simple, factual statements we are very much in the realms of controversy. At one end of the spectrum are the enthusiasts who point out that every muscle atrophies gradually if unused and stress the enormous importance of exercise or exercises. At the other end are the sceptics who point out that the indolent tortoise and the lumbering elephant are very long-lived, that some human centenarians have had very sedentary lives and that quite a number of athletes die young. As is so often the case, the truth probably lies somewhere between the two extremes.

If, without going to the extreme of making muscular fitness the be-all and end-all of life, we accept the desirability of reasonable daily exercise, we are still in the realm of controversy. A few health workers maintain that for the adequate exercising of various muscles we need the carefully selected and graded exercises of a keep-fit class. Many others hold that the main benefit of a keep-fit class is social, bringing together people who have a certain similarity of interest, and that exercise can be obtained in other and perhaps to some people pleasanter ways. One school of thought favours gentle but sustained exercise, e.g., a daily four-mile walk or a round of golf. Another group of workers advocate more vigorous forms of exercise, e.g., jogging. Yet another view that appears to be gaining strength is that activity should be strenuous enough to raise the pulse rate to over a hundred and that ten minutes of really vigorous activity are more beneficial than an hour of gentle exercise.

Perhaps the most important thing to be said about exercise is that adjustment should be gradual. It is a mistake for a youngster suddenly to discontinue physical activity when he leaves school and for the sedentary middle-aged man suddenly to take part in a strenuous set of tennis.

Mental stimulation. Very much the same can be said of mental as of physical exercise. Excess, either in quantity or in quality, can leave us exhausted and irritable, but a reasonable amount is essential for the well-being of the mind. Probably many of us have known an intelligent man, previously preoccupied with an interesting and mentally exacting job and rather devoid of intellectual hobbies or recreations, who rapidly deteriorated mentally after retirement, simply because of lack of stimulation.

Yet, as with physical exercise, there is

wide room for controversy. Some workers maintain that we are healthiest if we use our brains to the point of pleasant tiredness. Others hold that preservation of habit is what matters: that the brain-worker will deteriorate if he ceases to use his mental faculties but that the person who slides through life with a minimum of intellectual exercise is not necessarily the worse for it. Still others think that a person becomes little more than an animated vegetable if he loses his intellectual curiosity, his aesthetic appreciation and his capacity to reason.

For mental fitness, as for physical fitness, the truth probably lies somewhere between the extremes, and gradual adjustment is important. The youngster who suddenly discards all non-intellectual interests and concentrates solely on his university studies or on gaining promotions in his career is courting future illness; and the elderly professional worker who at retirement gives away his books and yet acquires no alternative intellectual interest is equally making a serious mistake.

Hobbies and recreations. In the words of an old proverb, 'All work and no play makes Jack a dull boy.' It seems obvious that a brain-worker should have some pastimes or recreations involving physical exercise and that a person who works with his hands should have some recreations involving the use of mental and aesthetic capacities. Yet many of us have known people who appeared fit enough although their hobbies resembled their work – the bus conductor or gardener who as a young man occupied his leisure in playing cricket and later in life became keen on bowling, or the university lecturer who spent his spare time in writing books or playing bridge. Perhaps, too, as increased mechanization makes early retirement the rule rather than the exception, it is important that some hobbies or recreations – intellectual or physical – should be of such a nature that they can ultimately form a partial substitute for work.

Long-term aims or beliefs. It is a little difficult to see how a person leading an entirely purposeless life can be healthy. The individual who is sustained by a sincere belief in a future existence (giving him a pre-designed code of behaviour and immediate answers to many moral problems), or the humanist sustained by a passionate desire to benefit humanity, or even the person with a strong ambition for himself or for his family, is in a position of advantage: his life has some purpose. Yet we are again entering into the realm of controversy. Do people who are genuinely religious or sincere humanists or ruthlessly ambitious have any real evidence that they are healthier or happier than those who adopt the Horatian maxim of living for the day, taking the pleasures of each day as they come? As so often on problems of keeping fit, we can say vaguely that a

purpose in life is probably desirable.

Short-term goals. The saint and the conqueror can perhaps sustain themselves simply by long-term aims. Most of us, however, are neither Joans of Arc nor Napoleons. We need the temporary and short-term satisfactions and gratifications created through the achievement of immediate aims. Examples are the ambitious person who decides to secure a promotion post within the next year (and derives great satisfaction from doing so) or the financially minded person who decides to pay off half the hire-purchase of his television set in six months (and again is delighted at his success).

These short-term goals carry with them, of course, the danger of short-term failure: the ambitious person may not secure his promotion or the money-minded person may not manage to make his payment. Also, some people appear to go through life successfully without setting themselves any short-term objectives.

Yet the present writer feels that the few psychologists (as opposed to the mass of gymnasts and exponents of physical culture) who have studied the complex problems of keeping fit have tended to neglect or under-value the importance of short-term goals.

Congenial and trusted associates. Man is a social animal. He needs trusted friends and people with whom he can discuss his problems and his interests on level terms and knowing that his statements will not be relayed to other people. The person who moves his home, loses touch with relatives and old friends and fails to make new friends is seldom mentally healthy.

Yet a minority of people seem to be able to endure a hermit-like existence without harm.

Satisfactory environment. Acceptance of the environment, domestic and working, is largely a matter of conditioning. Although, again, this area is controversial, it is perhaps true to say that mental, physical and social health is difficult to maintain if a person is forced into an environment worse than that to which he or she has been accustomed.

Facilities for treatment and prevention of disease. Untreated illness is manifestly incompatible with fitness. In the U.K. and various other countries an enormous advance towards the fitness of individuals has been made by the provision of facilities for treatment without any immediate payment.

An even greater advance towards physical and mental fitness has been the provision in many countries of services to promote good health and to detect and rectify deviations from health before they produce symptoms.

keloid. An overgrowth of scar tissue, occurring at the site of the scar and extending beyond its original limits, as a raised, hard, fibrous mass. Keloids may occur following burns, cuts, abrasions and surgical operations. They are not harmful or malignant, and are in general painless, but they are often unsightly. Surgical removal of a keloid is usually unsuccessful because the same conditions that permitted the initial overgrowth of scar tissue may well cause another overgrowth. Where the keloid is unsightly, shrinkage by radium or x-rays may be required.

Kenny treatment. A method of treatment for paralytic poliomyelitis pioneered and advocated by Sister Elizabeth Kenny (1886-1952) of Brisbane, Australia, and later of the U.S.A. The system involves hydrotherapy and active re-education of muscles.

keratitis. Inflammation of the cornea of the eye. It may be the result of injury or infection or of deficiency of vitamin A.

Symptoms include pain, undue sensitivity to light and in advanced cases impairment of vision through scarring of the cornea. While treatment varies with the cause, antibiotics are in general useful; but any inflammation of the eye lasting for more than twenty-four hours should have medical attention, and severe inflammation demands immediate attention.

ketogenic diet. A diet in which the fat content is increased at the expense of the carbohydrate content until incomplete products of fat digestion (ketones and acetone) appear in the urine.

kidney. The kidneys, which are an important part of the URINARY SYSTEM, are a pair of bean-shaped organs, lying high at the back of the abdomen on each side of the spine, opposite the last thoracic and the first three lumbar vertebrae. In the adult they measure roughly $11 \times 6 \times 4$cm. $(4.5 \times 2.5 \times 1.5$in.) Their main function is to filter out of the circulating blood certain waste substances – such as urea and excess water – and to excrete them through the ureters as urine, which is stored in the bladder until released.

Diseases. There are clearly two possibilities: (1) there may be deficient filtration of water (so that dropsy – usually called oedema – occurs) or of urea (so that there is danger of excess urea remaining in the blood: uraemia); or less commonly, (2) the filtering mechanism is exaggerated, so that for example, people with normal levels of sugar in the blood nevertheless have some sugar excreted in the urine and can be mistakenly thought to suffer from diabetes.

The actual diseases which can affect the kidney are so numerous that only a few can be mentioned here. It may be useful, however, to start with an exclusion. Frequency of need to pass urine, delay in starting and weakness of the stream may be due to cystitis (inflammation of the bladder) or in men to enlargement of the prostate, but are not signs of damage to the kidney.

Congenital abnormalities include cysts of the kidney which in some cases destroy so much kidney tissue as to prevent the baby from surviving.

In circumstances in which there has been a rapid loss of abdominal fat, the normal slight mobility of the kidneys may be increased so that the condition of MOVABLE KIDNEY or, if more severe, FLOATING KIDNEY, may occur.

Suppression of urine (anuria) may result from obstruction of the ureter of one kidney by a stone when the other kidney is out of action. The symptoms – drowsiness, muscular twitchings, etc. – are essentially those of uraemia, and are followed by death unless effective treatment is undertaken.

Acute nephritis occurs most commonly in childhood and adolescence and is usually caused by bacterial infection, especially by streptococci. The disease is in large measure preventable by adequate treatment of streptococcal infections with antibiotics or sulphonamides. The signs include puffiness of the eyes and face, swelling of the legs, scanty urine of high concentration and of high colour (because it contains blood) and in most cases headache and nausea. Treatment includes rest in bed and for a considerable period a diet low in protein, salt free, and high in carbohydrate. Most patients make a complete recovery.

Chronic parenchymatous nephritis is commonest in young adults. It may follow acute nephritis or arise gradually without obvious cause. The most prominent feature is massive oedema of the face, hands, trunk and legs, with pallor (from anaemia). Since the kidney is also swollen and pale, the condition is sometimes described as 'a large pale kidney in a large pale man'. The blood pressure is slightly raised. The urine is scanty and of high concentration but does not usually contain blood. A salt-free diet is worth trying for six weeks or so, but in most cases recovery is not complete and the patient has to adjust to permanently impaired kidneys – living a regular life without excesses, and avoiding excess of salt.

Chronic interstitial nephritis or 'granular kidney' is mostly a disease of the second half of life. It often accompanies arteriosclerosis. It is made more likely by a very strenuous life, prolonged excessive indulgence in alcohol, prolonged over-eating, lead poisoning, gout and syphilis. The symptoms are rather variable but often include headache and indigestion. The urine is scanty and watery, the arteries are thickened and the blood pressure is raised. The patient should live a quiet, regular life, with a light diet and occasional doses of diuretics to induce the passing of urine.

Until recent years the long-term outlook was poor, but it has been transformed by the introduction of renal dialysis, i.e., use of a KIDNEY MACHINE to enable the body to get rid of waste products that would normally be eliminated by the kidneys. In recent

blood leaves
patient's arm

pump

blood returns
to patient's arm

blood cells retained
in filtering tube as
they cannot pass
through the holes

waste matter
escapes from blood
through minute holes
in filtering tube

salt solution
circulating around
filtering tube

Kidney machine

years transplantation of a healthy kidney from a donor has also saved many lives.

kidney machine. Severe kidney disease may result in kidney failure. In this case waste products, instead of being excreted in the urine, are retained in the blood stream and, as they accumulate, will ultimately cause death from uraemia. Where the kidney is too diseased to pass waste products efficiently from the blood to the urine, a machine can be utilized as a substitute kidney. The patient is connected at suitable times to the machine by tubes inserted into blood vessels of his arm or leg, so that his blood, as well as circulating round his body, goes through this machine. The circulating blood passes over a thin, plastic membrane which is surrounded by a saline solution. Blood corpuscles are too big to escape through the membrane and so they duly return to the body; but waste products and excess water pass through the membrane into the surrounding solution.

Under suitable conditions a kidney machine can be installed in a patient's home, and a person with chronic kidney disease will need to spend perhaps ten hours three times a week linked to the machine but otherwise can lead a reasonably normal life.

The process of extraction of waste products through a kidney machine is technically called renal dialysis.

kidney stone. An accumulation of calcium oxalate, calcium phosphate or uric acid in the collecting cavity or pelvis of the kidney. Gout and infection of the kidney are among the causes.

The stone may remain in the kidney creating no symptoms; it may remain in the kidney and cause pyelitis; it may cause attacks of renal colic, characterized by sharp pain shooting downwards from the area of the kidney; it may obstruct the ureter, rendering one kidney functionless; or it may be passed into the bladder, where it sometimes causes cystitis but is more often passed with the urine. Treatment is initially directed to flushing away the stone by large quantities of alkaline fluid, and meantime using pain-killers if necessary. If these measures fail, surgical removal may be required.

kilojoule. A unit of energy increasingly used to measure food values. A joule is the amount of heat or energy generated by a current of 1 ampere flowing for 1 second against a resistance of 1 ohm, and a kilojoule (often contracted to kJ) is 1,000 joules.

In the past the energy of food was measured in CALORIES (written with a capital C) which were, strictly, kilocalories, each being 1,000 calories. Since 1978 food manufacturers in Britain and various other countries have been encouraged to use the new units when marking food. Conversion, however, is fairly easy since 1 Calorie is equivalent to 4.2 kilojoules. Thus a person on a strict slimming diet will aim at 4,200 kJ daily, instead of 1,000 Calories.

king's evil. An old name for SCROFULA.

kiss of life. See ARTIFICIAL RESPIRATION.

kleptomania. An irresistible desire to steal without regard to personal needs. Very often the articles stolen are of no value to the stealer but perhaps have a symbolic meaning, so that by acquiring them the person relieves his mental tension. Genuine kleptomania requires treatment, usually by psychoanalysis to uncover the root of the compulsion.

True kleptomania is quite a rarity, but four other conditions are often confused with it: (1) stealing by young children who simply lack understanding of the meaning of personal property and need guidance and explanation; (2) stealing by older children as a symptom of maladjustment, often undertaken with a view to giving the stolen articles to others in the hope of gaining affection, and sometimes done in response to a 'dare'; (3) deliberate and conscious shop-lifting, where the plea of kleptomania is offered in an attempt to mitigate criminal responsibility; and (4) a senile variety which is related to absent-mindedness.

knee. The hinge JOINT formed by the rounded ends, or condyles, of the thigh bone (femur) and the head of the tibia in the lower leg. The fibula, the other bone of the lower leg, does not enter into the formation of the joint. The joint is bound by very strong ligaments. In front of it, but not really part of it, is the PATELLA or kneecap, lying in the muscle tendon.

Injury. A common accident when the knee is twisted is dislocation of one of the cartilages within the joint, so that it is partially detached and nipped between the bones, causing a 'locking' of the joint, with pain and swelling. An anaesthetic may be necessary to overcome the locking. Thereafter rest and light pressure from an elastic bandage usually suffice. If recurrences are frequent an operation for removal of the cartilage may be needed.

knee, housemaid's. See HOUSEMAID'S KNEE.

knee jerk. When the leg is hanging free (e.g., crossed over the other), tapping the front just below the kneecap produces a jerking movement if the nerves from the knee to the spinal cord and from the cord to the knee are intact. The jerk is exaggerated in some diseases (e.g., disseminated sclerosis) and absent in some other diseases (e.g., severe neuritis). Hence the knee jerk is a useful diagnostic sign.

knock knee. A deformity in which the knees are bent inwards towards each other, otherwise known as genu valgum. The commonest cause was formerly rickets but as this disease has become rare in developed countries the condition is nowadays most often associated with flat-foot.

Massage and manipulation will usually help provided the condition is identified early. In cases diagnosed later operation may be needed.

Koplik's spots. Bluish-white spots on the mucous membrane of the inner lining of the cheek and gums, especially opposite the molar teeth. They appear only in the early stages of measles, often before the rash, and are therefore useful in the diagnosis of the disease.

Korsakoff's syndrome. A deterioration of the nerves and brain, characterized by memory blanks, poor mental co-ordination and pathological lying, – i.e., the construction of elaborate and completely motiveless untruths. The cause is serious deficiency of the B group of vitamins, usually as a result of chronic alcoholism: excess alcohol not only lowers appetite so that insufficient vitamins are eaten but also inactivates them. The condition improves greatly when treated by concentrations of the appropriate vitamins.

kwashiorkor. A disease, essentially of protein deficiency, common in children in developing countries.

kyphosis. See CURVATURE OF THE SPINE.

L

labia. The lips of the vulva (the external female genitalia). See REPRODUCTIVE SYSTEM.

labour. The process at the end of pregnancy during which the muscular contractions of the uterus expel the new-born child, the membranes and amniotic fluid surrounding it, and finally the placenta through which it derived sustenance during intra-uterine life. For a detailed account see CHILDBIRTH.

Premature labour is labour occurring after viability (6 to 6½ months), so that the child is capable of survival, but before full-term. Interruption of pregnancy before viability is usually called miscarriage or abortion.

False labour is the occurrence of colicky pains towards the end of pregnancy, mimicking real labour. These usually arise from irregular contractions of other abdominal organs but are characterized by lack of rhythm, by being felt in the abdomen rather than in the back, and by the absence, when it is gently felt by the hand, of any general contraction of the uterus. Investigation may disclose constipation or an infected or distended bladder. Appropriate treatment combined with sedatives will usually allay the symptoms.

laburnum. The pods and seeds of this tree contain an alkaloid, cystisine, which is also found in broom and lupin seeds. About an hour after eating the pods or seeds a child becomes pale, dizzy and anxious, and usually suffers from vomiting and diarrhoea.

Treatment consists mainly of giving the child warmth, adequate air, reassurance, and – if vomiting or diarrhoea are severe – liquid drinks to prevent dehydration. If there is little vomiting, an emetic to induce it (e.g., salt and water) may help to remove the poison from the stomach. If there is little or no diarrhoea, a laxative may assist in the elimination of the poison from the intestine.

laceration. A wound produced by the tearing apart of tissues. Severe lacerations are typical of machinery and traffic accidents and are generally associated with considerable bruising. Such wounds are usually irregular in shape; the skin around is torn and discoloured; there may be ingrained dirt or indriven portions of clothing; pain is often slight because of nerve-fibre destruction; similarly, bleeding may be minimal because injured blood-vessels become blocked by their torn walls.

Tissue-damage and the diminished blood supply reduces the ability to combat infections, and also means that the damaged tissues are liable to die or at least to slow delayed healing. Successful repair requires meticulous care with antiseptic cleansing, the removal of foreign matter and dead tissue, arrest of haemorrhage, assessment and repair of damage to deeper structures, and finally accurate suturing with provision for drainage. An anti-tetanus injection should also be given.

lacrimal. The eyes are continuously bathed by a watery fluid, the tears, produced by glands behind the upper eyelids, and entering the conjunctival sacs by multiple secretory ducts. Excess fluid leaves the sacs by drainage pores at the inner angles of the eyelids and is collected in a small reservoir which continues as a duct to the lower part of the nasal cavity. Lacrimal means 'pertaining to the tears', and is used to qualify the names of the successive parts of these lacrimatory arrangements as lacrimal gland, lacrimal secretion, lacrimal canals, lacrimal sac, and naso-lacrimal duct.

lactation. The period during which the mother secretes milk and the infant is suckled. See BREAST FEEDING.

lameness. The causes of lameness vary, from a blister or corn on the foot, or even ill-fitting or badly designed shoes, to a serious disease of the brain or spinal cord. In young children lameness may be an early sign of disease of the hip joint (e.g., tuberculous infection). In general, unless there is an obvious trivial cause, lameness requires medical investigation.

Langerhans, islets of. Clusters of cells scattered throughout the pancreas. In these cells INSULIN is produced.

laparotomy. The operation of opening the abdominal cavity either for the purpose of dealing with a diseased or damaged organ or for exploratory or diagnostic purposes.

laryngitis. Inflammation of the larynx and vocal cords resulting in dryness of the throat, hoarseness (sometimes going on to complete loss of voice), tickling cough and raised temperature.

Acute laryngitis is usually due to infection of the voice-box after it has been rendered susceptible by exposure to irritating vapours, or by exposure to cold (especially very cold air breathed through the mouth and therefore unwarmed), or by over-use of the voice. The four standard measures of treatment are rest, provision of an even temperature, cough sedatives and appropriate inhalations, such as a teaspoonful of tincture of benzoin in 0.5 litre (1 pint) of boiling water. Inhalations are very useful but the patient must remain for some hours in a warm atmosphere after each inhalation. Gargling, although often used, is of doubtful value. Generally recovery occurs within a few days, although occasionally the acute stage passes into the chronic one.

Chronic laryngitis, with similar symptoms and long-term swelling of the vocal cords, may follow an uncured acute attack, may be the result of habitual straining of the voice (clergyman's throat) or may occasionally result from excessive smoking. If the condition does not respond to ordinary treatment examination by a throat specialist is desirable.

larynx. The portion of the RESPIRATORY SYSTEM adapted for the production of VOICE and SPEECH.

Lassa fever. An acute and often fatal infectious disease first identified in Nigeria in 1969 and subsequently found in other countries in Central and Western Africa. The disease is caused by a virus which is carried by a particular type of African rat, but is also occasionally spread through direct personal or nursing contact with an infected person or his clothing or excretions. In general the disease occurs in countries in which the particular rat breeds.

The incubation period is seven to ten days and the main symptoms are fever, sore throat, complete exhaustion, toxic appearance and sometimes vomiting and chest pains.

Control measures include attempts to eradicate the particular species of rat, prevention of contamination of food by such rats, and early identification and rigorous isolation of suspected cases.

Treatment consists mainly of skilled nursing with attention to symptoms, although injection of plasma obtained from the blood of recovered or convalescent cases help, as does INTERFERON. As yet no antibiotic useful in treatment has been discovered and no vaccine for prevention is available.

laughing gas. Nitrous oxide, a colourless gas sometimes used for anaesthesia in dentistry. In relatively pure form it rapidly produces unconsciousness, but if administered with some air mixed with it, it gives rise to a kind of intoxication, often characterized by laughter or, less frequently, by weeping.

lavage. The washing out of any internal organ. Lavage is most commonly used for the stomach in cases of poisoning (other than corrosive poisoning) or conditions of dilatation with accumulation and fermentation of stomach contents, e.g., some cases of severe indigestion. A special rubber tube is passed through the mouth and gullet into the stomach. There is a filter funnel attached, and warmed water containing a little potassium permanganate is run into the stomach and siphoned off.

Colonic lavage is sometimes used in chronic constipation, and bladder lavage is occasionally recommended in chronic cystitis.

laxative. An 'opening medicine' alternatively known as an aperient employed in the treatment of CONSTIPATION.

In most cases a mild laxative is preferable to a stronger one, and the dose should be the minimum to produce an easy motion.

lead poisoning. The condition resulting from absorption of lead salts by the body. Despite many precautions the condition is still not infrequent in lead workers, such as painters, glaziers, potters, plumbers and makers of electric batteries; and it is sometimes found in children who have chewed articles painted with a lead-based paint. Since most lead water-pipes have now been replaced, lead poisoning from water is becoming a thing of the past.

Acute lead poisoning from a single large dose usually starts with cramp-like abdominal pain and obstinate constipation followed in severe cases either by intense headache, convulsions and sometimes coma (where the lead salts damage the brain) or by paralysis of the muscles of the fingers and wrists.

Chronic lead poisoning, from absorption of small amounts over a period, is commoner. Here the main symptoms are those of anaemia, (e.g., tiredness, weakness and pallor) with paralysis of wrist and fingers in due course, and sometimes with abdominal colic. A diagnostic sign, present in many but not all cases, is a blue line in the gums, not to be confused with the line sometimes seen between gums and uncleaned teeth. Where the diagnosis is in doubt, blood examination is helpful.

Prevention includes: (1) wherever practicable, substitution of non-toxic substances (e.g., plastics) for lead compounds; (2) where lead must be used the taking of appropriate steps to prevent the escape of dust and fumes; (3) personal cleanliness by workers, including the scrubbing of hands and nails before eating; (4) the use of protective clothing, including well-fitting overalls and including masks where processes are dusty; (5) periodical medical examination of employees in lead industries; and (6) diminution of the amount of lead in petrol (and consequently in fumes from vehicles).

In treatment calcium compounds have largely superseded older methods, because the main effect of lead absorption is to remove calcium. Morphia may be needed for the pain, though a high calcium diet – including two pints of milk daily – will usually end the colic within two days. Laxatives are necessitated by the constipation, and where paralysis of fingers and wrist persists electrical treatment may be useful.

left-handedness. Natural dominance of the left hand. The condition, which is probably inherited, is found in about one-tenth of children.

From school desks to adult tools society has been organized for the right-handed majority. Yet attempts to force left-handed children to use their right hands sometimes result in emotional disorders or speech defects and always result in poorer performance than would have been possible with the natural hand. It is now generally accepted that a child should be allowed to use his natural hand, but since our writing is from left to right some left-handed children at first tend to reverse figures and letters, e.g., confusing 'b' and 'd', and reading 'top' for 'pot' and 'was' for 'saw'.

leg. In anatomical descriptions the term is restricted to the portion from the knee to the ankle, the part from knee to hip-joint being termed the thigh.

The skeleton of the leg (in the anatomical sense) is formed by the tibia or shin-bone on the inner side and the thinner fibula on the outside. The fleshy calf of the leg is formed by the gastrocnemius and soleus muscles ending in the Achilles tendon which is inserted into the heel bone.

legionnaires' disease. A serious bacterial disease first recognized when an outbreak occurred at a gathering of members of the Pennsylvania State American Legion in 1976 at Philadelphia.

The disease, which has an incubation period of seven to ten days, usually starts with muscle pains, dry cough, shortness of breath and rising temperature, sometimes with rigors, and in a day or two produces signs and symptoms identical with those of pneumonia. It may well be that some cases diagnosed in the past as pneumonia were really cases of legionnaires' disease. Oxygen treatment helps the breathing and, although not all antibiotics are effective, adequate dosage of an appropriate antibiotic usually results in rapid cure.

In an established outbreak it is easy to treat the later cases with erythromycin or tetracycline (the most effective antibiotics) but the difficulty lies in diagnosing the early cases in time to reduce the 15 per cent risk of death, because clinically and radiologically the condition so resembles pneumonia that the existence of legionnaires' disease is unlikely to be suspected until several persons thought to have been suffering from pneumonia show a lack of response to normal treatment for that disease.

The method of spread is not yet certain but the majority of workers who have studied the disease believe that spread is through the air, perhaps in dust particles, or through contaminated water.

Legionnaires' disease raises many questions that are not at present answerable: for instance, where does the germ exist between outbreaks, are there human or animal symptomless carriers, how exactly does the disease spread, can a rapid method of diagnosis be evolved, and are there any useful and practicable preventive measures? At least the disease serves as a reminder that scientific knowledge is very far from complete.

leisure. See KEEPING FIT and RETIREMENT.

lens. See EYE.

leprosy. A mildly infectious disease of prolonged incubation and very prolonged course, characterized by nodules and ulcers both in the skin and beneath its surface, and by damage to nerves. The disease is caused by a micro-organism not unlike the germ that causes tuberculosis.

Leprosy is still widespread in Asia, Africa and Central and South America with a few cases still arising in other areas, e.g., Iceland and Northern Australia. The disease is spread by close and continuous human contact, especially in unhygienic conditions; but the medieval idea of its high infectivity is quite wrong and really due to confusion with other conditions. The incubation period is usually several years, and in some cases over ten years.

Although most cases are to some extent intermediate or mixed, the two main types are here outlined.

1. The nodular type usually begins with general discomfort, bouts of fever, pains over large areas of the body, and nodular swellings, especially in the face and hands. The swollen patches become thickened and painful, and they gradually spread to become insensitive so that pain disappears. As the nose becomes involved and flattened the face assumes a so-called 'leonine' appearance. Organisms may invade the eyes, causing blindness.

2. In the tuberculoid type sharply defined patches of the skin become raised on any part of the body, the buttocks being perhaps most commonly affected. The patches expand, becoming dry, pale and devoid of sensation. Involvement of nerves often results in loss of power and loss of sensation in the fingers and toes. Ulcers may occur and the tissues of the fingers and toes may die.

If untreated, the disease may continue to progress for thirty years with or without periods of partial remission, or it may become arrested at any stage.

Oil of chaulmoogra, for many years the standard treatment and definitely useful, is nowadays increasingly being replaced by dapsone (DDS), given by mouth or by injection for a prolonged period. Additionally, antibiotics or surgical treatment may be needed for the ulcers, and special attention should be given to the eyes. Since leprosy is only mildly contagious the old idea of very strict isolation is outmoded, although it is still desirable to remove a child from a leprous parent.

Lesbianism. A sexual relationship between women, corresponding to homosexuality in men (and strictly included in the latter term). Usually the physical side of such relationships amounts to mutual masturbation.

Possible causes of Lesbianism include genetic and environmental factors, which combine to make a particular woman predominantly masculine; prolonged sexual rivalry; and disgust at the roughness of the male approach to intercourse.

lesion. A general term indicating disease or damage in any part of the body.

leucocyte. A white blood corpuscle. Out of every 500 blood corpuscles about 499 are red and concerned with transport of oxygen and about 1 is white (or actually almost colourless), larger than the red cells, and concerned with defending the body against infection and engulfing invading foreign bodies. A cubic millimetre of blood normally contains about five million red blood corpuscles and nine thousand white blood corpuscles which are divisible into various types, e.g., neutrophils, eosinophils and lymphocytes.

An increase in the number of leucocytes in the blood is known as leucocytosis. A slight temporary increase occurs during digestion of food and an increase of longer duration is found in pregnancy. Normally, however, leucocytosis implies a reaction to the invasion of bacteria or other foreign bodies. It is a sign that the blood is 'on the defensive'.

Leucocytes of different types do not respond equally to any one invader. Thus eosinophils increase markedly in diseases due to animal parasites (such as various worms) and also in asthma and the early stages of scarlet fever; the number of lymphocytes rises markedly in tuberculosis; and neutrophils are increased in the majority of infections.

In any infection a leucocytosis, e.g., an increase from nine thousand to fifteen thousand per cubic millimetre, is a good sign, indicating that the white blood corpuscles are responding to the challenge. Conversely, no increase or inadequate increase in white blood corpuscles is an unfavourable sign.

leucocytosis. See LEUCOCYTE.

leucopenia. Diminution of the white blood corpuscles below the normal proportion of nine thousand per cubic millimetre of blood. Leucopenia is found in typhoid fever, measles and influenza; in some mosquito-borne infections such as malaria and kala-azar; in severe anaemias in which the red blood corpuscles are, of course, also reduced; and in some cases of exposure to x-rays or radium or atomic radiation.

leucorrhoea. Abnormal discharge of white fluid from the VAGINA.

leucotomy. An operation whereby an incision is made through the skull into the brain for the purpose of cutting certain nerve fibres and so removing the pathways between particular sets of stimuli and particular responses.

The operation has been extensively used to give relief in certain serious mental disorders, especially those associated with intractable mental suffering and anxiety. It is recommended in severe cases of schizophrenia and manic-depressive psychosis which have failed to respond to other methods of treatment. However, it is quite a serious operation, and there is no guarantee that it will not also result in the destruction of useful pathways.

leukaemia. A disease or group of diseases characterized by grossly excessive activity of either the bone marrow (in which many leucocytes are formed) or the spleen and lymph glands (in which lymphocytes are formed), resulting in an enormous increase in the number of circulating large leucocytes or of lymphocytes.

The acute forms, which occur in children and young adults, usually start with fatigue, raised temperature, haemorrhages from mucous membranes and enlargement of the spleen and lymph glands. These acute forms show symptoms which are identical with acute septicaemia and blood tests have to be carried out to distinguish the two conditions. Acute leukaemia was formerly always fatal, but corticosteroids and cytotoxic drugs have achieved some degree of success.

Chronic myelogenous leukaemia, in which the bone marrow produces vast numbers of immature leucocytes, usually occurs in young adults. Clinical findings include gross enlargement of the spleen, pain, progressive weakness, and haemorrhages from the nose. Remissions frequently occur, sometimes lasting for several months, but the condition is usually fatal, although x-rays and cytotoxic drugs sometimes effect a cure.

Chronic lymphatic leukaemia appears more in males above middle age. Symptoms are similar, except that there is much enlargement of lymph glands and less swelling of the spleen. Remissions are frequent and lengthy, and patients have been known to live for over ten years.

While a few cases of leukaemia have been caused by ionizing radiations and especially by the explosion of atomic bombs, and while a possible hereditary element has been suggested in lymphatic leukaemia, the main factors causing it are still unknown. Most experts regard leukaemia as being essentially a cancer of the blood-forming tissues.

libido. Psychological energy; the individual's innate drive for pleasure and satisfaction.

Freud uses the term as meaning fundamentally a drive for sexual gratification and for perpetuation of the species; but it has to be remembered that Freud groups together all forms of affection under this heading. Jung and other psychologists employ the term to include the drives for superiority, acknowledgement, affection, parental love, etc., as well as that for sexual gratification. As generally used in modern psychology it embraces all forms of vital energy.

Librium. A TRANQUILLIZER.

lice. The head louse (Pediculus capitis), the body louse (Pediculus corporis) and the crab louse (Phthirus pubis) are all variants of the same species. The eggs or nits are

actual size

Louse

cemented to hairs or clothing and hatch in seven to fifteen days, and the new lice become mature in about a fortnight.

Lice, traditionally associated with unclean heads or bodies, cause itching, discomfort and lack of sleep. They can also transmit the organisms of typhus fever and relapsing fever.

Prevention is essentially by cleanliness, though it has to be remembered that a person whose personal hygiene is perfect can be infected from a less clean associate. Treatment is normally by lethane spray or by a 2 per cent emulsion of DDT rubbed on the scalp.

In outbreaks of typhus a 10 per cent DDT powder can be sprayed through the openings in the clothing, and can thus save the very considerable time that would have to be spent if thousands of contacts and suspected contacts had to undress before receiving treatment for eradication of lice.

lichen planus. An extremely itchy skin condition, with shiny, flat-topped papules particularly affecting the front of the forearms and wrists, the inner aspects of the thighs and the front of the shins. The condition is probably due to a virus. Prednisone is perhaps the most effective drug, and sedatives are also usually needed until the intense itching subsides.

ligament. A band of tough fibrous tissue which binds together the component bones of a joint or helps to keep an internal organ in place. Much of the strength of such joints as the knee and the ankle derives from the ligaments. When a ligament is unduly stretched or very suddenly stretched its fibres may be ruptured, causing a SPRAIN.

lipoma. A slow-growing, non-malignant tumour composed of fat. Lipomata are usually rounded and have well-marked capsules from which they can be shelled out if need be.

By far the commonest variety is the subcutaneous lipoma, occurring under the skin of the neck, shoulder, back or buttocks. It is quite painless and causes inconvenience only by its size or appearance. Less frequently lipomata occur within muscles or within the capsule of a joint. Often several lipomata develop near each other.

Small lipomata are usually best left alone. If a large lipoma causes disfiguration or creates' pain through pressure, surgical treatment consists simply of opening the capsule and shelling out the fatty material. Recurrence is almost unknown.

lips, disorders of. Lip disorders, because they cause cosmetic disfigurement, are generally recognized promptly and treated vigorously.

Cleft or HARE-LIP is the most important congenital lip disorder. About two-thirds of cases are associated with cleft palate. Treatment is by surgical repair.

The commonest cause of lip swelling is a mucous cyst, resulting from blockage of a mucous gland. It should be removed by a small operation.

Chapping of the lips, with a crack in the middle of the lower lip which frequently bleeds, is a common complaint in cold weather. Treatment and prevention include the application of glycerine and bland lip protective ointments.

Herpes simplex cold sores are common, and are self-healing or responsive to simple treatments such as application of ointment or spirit, but they are liable to recur.

The lips are the commonest place, outside the genital area, for syphilitic chancre. Treatment is with penicillin in substantial and maintained dosage.

Cancer of the lips is commonest in old men who have followed an outdoor occupation; prolonged exposure to bright sunshine is thought to be a factor in its development. The tumour is slow-growing and generally curable by surgery or radiotherapy.

Lister. Joseph Lister (1827-1912), later Lord Lister, an English surgeon and the founder of ANTISEPSIS in surgery.

lithiasis. A condition characterized by the formation of CALCULI (stones) of any kind, especially in the bile ducts or in the urinary tract. Treatment varies according to the site and duration of the disorder, but may include surgery.

lithotomy. The incision of a duct or organ, particularly of the bladder, to remove a stone.

In the lithotomy position, commonly employed for gynaecological examination and operation and for childbirth, the woman lies on her back with legs apart and with both the hips and the knee joints well bent.

liver. The largest gland of the body lying

lobectomy

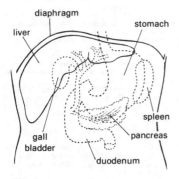

The liver

beneath the diaphragm in the upper right of the abdomen, with an important role in the body METABOLISM. It has a double blood supply, from the hepatic artery, bringing oxygenated blood from the heart via the aorta, and the portal vein, bringing blood from the stomach and intestine, rich in absorbed foods which the liver processes. It secretes BILE, destroys old red blood cells, converts most sugars into glycogen which it stores, and plays a large part in fat and protein metabolism as well. It is responsible for the control of catabolism (i.e. decomposition) of the ammonia produced as a by-product of protein breakdown in the gut.

In addition it is the body's main defence against potentially dangerous substances: many drugs (e.g., alcohol), which would otherwise accumulate in the body, are broken down to simpler non-poisonous constituents by the liver. It acts similarly in respect of the body's own hormones.

The liver of some animals is used as food.

Diseases. Because of its major role in metabolism the liver is particularly liable to blood-borne infection by diseases in other parts of the body, whilst disturbance of its own normal function by disease may have widespread serious consequences.

Infective hepatitis, caused by virus infection of the liver itself, is the commonest cause of JAUNDICE in adults. The condition gradually clears up without specific treatment, but it is usually necessary to treat the symptoms (e.g., itching of the skin).

Bacterial infection from other abdominal organs, formerly common, is now rare, due to improved diagnosis of abdominal sepsis and the widespread use of antibiotics.

Amoebic abscess, caused by the organism responsible for amoebic dysentery, is common in tropical areas with poor

sanitation. Treatment is not easy but several drugs exist that act specifically against the amoeba. Hydatid disease of the liver, caused by a dog tapeworm, requires surgical removal.

Primary cancer of the liver is rare in Europeans, but common in Africa and the Far East and known to be associated with certain items of diet. Drug treatment and surgery are employed. Prevention by change of diet may be possible. The spread of cancer from the gut, lung, breast, etc. to the liver is common, and difficult to treat.

Cardiac failure, alcoholism, and other diseases of the body function have specific effects on the liver and require treatment of the original disease for their relief.

lobectomy. The surgical operation for the removal of one of the lobes of a lung. The lungs are divided into sections called lobes – three in the right lung and two in the left – and each lobe is almost completely separate with its own airway and blood vessels. Using modern methods of anaesthesia, lobectomy is now a routine procedure for the thoracic surgeon.

The operation is principally used in such conditions as bronchiectasis, chronic lung abscess, cysts of various kinds, and in cancer of the lung. Careful investigation of the extent of the disease is required beforehand, in order to find whether it is likely that the affected area can be completely removed.

lobotomy. Another name for LEUCOTOMY.

lockjaw. A firm closing of the jaw due to spasm of its muscles. Also known as trismus, it is usually associated with TETANUS and caused by the toxin produced by the tetanus bacteria. Treatment is directed towards maintaining respiration. Prevention is achieved by immunization with anti-tetanus toxoid.

locomotor. Pertaining to or capable of movement.

locomotor ataxia. A formerly common but now very rare disease of the spinal cord, occurring as a late complication of syphilis some five to twenty years after the original condition. An alternative name is tabes dorsalis. See SYPHILIS.

longevity. The achievement of long life, beyond 75 or 80 years of age.

The nature of the AGEING process, though the subject of increasing research, is still imperfectly understood. Nevertheless, formulae and elixirs for prolongation of life have abounded throughout history. A modern formula might well include the following items: rural residence and lifestyle, with physical work begun early in life and continued to a late age, a long marriage, abstinence from tobacco, moderate intake of a mixed diet, and half a bottle of wine a day with meals.

lordosis. See CURVATURE OF THE SPINE.

LSD. An abbreviation for lysergic acid diethylamide, a hallucinogenic drug, i.e., one which causes hallucinations. It was originally derived from ergot but was synthesized in 1938. Drug users refer to it as 'acid', 'sugar' or 'zen'. It is one of a class of drugs known as psychotomimetic (simulating mental illness) and such substances have been used by primitive races from time immemorial, being taken during tribal rites to induce frenzy and illusions of supernatural power. Other examples are mescalin, obtained from the Mexican agave, bufotenin, a skin-secretion of toads, and also marihuana.

LSD has been employed therapeutically in mental illness to improve the attitude of patients to psychotherapy, but its unauthorized use in 'taking a trip' is both illegal and very dangerous. Devotees claim that the episodes of hallucination and temporary insanity, produced by even minute amounts of the drug, are an enlargement of experience because of the profound alterations which occur in their perceptions and emotions.

There is however substantial risk of causing a prolonged psychotic illness resembling schizophrenia or toxic psychosis, and of inducing delusions and impaired judgement which may lead to fatal results. There have, for instance, been incidents in which individuals have thrown themselves from a height under the delusion that they were able to fly. There is also evidence that the drug can produce genetic damage with effects on subsequent children.

The hallucinogens are not drugs of addiction leading to dependence, but they are more immediately harmful because of their effects on the brain and the transmission of nerve-impulses.

lumbago. Any pain in the small of the back is commonly called lumbago but the causes may be diverse and include specific lesions such as lumbar strain, osteoarthritis and prolapsed inter-vertebral disc. The term is best reserved for the condition of fibrositis affecting the muscles and their associated fascial structures in the lumbar region of the back, which is immediately below the waist.

The symptoms, which may be acute or chronic, are predominantly pain and muscular spasm. In acute lumbago the pain and disability may be very severe, the patient being quite unable to straighten his back from a semi-stooping position.

Immediate treatment includes rest, warmth and physiotherapy, coupled with the use of analgesics to relieve the pain. Prevention of recurrence requires the removal or correction of pre-disposing factors and the treatment of any identifiable general disease.

See also BACKACHE; RHEUMATISM, MUSCULAR.

lumbar puncture. The tapping of the space between the spinal cord and its enveloping membranes in the lumbar region for diagnostic or therapeutic purposes in cases of injury or disease of the CENTRAL NERVOUS SYSTEM. The fluid in the space is drawn off through a hollow needle. Also known as 'spinal tap', the procedure is practically painless in skilled hands.

The pressure with which the cerebrospinal fluid emerges, its appearance, its composition, and its bacteriological state are all of diagnostic significance and provide evidence about the brain and spinal cord, the presence of fresh or old haemorrhage, and the presence and nature of any infection.

In certain infections the lumbar puncture (intrathecal) route is the best for the administration of selected drugs.

lungs. The pair of organs in the RESPIRATORY SYSTEM where the oxygenation of the blood takes place.

lupus. Originally used to describe a chronic degenerative skin condition with swelling and ulceration, the term is now always used with a second term specifying the type. For example: (1) lupus erythematosus is a general illness which may be chronic (with skin lesions alone), subacute, or disseminated, in which there may be involvement of blood vessels or nerves; (2) lupus vulgaris is a form of tuberculosis of the skin.

lymph. A transparent fluid, sometimes slightly yellow and opalescent, collected from the tissues throughout the body. It flows through the LYMPHATIC SYSTEM and comprises a clear liquid portion, varying numbers of white blood cells and a few red blood cells.

lymphadenoma. See HODGKIN'S DISEASE.

lymphatic system. The capillaries, collecting channels and trunks that collect LYMPH from the tissues and carry it via the main lymph vessels, the thoracic duct and the right lymphatic duct into veins at the base of the neck.

The lymphatic vessels are absorbent in function, preventing the accumulation of excess fluid in the tissues, and carrying in the lymph a good deal of the fat absorbed during digestion into the blood stream. The lymphatics play an important part in drainage from an infected area, the lymph nodes acting as a filter against the spread of infection. The long-held view that the lymphatics contribute only to the spread of malignant disease is being modified in the light of considerable current research into the nature of body defences against cancer.

Lymph glands. Numerous flattened, oval or rounded structures located along the course of lymphatic vessels. They vary greatly in size, from 1 to 25 mm. in diameter. Several lymph vessels enter on one side of the gland and usually a single vessel leaves from the opposite side, the gland acting as a filter against the spread of infection. Normally, the lymph passes through one or more lymph glands or nodes on its way to the blood stream, and the glands are particularly numerous in the neck, pelvis, abdomen and around the lungs. They consist of masses of lymphocytes enclosed in a fibrous capsule. The lymph nodes are important in the body's system of defence against disease, both because of their filter action and also because they produce lymphocytes, a form of white blood cell, which help combat infection.

Diseases. These generally take the form of a swelling of the glands, with or without pain.

Acute infection is often associated with painful enlargement of the local lymph glands, while chronic inflammation occurs particularly in tuberculosis and syphilis, in which it is painless. In all cases of infection treatment is by attention to the original cause, with appropriate antibiotic therapy.

Primary cancer of the lymph nodes is not common, but secondary deposits of a malignancy are a frequent cause of lymph node enlargement.

In HODGKIN'S DISEASE and LEUKAEMIA the lymph nodes are usually involved.

lymphogranuloma venereum. An infectious disease spread by sexual contact and affecting the lymph channels and lymph glands related to the genitalia. It causes enlargement of glands in the groin and this may be followed by the development of pus and ulcers on the overlying skin. Other complications are stricture of the rectum and coarsening of the skin. There may also be general disturbance with fever, chills, headache and loss of appetite.

The condition is due to a minute organism of the genus *Bedsonia;* it occurs chiefly in tropical and sub-tropical regions and may be both protracted and disabling. The incubation period is very variable, from a few days to several months, and the individual is infectious as long as there are active lesions.

Treatment by sulphonamides or the

inguinal nodes filtering lymph from leg and abdominal wall

cervical nodes filtering lymph from scalp, face, tonsils and tongue

axillary nodes, filtering lymph from arm and chest wall

The superficial lymphatic system

tetracyclines is effective but one attack does not confer immunity.

M

McBurney's point. A rather vaguely defined position low down on the right of the abdomen. It lies about one-third of the way along an imaginary line from the front spine of the right hip bone to the umbilicus. In a typical case of appendicitis, tenderness on pressure is maximum at this point.

macule. A spot or blemish on the same level as the surrounding skin, as contrasted with a papule which is raised above the surface. A rash is commonly described, according to the position of the spots, as being macular or papular.

maladjusted child. A child who shows evidence of emotional instability or psychological disturbance in ways that have a bad effect on himself or his companions and who cannot, without expert assistance, be helped by his parents, teachers or other adults with whom he ordinarily comes into contact.

It has been estimated that between 5 and 10 per cent of children of school age are maladjusted although no simple criteria of diagnosis exist. Maladjustment may show itself through the child's return to more infantile patterns of bowel and bladder control, by timidity or a withdrawal into fantasy, by failure to make progress in class or a sudden deterioration in school work, by playing truant, by temper tantrums, or by dishonest, aggressive or destructive behaviour which may end in delinquency. The variety of symptoms suggests that there is no single cause.

It is often said that NEUROSIS is responsible for a large proportion of maladjusted children with PSYCHOSIS accounting for some cases and yet others attributed vaguely to personality disorder. Clearly there are many factors involved: the child's genetic inheritance may make him more able or less able to endure stresses without damage to his personality; long-term psychological and social factors may deprive him of the affection and security needed for personality development; over-forcing by ambitious parents, over-strictness and over-indulgence may play parts; occasionally a sudden event that utterly shocks the child may be a precipitating factor; and perhaps a minor degree of maladjustment is part of the normal process of growing up – with the child increasingly seeking to decide his own actions but lacking an adult's experience of life. Broadly, long-term deprivations seem more important than single shocking events; and study of maladjusted children reveals that many of them come from broken homes or homes in which marital disharmony is marked.

Identification of the maladjusted child depends largely on the awareness and understanding of teachers, school doctors and school nurses, but also on their belief that available treatment facilities are really useful. So the provision of an efficient child guidance clinic in an area may actually appear to increase maladjustment.

Anti-social behaviour among boys tends to come more to notice than among girls, at least until the age of puberty. Hence far more boys than girls receive treatment for maladjustment. Again, teachers and school nurses concerned with secondary education come to expect a little abnormal behaviour among adolescents and to regard it in most cases as not needing prolonged skilled treatment. So there are roughly four times as many referrals of primary as of secondary children to child guidance clinics.

The child guidance clinics of the school health services provide the corner-stone of treatment of maladjusted children. A full investigation of the child by a team consisting of a child psychiatrist and specially qualified medical officer, a psychologist and a psychiatric social worker is normally carried out. When the investigation, which is often long and involved, is completed, the same team institutes treatment. Though a day or residential school for maladjusted children may be recommended it is felt that most children are best helped by being treated in their usual school and home environment. In all cases, the child's psychological disorders require appropriate treatment, and his home circumstances careful assessment and possible adjustment. Treatment is often prolonged and difficult. Reliable estimates of success and failure rates do not exist. In any case, the child often requires support into early adult life.

Although a sizeable slice of the work of health visitors in Britain and public health nurses in the U.S.A. consists in trying to create stable emotional conditions for children and in seeking to educate parents about children's requirements for mental and social development, the general improvement in children's physical health and physical environment does not appear to have been accompanied by a similar reduction in maladjustment. There are at least two possible explanations: (1) that external stresses acting on parents (e.g., wars, unemployment and fear of redundancy) have adversely affected the domestic environment of children; and (2) that standards of diagnosis have altered, so that a child who would have been regarded merely as 'highly strung' twenty years ago is now classed as sufficiently disturbed to need treatment at a child guidance clinic. Probably both explanations contain a considerable element of truth.

malaria. A tropical or sub-tropical disease caused by the presence of the parasite *Plasmodium* in the red blood cells. It is transmitted by the bite of an affected female mosquito of the genus *Anopheles* which has previously sucked the blood of a malaria sufferer. The plasmodia reproduce in the human at frequent intervals, each entry of a new generation of the parasite into the red blood cells giving rise to a further acute malarial attack. Such an attack consists of a chill, accompanied and followed by a fever and general symptoms, and terminates in a sweating stage. Attacks recur at 48-hour, 72-hour or less definite intervals, depending on which of the four species of *Plasmodium* known to affect man is responsible. An attack of malaria may simply end in recovery quite spontaneously (with or without subsequent relapses months or years later), or it may, in the case of *Plasmodium falciparium* malaria, proceed to involve the brain and also, possibly, the kidneys, leading to severe illness and frequently death.

Those raised in malarious areas develop quite a strong immunity to the more severe forms of the disease, but generally at the cost of being anaemic, emaciated, and depressed as a result of repeated attacks.

Malaria may be prevented by the elimination of anopheles mosquitoes from areas of human habitation by use of insecticides and draining of swamps and marshes. Hundreds of millions of people have thus been freed, in the last twenty-five years, from the possibility of malarious attack, though permanent watchfulness has to be maintained to prevent the re-establishment of the mosquito. Where the mosquito continues to breed, protection against malaria is obtained by using insect repellents, fitting window screens, etc. to reduce the possibility of being bitten, and above all by the regular use of appropriate anti-malarial drugs. Those visiting a possibly malarious area, however briefly, must take suppressive drugs throughout the visit and for the following four weeks.

Chloroquine has long been the most useful of a number of drugs for the treatment of acute and chronic cases of malaria. It has mostly replaced quinine.

Research into the possibility of immunization against malaria is well advanced.

male climacteric. See CLIMACTERIC.

malignant. The term is applied to those tumours (such as cancer and sarcoma) which spread so that the disease appears in other parts of the body. This is in contrast with benign tumours which do not give rise to these 'secondaries' and cause

trouble merely by pressure. The term is also applied to abnormally serious forms of disease, e.g., malignant hypertension.

malingering. Deliberate feigning or exaggeration of illness or injury, usually for one of three reasons – to avoid work especially unpleasant tasks; to obtain compensation for an injury; or to secure sympathy. Malingering involving physical signs can generally be detected because the person counterfeiting an illness seldom knows or can imitate all its signs and because prolonged maintenance of a sign is difficult: for instance, the person feigning pneumonia may deliberately speed his respiration and may take a drug to quicken his pulse rate, but when he falls asleep the respiratory rate drops immediately. Where the malingerer relies on symptoms, diagnosis is much more difficult: for example, nobody except the victim can be certain whether the suspected case of appendicitis really feels abdominal pain and actually experiences tenderness when a finger is pressed on McBurney's point. In many cases of malingering there is some existing pain or disability which the patient exaggerates and to differentiate between malingering and a genuine incapacity to work in such circumstances is one of the most difficult tasks confronting a doctor, especially as people have widely differing degrees of susceptibility and sensitivity to pain. A doctor who suspects malingering is wise to carry out extensive tests and to seek a second opinion before making an accusation; and even where a person is definitely malingering there may be need for treatment of the psychological condition that causes him to seek to avoid work or to crave for sympathy.

malleolus. The bony projections on the sides of the ankle, formed by the ends of the tibia and fibula respectively.

malnutrition. The end result of eating too little of the right kinds of food. Strictly, its use should be restricted to those nutritional disorders, such as rickets and scurvy which are due to lack of specific nutrients in the diet. However, it is generally taken to include the results of general underfeeding.

The primary causes of most malnutrition occurring in the world are poverty and ignorance. Thus even in affluent, developed countries a comparatively small minority of the population is affected through failure to maintain a good DIET; these include the elderly, migrant workers and their families, the lowest paid and the chronically unemployed. Severe malnutrition in such countries is uncommon (though it has been estimated that up to 2 per cent of the total population of the U.S.A. suffers from malnutrition, and the percentages in certain groups such as the Eskimos and Indians may be extremely high). In virtually all the underdeveloped countries the overwhelming majority of the population is subject to malnutrition. Uneducated in nutritional requirements, ill-versed in agricultural techniques (or landless and unemployed), and racked by intestinal parasites, hundreds of millions of people are frankly under-nourished or become so with the failure of even one harvest and its attendant food-price inflation.

By far the most important dietary deficiency disease is protein-calorie malnutrition, which affects tens of millions of children in Asia, Africa, the Middle East, the Caribbean, and Latin America. Its effects range from those caused mainly by protein deprivation, i.e., kwashiorkor, to marasmus, caused by severe continuous restriction of calories, protein and other nutrients. Intermediate states are generally found. When protein and energy requirements are most needed to meet the demands of growth, as in infancy, childhood, and at puberty, insufficient protein in the diet, generally accompanied by restricted calorie intake, leads to the development of kwashiorkor. In populations living on minimal protein and calorie intake, kwashiorkor epidemics may be precipitated by outbreaks of feverish illness such as malaria or measles, or by infestation with malarial parasites. The disease may affect people of all ages, but is commonest in children between the ages of 1 and 4 years, occurring after weaning from the breast to an unsuitable diet low in protein and calories, such as maize porridge. Marasmus, by contrast, principally affects infants under one year of age. It generally follows the early failure or deliberate ending of breast feeding and its replacement by dilute milk, milk products or other diet low in both calories and protein. In addition, unhygienic preparation of such food leads to repeated gastro-intestinal infections, which the mother all too often treats by virtual starvation for long periods.

Protein malnutrition carries a high death rate even amongst those who receive skilled treatment. And though even children with very severe kwashiorkor or marasmus may be 'cured' through careful dietary measures, education of the mother in sound nutritional practice is equally vital if relapses are to be prevented. Treatment should thus include a minimum of modern medical technology, and the maximum opportunity for learning through practice.

Prerequisites for the prevention of protein malnutrition are: general health and nutritional education, the abolition of urban poverty, the introduction of appropriate agricultural technology, malaria and measles prevention programmes, and effective population control. Similarly, the prevention of most nutritional disorders amongst the potentially affected groups in affluent countries requires combined health educational and social measures.

There are a number of medical conditions which cause malnutrition in spite of a good diet. These include steatorrhoea which limits the absorption of calcium and fat-soluble vitamins, cirrhosis of the liver which may interfere with the proper utilization of nutrients, and a kidney disorder in which there is loss of protein in the urine.

In addition, insufficiency of MINERAL SALT causes disease, e.g., anaemia resulting from lack of iron or goitre from lack of iodine; and there are a considerable number of DEFICIENCY DISEASES, caused by insufficiency of one or more of the specific vitamins.

Malta fever. See BRUCELLOSIS.

mammary glands. The BREASTS.

mammography. Examination of the breasts by infra-red rays or x-rays. This can often reveal the existence of a tumour or cyst at an early stage when treatment is easier and more effective than if diagnosis is not made until the swelling can be seen and felt.

mania. Often used as a loose term, applied to any form of mental disorder or even a strong preoccupation, such as stamp collecting, religion, etc.; the medical definition of mania, however, is the manic phase of a MANIC-DEPRESSIVE PSYCHOSIS.

manic-depressive psychosis. A disorder of mood in which excitement and mania alternate with periods of depression; delusions are prominent and suicide is relatively common. A specific cause has not been identified. Inheritance plays some part, about 5 to 10 per cent of sufferers having had a parent similarly affected, but many other factors are also recognized: childbirth, the climacteric, head injury, severe infection (particularly influenza), bereavement, financial problems, and difficulties in personal relationships. These factors may act alone or together; but on the other hand often no cause can be identified.

The depressive phase of the illness usually begins and ends gradually, though abrupt transitions may occur. It is characterized by a general slowing down of all the faculties. Appetite and sexual desire are diminished. Sleep often ends at 3 or 4 a.m., to be followed by hours of fitful dozing. Confidence and interest are lost, as is the ability to experience pleasure. Slowed down in this fashion, the person's life often becomes filled with preoccupations and worries from which he is unable to escape. Such an attack may last for weeks or months. If more severely affected, the person may become obsessed by past failure and misery, and profoundly pessimistic about the future. Filled with self-reproach and self-depreciation he may develop delusions of poverty, or of his own wickedness, or even that he is dead. Suicidal ideas may be present, and suicidal attempts may occur in any person with more than a mild degree of depression so that some cases do end in suicide. Most, however, gradually recover spontaneously, though a few pass into the manic phase. A substantial number have repeated attacks and a few develop chronic depression. Mild cases may be treated in their own homes with anti-depressant drugs by day, sleeping pills by night, and the pursuance of a regular, undemanding daily routine, including work where possible. The more severely depressed are admitted to hospital and generally receive electro-convulsive and drug therapy.

The manic phase of the illness is uncommon. It is characterized by an increase in activity with lessened self-restraint. Work efficiency is generally unaffected in the mild early stages of an attack, but the person may be indiscreet and extravagant, and unpersuadable, through loss of insight, of the abnormality of his behaviour. If he passes into mania his activity gets out of hand; with incessant speech, shouting and singing, and apparently purposeless activity his state of excitement becomes socially unbearable. Often neglecting his food, he may be unable to sleep, and may have increased sexual desire and decreased sexual restraint. Manic attacks are usually shorter than depressive ones, and most recover spontaneously, but relapse is common and a few patients develop chronic mania. Treatment is generally undertaken in hospital and includes the use of tranquillizers.

In all cases of manic-depressive psychosis, consideration of a patient's underlying personality and environment is vital in providing treatment. During the recovery period attention has to be given both to improving his adjustment to life and to making changes in his domestic, work and social environment.

Manic-depressive psychosis occurs in about one person in a hundred throughout a lifetime, affecting women about twice as frequently as men.

manipulation. A rather vague term that covers the setting of broken bones, the replacement of dislocated joints, the breaking down of adhesions that have rendered active movement of a joint difficult, and the treatment of various diseases by movement of the spine.

The placing of the broken ends of a fractured bone in the best position for successful healing is a very ancient part of medical treatment and has given rise to the modern speciality of manipulative surgery, while assisted movement of joints stiffened by disease or injury has similarly given rise to physiotherapy.

Outside orthodox medicine lie two systems of manipulation: chiropractic, which is based on the idea that many (or all) diseases are caused by pressure on nerves and can be cured by appropriate manipulation of the spine; and OSTEOPATHY.

Mantoux test. See BCG VACCINATION.

MAO. See MONOAMINE OXIDASE.

marasmus. A disease of MALNUTRITION.

marihuana. A form of the drug CANNABIS.

marital disharmony. Discord in marriage which may be overcome or go on to complete marital breakdown. The extent of marital disharmony in our society is unknown. The statistics of such bodies as the Marriage Guidance Council refer only to the minority who seek their help, while divorce statistics refer only to those marriages which end in the divorce courts. Furthermore, causes of marital breakdown accepted by divorce courts – adultery, desertion, cruelty, and so forth – tell little about the underlying causes of disharmony, many of which reflect individual and social expectations of marriage and the extent to which these are unfulfilled. For example, in a society such as our own, which places great emphasis on romantic love and sexual exclusiveness within marriage, a single sexual peccadillo has often been enough to precipitate complete marital breakdown. By contrast, until modern times at least, middle class marriages in France were more often arranged with considerations of birth and fortune in mind, and discreet extra-marital liaisons, albeit only by the husband, were tolerated.

The main causes of contemporary marital disharmony are probably emotion-al immaturity and sexual dissatisfaction. The younger the age of the couple at marriage the greater is their chance of appearing in the divorce courts. Teenagers are rarely equipped to cope with the demanding relationships of marriage, and seldom have the capacity for sexual relationships mature enough to give their marriage a good start. Husband and wife often develop in conflicting directions as they emerge into emotional adulthood, and the arrival of a baby may mean that the young mother becomes preoccupied with the child while the young father seeks other interests. There is much evidence to suggest that marriage (and, with it, parenthood) should be postponed until the mid-twenties.

As the expectation of sexual fulfilment in marriage – the giving and receiving of delight which deepens and reinforces the bond between the partners – has increased, so has the disharmony consequent upon sexual dissatisfaction. This dissatisfaction, e.g., when the women has pain on intercourse (usually capable of remedy) or where the man reaches his climax early (again often remediable), is an important cause of breakdown in marriages in which joint conjugal roles operate (see MARRIAGE). Such breakdown generally occurs in the early years of marriage.

Disharmony in segregated-role marriages most often centres around cruelty and financial irresponsibility, particularly by the husband. Here, if breakdown occurs it is usually later, when the children are physically more independent. Though it is generally recognized that harm may be caused to children by the divorce of their parents, many underestimate the potentially harmful effects of continued upbringing by constantly bickering parents.

The appearance of marital disharmony generally calls forth an informal network of advice from relatives and friends, usually to the partners individually. They may usefully seek the help of their family doctor, their minister of religion or a marriage guidance organization. Though most instances of marital disharmony are thus resolved some inevitably result in DIVORCE, the number of divorces in a society being more a reflection of the liberality of its divorce laws and the cost of obtaining a divorce than an accurate statement of the number of marriages irretrievably broken down. Something like 20 per cent of British marriages end in divorce.

marriage. A union between a man and a woman such that the children borne by the woman are recognized as the legitimate offspring of both spouses. Polygamy (as practised in Islamic countries) is not considered in this article, which deals only with monogamy.

Choice of spouse. In all societies premarital sexual relationships are strictly coded, choice of spouse is bound by certain rules, and anti-adultery customs are widespread. The taboo against incest appears to be universal nowadays, though cousin marriage is still commonplace in many societies. The desire to limit the occurrence of x-linked and autosomal recessive hereditary disease provides contemporary scientific support for the widespread custom of marrying out of both the family and, very often, the community.

The choice of spouse may be made by the parents or other close relations of eligible persons, by recognized marriage brokers within the community, or by the couple themselves. The latter is the almost universal practice in modern societies and is, at a greatly varying rate, coming to replace arranged marriages in almost all societies in which these take place. For all its appearance to the contrary, even the arrangement of marriage by the couple themselves operates within strictly defined limits. Because of the basic necessity that the couple have to meet each other, geographical and social limitations operate: thus people tend to marry those of their own district, religion, race, social class, and educational level. Amongst university graduates the last consideration appears to be the most important, whilst the development of greater geographical mobility and the drift towards a single world culture seems gradually to be making the other factors less important.

Conjugal roles within marriage. These are determined by the social, legal and religious frameworks within which marriage takes place, as well as by the families of origin of the spouses and their own personal attributes. Marriage roles

adapt and develop as children are born and the family develops, and particularly as the changes in the social standing and activities of women develop.

In pre-industrial societies the conjugal roles of men and women are separate, distinct and forbidden to one another. The husband provides, takes risks, or performs heavy labouring tasks, and he may indeed, without outraging social conventions, enforce his authority by chastising not only his children but also his wife. Meanwhile the wife keeps house and bears and rears children. In modern industrial society most women engage in wage earning before marriage and after their period of childbearing and pre-school child-rearing is over. Decision-making has come to be a shared function, with neither partner dominant, although on any one matter the couple may recognize that one member has greater expertise or experience, e.g., that on failure to reach agreement they will normally accept the husband's view of the best lawnmower or the wife's view of the best cooker to buy.

Yet in spite of their increased economic value to society as a whole, and to their marriages in particular, the ability of women to exercise their rights is limited by their childbearing function, by their exclusion from some traditional male occupations, and by the persistence of traditional attitudes and values. These however are adjusting, though unevenly, where they conflict with new industrial and social developments.

It is sometimes alleged that a common cause of MARITAL DISHARMONY in persons of differing backgrounds or different races is unharmonized ideas of conjugal roles, as when the husband enters matrimony with the idea that he is the dominant partner while the wife starts marriage with the concept of equality. Difficulties of conjugal roles are also liable to arise where one partner is absent for a long period (e.g., the soldier returning from war service) so that, by the time of the return the other partner has become accustomed to making the decisions for the household.

Contemporary patterns of conjugal roles reflect the uneven pace of change in different groups in modern society. The evolution of 'joint' conjugal roles is progressing rapidly throughout the world, with husbands sharing domestic work and child-rearing as wives share the role of provider. However, such tendencies are still poorly developed amongst the lower-paid and less educated, where 'segregated' conjugal roles are usual – with wives responsible for housework, child care and budgeting, and husbands for providing basic housekeeping money, doing occasional arduous tasks about the home, and being the ultimate child disciplinarian. Those in joint-role marriages more often take their relaxation in the home, together and with friends of both sexes, and have greater expectations of the sexual satisfactions to be obtained from marriage. Joint- and segregated-role marriages are extreme types; most marriages are intermediate with a bias towards one type or the other.

Trends in marriage. Although marriage generally takes place later amongst the better-off and better-educated, for a long time the age at marriage has been dropping amongst people of all social origins. The consequences of early marriage are manifold. Divorce rates are much higher amongst those married in their teens and child management is sometimes poor where the parents are themselves hardly mature. On the other hand the advantages of early completion of families, which accompanies a lower age of marriage, include fewer complications of childbirth and a lower risk of producing a mongol child. Marriage appears to be conducive to better health and, on average, married people who are admitted to hospital are discharged sooner than unmarrieds, marriage providing a valuable social support system. Throughout this century the prevalence of marriage, and the esteem in which the married state is held, have increased steadily. The consequent eagerness of people on the one hand to enter marriage, and on the other to expect to achieve contentment as of right, is reflected in the increasing number of marriages which fail. The considerable liberalization of divorce laws in most industrial societies allows partners in failed marriages to dissolve their marriage contract and become available for re-marriage. In consequence divorce rates are also rising rapidly, and an increasing number of young people reaching marriageable age are the products of marriages which have failed. This cannot but influence the pattern of marriage of the future.

masochism. A sexual PERVERSION or deviation in which the person derives pleasure from being beaten, punished, humiliated or abused, usually by someone of the opposite sex. It is in many ways the opposite of SADISM.

In the typical form the individual is controlled by the idea of being completely and unconditionally subject to the will of an attractive person of the opposite sex; he often spends much of his time in fantasies of being whipped or abused, with generally one form of punishment (e.g., beating on the buttocks) and one imagined punisher predominating; he tries to realize these fantasies with the person of his choice or with a substitute; he obtains his sexual pleasure from this experienced (or sometimes imagined) passively endured violence; and he is incapable of finding sexual satisfaction in normal ways. In many cases, however, the desire for punishment never goes beyond the fantasy level, and where the fantasy is realized the whipping is often a preparation for sexual relations rather than a substitute for them.

Early investigators often termed masochism a female characteristic, but it has been shown that it is also very common in men.

Some cases of masochism undoubtedly originate in a child being beaten for masturbating and coming to associate the humiliation and pain of the beating with the pleasure of masturbation. It is sometimes alleged that the deviation may start with the sensuous excitement in childhood when a mother embraces the child and gently pats its buttocks. On the causes of masochism we have a great deal of psychological theorizing and very little proved fact.

While a sadist is potentially dangerous to others, since he enjoys inflicting pain and may do serious damage, a masochist is not dangerous. The pain is inflicted on himself and there comes a point in which the initial pain-pleasure feeling is destroyed by the intensity of the pain, so that the masochist seeks the cessation of the punishment.

The term is coming to be used in a wider sense that implies enjoying one's own helplessness or suffering, or deliberately denying oneself enjoyment and success, or punishing oneself (e.g., by excessive work perhaps as a reaction to forbidden desires). It is also increasingly held that sadism and masochism are only the extremes of the spectrum of human attitudes: while few of us would normally enjoy inflicting pain on others and while relatively few of us would enjoy being whipped by an attractive member of the opposite sex, perhaps most of us have a mild streak of sadism (and occasionally enjoy dominating and mastering) and also a mild streak of masochism (so that we at times relish being 'ticked off' by our partners).

massage. Treatment by stroking, rubbing or kneading the superficial parts of the body with the hand or with an instrument, for such purposes as restoring the power of movement, breaking up ADHESIONS, improving the circulation, aiding digestion, or simply in order to produce a sense of relaxation and well-being. Massage is commonly employed in physiotherapy as an important part of an integrated physical rehabilitation programme.

mastitis. Inflammation of the female breast. It occurs generally in the early weeks of breast feeding as a result of infection developing in stagnant milk which is lying in the broken surface of uncared-for, cracked nipples. Part of the breast becomes hard and tender and the overlying skin reddened. Treatment is by antibiotics, prevention of milk accumulation by proper care of CRACKED NIPPLES, and kaolin poultices. Breast feeding need only be interrupted if pus is present, in which case incision and drainage is required. Mastitis rarely occurs when the simple rules of breast care and hygiene are observed.

mastoid disease. A complication of otitis

media (middle ear infection), in which infection spreads from the middle ear to involve the mastoid bone behind the ear, leading to pain, increased discharge or its sudden cessation, increasing deafness and general debility. As permanent deafness, meningitis, or even brain abscess may result from neglected mastoid disease, the doctor's advice should be sought if earache is troublesome. Treatment is by antibiotics and sometimes an operation is necessary. Mastoid disease is prevented by prompt recognition and adequate treatment of otitis media. It is now rare in Britain, but still common in underdeveloped countries.

masturbation. Attempted satisfaction of one's sexual urges alone and unaided. Commonly the hands, fingers and thighs are used to stimulate the head of the penis or the clitoris. This generally results in orgasm within a few minutes. It is widely practised from early childhood onwards, and is a harmless substitute for sexual intercourse except when it interferes with the establishment of normal heterosexual relations, or when feelings of guilt resulting from it lead to personality conflicts. Unfortunately, as a result of erroneous opinions expressed by doctors and others in the past, these guilt feelings are quite widespread.

maternal and child welfare. An omnibus term – nowadays often altered to maternal and child health – for services designed to promote the physical and mental health of both mother and child, and to prevent, recognize and treat departures from health in the expectant and nursing mother, the unborn child, the infant, and the pre-school child. Broadly the term includes antenatal, post-natal and child health clinics, the work of obstetricians and midwives, much of the work of health visitors and part of the work of paediatricians. Essentially the services aim to improve the health of mother and child, so that the mother gives birth to her child with the minimum danger and discomfort and without deleterious effects on her own health, while the child is born healthy and receives adequate care until he starts school.

Achievements of maternal welfare services. The greatest achievement has undoubtedly been to cut maternal mortality from around 10 per cent in mid-Victorian times to 0.2 per cent by the early 1940s with subsequent further reduction in the era of chemotherapy and antibiotics, which completed the virtual eradication of sepsis.

Achievements of child welfare services. The development of child welfare services in Britain roughly coincided with other changes likely to improve the health of children – decreased family size, improved living standards and introduction of effective treatment. Nevertheless, many studies have shown beyond a shadow of doubt the enormous value of child welfare services, e.g., sharp reduction of infant

deaths in areas that had increased their health visiting staffs and their clinics without any similar reduction in deaths in comparable areas that had not achieved increases, and in due course a fall in deaths in the latter areas after they had belatedly extended their staffs. Broadly, these services have been responsible for almost all the education carried out on infant health and well-being from nutrition to requirements for mental development, and from prevention of burns and scalds to encouragement of immunization. Some visiting of apparently healthy children remains necessary, to maintain rapport with parents, to identify the beginnings of departure from physical or emotional health, and to ensure that a parent to whom such departure is not yet obvious has enough confidence in the health expert to accept advice.

measles. A very infectious virus disease which few children escaped before widespread vaccination became available. One attack usually leaves the individual immune to further attacks. It is acquired by inhaling infected droplets and, after a ten-day incubation period, produces a chest infection, a rash, and conjunctivitis. It is more serious in children under 3 years who are badly nourished or suffering from other diseases. The most common complication is bronchopneumonia which may be fatal. Otitis media is also common, while measles encephalitis, though rare, is also sometimes fatal. Treatment is essentially directed to relieving symptoms: fourteen days' isolation should follow the appearance of the rash, and antibiotics are prescribed for the treatment of complications. Prevention is obtained by a single injection of measles vaccine during the second year of life.

median. In anatomy and pathology, midline or central. The median plane divides the body into right and left halves. The median nerve runs down the arm and supplies the muscles that bend the wrist and some muscles of the thumb.

mediastinum. The collection of tissues and organs separating the two lungs, between the breast bone or sternum in front and the vertebral column behind, and from the base of the neck above to the diaphragm below. It contains the heart and great blood vessels, the trachea, oesophagus, thymus gland, lymph nodes, and other structures and tissues.

medical officer of health. In countries in which some or all aspects of community health are the responsibility of a local authority or a local health board (as opposed to being a national or state responsibility), the medical officer of health is the doctor in administrative charge of the health services provided by a county, town or district.

In Britain until 1974 the medical officer of health directed and coordinated the work of public health doctors, health visitors, midwives, sanitary inspectors, home nurses, and (until 1948) the staffs of over two-thirds of the country's hospitals. His functions included the control of infectious diseases, the provision of a healthy environment, organization and development of school health services, health education, responsibility for fever hospitals, mental hospitals, maternity hospitals, and in many districts responsibility for home helps and for the provision of old people's homes. He was essentially a mixture of administrator, epidemiologist, sociologist and health educator, concerned with all matters pertaining to health.

Removal of hospitals from control in 1948 gave him increased opportunity to concentrate on prevention of disease and promotion of health, but during the next twenty-five years it became increasingly obvious (1) that health visitors, social workers and sanitary inspectors were aquiring full professional status and could not forever be directed by a doctor, and (2) that there was a need for integrated planning of hospital and community health services. So in 1974 health boards were created (with as top managers a medical officer, a nursing officer, an administrator, and a finance officer). The MOH disappeared: the portion of his work concerned with co-ordination and deployment of health visitors and home nurses passed to the chief nursing officer of the health board, the health education component passed to the chief health education officer (although he was made responsible to the board's chief medical officer), the sanitary portion went to the director of environmental health of the district local authority, and the strictly medical part passed to the chief administrative medical officer of the board.

medicines. Substances taken by mouth, or otherwise put into or on the body, specifically for the prevention or treatment of disease. See DRUGS.

megaloblastic anaemia. Anaemia in which the blood contains underdeveloped red blood corpuscles termed megaloblasts. By far the commonest of such anaemias is PERNICIOUS ANAEMIA but a similar anaemia occasionally occurs in infants given a diet with insufficient folic acid.

megalomania. Preoccupation with ideas of exalted power or wealth, commonly called 'delusions of grandeur'. Minor degrees are common in everyday life and generally represent an over-compensation for a feeling of inferiority. The types of medical interest are essentially those in which ideas of power co-exist with feelings of persecution.

In PARANOIA and the paranoid type of SCHIZOPHRENIA megalomania is often accompanied by delusions of persecution which are systematized, i.e., if a single false belief for instance that relatives and associates are conspiring to deprive the sufferer of a fortune or are plotting to

Keep all medicines out of the reach of children

murder him) is accepted as correct, the delusions appear consistent and logical. In this form of mental illness the patient living in an atmosphere of suspicion and surrounded by imaginary 'enemies' perhaps indulges in the delusions of grandeur in an attempt to maintain self-respect. Until the disease becomes advanced it is difficult to differentiate this dangerous condition from the paranoid reactions discussed later. Yet diagnosis is important because the insane person may seek to kill or injure his 'persecutors' in imagined self-defence.

Commoner are paranoid reactions in which most of the personality remains comparatively intact though rigid and suspicious, but on one particular aspect there are systematized delusions of grandeur or of persecution or often of both. Here the sufferer from megalomania while perhaps earning his living by normal work, may have delusions of a religious mission, often of a messianic nature, of vast political or social reforms, or of amazing inventions. Religious paranoiacs for example, may believe that they have been sent by God on a mission of human salvation and may spend much of their time preaching to attract converts to their cause. Their sermons are frequently filled with dire threats of eternal damnation and similar consequences of non-conversion. Many paranoiacs become attached to political parties, often to extremist movements, becoming tireless and fanatical and often self-righteous, and frequently do more harm than good to their cause, though they occasionally acquire enormous influence and massive followings. Some paranoiacs invent remarkable devices which they experience great difficulty in marketing. They then become increasingly convinced that they are the victims of a conspiracy to steal their invention or even the subject of a plot to damage their country by denying it the benefits of their great talents.

Thirdly, there occur paranoid states, usually transient and with spontaneous recovery. Here the individual is initially suspicious or boastful or both, but temporary delusions of grandeur or of persecution are precipitated by a situation causing acute mental stress.

Whether we think of megalomania or of ideas of persecution, the paranoid state is a temporary, abnormal state, caused in susceptible persons by a stressful situation and with complete recovery highly probable. The paranoid reaction is long-lasting but does not usually necessitate admission to mental hospital, but paranoia or paranoid schizophrenia is a very serious mental disease.

meiosis. See GENETICS.

melaena. Black, tarry motions, a result of the swallowing of blood, e.g., from bleeding of the nose, or of bleeding from the stomach or intestine. Irrespective of the cause, the blood has remained in the digestive system long enough to be acted on by the digestive juices, and the iron of the haemoglobin has been largely converted into iron sulphide.

By contrast the passing of red blood indicates bleeding near the anus, e.g., from haemorrhoids.

melancholia. A depressed emotional state with abnormal mental sluggishness, apathy, and indifference to one's surroundings.

membranes. (1) A synonym for the amniotic sac; see CHILDBIRTH. (2) Mucous membranes are mucus-secreting membranous structures that line body cavities or passages that are open to the external environment, for example, the lips, mouth, throat, windpipe, etc.

memory. That faculty of mind by which sensations, impressions, and ideas are recalled. Since the brain has to process and co-ordinate information available to it from the external environment, to analyse the best course of action to take on the basis of this information, and to instruct the remainder of the organism to act on the basis of this analysis, it requires to have some way of comparing the information reaching it at any time with that previously encountered describing comparable situations, the responses made to these situations, and the outcome of these responses. It is the mechanism of recording, storing, sifting and comparing information which is referred to as memory.

The process of fixation of the memory takes place in at least two stages. New information arriving at the brain is placed first in a short-term memory store, probably situated just below the cerebral cortex. It is easily lost from this store. That which remains is transferred after some minutes or hours to a permanent long-term store situated in the cortex itself. The natural loss of memory from the short-term store may be increased by shocks to the brain caused, for example, by convulsions or concussion which are known to lead to memory loss for the events immediately preceding them. Memories in the permanent store are not lost in this fashion.

Disorders. Memory is referred to as disordered when recall is disturbed. It often gives the appearance of being disordered when the real problem is loss of attention, as in depression or during hallucinations.

Disorders of memory are commonly divided into amnesias, paramnesias and hyperamnesias. Amnesia, or absence of memory, may be complete or partial: amnesia confined to recent events is characteristic of senile cerebral degeneration and its increase may be prevented by supply of vitamin B_1, while in brain damage there is often persistent amnesia for events immediately preceding and following the accident. Paramnesia, false recollection, may co-exist with amnesia in organic psychoses. Hyperamnesia denotes excessive retention of detailed memories, and is found in some prodigies and in certain mental disorders.

Mendel. Gregor Johann Mendel (1822-1884), a Moravian monk, botanist, and the pioneer of modern GENETICS.

Ménière's disease. See HEAD NOISES.

meningitis. Inflammation of the membranes (meninges) which cover the brain. Sometimes the inflammation is caused by the spread of infection from a compound fracture of the skull or from chronic middle ear or mastoid disease. More frequently it is caused by micro-organisms that spread in the sub-arachnoid space between the two inner membranes. Meningitis is classified according to the responsible micro-organism, e.g., meningococcal or cerebrospinal fever (the commonest), tuberculous (inevitably fatal until after the discovery of the antibiotic, streptomycin) and viral (usually the mildest).

The term meningitis, used without any qualifying word such as 'tuberculous' generally means infection by the meningococcus which causes cerebrospinal fever. The germ can be transmitted by the breathing of infected droplets from cases or more frequently from carriers. The onset of this disease is usually abrupt after a short incubation period of one to three days, with high temperature, rigor, headache, delirium and muscular stiffness particularly of the neck and back muscles which in severe cases may lead to arching of the body. Haemorrhagic rashes also sometimes occur and are the basis for the synonym 'spotted fever'.

Precise diagnosis in cases of meningitis depends on examination of the cerebrospinal fluid, samples of which are obtained by lumbar puncture.

Meningitis of all types was formerly a grave condition with a high death rate but the outlook has greatly improved since the introduction of antibiotic drugs. This is even true of tuberculous meningitis, formerly a relatively common and invariably fatal condition in infants and children, but now less often encountered because of the general decline in the sources of tuberculous infection.

menopause. The stage of life in women at which menstruation ceases. It is also known as 'the change of life' or the female climacteric. The menopause usually takes place between the ages of 45 and 50 but there is a considerable range of variation related to race and inheritance. An early onset of menstruation (menarche) is frequently associated with late cessation, and a premature menopause in the fourth decade of life is not very unusual.

The menstrual periods normally cease in one of three ways. They may stop abruptly and never recur; they may continue rhythmically as before with blood loss gradually diminishing to zero; or the regular monthly cycle may progressively lengthen to several months and finally terminate. Any departure from these typical histories should be regarded as pathological and any form of irregular haemorrhage in women of menopausal age requires careful investigation.

The menopause is due to a decline in activity of the ovaries and this produces various other effects. The sexual organs undergo atrophy and retrogression; e.g., the breasts shrivel and the vagina becomes smaller and its secretion diminishes. This may cause pain on intercourse and diminished resistance to infection. Within the pelvis the tissues become lax and support to the uterus is diminished so that displacement may occur.

In addition there may be general symptoms related to alterations in the balance of the ENDOCRINE GLANDS, such as increased deposition of fat, atrophy of skin, growth of facial hair, and disturbances of the cardio-vascular system. The latter are responsible for the very characteristic menopausal symptoms of 'hot flushes' and excessive tendency to perspire. There may also be headaches, irritability, and depression which occasionally develops into melancholia. In most cases a more normal hormonal balance is gradually re-established and the adminstration of preparations of oestrogen can be reliably expected to relieve the more distressing symptoms of discomfort until this occurs.

In most women the stresses of the menopause are not extreme and they soon subside. Well-being is restored, sexual desire is retained, and there are compensations in the loss of pre-menstrual tension and the recurrent discomforts of menstruation. Occasional cases of continued emotional distress require psychiatric advice.

A parallel but slower and more gradual CLIMACTERIC, with waning of fertility, sexual activity and general vitality, occurs in men, sometimes accompanied by irritability, depression and reduced mental concentration.

menorrhagia. See FLOODING.

menstruation. Throughout that part of her life when a woman is capable of bearing children, her sex-organs undergo a regular monthly cycle of events. This is marked by bleeding from the uterus occurring about every twenty-eight days and lasting for four or five days, and is known as menstruation or the menstrual period.

The menstrual cycle is controlled by the ovaries. At the start of the cycle, on about the first day of a menstrual period, a small mass of special cells, known as a Graafian follicle and enclosing an individual egg cell or ovum, begins to enlarge and ripen and project on the surface of the ovary. About the fourteenth day of the cycle the follicle ruptures (ovulation) and the egg cell then enters the Fallopian tube of the uterus and makes its way to the body of the uterus. The Graafian follicle, after it ruptures, undergoes further changes and secretes a hormone called progesterone. This stimulates the lining of the uterus to thicken and develop in readiness for the ovum to become embedded in it, in the event of it being fertilized. The climax of the process is reached on about the twenty-eighth day of the menstrual cycle. If fertilization has not occurred the developed uterus wall breaks down to cause the menstrual flow, carrying the unfertilized ovum with it. The whole cycle then starts again. If the ovum is fertilized the uterus wall is ready to receive it and there the EMBRYO will develop.

Ovulation and entry of the ovum into the Fallopian tube occur about the fourteenth day of the cycle. This is the best time for fertilization, a fact which forms the basis of the 'rhythm method' of BIRTH CONTROL.

During the menstrual period hygiene is important. The flow may be absorbed by sanitary towels or by an internal tampon, and a daily bath is no longer regarded as unsuitable.

Menstruation may be accompanied by some minor pain and discomfort but this can usually be relieved by rest, warmth and analgesics.

Premenstrual tension. While in many women menstruation starts each month without any previous symptoms, it is not uncommon for the onset of menstruation to be heralded by a few days of irritability, nervousness, feelings of depression, headaches and increased liability to minor accidents. The symptoms are thought to be related in part to retention of fluid. In general a modicum of rest, restriction of salt intake for four or five days and mild analgesics such as aspirin cope with the condition, but in serious cases medical advice should be sought.

Disorders related to menstruation are described under AMENORRHOEA, DYSMENORRHOEA and METRORRHAGIA.

mental deficiency. There are in any population individuals who vary quite widely in their personalities, skills and abilities but who nevertheless can be regarded as normal. Standard INTELLIGENCE TESTS are so constructed that the average intelligence quotient (IQ) is 100 but an actual score which reaches at least 70 to 75 is regarded as still being within the limits of normality.

Individuals who cannot reach even this level of performance are said to be mentally defective or to suffer from mental handicap. It is important to draw a distinction between mental deficiency and mental illness because the latter is a state of abnormal mental function afflicting persons who are usually otherwise of normal mental capacity.

Legally, mental deficiency is defined as a condition of arrested or incomplete development of mind existing before the age of 18 years, whether arising from inherent causes or induced by disease or injury. The usual classification is (1) mildly mentally handicapped with IQ 50 to 70 and (2) severely mentally handicapped with IQ below 50.

The overall proportion of all types of mental handicap in the community is probably about 25 per thousand. Of these only about 4 per thousand can be classified as severely handicapped. Most of the others although regarded as mildly handicapped within their school environment usually prove to be capable of living independently in the community without the aid of many special services, partly because of their ability to undertake successfully work which does not call for skill and partly because their abilities continue to develop during a substantial part of young adult life.

Those who are severely handicapped present a greater problem. Very many are in special hospitals not only because of their subnormal intelligence but because of social incapacity and deviant behaviour, or very often because there is simply no suitable provision for them elsewhere. A recent survey showed that at least three-quarters were continent, ambulant and had no behavioural problems and that only a few actually required the skilled medical and nursing attention which a hospital provides.

Apart from these facts, there are other considerations such as the effect on personality of the regimentation of hospital life, loss of identity, and under-activity. There is therefore a growing appreciation that large mental sub-

The menstrual cycle

normality hospitals are 'anti-therapeutic' and that cases of this kind would benefit from being returned to the community and accommodated in small hostels so that they might be enabled to lead as happy and fulfilling a life as possible.

Causes. Many cases are genetically determined. The best known of these are mongolism, due to chromosomal abnormality, and phenylketonuria, a metabolic defect. Others are related to the mother's health during pregnancy, to obstetric complications, and to the condition of the child at birth, particularly if premature. After birth various cultural and material factors influence development. Amongst these are social practices, education, family size and structure, family stability, housing, and poverty.

Prevention of mental retardation. Causes related to GENETICS can be minimized or avoided by GENETIC GUIDANCE; mongolism can be detected through examination of the amniotic fluid and abortion considered in positive cases; there are also tests for phenylketonuria and similar metabolic conditions. There is still scope for better antenatal and obstetric care and improved post-natal and child health services. Immunization against rubella (German measles) and the detection and treatment of Rhesus incompatibility, mycoplasma infections, and placental insufficiency are recent developments which are contributing to a reduction in mental damage. During later development there are opportunities for better child care, with early detection of abnormalities and retardation, backed up by 'preventive education' and organized social care. Measures of this kind can identify children at risk and provide for their special needs before their behaviour and development deviate too irretrievably from acceptable normality.

mental diseases. Mental disturbances fall into two categories: PSYCHOSIS and NEUROSIS; and there is also a borderline between psychiatry and medicine known as PSYCHOSOMATIC DISEASE.

mental efficiency. The capacity to cope competently and without excessive strain with ordinary occupational, domestic and social happenings.

Estimation. Although we all have a rough idea of what the term means, exact measurement is extraordinarily difficult. We could start with an intelligence test, on the assumption that it really measures intelligence and not the particular parts of intelligence needed for the test, and could seek to grade mental efficiency simply according to intelligence. Yet some people of very low intelligence appear to manage their affairs well, and conversely some people who have demonstrated high intelligence, e.g., by obtaining degrees and even higher degrees, show a lack of competence in matters of everyday life. Clearly mental efficiency is not just intelligence.

Again it is obviously related not only to the person but to the relevant circumstances or events. A man may display considerable mental efficiency when occupying one post but may show incompetence or excessive strain when promoted to a more difficult post. A woman may appear an efficient housewife and mother in a normal two-parent family but be quite incapable of coping if her husband dies suddenly.

In the present state of our knowledge it is probably desirable to limit the estimation of mental efficiency to particular existing or hypothetical circumstances, e.g., to ask, 'is this elderly doctor alert enough to diagnose my illness?' or 'does this woman have the common-sense and stability to handle the office during my absence?'

Improvement. Even though we cannot yet measure mental efficiency with any degree of accuracy we know many factors that affect it. Of these a few are mentioned below.

1. Physical health. Body and mind are intimately connected, and mental efficiency presupposes reasonable mental health. A person who has been deprived of adequate sleep for several successive nights, who is undernourished and hungry, who is physically exhausted, who is in a high fever or suffering from considerable pain is not mentally efficient. Clearly the maintenance of good physical health is important for mental efficiency; and obviously it is sensible to try to avoid taking important decisions at a time when our health is below par.

2. Drugs, etc. The effect of dangerous drugs in decreasing mental efficiency is obvious, as is the effect of excessive alcohol, although the borderline of excess may be arguable. Clearly avoidance of these drugs and of too much alcohol is conducive to mental efficiency. When we leave the obvious points, however, much is unknown. To give an example: it is questionable whether the efficiency of a poor sleeper is increased or decreased by a mild sedative at night.

3. Mental exercise. Just as muscles grow weak from lack of use, mental capacities decline if unexercised. While excessive mental effort is as harmful as excessive physical effort, it is good for us to have a reasonable amount of cerebral activity.

4. Cultivation of mental poise. Strong emotions and prolonged worry deplete one's stores of mental energy and therefore impair efficiency. Unfortunately, while it is easy to advise people to avoid excessive anger, fear, worry and jealousy in the interests of both mental and physical health, it is much more difficult to suggest methods of avoiding these things. Certainly a man can strive to face up to the reasonably worst happening that might arise out of his fears and worries, and he will often find that it is much less serious than his vague fears had suggested. Again

he can, in the old phrase, 'count his blessings': there are many good and pleasant things in the lives of all of us. Or he can discuss his problems with somebody whom he trusts, not simply to secure the advice of a more emotionally detached person but also to gain relief by bringing his fears and worries to the surface. Not least, he can try to force himself to devote part of his mental attention to the well-being of another person or organization, thus temporarily detaching himself from his own problems.

5. Achieving satisfactions. Probably nothing is more harmful to mental efficiency than continued lack of satisfactions, e.g., the man who feels that he is becoming too old for promotion, that his children have gone their own way, that his wife is much more interested in her job than in him, that he lost his sole recreation when he became too stiff for tennis and that his one attempt to serve the community failed when he stood for a local council and was not elected. Some experts advocate the pursuit of limited satisfactions, living for the day or the week, e.g., deciding 'I'll complete this particular piece of work today and tomorrow' (and mildly luxuriating in having achieved the goal). Others advise the sustained pursuit of larger and more long-term goals. In any case some satisfactions are essential for mental efficiency.

6. Cultivating relationships. The human being is a gregarious animal, and the person who lives entirely for himself and by himself is seldom mentally efficient. For emotional health most of us – though there may be a few exceptions – need the companionship of congenial persons with whom we can discuss joys, sorrows, triumphs and losses. In selecting such congenial persons, initially on grounds of similar views, ideas, tastes or backgrounds, we must of course realize that companionship is a two-way process. People are unlikely to be interested in our ideas or problems unless we can take some interest in theirs.

See also KEEPING FIT.

mental health. In Great Britain the treatment of mental disorder absorbs about one-eighth of health service expenditure and occupies nearly half the total complement of hospital beds. The suicide rate of the community averages about 10 per 100,000 each year, and mental, psycho-neurotic and personality disorders are responsible for fully 10 per cent of the total working days lost through certified incapacity for work.

In developed countries the prevalence of mental disease is about 6 persons per thousand of the population, and mental defectives number as many as 25 per thousand. Although comparable figures for under-developed countries are difficult to obtain with any degree of accuracy they are probably much lower. The reasons

suggested for the difference are somewhat speculative but they illustrate some of the factors contributing to the present massive burden of mental disorder and mental ill-health which constitutes not only a community and individual source of distress, but also a serious drain on economic resources.

Since some psychoses and some types of mental deficiency are genetically determined, the basic prevalence of these should not vary much, though one effect of better child health services is to ensure the survival of many more mentally handicapped children. In senile psychosis it is obvious that its prevalence must vary with the age-constitution of the population. If the benefits of civilization ensure more general survival to later ages it is inevitable that more persons will show symptoms of mental disorder resulting from degenerative changes in their brain and blood vessels. However, it is when we leave these clearly recognized conditions and turn to the wide range of other mental illness included in such terms as psycho-neurosis, psychosomatic disease and personality disorder, as well as mere social inadequacy, that we find the greatest difference. It may be that these are more obvious in a civilized environment, but since they are related to stress it is not unreasonable to assume that they will be much more prevalent as a result of the pressures imposed by an increasingly demanding, complex, and changing society.

The factors responsible can be related to culture and social interaction operating in society as a whole, within the family, and at work. Developed countries impose more exacting standards in which the pressures for conformity arouse either rebellion or anxiety and provide innumerable opportunities for conflict not only in personal relationships but in relation to choice of action. There continues to be a decline in religious belief, and faith has been replaced by perplexity, uncertainty, and insecurity. At a more individual level cultural differences between the generations are often irreconcilable. Smaller families weaken the power of kinship. There are not so many aunts and uncles as there once were and the tasks of caring for the aged fall to fewer hands. Housing shortages lead to overcrowding and shared accommodation with all the resulting deterioration in inter-personal relationships. Family ties are loosened by rehousing in distant areas remote from grandparents, relatives and friends. High flats cause social isolation followed by loneliness and depression.

In industry frustration develops from repetitive tasks and lack of creativity; anger is aroused by unsympathetic foremen and uncaring management; anxiety results from considerations of job security.

To these and similar difficulties individuals react in many ways – by rebellion, by 'opting-out', by anxiety, or by developing symptoms of illness. Psycho-neurosis or psychosomatic disease shows as an unconscious escape mechanism, and the possession of a medical certificate of incapacity equates with the former ability of the peasant largely to please himself and not to worry about the problems of maintaining artificial standards and of conforming to a pattern of life with which he was out of sympathy. There is no ready prescription for curing the symptoms of mental distress which stem from the ills of civilization, and perhaps no final solution is even possible. All progress is striving and the less competent members of the community tend inevitably to get hurt.

We live however in a period of great secular change during a transition between feudalism and egalitarianism. Ultimately there may emerge a future of greater tranquillity but there is little certainty of this as we contemplate the great problems of over-population and dwindling resources of food and raw materials.

Nevertheless there are still goals to be achieved in the short term: education; improvement of living and working conditions; encouragement of family integrity; adaptation of industry to provide security, satisfaction and a sense of participation; the pleasurable and intelligent use of leisure; and the provision of adequate care services for all kinds of social and medical problems – all these still provide opportunities for great and beneficial advances.

Perhaps the most immediate lines are (1) genetic guidance, coupled where necessary with contraception, to reduce hereditary mental and physical diseases; (2) child health services designed to reduce by timely advice such detrimental factors as over-strictness, forcing, over-indulgence and inconsistency; and (3) education, fitted to the needs and aptitudes of the individual child, and preparing him for leisure as well as for work.

mercury poisoning. Breathing in or swallowing the vapour of metallic mercury is an industrial hazard as most of its compounds are intensely poisonous. In the past most cases of acute poisoning were due to absorption of mercuric chloride (corrosive sublimate) used as an antiseptic douche or lotion, or to its accidental or deliberate swallowing. Symptoms were severe with damage to bowel and kidneys, and death not infrequently followed.

Chronic mercurial poisoning occurs as an industrial disease in such occupations as thermometer, meter, and mirror making, which use metallic mercury; in the fur felt trade which uses mercuric nitrate; and in the manufacture of detonators (fulminate of mercury). The effects are inflammation of the mucous lining of the mouth, increased flow of saliva, loosening of the teeth, and various nervous symptoms such as optic neuritis, minor epilepsy, tremors and mental disturbance. Strict measures of industrial hygiene must be enforced.

Mercury is also becoming an ecological hazard. Outbreaks of acute poisoning (Minamata disease) have occurred in Japan through eating tuna fish caught in waters contaminated by methyl mercury, an industrial waste. Methyl mercury is also used as a fungicide in the treatment of seed-corn and there have been serious incidents causing many deaths where such grain was eaten instead of being sown.

mescalin. A HALLUCINOGEN obtained from the Mexican agave, with similar effects and dangers as LSD.

mesentery. The mesenteries are folds of peritoneum which hang loosely from the back of the abdomen, join the different parts of the intestine and in effect sling them to the back abdominal wall. The mesenteries also contain numerous lymph glands and vessels, and contain the mesenteric blood vessels which supply blood to the intestine. The mesentery of the small intestine is a roughly fan-shaped fold.

mesmerism. An alternative name for HYPNOSIS.

metabolism. To sustain its vital processes every living organism requires to extract and use the energy stored in FOOD. By digestion food is broken down into simpler substances which are absorbed into the blood stream and thereafter undergo chemical reactions in the body. These reactions provide for the growth and repair of tissue, the production of heat and energy, the activity of muscle and nerve, the manufacture of essential secretions, and finally the passing of waste-products.

These interdependent activities are collectively called general metabolism. When complex substances are broken down the process is catabolism; their chemical conversion is anabolism. Special metabolism is an account of the changes affecting a particular constituent of the diet.

Chemical reactions may be such as to absorb heat (endothermic) or to give out heat (exothermic). Most of those occurring in the body are exothermic. Even when the body is at rest it has a minimum need for energy to maintain its circulation, muscle-tone, and temperature. This energy, derived from food and food-stores, ultimately appears as heat. Since heat is produced by the 'burning' of food, with absorption of oxygen and elimination of carbon dioxide, it is possible to measure the uptake and output of these gases and then calculate how much heat must have been evolved. This procedure is used to determine the basal metabolic rate (BMR), and for purposes of comparison between persons of different sizes this is expressed as Calories per square metre of body-surface per hour. (When considering diets it is the Calorie requirement per day which is quoted.)

Since by far the biggest expenditure of energy during complete rest is on maintenance of bodily warmth, the amount needed varies not only with weight but with the amount of body surface through which heat can be lost. The smaller an animal the greater is its proportion of body surface to weight. Thus a man of average height and bulk, weighing about 70 kg. (11 stone) requires approximately 1,100 Calories daily for basic metabolism, or roughly 1,000 Calories per square metre of body surface, while a rabbit, weighing 3 kg. (6 lb.), needs about 150 Calories, or again roughly 1,000 per square metre of body surface.

Basal metabolism varies inversely with fatness, because the stouter the person the greater his total body surface. Thus a fat man whose basal metabolism uses 1,400 Calories daily will at first lose weight rapidly on a 1,800 Calorie diet, because the remaining 400 Calories are clearly insufficient to balance even the mildest of normal activities; but after some weeks of obtaining balancing energy from his own fat and muscular tissues, he becomes appreciably slimmer, has a lessened bodily surface, and perhaps has a basal metabolism of only 1,250 Calories, so that his weight loss on 1,800 Calories daily becomes much slower.

During the first year of life the BMR is about 50, declining to 40 at age 20 for normal adult males and continuing to fall gradually to 36 in old age. Physiologically, BMR is increased by muscular exercise, low environmental temperatures, and by the intake of food, especially protein. Conversely BMR is reduced by rest, warmth, and starvation, and it falls by about 15 during sleep. Pathologically, BMR is raised by fevers and by hyperthyrodism and lowered by hypothyroidism, under-nutrition, and certain disorders of the adrenal and the pituitary glands.

The special metabolism of various foods in the diet is complex and is dealt with under DIGESTION.

Diseases. Metabolic diseases may result from (1) disturbance of the acid-base balance which normally keeps the blood and tissues slightly alkaline; (2) endocrine disorders and defects in metabolizing specific dietary constituents; and (3) excess or deprivation of essential food elements.

1. The acid-base balance may become altered towards acidity or alkalinity. Since blood and tissues are mostly composed of water it is convenient to consider pure water first. Water is composed of hydrogen (acid) and hydroxide (base) ions, in chemical symbols H and OH. If carbon dioxide (CO_2) is added to water it combines with some of the hydroxide to produce a weak acid, carbonic acid, so that the water becomes slightly acid. In blood a change of acid-base balance is a little more complicated because blood contains certain 'buffer' substances such as sodium bicarbonate which tend to neutralize carbonic acid. But if enough carbon dioxide passed into the blood to form more carbonic acid than the buffers could deal with, the blood would become slightly acid. Normally carbon dioxide is breathed out from the lungs, but if respiration is impaired (e.g., by the deliberate holding of the breath or by any respiratory disease) it accumulates in the blood and, when the carbonic acid produced by the action of carbon dioxide on the water of the blood is enough to overcome the buffers, the blood becomes slightly acid (acidaemia). A similar situation can occur when a disturbance of carbohydrate metabolism produces excess of aceto-acetic acid, or when inefficient kidneys fail to excrete sufficient of this acid. Conversely, the blood may become too alkaline (alkalaemia) through overdosage of alkalies (antacids) taken for indigestion, or in persistent vomiting with loss of the normal hydrochloric acid from the stomach, or in over-breathing at high altitudes with excessive loss of carbon dioxide.

2. Various endocrine disorders affect the metabolic rate, e.g., insulin deficiency (causing excessive sugar in the blood), and diseases of thyroid secretion (excess raising the metabolic rate, and deficiency lowering it). Examples of defects in the breaking down of specific dietary constituents include gout (in which uric acid accumulates in the tissues), phenylketonuria (in which the body cannot deal with the amino-acid phenyl-alanine), and coeliac disease (in which the body cannot cope with gluten).

3. Excess or deprivation of any food element affects metabolism, e.g., too much carbohydrate and fat causes obesity, severe protein deficiency produces kwashiorkor, and carbohydrate insufficiency – whether from low intake or from inability to use it (as in diabetes) – produces acidaemia. See also DEFICIENCY DISEASES, VITAMINS and MINERAL SALTS.

metastasis. The transfer of disease from one part of the body to another by movement of disease particles either in the blood stream or in the lymphatic vessels. In particular in cancer there is a serious danger of a few cells becoming dislodged from the primary growth and giving rise to a secondary cancer elsewhere in the body. Clearly this danger makes it important that cancer is treated early, before any metastasis has occurred.

metazoan parasites. See TROPICAL DISEASES.

metritis. Inflammation of the uterus. Apart from cases due to gonorrhoea, acute metritis is usually the sequel of septic infection occurring after childbirth or abortion, especially in cases induced without proper aseptic precautions. Chronic metritis may occasionally be due to other pelvic infections.

The symptoms of irregular haemorrhage and discharge, with backache and a bulky uterus persisting after childbirth, are considered to be due to dysfunction of the ovaries and are treated accordingly.

metrorrhagia. Irregular haemorrhage from the uterus. The condition is sometimes divided into (1) menorrhagia, excessive blood loss during the menstrual period; (2) strict metrorrhagia, bleeding between the periods; and (3) bleeding occurring after the menopause. However, the first two often overlap.

Such bleeding is due to some condition of the vulva, vagina or uterus and calls for expert gynaecological investigation. The commonest causes are uterine polyps (fibroids) or other types of tumour. There should be no delay in seeking advice and treatment.

microbe. A general name for all micro-organisms too small to be seen by the naked eye. In broadly descending order of size microbes can be classified as protozoa, fungi, bacteria, rickettsia and viruses.

microscope. An optical instrument with a magnifying lens or combination of lenses for inspecting objects too small to be seen in detail – or at all – by the naked eye. The electron microscope gives vastly higher magnifications.

micturition. See URINATION.

middle ear disease. See EAR, otitis media.

migraine. A paroxysmal nervous disturbance with headache, nausea, vomiting and some sensory disturbance usually related to vision. The headache tends to be limited to one side or part of the head. The visual phenomena experienced may take various forms such as mistiness of vision, flashes of light, dark or bright spots, and usually precede the onset of headache as an AURA.

Although this is the classical description of migraine any recurrent headache is frequently so-called. Many cases respond quite well to a simple 'headache-powder' containing aspirin, phenacetin and caffeine, especially if given early in an attack. A preparation of ergot (ergotamine tartrate) has some reputation as a remedy either given by injection or in a larger dose by mouth.

The condition, common in adolescents and young adults, often disappears around the age of 50.

milk. A whitish liquid which is the normal secretion of the mammary glands of female mammals and is intended to provide for the nutritional needs of their offspring until weaned.

It consists of a watery solution of protein, lactose (milk sugar) and mineral salts, with small suspended globules of fat forming an emulsion. The relative proportions of these constituents vary in different animals; in particular the amount of protein varies roughly in proportion to the rate at which the offspring grows.

In milk the protein consists mainly of casein and lactalbumen with some enzymes. Milk sugar is lactose, which is easily broken down into glucose and galactose; it is the only source of the latter, which is a constituent of brain and nerve tissue. Milk fat is a variable mixture of glycerides – combinations of glycerin with a fatty acid. The principal fatty acid is butyric acid. Milk is also a very good source of essential minerals, especially calcium and phosphorus, but it is deficient in iron. Other minor constituents are phospholipids, cholesterol (an alcohol which helps to maintain stability of the fat emulsion), pigments, and vitamins. Usually the latter are all represented to some extent and especially c and D, but it is not a rich or reliable source of these and infants should be given supplementary supplies.

Raw milk is a potential danger as a common vehicle of disease and should always be pasteurized. or sterilized.

milk diet. See DIETS, SPECIAL.

mind. The nature of the mind is something which has engaged the attention of philosophers ever since man began to think about his place and purpose in the universe.

It is now generally accepted that mind is not a thing but an activity of the brain and on this basis there has been built a scientific discipline which seeks to explore, catalogue, and explain this activity. This is PSYCHOLOGY or the science of mental life.

mind and body. The nervous system is an instrument of adaptation. Its purpose is to adjust the organism to its environment; and the ultimate object of any sensation, emotion or thought-process is to produce some sort of action appropriate to the circumstances at any given time. Any disturbance received from the environment is technically a stimulus and the action evoked is a response.

Stimuli operate at various levels. Most simply they may produce a reflex action without the mind being involved at all. If for instance a person incautiously touches a hot object the hand is snatched away automatically by a spinal reflex action and closer examination would show that this painful stimulus had also produced physical effects, e.g., in the abdomen. If in addition the person had received a 'fright' from a painful experience of this kind there would be a conscious emotional response, with such symptoms as increased heart beat, sweating, nervous tremor, or by 'shock' with feelings of tiredness, faintness or collapse. Subconsciously the mind might respond by learning as illustrated in the proverbial saying that 'a burned child dreads the fire'.

It is when stimuli produce effects upon consciousness or the subconscious that we can expect adverse reactions between mind and body. In short, emotions profoundly affect the characteristics of bodily adaptation to stress.

The primitive emotions include anger,

fear, anxiety (which is a kind of fear), love, and the need to be loved. All of these are accompanied by bodily reactions which prepare the body for action and which may produce either conscious or subconscious effects. Under conditions of civilization the appropriate action cannot always be taken, and so inner tensions develop. These provide the causes for two main groups of diseases: PSYCHOSOMATIC DISEASES and neuroses (see NEUROSIS).

Conditions of both kinds constitute a very large part of any general medical practice. The treatment which they are accorded is generally only symptomatic and does not influence the root-causes of disability although it may give a measure of psychological support.

Illnesses of these kinds can only be permanently alleviated or relieved by removal of the origins of stress or by psychoanalysis to identify the cause and then to persuade the individual to recognize the causes, to appreciate and understand how they have produced his illness, and to induce him to make the calm and resolute efforts necessary to alter his way of life.

Measures for this alleviation or relief are highly important, but clearly removal of the causes of stress (not easy) and successful persuasion of a patient to alter his pattern of living (again not easy) will not reduce blood pressure already dangerously high, nor remove a peptic ulcer that has already eroded the coats of the stomach, nor fully remove a tendency to over-anxiety that has existed for forty years. So, as knowledge of mental factors improves, it becomes more and more important to deal with the causes of psychosomatic and neurotic diseases before the diseases have became established. The fostering of good mental and emotional health is perhaps the biggest task facing health workers today.

mineral salts. A well-balanced DIET must provide not only sufficient FOOD for the energy needs of the body and adequate amounts of fluid and vitamins but it must also supply certain mineral constituents. The basic essentials are salts of sodium, potassium, and magnesium, but these are always present in any reasonable diet and no special measures are required to ensure their adequacy. Next in importance are phosphorus and sulphur which are mainly derived from protein and which play an essential part in various enzyme reactions. They too are unlikely to be deficient if the diet otherwise contains sufficient protein.

The minerals most commonly lacking are calcium, iron and iodine. Calcium is particularly required for the formation of bones and teeth, and infants with calcium deficiency may show symptoms of tetany. Children require at least 1 g. of calcium per day and pregnant and nursing mothers about twice that amount. Milk is by far the best and most readily assimilable source.

Iron is necessary for the synthesis of haemoglobin, the oxygen-carrying pigment of the blood. The daily requirement is from 15 to 20 mg. Deficiency leads to anaemia and the best sources are liver, meat, eggs and some cereals and vegetables including spinach, beans, peas, whole-wheat and oatmeal.

Iodine is an essential constituent of thyroid hormone, and goitre results if intake is insufficient. Sea foods are the chief natural sources but most table salts contain small quantities of sodium iodine (1 in 100,000). The daily requirement is about 15 micrograms. Apart from these well-recognized requirements evidence is accumulating of the importance of 'trace elements', e.g., copper, cobalt and manganese.

miscarriage. The accidental termination of pregnancy before the unborn child has become viable i.e., developed sufficiently to live. The border-line from premature labour is generally taken at twenty-eight weeks after the first day of the last menstrual period, although some children born before that date survive and many born slightly after it die. In contrast to miscarriage the word ABORTION is increasingly associated with deliberate termination of pregnancy.

It is commonly said that about 15 per cent of pregnancies end in miscarriage but reliable figures are hard to maintain because an early miscarriage may be mistaken for a menstrual period. The real figure may well be as high as 20 per cent.

Causes of miscarriage include (1) haemorrhage into the thickened uterine wall or into the foetal membranes, causing separation of the fertilized ovum or death of the foetus; (2) death of the foetus from disease or malformation; and (3) stimulation of the uterine centre (equivalent to the starting of labour), for example through trauma, surgical operation, violent emotion or extreme exhaustion. Among the many predisposing causes may be mentioned endometritis, syphilis, toxaemia of pregnancy, nephritis and uterine malformations.

The main indications of miscarriage are bleeding, usually beginning as a slight staining and becoming more profuse, and sometimes (but not always) pain, radiating round from the back.

In threatened miscarriage, where the bleeding is only slight and the pains are moderate and infrequent, rest and sedatives may permit the pregnancy to continue; and in cases of doubt bleeding in any wanted pregnancy should at first be treated as threatened miscarriage. If miscarriage is inevitable and there is serious bleeding and severe pain the operation of curettage may be needed to complete the process quickly and so end haemorrhage which, if continued, might endanger the mother's life.

Some women are subject to repeated miscarriages, and various measures such as prolonged rest, the administration of hormones, and the treatment of any disease or other conditions which are present may help to secure a more successful outcome. Expert advice should be sought, and good antenatal care is important.

mites. Tiny, eight-legged arthropods, rather similar to ticks, many of which live as parasites on animals or plants, or on decaying organic matter.

Perhaps the best known are the *Sarcoptes scabie* which is responsible for scabies, the *Demodex follicularis* which causes a form of mange in dogs, and the common harvest mite which on occasion causes itching and blisters. A form of typhus – scrub typhus – is caused by a mite.

mitosis. See CELL.

mitral disease. See HEART.

Mittelschmerz. Pain occurring in the middle of the interval between menstrual periods, not yet fully understood but thought to be connected with ovulation. On occasion acute appendicitis has been mistaken for *Mittelschmerz* with tragic results.

mongolism. A common type of permanently retarded growth and mental development in which the face is short and broad, the skull round and rather small, the eyes slightly slanted and often without eyelashes, the tongue large and often protruding, the hands broad and clumsy, and the fingers short. Sufferers from this congenital condition tend to have, when adult, an intelligence roughly equivalent to that of a child aged 3 to 7 years. They are cheerful, amiable, likeable and more lively than most other types of mentally handicapped person.

Mongols require continuous supervision and protection throughout their life, and they should be provided with interests adapted to their capabilities through occupation centres.

The condition, which occurs in about 1 in six hundred live births, is found most commonly in children born to mothers over the age of 40 years. It is sometimes due to the possession of an extra chromosome (forty-seven instead of forty-six), and in other cases due to an abnormal arrangement of the chromosomes. The condition was generally termed mongolism until about 1960 because of the slanting of the eyes, but in recent years 'mongolism' has tended to disappear in scientific usage. Mongols – now called sufferers from Down's syndrome – constitute about one-quarter of all mentally handicapped children.

monoamine oxidase. An enzyme, commonly abbreviated to MAO, which facilitates the oxidation of adrenalin in the body and thereby reduces the activity – e.g., increased pulse rate and respiration – that would otherwise take place from excess of adrenalin.

One theory of depression is that it is due to deficiency of adrenalin or of a similar substance (a pressor amine). Hence drugs that suppress the production of monoamine oxidase (MAO inhibitors) and so preserve the body's adrenalin are extensively used in the treatment of depression. These inhibitors should not be used in various diseases of the heart and liver and must be taken only under strict medical supervision; but, so taken, they have a considerable record of at least partial success.

morbidity. The prevalence of disease in a community.

morning sickness. Many but by no means all pregnant women experience feelings of nausea on rising in the morning, usually between the second and fourth months of pregnancy. In some cases there is actual vomiting of a small amount of mucus. In the absence of any signs of toxaemia or other abnormality this 'morning sickness' can generally be regarded as of no important significance. Symptomatic treatment by gastric or nerve sedatives is often prescribed or vitamin intake increased by large doses of vitamin c and the vitamin b complex.

Occasionally the condition may progress to the more serious condition of hyperemesis gravidarum but usually in such cases a toxic element is demonstrably present to provide a basis for more rational lines of treatment.

moron. An American term for a mentally defective person corresponding to the British classification 'feeble-minded', with an intelligence quotient between 50 and 75.

morphia. Morphia or morphine is the chief alkaloid contained in opium. An extremely effective pain-killer, it is one of the most valuable of drugs.

In ordinary dosage it produces a very short period of restlessness and excitement (probably due to removal of the inhibitory effect of the higher nervous centres) and thereafter a dulling of the perceptive faculties, a loss of the sensation of pain and indeed a decreased activity of all sensations, and a state of drowsiness. A characteristic feature – useful for the diagnosis of morphine poisoning – is contraction of the pupils.

The normal dosage for an adult is 16 mg. by injection but children are abnormally sensitive to the drug, so that the dosage has to be far less in proportion to their weight. Many paediatricians consider that morphine should in no circumstances be given to children under 2 years.

The dangers of this extremely useful pain-killer are twofold. (1) It causes depression of the respiratory centre (and therefore shallowness of breathing), of the circulatory system (and therefore lowered blood pressure), and of the alimentary system (and therefore constipation), and in excess the depression of the respiratory centre can lead to death from asphyxia. (2) It is very much a drug of addiction: even three or four doses at intervals of eight hours can lead to appreciable desire for it, and continuation of dosage for a few days can lead to definite craving. Hence the use of the drug has to be strictly controlled.

In morphine poisoning – identified by pinpoint pupils, shallow breathing and cold skin – the patient should be kept moving and should be given strong coffee if able to drink, and a doctor should be promptly summoned.

mosquito. A general name for gnat-like insects of the family *Culicidae*. They are important in medicine as transmitters of certain tropical diseases because of their propensity for biting and blood-sucking. They include *Anopheles*, many species of which convey malaria, and *Aedes*, whose members transmit yellow fever. *Culex* species are responsible for the spread of filariasis and dengue fever.

Mosquitoes of the *Anopheles* and *Culex* genera occur also in temperate climates but do not spread disease because of the absence of initial infection.

mould. See FUNGUS.

mouth. The uppermost part of the DIGESTIVE SYSTEM. Its function is the ingestion and mastication of food and it also plays a part in speech production.

Inflammation of the mouth is known as STOMATITIS.

Mouth dryness. Dryness of the mouth (xerostomia) is due to deficient secretion of saliva and is a common symptom of any acute feverish illness. It is indicative of loss of body fluid (dehydration), a condition which must be corrected promptly by the administration of additional fluid either by mouth or by injection.

Of less important significance is the dryness of the mouth experienced by mouth-breathers in whom the normal amount of salivary secretion is insufficient to counteract evaporation to the air-flow. Dryness of the mouth may also occur as a result of strong emotion, especially fear. Mouth dryness from minor causes may be helped by the use of chewing-gum, acid sweets or by bitter tonics given before meals.

mouth-breathing. Habitual mouth-breathing results from chronic nasal obstruction. In children this tends to produce deformity of the face, naso-pharynx and chest. In most instances it is primarily due to persistent infection and enlargement of the ADENOIDS.

In adults nasal obstruction may result from deflection of the nasal septum (either as a congenital defect or acquired through injury), from chronic infections of the nose leading to swelling of the nasal mucous membrane and sometimes to the formation of bulky growths known as polypi; or from infection and suppuration in the nasal sinuses.

Specialist advice and treatment are generally needed.

mouth-to-mouth breathing. See ARTIFICAL RESPIRATION.

mouth washes. Antiseptic solutions for rinsing the mouth and throat to allay the pain and irritation of septic and inflammatory conditions and to encourage healing. Gargle is a practically synonymous term and gargling is a procedure employed in an attempt to reach the tonsils and pharyngeal wall where infection is common.

Although mouth washes give temporary relief it is doubtful if they have any great effect on infections, which really require specific therapy, and their mechanical cleansing action may be equally well obtained from a simple solution of common salt (one teaspoonful in a tumblerful of warm water). They do, however, have a useful place in dentistry, particularly after extractions, since astringent and antiseptic properties can help to minimize or arrest haemorrhage and combat socket infection.

movable kidney. The kidneys are situated high in the loin on each side of the vertebral column and are kept in position by an envelopment of fatty tissue and by the anchorage afforded by their main blood vessels. Although they move slightly up and down with respiration their lower poles cannot normally be felt through the abdomen. When a kidney has greater mobility than this it can be felt and is said to be movable or floating according to degree. The medical term is nephroptosis. The condition tends to occur in circumstances which cause loss of fat and muscular tone – emaciation for various reasons or repeated pregnancies – and is much more common in women and on the right side because of the longer renal artery.

Symptoms are usually of vague dragging abdominal pain often radiating downwards. Occasionally, more acute colicky attacks occur because of torsion and kinking of the ureter, the duct carrying urine to the bladder. Such an incident may be accompanied by blood in the urine.

Patients are very apt to become neurotic about the presence of a movable kidney. If treatment has to be considered a properly fitted abdominal support relieves most cases.

mucous membrane. See MEMBRANES.

mucus. The slimy protective secretion of the mucous MEMBRANES.

multipara. A woman who has given birth to more than one child.

multiple sclerosis. A chronic disease of the nervous system in which patches of defective and hardened tissue appear at random in the brain and spinal cord and interfere with the normal function of the affected parts. The condition is also called disseminated sclerosis. Its cause is unknown.

The disease usually starts at 20 to 40 years (practically never after 50), and its course is progressive with increasing disability, although temporary remissions are a feature. The typical symptoms are weakness, uncoordination, rigidity and paralysis of the lower limbs (spastic paraplegia) together with the very characteristic and often associated occurrence of nystagmus, tremor of the arms, and a peculiar scanning or syllabic speech.

There is no effective treatment but it is important to maintain general nutrition and limited activity. Massage and passive movements can help to prevent painful and deforming contractures.

mumps. An acute infectious disease of sudden onset, caused by a virus. It is characterized by fever and by swelling and tenderness of the salivary glands. Usually it is the glands situated in front of the ears which are most affected, so that the resultant swelling produces the typical swollen and distorted facial appearance.

The incubation period is twelve to twenty-six days; the incidence is chiefly in children aged 5 to 15 years; in older persons the testes or ovaries may be affected and symptoms of meningitis or encephalitis occasionally occur. Spontaneous recovery is usually complete within ten days and second attacks are uncommon. Vaccination is available but the immunity is short-lived and it is not generally advised except in special circumstances.

muscle. A type of tissue which has the ability to contract in response to nervous stimuli and which thus provides power for movement.

It occurs in three forms: (1) voluntary, skeletal or striped muscle; (2) involuntary, visceral or unstriped muscle; and (3) cardiac muscle. The term 'striped' refers to the appearance of voluntary muscle under the microscope when the fibres show alternate light and dark cross-banding.

In general, skeletal muscles are either elongated with a roughly cylindrical or spindle shape, or broad and flat. They are connected to the bones, cartilages, ligaments or skin either directly or by means of tendons. The end of the muscle which is attached to a point relatively more fixed is known as the origin, and its other end is its insertion. When the muscle contracts origin and insertion are necessarily brought closer together and the desired movement results. However, when a muscle is required to contract, its opposing muscle must relax in order to enable it to do so; it may therefore be said that muscles work in pairs.

Visceral muscle forms the walls of hollow organs and ducts including the blood vessels. Cardiac muscle is found only in the walls of the heart.

Voluntary muscles are under the control of the individual and their contraction can be initiated, controlled or inhibited at will. Visceral and cardiac muscle are not subject to such control and react automatically to stimuli from the autonomic nervous system.

Diseases. Paralysis and atrophy of muscle usually result from damage to the

biceps contracts to bend elbow

triceps relaxes to allow it

triceps contracts to straighten elbow

biceps relaxes to allow it

Diagram showing how muscles work in pairs

nerve caused by infections such as poliomyelitis, by damage to blood vessels affecting the nervous system or by multiple sclerosis and other diseases of the actual nerves.

Violence may produce rupture of muscle fibres to cause a strain treated by rest and support. CRAMP is a painful spasmodic muscle contraction due to over-exertion or insufficient blood supply. Some cases due to arterial disease may be helped by drugs which dilate the blood vessels. Occupational cramps (writer's, telegraphist's and piano-player's) are caused by constant repetition of small movements. Myalgia is a painful condition in which muscles and their fibrous components and attachments become inflamed by strain and exposure; common varieties are lumbago, pleurodynia (rib muscles) and the stiff neck of acute torticollis. Rest and heat treatment usually relieve symptoms.

Apart from these common conditions there are certain rarer and less well-understood muscular diseases which are often inherited. Myotonia congenita is a disease of childhood characterized by slowness of relaxation after voluntary contraction, and myotonia atrophica is a similar condition of middle age, with wasting of muscle tissues. Familial periodic paralysis is marked by recurrent attacks of extensive paralysis. It occurs mostly in adolescents and tends to improve with age. Myasthenia gravis is characterized by rapid exhaustion of the muscles when movements are rapidly repeated.

Muscular dystrophy (myopathy) affects children and young people as several different clinical types. Most cases are hereditary and x-chromosome linked (see GENETICS) which means that males are mostly affected. Female carriers of the defective gene can be detected by an enzyme test. The condition is one of muscle degeneration. There is no known effective treatment and severe cases may not survive beyond young adult life. Massage, physiotherapy and orthopaedic appliances help to minimize disability.

muscle relaxants. Drugs which, if injected into the bloodstream, prevent muscles from contracting. They are useful before certain surgical operations.

muscular rheumatism. See FIBROSITIS.

mushroom poisoning. The edible mushroom of commerce is *Agaricus campestris.* It is also found growing under natural conditions, but the gathering and eating of wild mushrooms is fraught with considerable risks unless the collector has sufficient botanical knowledge to ensure that poisonous fungi are not included by mistake. There are at least a dozen species which can cause serious illness or death. The most fatal are death cap mushroom (*Amanita phalloides*) and the fly agaric or scarlet fly cap (*Amanita muscaria*).

Eating a poisonous type of mushroom is quickly followed by severe abdominal pain and by vomiting and a cholera-like type of watery diarrhoea which may be blood-stained. The pulse is slowed and there are effects on the nervous system shown by disturbance of vision, dilated pupils, restlessness, and delirium.

Immediate treatment includes repeated stomach washes and the giving of large doses of atropine which is a specific antidote to the poisonous agent muscarine. There is generally severe and prolonged prostration and in fatal cases the victim gradually sinks into a coma which leads to death within a week.

myasthenia gravis. A disease characterized by rapid exhaustion of the MUSCLES under voluntary control when movements are carried out repeatedly in close succession. With rest, normal power slowly becomes restored although this ability to recover may be lost in later stages. The condition occurs mainly in young adults and the sexes are affected equally. The muscles involved in order of frequency and severity are those in (1) the head and face, especially the ocular muscles, (2) the neck, (3) the respiratory system, (4) the limbs and trunk. In progressive cases death may occur from respiratory paralysis.

Muscular contraction depends on acetylcholine at the point where the nerve-ending contacts the muscle itself. Its action is limited by the enzyme acetylcholinesterase. By injecting the substance Tensilon (edrophonium chloride) the enzyme is inhibited and the action of acetylcholine is prolonged. This procedure is used as a diagnostic test for myasthenia gravis and temporarily abolishes the muscle exhaustion.

Various other longer-acting anti-cholinesterases are available for treatment, and some cases are also treated by removal of the thymus gland.

mydriatic. A drug which dilates the pupil of the eye. Such medicaments are used in both the diagnosis and treatment of eye diseases. They act by temporarily paralysing the endings of the nerve supplying the muscle which controls the iris. A large dilated pupil facilitates examination of the inside of the eye, and since the power of accommodation or focusing is also rendered inactive, any errors of refraction which could be corrected by spectacles can be more easily and accurately measured.

In treatment the main indication for the use of a mydriatic is IRITIS, in which it is necessary both to rest the iris and to ensure that it neither adheres to the lens in a contracted position nor causes inflammatory deposits on the lens which would damage the sight.

myelitis. An inflammatory or degenerative condition of the SPINAL CORD.

myelogram. An x-ray of the spinal cord after injection of a radio-opaque oil by lumbar puncture.

myocarditis. Inflammation of the muscle of the HEART. Acute myocarditis is relatively uncommon and occurs as a sequel to various generalized infections.

myocardium. The specialized muscle which forms the walls of the HEART.

myopia. A defect of EYESIGHT, commonly known as 'short sight', in which, although objects held near the face are seen clearly, distance vision is blurred.

myxoedema. The condition which results from a deficiency of thyroid secretion. In cases which arise spontaneously the gland is small, rather wasted and fibrosed. It occurs chiefly in women of menopausal age. The signs and symptoms of myxoedema are very characteristic: the features become broadened and bloated with puffy drooping eyelids; there is swelling and thickening of the tissues under the skin (solid oedema); the skin becomes dry and rough with absence of sweating; the hair becomes harsh, sparse and dry; movements and mental activity become slowed; the basal metabolic rate is low and the patient always feels cold. The condition can be effectively treated by the administration of thyroxin.

Myxoedema due to congenital deficiency of the thyroid gland is known as CRETINISM.

N

naevus. The medical term for a BIRTH MARK.

thumb-nail
cut to
a curve

great toe-nail
cut straight

**Fingernails and toenails should be cut
in different styles**

nail. The visible, horny part of the nail
consists of hardened and bony epidermic
cells, and the nail grows from the nail-bed
or matrix which is overlapped by a fold of
skin. The half-moons at the base of the
nails appear pale because they are not
firmly attached to the underlying tissues.

Excessive paring, especially at the
edges, can lead to cracks and bruising with
subsequent formation of nail abscesses and
whitlow. Painful cracks (hangnails)
occurring in the skin at the sides of nails in
winter are due partially to insufficient
blood supply through the blood vessels
being constricted by cold, and partially to
insufficiency of natural oil in the skin. See
also NAIL, INGROWING.

nail-biting. A common compulsive symptom
of frustration or repressed aggression. A
child, jealous of a younger brother or sister
or insecure because of real or apparent
lack of parental affection, is unable to vent
his aggression on others and gets rid of it
by biting his own nails, achieving some
satisfaction from his ability to see and feel
the results of his actions. In at least a
proportion of cases nail-biting having thus
started, persists as a habit after the initial
cause has disappeared.

Prevention is essentially the avoidance
of insecurity and severe frustration.
Nagging and punishment are usually
ineffective. There are essentially two
hopeful lines of treatment. (1) Where the
initial cause is still operating, careful
assessment of parent-child relationships
and sometimes of child-school
relationships, and thereafter removal of
the cause. (2) Where nail-biting has
become essentially a habit, an attempt to
instil pride in the hands by careful
manicuring and nail-cutting.

nail, ingrowing. A condition, mostly of the
great toe, in which the nail grows into the
flesh on one side or the other, creating
considerable pain. The two common
causes are badly fitting shoes with
pressure on the nail, and cutting the toe-
nails in a curve (as is normal with fingernails). Prevention consists in careful
selection of comfortable, well fitting shoes
and in cutting the toe nails straight across,
with the sharp points at the side either
filed or finely clipped. Where the condition
has occurred, treatment usually involves
surgical removal of a v-shaped piece from
the middle of the top of the nail (so that,
instead of growing sideways, it will grow to
fill the gap) and the temporary placing of a
dressing soaked in collodion between the
nail edge and the flesh. If this treatment
fails, removal of the nail may have to be
considered.

napkin or **nappy rash.** Dermatitis of the
area covered by an infant's napkin,
through irritation by urine. Soothing
ointments are needed, and the napkins
should be sterilized by boiling.

narcissism. Excessive love of oneself.
Basically narcissism represents a fixation
at (or a regression to) an infantile
emotional level, occurring in persons
whose intelligence is normal or sometimes
above average. Complete narcissism is a
form of NEUROSIS and certainly requires
psychiatric treatment; but there are many
intermediate stages in which a person is
self-centred to more than an average
extent and is rather childlike in his or her
emotional attitudes to life. Whether
treatment is necessary depends on the
degree of self-centredness. Whether
treatment, if needed, is acceptable
depends on the extent to which the
individual has – or can acquire – insight
into the condition.

narcolepsy. A disorder in which a person is
subject to uncontrollable drowsiness
unrelated to actual fatigue, such as falling
asleep while delivering a lecture or
immediately after laughing heartily at a
joke. In some cases investigation shows
that the cause is damage to the
hypothalamus of the brain, e.g., from
tumour or head injury or following
encephalitis; but in quite a proportion of
cases clinical and x-ray examinations fail
to identify a cause. Apart from treatment
of the cause if found (e.g., removal of a
tumour) most victims respond well to
dosage with amphetamine sulphate, but in
general this is a palliative rather than a
cure: in other words, the attacks of
drowsiness or actual sleep recur if the
amphetamine is discontinued.

narcosis. Dulling of consciousness or deep
sleep, produced by the action of (1)
narcotic drugs such as morphia, and (2)
anaesthetics. Continuous narcosis is a

method of preliminary or temporary treatment sometimes used in mental disorders associated with excitement or great agitation: the patient is rested in preparation for later treatment by being kept asleep or almost asleep for several days, being awakened only for meals and for the performance of natural functions.

nasal catarrh. See CATARRH.

nasal feeding. A method of feeding a person who cannot swallow. A thin tube is passed through nostril, throat and gullet to the stomach, and liquid is then poured slowly into a funnel attached to the tube.

National Health Service. See HEALTH SERVICES.

natural childbirth. Childbirth without anaesthetics or analgesics.

It is based on the theory that the pain is primarily due to fear and can be removed by rational explanation and the teaching of relaxation exercises, generally termed psychoprophylaxis.

Some obstetricians deny the pain can be so removed, but many thousands of women claim to have derived benefit and in many cases to have given birth without requiring any form of anaesthesia. In the present state of knowledge it would seem advisable for expectant mothers to attend health education and psychoprophylaxis classes, to use the exercises in the early stages of labour, but to have anaesthetics available for such women as do not find the measures fully effective.

naturopathy. A superficially attractive system of health care by simple, 'natural' diet, regular exercise, the avoidance of all 'artificial' foods including foods grown with chemical fertilizers, and the rejection of drugs and medicines, although some naturopaths will accept drugs produced from plants but not synthetic drugs. Clearly there are certain advantages in a system that succeeds in avoiding over-eating, under-exercise, cigarette smoking and the over-use of medicines to which many of us are prone. Yet in attributing all disease to artificial foodstuffs and artificial ways of life and in seeking what is essentially a return to nature the naturopaths conveniently forget that primitive tribes suffer from a mass of infectious and nutritional diseases, that their members are quite often stunted or deformed and that in such communities early death is the rule rather than the exception.

Food, however pure, can neither prevent nor cure invasion of the body by a droplet-borne bacterium or virus; a natural way of life cannot stop the carrier of a hereditary defect from passing it to his offspring nor incite a failing pancreas to produce enough insulin for the body's needs; avoidance of artificiality cannot prevent the development of allergy to a particular pollen or remove the pain of a wound or burn. Moreover, if we turn to such naturopaths as accept 'natural' drugs, there seems little difference between

treating malaria with the 'natural' bark of the cinchona and treating it with quinine 'artificially' extracted from that bark (except that in the latter case the dose is much more accurate), and little difference between supplementing a winter diet that is deficient in vitamin c with 'natural' lemon juice or supplementing with an equivalent amount of synthetic ascorbic acid.

Every species that has survived has done so by a process of continuous adaptation. Such things as canned foods and artificial heating that enable man to exist under arctic conditions, vaccines and antibiotics that allow him to combat infection, and contraceptives that enable him to cope with the population explosion are all parts of the process of continuous adaptation. The naturopath philosophy, resisting and rejecting adaptation, would, if universally adopted, result in the regression of mankind to its primitive state.

nausea. A feeling of impending vomiting. This may occur as a result of emotional disturbances (especially fear), unpleasant sights, smells and tastes, indigestion and gastritis, food-poisoning, or severe eye-strain. It may also appear as an early symptom in an attack of migraine, in the early stages of many fevers, in sea-sickness, and in the morning sickness of early pregnancy. In many of these conditions nausea precedes actual vomiting.

navel. The umbilicus or navel is a depressed, button-like scar in the central line of the abdomen. It is the scar resulting from the cutting of the UMBILICAL CORD which originally united the unborn child to the placenta.

near-sight. Short-sightedness or myopia. See EYESIGHT.

neck. The neck is supported by seven cervical vertebrae which are braced by strong muscles that enable the head to be freely moved. The muscles on each side which stand out prominently when the head is turned are the sternomastoids. In the front of the neck from above downwards are the hyoid bone, the larynx and the trachea (windpipe), with the oesophagus (gullet) lying behind the trachea, and the thyroid gland situated in front of the larynx. The main blood vessels in the neck are the carotid arteries and the jugular veins.

Swellings in the neck are most commonly due to enlarged glands, arising from septic tonsils or teeth, from tuberculosis, or from glandular fever. Swelling in the front of the neck is generally due to enlargement of the thyroid gland. See GOITRE. Pain in the neck muscles may result from inflammatory causes, but probably the commonest is rheumatic wry neck or torticollis.

necrosis. Death of a limited portion of the cells or tissues of the body. It may occur from cutting off the blood supply to the affected area, in bacterial poisoning or after severe burns or other injuries. The dead tissue may be discharged to the surface with pus, or may remain and cause prolonged suppuration and so necessitate surgical removal, or may remain and become converted into a harmless lump of bony or fibrous tissue.

negativism. A phase, common around 2½ years, in which requests or commands are bluntly refused. See CHILDHOOD, PSYCHOLOGY OF.

Negativism is also sometimes found in old people who use it as a convenient method of stressing their importance. It usually disappears if the old person is given a little more attention and helped to find interests.

neoplasm. The medical term for a TUMOUR.

nephritis. Inflammation of the KIDNEY.

nephrosis. A condition in which the filtering mechanism of the KIDNEY is damaged.

nerve. A bundle of conducting fibres through which impulses pass between the brain and spinal cord and other parts of the body. See NERVOUS SYSTEM.

nervous breakdown. A common term for any emotional illness which makes it impossible for a person to cope with the stresses and strains of life. The corresponding medical term is NEUROSIS, but the two words tend to differ in breadth of meaning. Neurosis includes also milder forms of emotional disorder in which the person feels tired or depressed or inadequate or persistently anxious or suffers from obsessions, but still manages to carry out his normal work. The non-medical term, nervous breakdown, generally indicates a neurosis that has progressed to a stage at which the victim can no longer carry out the duties for which he has been trained, or can no longer be deemed a responsible member of the community.

nervous child. The terms 'nervous' and 'maladjusted' are both used to indicate children with psychological difficulties, though the second term implies that the instability or disturbance is too severe to be remedied by parents and teachers, while 'nervous' causes no such implication. The difficulties usually manifest themselves in one of four main ways: (1) as behaviour disorders, e.g., temper tantrums, aggressiveness, bullying, stealing and sex difficulties; (2) as habit disorders and physical symptoms, e.g., stammering, thumb-sucking, nail-biting, bed-wetting and sleep-walking; (3) as neurotic disorders, e.g., pathological anxiety, phobias and compulsive acts; (4) as educational and vocational difficulties, e.g., school failure, school phobia, and frequent day-dreaming. Psychotic behaviour (such as extreme withdrawal or manifestations of hallucinations) is not usually classified under the heading of nervous disorders.

In most cases the difficulties originate at home – in parental over-strictness and over-discipline, in over-indulgence, in inconsistency, in lack of demonstrated affection, in quarrels between parents, or in situations creating jealousy of a younger or older brother or sister. Less frequently their origin is in school circumstances.

Prevention is largely a matter of parents becoming aware of a child's need for physical and emotional security, demonstrated love, reasonable parental consistency, freedom to explore and investigate coupled with a kindly, guiding authority, and provision of playthings and playmates appropriate to the stage of development. Most people, however, are occasionally inconsistent or thoughtless, and parents should appreciate that children have considerable resilience. Errors in child management have to be continued or repeated to produce child maladjustment. The advice of the family HEALTH VISITOR can be of great value to parents, e.g., anticipatory guidance about the next stage of development and its problems, current guidance about the handling of existing difficulties, and, not least, reassurance of needlessly worried fathers and mothers.

Where a child's behaviour is for an appreciable time inappropriate to his age and stage of development, detailed investigation and prolonged treatment may be needed. See CHILD GUIDANCE and MALADJUSTED CHILD.

nervous system. The mechanism primarily responsible for the co-ordinated activity of the body as a whole.

A typical nerve cell (or neurone) consists of a small nucleated body, many tiny branching filaments (dendrites), and a long branch (the axon) which in turn ends in branching filaments. Essentially a neurone is a long fibre that collects impulses from the delicate filaments at one end and transmits them to the filaments at the other end; and a nerve is a bundle of such fibres. A single nerve may consist solely of sensory fibres that carry impulses of sensation from the periphery towards the brain, or solely of motor fibres that carry instructions outwards towards the muscles, or of a mixture of motor and sensory fibres.

The transfer of sensory information (e.g., about pain, heat, or cold affecting a toe) to the brain and of instructions back to the relevant muscles is achieved not by a single sensory fibre and a single motor fibre, but by two series of fibres with interlacing endings. The message, whether sensory or motor, can be considered as an electrical impulse which runs along the fibre and then 'sparks the gap' between the ending of one neurone and the beginning of the next.

The cerebrospinal system is said to have two parts: central and peripheral. The central nervous system consists of the BRAIN and the SPINAL CORD. The brain receives information from the cranial nerves (e.g., those serving the eyes and nose) and the spinal nerves (e.g., those receiving impulses from the limbs). The cranial and spinal nerves together constitute what is known as the peripheral nervous system. The brain processes the information and sends out appropriate instructions along the motor nerves (e.g. telling the leg muscles to move the body nearer to an object that the eyes have seen). The spinal cord is the main nerve trunk between the brain and the arms, legs and trunk.

By no means all messages, however, make the full journey to the brain and back. On a level with every pair of nerves leaving the spinal cord there is an alternative system for relaying the impulses within the spinal cord itself without the necessity of involving the brain; this mechanism is known as the reflex arc and is responsible for maintaining the muscle tone as well as for very specific muscle responses known as REFLEX ACTIONS. For instance, if the hand touches a very hot object the sensory impulse (conveying the awareness of pain) results in an instruction at spinal cord level for the muscles of the arm to take appropriate action, so that the hand is actually removed from the hot object before the brain receives the impulse which it interprets as pain.

The *autonomic nervous system* conveys messages to involuntary muscles and secreting glands, which is to say that it regulates functions not under the control of the brain, e.g., heart-rate, blushing, sweating and control of digestion. Functionally the autonomic nervous system is divided into two parts. The *sympathetic nervous system* is connected with the thoracic and upper lumbar spinal nerves, while the *parasympathetic nervous system* is connected both with the vagus (tenth cranial nerve) and with the sacral nerve.

Activity of the sympathetic nervous system mobilizes the body to meet physical danger – dilating the pupils and to some extent raising the hair (creating a frightening appearance), widening the coronary and other major arteries (and so increasing the flow of blood to the muscles), constricting skin blood vessels (and so ensuring less blood loss from a superficial wound), increasing the force of the heart beat (thus again making more blood available for the muscles), dilating the bronchi and bronchioles (and so allowing more air into the lungs), and decreasing the activity of digestive organs (for digestion can be postponed until the danger is past). Essentially these nerves release additional amounts of the hormone adrenalin, so that an injection of adrenalin has similar effects.

By contrast the parasympathetic nerves restore peace after the emergency has been tackled, by slowing down the heart, reducing the blood flow, restoring digestive activity, and allowing the sphincters of bladder and anus to relax and permit

1 brain, which receives information from sensory nerves and transmits instructions via motor nerves
2 spinal cord, protected by the spinal column, which is the nerve pathway to and from the brain
3 spinal nerves, sensory and motor, branching to all parts of the body

The nervous system

urination and defaecation. Both these systems are greatly influenced by the ENDOCRINE GLANDS and they both influence and are influenced by the emotions.

nettle rash. An allergic condition characterized by the rapid appearance of weals and blisters, usually lasting for only a few hours, and accompanied by intense itching. Its technical name is urticaria.

The rash resulting from actual nettle stings appears to be due to the injection of histamine and acetylcholine; and so-called nettle rash from other causes (e.g., after the eating of a food to which the individual is sensitive) is thought to be due to release of histamine in the tissues. Antihistamine drugs are generally effective, and calamine lotion will relieve the itching until the drug takes effect.

Where the condition recurs a careful search for the cause is desirable, but the fewer the number of attacks the less the likelihood of identifying the source.

neuralgia. Shooting pain, usually occurring in paroxysms, along the course of any nerve, but most commonly arising in the nerves of the face and head. The condition is often caused or precipitated by a cold draught, or may arise from pressure on a nerve or from irritation of a nerve by disease in its vicinity. In many cases no cause is found.

Hot fomentations usually give some relief, and aspirin and phenacetin are useful, although both merely give temporary relief and allow time for spontaneous cure to occur.

neurasthenia. A vague term denoting an irritable, hypersensitive weakness and depression. A person suffering from the condition feels exhausted and unhappy, cannot concentrate for long, is constantly beset by worries, and is very concerned about symptoms which often include headaches, muscular pains, fullness in the abdomen and tremor of the hands.

Freud regarded neurasthenia as a result of repressed auto-eroticism, or self-love, which finds expression in sexual conflict or sexual difficulty, and so creates exhaustion. Probably that is not the only explanation, but in all cases neurasthenia originates in a disturbance of the mind. Hence, while tranquillizers may play a part in the treatment of mild cases of short duration, for most serious cases some form of psychological treatment is essential, including an attempt to identify and remove the underlying causes.

Traumatic neurasthenia is a similar or identical condition which develops after an injury, e.g. in a traffic accident, with the weakness and proneness to fatigue persisting long after the physical injury has healed. 'Compensation neurosis', as it is sometimes called, does not imply malingering or deceit. To the victim it is absolutely genuine. Yet in most cases it clears up rapidly after the amount of compensation has been settled.

neuritis. Inflammation of a nerve (localized neuritis) or of several nerves (polyneuritis).

The symptoms vary according to whether the inflammation is of the nerve sheath or of the actual nerve filaments themselves and according to whether the nerve is irritated or incapacitated. Early signs may include numbness (most commonly of the 'glove and stocking' areas) and loss of sensation, or pain and muscle weakness and tenderness. If the condition progresses the skin of the affected area often becomes cold and shiny, while the muscles waste.

Causes of localized neuritis include (1) exposure to cold, found most commonly in Bell's palsy and sciatica; (2) pressure, e.g., from a tumour; (3) poisoning, e.g., lead particularly affects the wrists; and (4) diphtheria, formerly a very common cause of temporary neuritis. Treatment consists largely of identifying and removing the cause, although electrical treatment and counter-irritation may help.

Causes of multiple neuritis include various acute fevers, diabetes, beriberi (the deficiency disease caused by lack of vitamin B_1), and poisoning by alcohol, arsenic and lead. Alcoholic neuritis, commonest in middle-aged women, is probably not so much due to poisoning as to destruction of vitamin B by alcohol (so that it resembles the neuritis of beriberi). It affects the legs mostly, causing foot-drop and poor sensation in the feet, and a compensatory high-stepping gait. Treatment involves identification and removal of the cause, rest, massage and electricity.

neurosis. A very common but rather ill-defined group of psychological abnormalities (also known as psychoneurosis), including excessive anxiety, anger, fear, hate, jealousy, hysterical states and the states associated with phobias and obsessive actions. The distinction from PSYCHOSIS (mental illness) is clear: the psychotic's personality is unbalanced and disorganized, on certain matters he is out of touch with reality and cannot reason properly, and he is usually unaware that he is ill; the neurotic is in full touch with reality, can reason normally and is very worried about his illness. It is more difficult to indicate the border between neurosis and the edge of normality: there is no sharp boundary between the over-anxious person who tends to worry too much and the victim of anxiety neurosis. Broadly, if extreme tidiness, or concern with detail, or anxiety, reaches the stage where it is interfering with work performance and social relationships, it is a neurosis.

While heredity may play a small part, neurosis is in the main due to a combination of unfortunate happenings in childhood and adult stresses. As Freud showed, neuroses originate in unresolved conflicts (e.g., between innate tendencies and parental precepts), and mostly represent a flight from the particular conflict; and the pre-neurotic person (less secure or more apprehensive than others, or described as 'rather a perfectionist' or 'a bit jealous') is precipitated into full neuroticism by the stresses of adolescence, by work strain or by marital problems.

Prevention would seem to lie in the education of parents, and also of teachers and others concerned with children, about the emotional and psychological requirements of children for adequate development of personality, so that a sustained attempt may be made to build personalities capable of standing up to the strains and tribulations of normal life. Some workers claim that, now that most infectious diseases and many physical diseases of children have been brought under control, the teaching of mental hygiene is the main task of the modern health visitor.

The neurotic is unhappy and incapable of good work, and his symptoms are genuine. He badly needs help, and there is no point in advising him to 'pull himself together'. If he could do so, he would not be a neurotic.

One form of treatment is to supply tranquillizers and to take such steps as may be practicable to lessen current worries or problems – in other words to seek to restore the patient to his pre-neurotic state in which he managed to cope fairly well with his difficulties. Where the precipitating strains were heavy and can be removed or lessened, and where the underlying conflicts are not too extreme, this may be all that is needed.

Alternatively or additionally, an attempt may be made to discover the underlying factors, to bring the conflicts to the patient's consciousness and to help him to resolve them in a way satisfactory to himself. This may involve a full course of psychoanalysis.

Many American experts believe that the first form of treatment alone is inadequate, and that it is essential to help the patient to find his problems and improve his capacity for problem-solving. Many British experts hold that detailed psychological investigation is unwarranted unless simpler methods have failed.

Neurosis is not only very common, but is also particularly common in persons of high intelligence and ability. Hence both prevention and treatment are important, not only for the sake of the unfortunate persons but also in the interests of the community.

neurosurgery. The branch of surgery which deals with operations performed on the brain, spinal cords or nerves, e.g., to remove a tumour of the brain or to treat a prolapsed vertebral disc.

nicotine. An alkaloid in tobacco which is responsible for the nausea, sickness, faintness, etc., sometimes experienced at the initial smoking experiment. In habitual smokers it causes increased pulse rate and raised blood pressure, and it may be the factor in tobacco that contributes to diseases of the arteries.

Nicotine is used as an insecticide, and can be inadvertently swallowed. A toxic dose produces a burning sensation in the mouth, followed by vomiting and diarrhoea, violent excitement, and presently exhaustion, loss of consciousness and sometimes death. Treatment consists of rapid emptying of the stomach by stomach tube or by emetic, injecting a small dose of atropine, and, if respiration is becoming difficult, using artificial respiration.

night blindness. Inability of the eyes to adapt to partial darkness. While the normal person experiences at dusk a gradual diminution of vision, a person with night blindness passes suddenly from daylight to complete darkness. The common cause is deficiency of vitamin A,

but night blindness also occurs as a hereditary condition and in some diseases of the retina and choroid.

nightmare. A dream marked by very acute fear, anxiety or other unpleasant emotion. In most cases nightmares reflect, often in distorted form, difficulties and emotional disturbances in waking life. See NIGHT TERROR.

night terror. The fundamental difference between a nightmare and a night terror is that in the former the frightening dream is recalled and fear departs when the person reaches full consciousness, whereas in night terror the person wakens suddenly in a state of panic but can give no reason for his fears.

Night terrors sometimes occur in adults but are mostly found in nervous children, especially after unusual excitement or fatigue. For most cases three negative measures prevent recurrences: avoidance of excessive excitement and fatigue, especially in the evenings; adjustment of meal-times or amounts so that no heavy meal is eaten within two or three hours of going to bed; and avoidance of needless or excessive frustration at home and school. Where night terrors persist despite these measures the child should be referred to a child guidance clinic.

nipple. The teat of the female breast; the protuberance from which the milk ducts discharge. During pregnancy the nipple enlarges, simultaneously with the whole breast, and becomes more pronounced and darker in colour. Pigment is also deposited around the nipple during pregnancy and thereafter never entirely disappears.

Cracked nipples are not uncommon during the period of breast feeding. They are painful and can form a channel whereby infection passes to deeper tissues. Careful washing and application of friar's balsam often remedies the condition, and a metal shield worn between feeds can be useful.

Leaking nipples usually indicate lack of muscle tone, rather than excess of milk. The breasts can be toned up by alternate hot and cold sponging and by gentle massage. Attention to general health and to diet is also necessary.

Paget's disease of the nipple is essentially a cancer of the milk ducts. The affected nipple becomes scaly, thickened and smaller than the other nipple. Treatment is by surgical removal of the breast.

Eczema of the nipple superficially resembles Paget's disease but the nipples remain equal in size. The condition may be caused by scabies or may be allergic in origin. Treatment varies with the cause.

nitrogen. An inert gas which is the largest component of air and also an essential element in all living animals.

Soil bacteria and certain plants utilize nitrogen from the air to synthesize proteins which are the only foodstuffs containing nitrogen. The proteins are broken down in the digestive systems of persons and animals, and in part re-synthesized for replacement of tissue, while waste nitrogen is excreted by the kidneys, mostly as urea.

nitrogen mustards. A group of drugs which delay the multiplication of rapidly dividing cells. In such conditions as Hodgkin's disease and chronic leukaemia they do not constitute a cure but they may appreciably prolong life.

nits. Eggs of LICE. They are coated with a sticky substance and adhere firmly to hairs or clothing.

nocturia. Passage of urine during the night. In a healthy young adult the kidneys are relatively inactive during sleep, so that the bladder does not require to be emptied during the night. Older people often have to rise once nightly, but more frequent need to pass urine constitutes nocturia.

Causes include: (1) various diseases of the kidney resulting in increased secretion of dilute urine; (2) diseases of the bladder, such as cystitis; (3) in men, disorders of the prostate gland; and (4) in pregnant women, pressure on the bladder by an enlarged uterus. Unless the cause is obvious nocturia needs medical investigation.

nocturnal emissions. Involuntary discharge of sperms and fluid from the prostate gland during sleep. The discharge is sometimes, but by no means always, accompanied by erotic dreams, and so the term 'wet dreams' is often used.

During adolescence these discharges often distress boys and sometimes distress their parents. However, they are normal physiological happenings and should be so regarded. They do not harm the person in any way. Where they are frequent (more than about twice monthly) attempts may be made to reduce their frequency by plain living, avoidance of circumstances likely to lead to sexual stimulation and efforts to concentrate the youth's attention on non-sexual matters.

Nocturnal emissions also occur in some celibate men who lead continent lives, and in men subjected to sexual stimulation without gratification.

normal saline. A solution of common salt in sterile water made to exactly the same strength as in the cells of the body, i.e., 0.9 per cent. A rough approximation can be made by dissolving a level teaspoonful of salt in two tumblerfuls of recently boiled water. For purposes like bathing an eye or washing a wound this solution is much more soothing than simple sterile water.

nose. Although normally regarded as the organ of smell because of the olfactory receptors in its upper part, the nose is primarily the organ that warms, moistens and filters air before it passes to the lungs.

Internally the nose is divided into two parts by a cartilaginous septum. Entering each half through a nostril the air passes over a series of folded cartilages lined with mucous membrane and is thus warmed and moistened before travelling on to the

Anatomy of the nose

nasopharynx. The air is also filtered by minute hairs.

Diseases. Common symptoms of diseases of the nose include discharge ('running nose'), obstructed breathing ('stuffed nose') and impaired or lost sense of smell. Frequent diseases include colds, catarrh, adenoids and polypi.

There are paths of communication between the nose and the hollows (sinuses) in the neighbouring bones of the skull, so that an infection of the nose can pass to the sinuses.

Foreign bodies. Small children quite often insert foreign bodies into their nostrils, and this cause of nasal symptoms should never be ignored in the young. Vigorous blowing of the nose often dislodges the object, or, if it is within sight, it may be removed with small forceps. If it is not in sight and cannot be dislodged by nose-blowing expert attention is required.

Fractures. These are not uncommon as a result of direct violence, e.g., a blow, or impact of a cricket ball. There is generally considerable bruising, nose bleeding and displacement of the nose to one side. Immediate treatment includes keeping the patient's head up and applying cold water to the nose. Medical attention is important because without it the fracture will tend to heal with the displacement unconnected.

nose bleeding. Nose bleeding, from rupture of a small blood vessel inside the nose, has many causes. In a child it may follow obstruction by a foreign body, result from a blow on the nose, mark the onset of a severe fever, be due to nose picking, or have no discoverable cause. In an adult most of these causes may operate, but nose bleeding may be a release mechanism in persons with high blood pressure or excess of blood, and it may occur because of exposure to high altitudes.

Immediate treatment is to get the patient sitting with head thrown back and breathing through the mouth, to loosen constricting clothing (e.g., collar) and to pinch the nostrils together for several minutes. If the bleeding continues an ice-bag should be applied to the nape of the neck and another to the bridge of the nose. If the bleeding still continues, medical attention is required.

nose douching. A formerly common method of seeking to get rid of a thick or persisting nasal discharge was by gently douching twice daily with a solution of common salt or sodium bicarbonate, one teaspoonful to a glass of warm water. Douching, however, is not free from danger: the presence of an unpleasant discharge normally implies infection, and douching may push the infection to the air sinuses or to the Eustachian tubes and thence to the middle ear. In general, therefore, douching has been abandoned in favour of more modern methods of treatment.

notifiable diseases. In virtually all countries there are arrangements for notification of specified infections to a person charged with responsibility for their control, so that he can institute measures for the prevention of an outbreak, the protection of the community, the treatment of persons suffering from the condition and the further study of the causation and prevalence of the disease.

Health education, better hygiene, immunization facilities and improved living standards have made most infections rarities, so that the need for notification is sometimes questioned. Essentially it is required for the following reasons. (1) A general practitioner has no power to deal with contacts who are not even on his list of patients: he cannot, for example, offer them vaccination and keep them under surveillance. (2) Even in respect of his own patients the practitioner has no legal power: he cannot stop the infectious person from attending school, church or cinema. (3) He cannot institute such measures as chlorination of water in a suspected water-borne outbreak or temporary closure and investigation of a suspected bakery in a food-borne outbreak. (4) Where a disease normally occurs sporadically but occasionally becomes epidemic, an outbreak may be quite widespread before any one practitioner is aware that the few patients that he is seeing represent more than normal prevalence of the disease. (5) If thirty practitioners each see anything from one to ten cases in the early stages of an outbreak, no one of them is in a position to estimate requirements, for example in respect of additional hospital beds, extra laboratory facilities, additional nurses or extra supplies of vaccines or antibiotics (6) As some infections become rare they are easily missed by doctors who seldom encounter them: it is therefore important that there should be one doctor with full knowledge of the infectious situation and able either to alert his colleagues to the presence of a particular disease or to decide that the circumstances do not give rise to such risk as would justify such alerting. (7) Since diseases like cholera and typhoid create much public alarm it is important that there should be a recognized person who can not only tell the public what safety precautions to take but can also allay needless anxiety.

The infections currently notifiable in Britain are: cholera, diphtheria, dysentery, encephalitis, food poisoning, infectious jaundice, malaria, measles, meningitis, ophthalmia neonatorum, paratyphoid, plague, poliomyelitis, relapsing fever, scarlet fever, smallpox, tuberculosis, typhoid fever, typhus fever, whooping cough and yellow fever.

numbness. A state of altered sensation usually arising from pressure on a nerve, inflammation of a nerve, application of certain drugs to the skin, e.g., carbolic acid, or impact of intense cold on the skin. The altered sensation often begins with 'pins and needles' but rapidly progresses to absence of sensation.

Numbness of the hands and feet may arise in osteoarthritis or may be an indication of impaired circulation, but may also be due to any of the factors mentioned above. Treatment varies with the cause.

nurse. A person professionally qualified in the giving of personal nursing care to persons who are sick or infirm, whether in hospital or at home, and in the teaching of patients, relatives of patients, potential patients and the general public as to the preservation or improvement of health, the prevention of disease and the reduction of relapses and recurrences. For the sick patient the nurse's role is commonly thought of as consisting of doing things for the patient, using technical and ministration skills with, of course, full knowledge of related physical and emotional factors: but it also involves creating an atmosphere of confidence and inducing the patient to try to do things for himself. On the community side, whether engaged in preventive (health visiting) or curative (home nursing) work, the nurse is not merely acting for individuals or families, e.g., intervening between them and the stresses of physical environment and social climate, but also striving to induce them to act and behave in ways that will improve their physical, emotional and social well-being.

Florence Nightingale in her *Notes on Nursing* (1859) declared that nursing 'ought to signify the proper use of fresh air, light, warmth, cleanliness, quiet and the proper selection and administration of diet – all at the least expense of vital power to the patient', and a few years later she stressed the teaching role of the newly created health visitor. To these necessary but rather obvious qualities have to be added a highly developed and accurate observation, technical and ministration skills, capacity to set aside one's own feelings and needs because of the urgent needs of the patient, skill in the use of complicated equipment, insight into cultural and value systems, ability to communicate successfully, and professional ethical standards, together with – for a proportion of nurses – administrative and organizational skills (for the chief nursing officer of an area has to deploy and organize a professional staff numbering thousands), and knowledge of educational psychology and teaching methods (for a tutor has exactly the same functions as has a university or college of education lecturer).

Nursing is often thought of as a feminine profession, but the number of male nurses is increasing steadily.

nursing. Since it takes three years of full-time professional education to convert an intelligent young person into a qualified nurse, with further full-time preparation required for entry to various branches (e.g., health visiting, midwifery and home nursing), and since the complexity of a nurse's duties and responsibilities increases with almost every development in the various health sciences, it is no more possible to set down the essentials of nursing in a single article than it would be to specify the fundamental principles of accountancy or personnel management. Yet, just as many people have to invest money and prepare tax returns without being accountants or to co-ordinate groups of staff without being qualified personnel managers, so many people have – without specialized nursing education – to care for sick relatives at home.

A few basic points are therefore mentioned here. For simplicity the patient is called 'he' and the unqualified nurse 'she', but of course either could be of either sex.

Attitude. Probably the most important requirements for home nursing of a relative are sympathetic understanding and genuine interest, emotional self-control, alert observation, and respect for the judgment of visiting experts. The patient who is ill and in pain lacks his normal control of himself, he may be very irritable and unkind, he may seek to leave his bed long before it is safe for him to do so, or he may plead for his pain-killer considerably before it is due. It is vital that the person nursing him meets his irritability and difficult behaviour with kindly patience and a judicious mixture of sympathy and firmness. The patient who is beginning to recover is often bored and disgruntled. It is important that the nurse finds means of securing and maintaining his interest. She may be very worried about the serious nature of his illness, distressed about his pain, hurt by his unkind remarks and anxious about her own ability to carry out a particular treatment, but she needs to conceal these feelings. For the time being she is his main contact with the outside world and the person on whom he depends, and she must convey to him an atmosphere of calm confidence.

She sees the patient for hours on end whereas any visiting doctor or nurse sees him for minutes. So it is important that she uses her observation in order to report anything that might have a bearing on the diagnosis or on the treatment.

However skilled she may be in her own professional or commercial field she has to remember that she is an amateur in nursing and that the visiting doctor or visiting nurse is an expert, and that the expert's instructions must be carried out completely: the amateur nurse is taking part in a battle for the patient's life or for his health, and a soldier cannot argue with the commander in the middle of a battle. She has to realize, too, that the doctor's expertise and the nurse's expertise are different: a busy doctor or busy nurse can sometimes be induced by a persuasive amateur to concur in an opinion relating to the other person's expertise, but such reinforcement of the amateur's view is seldom beneficial to the patient.

Sick-room. To such extent as choice is possible the room should be of adequate size, reasonably warm but well ventilated, though with the bed out of all cross-draughts; and quiet with regard both to outdoor traffic and to indoor noises. The bed should be accessible from both sides. If light disturbs the patient's sleep a screen may shield the window or a partial shade may dim the electric light, while leaving the nurse enough light to see the patient and to read or write. A small table at the bedside for the patient's use and another table for the nurse's use are desirable, and if the bathroom is at some distance a washstand can be very useful. Since the nurse will be present for many hours, it is important that there is a comfortable chair for her use: reasonable comfort is essential for her continued efficiency, but this point is often forgotten by willing amateurs whose initial thoughts, naturally, are concerned with the well-being of the sick relatives. Apart from these items, the less furniture there is in the room the better.

The patient. When removing clothing from an injured patient or putting garments on him it is useful to tackle the uninjured side first, so limiting movement. In most illness the patient should be washed daily all over with warm water, the ordinary bedclothes being removed before the washing and the patient covered with a blanket, and the blanket being raised over individual parts of the body while these are washed and dried. The back should be examined daily for reddening and treated promptly if redness appears, so preventing bed-sores. In some cases various manipulations – such as changing of garments, washing, bed-making, feeding and toileting – cause some discomfort or actual pain, and both gentleness and quiet encouragement are needed.

The bed. Where available a single bed is better, both for the comfort of the patient and for the convenience of the nurse. The bedclothes should be light and changed frequently: as already mentioned the room should be warm and additional heat can be supplied by hot water bottles with, if the patient is too ill to complain of excessive heat, external wrapping. The sheet under the patient should be firmly tucked under the mattress all round, otherwise the patient in bed all day will quickly get it creased, producing discomfort and danger of bed-sores. If there is any likelihood of incontinence or if the patient is too ill to move from the bed to the toilet, a draw-sheet and rubber mackintosh are essential.

Bedmaking. To make a bed with the patient lying in it is a skilled art, but bed-making should be done twice daily for the patient's comfort. In general the guidance of a qualified nurse should be sought at first, and when the attendant feels competent for the job the help of a second person should be enlisted if possible. Probably the simplest method is to place a chair at the foot of the bed, to lift each blanket or sheet separately from the top and fold it over the chair, and when only one sheet remains over the patient for one person to raise him gently while another person straightens the sheet (or draw-sheet) under him. If the patient cannot lie for a minute without pillows he may have to be supported while the pillows are changed.

Temperature and pulse. These are important indications during illness. The person nursing a patient should learn to read a thermometer and record the temperature, always remembering to shake the thermometer down after use, to take the temperature in the same place (the mouth which is slightly higher or the armpit which is slightly lower) and not to record the temperature immediately after a meal or a hot drink or a hot bath. Similarly she should learn to take the pulse at the wrist, placing the tips of her first and second fingers over the artery on the thumb side of the wrist and counting the beats for thirty seconds. In some illnesses counting the rate of respirations can also be useful.

Medicines. Medicines should be kept in a different part of the room from fluids intended for external application, and the nurse should school herself never to pour out a dose without reading the label on the bottle. When one is tired – and home nursing is a fatiguing job – mistakes can occur easily.

Liquid food and solid food. It is important to appreciate the risk of dehydration and to ensure that the patient has sufficient liquid in a form that he is willing to take. In some illnesses the amount of fluid consumed has to be measured. Solid food is relatively unimportant in a very short illness but is clearly important in any prolonged illness. Attractive serving of food, attention to the patient's likes and dislikes and gentle persuasion may make the difference between food being accepted and refused.

Relief for the attendant. Apart from 'on call' duties (where they may be relaxing or sleeping but available at need) a qualified doctor or a qualified nurse is usually prepared during a prolonged emergency such as a major epidemic, to work for about fifty-four hours a week (or nine hours a day for six days a week), but judges that efficiency falls if it proves necessary to exceed these times. The same sort of maximum has been established in industrial work during the pressures of wars or civil calamities. The amateur nurse undertaking the care of a sick relative is tackling an unfamiliar job and is emotionally involved. It is therefore unlikely that, in an illness lasting more than a few days, she can cope efficiently with spells of duty longer than those acceptable to qualified professionals. A common mistake during the illness of a much-loved relative is to be 'on duty' for thirteen or fourteen hours a day for well over a week before seeking help. By that time observation has become less acute (and important signs may be missed), self-control is lessened (so that the patient may become conscious of worries and fears), toleration of unkind remarks or harmful behaviour is reduced, and the possibilities of mistakes over medicines are increased. In other words the amateur nurse's attempt to cope for too long may harm the patient as well as herself. Where a serious illness nursed at home looks like extending substantially over a week it is therefore sound common-sense to start considering what relief can be provided by relatives, friends, paid help or services available from the state.

nutrition. The term is used both for (1) the process whereby FOOD is converted into energy and living tissue, and (2) the state of a person with regard to his absorption and assimilation of appropriate foods.

Each species of animal appears to have its own requirements of food: some, like cattle, are strict vegetarians; carnivorous animals eat only animal flesh; and some – like man – are omnivorous, both meat and vegetables being included in the DIET.

In primitive communities qualitative or even quantitative under-nutrition is common: man has discovered which foods are edible, but depends on successful hunting of animals or successful growth of plants, with winter feeding an annual problem and famine a recurring danger to life. In highly developed communities food production and food preservation have normally removed all dangers of winter shortages, a wide choice of varieties of food is available, over-nutrition is common among the affluent, and people have had leisure to develop many irrational prejudices and taboos, so that under-nutrition can occur either from poverty or as a result of food fads. In the twentieth century, as population growth outstrips increase of food production, under-nutrition becomes commoner, and fully half of the world's population today are appreciably under-nourished.

FOOD is needed to supply energy not only for work and movement but also for such purposes as maintaining the bodily temperature and keeping the heart beating; to provide material for growth and for repair of tissue, with the amino-acids of proteins particularly required; and to provide substances - e.g., vitamins and trace minerals - for chemical processes that take place in the body.

While manual work manifestly increases food requirements it used to be said that mental work did not do so, but in recent years it has been established that mental activity does consume some energy.

The nutritional requirements for health are subject to many variations. To take some examples: in cold weather we use more Calories in maintaining our bodily temperature than in hot weather. Alcohol is a good source of Calories and therefore reduces our need for carbohydrate, but conversely it increases our need for vitamins of the B complex. In various infections the metabolic rate is speeded up so that we need more food, but paradoxically many foods are poorly digested, so that - to take one essential substance as an instance - by the time we have recovered from a severe infection our bodily stores of vitamin C are badly depleted.

Good nutrition is essential for health. Particularly vulnerable groups in respect of under-nutrition are: babies; rapidly growing children and adolescents - with the transition from school to work often a point of maximum danger; expectant and nursing mothers; old people - who often have deficiencies of protein, minerals and vitamins; immigrants - who may have difficulty in obtaining foods familiar to them and be reluctant to accept the diets normal in their new country; the very poor - who may have difficulty in affording expensive protein foods; and, commonest of all, the ignorant - whose food purchasing is often faulty and whose food preparation may destroy vitamins and lose minerals. Particularly vulnerable in respect of over-nutrition are persons whose occupations tempt them to over-eat, e.g., cooks and persons travelling on expense accounts.

nymphomania. Abnormally strong and frequent sexual desire in a woman. The parallel desire in a man is termed

If over 60, eat the following daily:
0.5 litres (1 pint) of milk if possible but not less than half this amount.
1 helping of 55g. (2oz.) of meat, fish, poultry (once a week eat liver and oily fish)
1 egg
28g.(1oz.) cheese
1 tomato or half an orange
1 helping of **root** vegetables or **green** vegetables
1 helping of potatoes
3 to 4 slices of bread (often wholemeal)
1 helping of porridge or breakfast cereal
40g.(1.5oz.) margarine or butter

Nutrition: good food

satyriasis. Nymphomania and satyriasis may become so severe that ethics and will-power lose their controlling influence and the need for relief by the sexual act dominates the imagination, but with actual intercourse providing less satisfaction than in the case of normal people.

The conditions used to be attributed to abnormalities of hormone secretion, but the modern view is that they have a deep-rooted psychological basis and that, while tranquillizers may temporarily subdue the extreme sexual drive, a full course of psychotherapy is usually needed.

nystagmus. Involuntary rapid and jerky movements of the eyeball, from side to side or up and down. Both eyes are usually affected. In children it may arise from diseases of the nervous system, congenital cataract, or inflammatory diseases of the eye. In adults it may appear in multiple sclerosis and cerebellar disease, and it is also found – without other signs of disease – in miners who work underground in semi-darkness. In general its presence suggests the need for immediate expert investigation.

nystatin. An antibiotic obtained from the bacterium *Streptomyces noursei*. It is used in the treatment of infections caused by certain fungi, especially *Candida albicans*. It is used in various forms: as a cream for skin infections, as an oral preparation, as eye-drops, and as pessaries or suppositories.

O

obesity. The condition of being overweight with excessive fat stored in the body.

In addition to being unattractive, appreciable excess of weight is dangerous: it forces the heart to work harder, because a greater volume of tissue has to be supplied with blood; it increases liability to pneumonia and other respiratory infections; it raises the chance of diabetes and arteriosclerosis; and because the stout person is in effect carrying an extra stone or half-stone whenever he moves, obesity increases the likelihood of arthritis, backache and flat feet. Not least, obesity decreases the expectation of life.

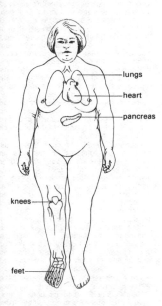

Obesity may be harmful to various parts of the body

The exact borderline of obesity is hard to define. A professional boxer usually knows his best weight – below which he loses strength and above which he loses speed – but most of us can only hazard a guess at our optimum weight. Attempts were formerly made to assess ideal (unclothed) weight by a simple formula.

However, bone structure varies. A man of 172 cm. (5 ft. 8 in.) and heavy frame may be underweight at 68 kg. (150 lb.) while another man of the same height and light frame may be overweight at 63.5 kg. (140 lb.). Modern attempts to divide adults into heavy, medium and light bone structure for each height are more useful, but even these are merely approximations, and rigid application of such tables (see HEIGHT AND WEIGHT) suggests, rightly or wrongly, that about half the adults in Britain are overweight.

Perhaps more important than any hypothetical ideal weight is whether a person's weight is rising or remaining stationary. Prolonged consumption of rather more food than is needed leads to production of more tissue, but the slightly corpulent person expends more energy in supplying blood to the extra tissue and because he carries additional weight, uses more energy in each physical activity. If his weight becomes stationary he is probably not unduly at risk. If, on the other hand, his weight is continuing to rise, his life and his health are in danger.

Obesity is commoner in some races, for instance, Eskimos, living in icy climates, need a thick layer of adipose tissue. It is occasionally associated with endocrine or glandular abnormalities (e.g., hypothyroidism or hypopituitarism) which reduce the rate of energy expenditure. But in general it represents simply a prolonged disproportion between the quantity of Calories ingested and the quantity utilized by the body. Certainly some people have bodies that use food inefficiently, excreting the excess in faeces, urine, sweat and breath without gaining weight; but in persons whose bodies make efficient use of food, weight gain indicates prolonged over-eating.

Over-eating proteins plays little if any part in obesity: increase of protein foods (e.g., lean meat and white fish) raises the rate of combustion in the body, and excess is excreted rather than stored. Fat plays little part: a disproportionate amount of fat leads to indigestion. The real culprit is excess carbohydrate (starches and sugars) which is stored in the body as fat. Lack of exercise may play a part in persons transferring from heavy manual work (in which many Calories are expended) to sedentary occupations, but it is more often a result than a cause of obesity: to lose one pound by exercise a man would have to walk fifty miles and disregard the increased appetite produced by his exertions.

Causes. The overeating that leads to obesity usually results from specific causes.

1. Over-feeding, especially excess of carbohydrates, in infancy and childhood, with subsequent persistence of the habit of eating too much. Fat babies tend to become fat children and in due course corpulent adults. Parents who systematically over-feed their young children are unknowingly shortening their lives. Obesity is commonly regarded as a problem of middle life, but at least half the cases start in infancy or childhood. In this connection it should be noted that, while obesity is often described as characteristic of affluent societies or of favourably placed groups in mixed societies, it can also occur in the poor because carbohydrate foods are usually cheaper than protein or fatty foods.

2. Psychological disturbances either in childhood or in adult life. The person who is lonely, bereaved, frustrated or otherwise disturbed eats in substitution for some other ungratified emotion. The emotional factors in obesity are only now becoming recognized. To treat a case of excessive weight without attention to emotional factors if they are present means either that the treatment will fail or that, if it succeeds in respect of reducing the amount of eating, it will leave the patient in a worse condition by removing his substitute for the unsatisfied emotion.

3. Nature of work. For instance, it is not unusual for cooks to be stout.

4. Failure to adjust food intake to changing circumstances. A retired athlete often puts on weight, as sometimes do people who move from physical to mental occupations. The elderly are usually less active than they were in their younger days and so require less energy (Calories) from their food.

Prevention. Just as obesity starts in childhood, so should its prevention. Essentially parents should be made aware of the dangers of over-feeding children, and especially of giving them excessive carbohydrates; health workers should seek to prevent or alleviate mental disturbances at all stages of the lives of their clients; and all concerned with health education should point out that even a small additional daily intake – a single extra slice of bread or three extra lumps of sugar – can in time create a considerable burden of overweight.

Treatment. Established obesity inevitably demands a rigorous DIET, with rigid restriction of amounts of bread, cakes, biscuits, milk puddings, sweets, cream and potatoes, limitation of alcohol, avoidance of eating between meals, and weekly weighing. Such a diet by itself almost always fails. To have any hope of success the person who is trying to lose weight also needs much reassurance and

encouragement, in addition to attention to any relevant emotional factors. Appetite depressants are sometimes used to help patients to endure restricted diets, but the amphetamines cause excitement and sleeplessness, and undue reliance on drugs often results in reversion to the previous weight after the drug is ultimately discontinued.

obsessional neurosis. An emotional disorder in which the victim's consciousness is dominated by certain ideas or impulses and by resistance to them. The sufferer is aware that his obsession is senseless and undergoes considerable mental anxiety during his fruitless efforts to gain freedom from the particular fear, preoccupation or impulses.

The causes are not fully understood. There appears to be a considerable amount of parental influence involved: in fully one-third of cases a parent has also been obsessional, and in many other cases a parent has been over-conscientious, excessively orderly, abnormally concerned with cleanliness or a stickler for precision. In such cases the origin of the disorder is probably less a matter of heredity than of the development of personality being impaired by the parental attitudes and behaviour. In other cases the source seems to lie in painful or disturbing experiences. In others, again, the psychoanalysts' explanation of obsessions as symbolic self-reproaches for earlier sexual misdemeanours is almost certainly true. However, some obsessionals have not had neurotic parents, have not experienced any series of painful happenings and have not indulged in conduct that weighs on their consciences.

The obsessions may consist of ideas, questionings, impulses, phobias or a mixture of these. Ideas vary from tunes 'running in the head' for prolonged periods to obscene associations, such as every hole or cleft reminding the patient of a vulva. Questionings include a persistent and senseless 'Why' about relevant and irrelevant matters, with often a preoccupation with religion or philosophical questions. Impulses may be aggressive or suicidal, or merely a compulsion to count every step walked or to touch every lamp-post passed. Phobias include fear of open spaces, of enclosed spaces, of darkness and of dirt.

Many apparently normal people have persisting ideas, questioning natures, senseless impulses and irrational fears. What differentiates the obsessional from the normal is the domination of the particular fear or idea and the painful effort made to get rid of it.

Treatment involves frank discussion with the patient, avoidance of situations in which the obsession is most marked and where practicable a change of environment. Psychoanalysis, hypnosis and suggestion help in some cases. Where the obsession is severe, and especially where it is dangerous either to the patient or to others, pre-frontal leucotomy may be considered, though the current tendency in such cases is to try appropriate drugs and to regard leucotomy as a last resort.

obstetrics. The branch of medicine concerned with pregnancy and childbirth.

occiput. The back and lower part of the skull pierced by the foramen magnum through which the spinal cord passes from the brain.

occlusion. The term is used in four different ways, all connected with the derivational idea of shutting. (1) Closure of the eyes by drawing the eyelids over them. (2) Blockage of any hollow tube, e.g., in coronary occlusion one of the arteries that supply blood to the heart is blocked by a clot. (3) Temporary closure of the vocal passage in speech, as in formation of the stop consonants. (4) The coming together of the upper and lower teeth in the process of biting. The converse term, malocclusion, is used only in the fourth sense and means inability of the teeth to meet correctly.

occupational diseases. In Britain fourteen industrial diseases are now notifiable to the Chief Inspector of Factories. They are lead poisoning, phosphorus poisoning, arsenical poisoning, mercury poisoning, manganese poisoning, carbon bisulphide poisoning, analine poisoning, benzene poisoning, anthrax, toxic jaundice, compressed air illness, epitheliomatous ulceration, chrome ulceration and toxic anaemia. Following improvement in working conditions all have now become rarities, although chrome ulceration, epitheliomatous ulceration, and lead poisoning each amount to about one hundred to two hundred notifications a year in Britain.

The commonest occupational diseases of today are of the skin, lungs and muscles.

Occupational dermatitis – clinically indistinguishable from any other form of DERMATITIS - may occur through the skin becoming sensitive to a particular solvent, oil or dye. Barrier creams carefully applied before work can help to prevent the condition.

Dust diseases of the lungs include pneumoconiosis (in coal miners, graphite workers and boiler scalers), byssinosis (due to inhalation of cotton dust), asbestosis, and silicosis. Preventive measures include substitution of a toxic substance by a harmless one, reduction of exposure to the dust by exhaust ventilation and scrupulous cleanliness, and the use of respirators to prevent inhalation of dust and fumes.

Occupational palsy or *cramp* is a condition of discomfort, pain and fatigue arising from habitual use of one set of muscles in finely coordinated movements; WRITER'S CRAMP and musician's cramp are examples.

occupational pyrexia. A condition, quite common thirty years ago but relatively uncommon today, occurring in workers in textile factories, and characterized by bouts of feverishness, headache, nausea, general weakness and disinclination for food. It is found more in recently appointed workers than in those with long service, and is almost certainly allergic, a hypersensitivity to some of the constituents of the raw materials. Treatment is essentially as for any other ALLERGY with change of work necessary in some cases. An alternative name for the condition is mill fever.

There are at least two explanations of the decrease in occupational pyrexia, both partially correct. Firstly, better ventilation and better hygienic standards generally have made it likely that people with only a mild hypersensitivity to a particular constituent will escape; and secondly, in the past mill fever was a convenient name under which to lump a number of different diseases, such as aspergillosis.

occupational therapy. Treatment of the physically or mentally ill by engaging them constructively in selected activities.

The term was originally used to denote the occupational methods adopted for the relief and treatment of nervous and mental illness, but has come to include similar methods in all forms of prolonged illness. In certain conditions particular forms of occupation are physically desirable to strengthen weakened or unused muscles; and in most illnesses occupational therapy has a considerable psychological effect, restoring the patient's confidence in himself and in his ability to do things.

Properly undertaken, occupational therapy involves attempting to discover the patient's aptitudes, talents or abilities, exploiting these in suitable occupation, and so building up a sense of achievement and satisfaction. This does not merely relieve the tedium of a long spell in hospital but also actively promotes recovery.

Weaving, raffia and basket work, needlework, toy-making, book-binding and painting are well-established forms of occupational therapy; but in general the occupation has to be geared to the patient, not the patient to the available occupation.

Occupational therapy, which gives the patient something useful and interesting to do, slides imperceptibly into vocational rehabilitation, in which a person who has become permanently unfit for his former occupation learns new skills in preparation for a job suited to his restricted abilities.

oedema. Abnormal accumulation of watery fluid in the body tissues or cavities. Oedema is not a disease but a symptom of disease of the heart, kidney or liver. Perhaps the commonest form of oedema is the slight swelling of the ankles that many people experience after prolonged standing. While this may be an indication of cardiac or renal disorder, it has various other causes, e.g., constriction of veins by tight garters. See DROPSY.

Oedipus complex. During the insecurity of infancy many boys pass through a stage in which they are more attracted to their mother than to their father and are even a little jealous of him. Where this stage persists and becomes exaggerated into a neurosis it is termed the Oedipus complex, named after a legendary Greek who married his own mother without being aware of her identity.

The explanations of Freud undoubtedly cover the fully developed complex and in such cases psychoanalytic treatment can be useful. Much commoner, however, is the almost latent variety in which the young man subconsciously looks for a bride who resembles his mother physically and mentally, compares his wife disadvantageously with his mother, resolutely declines to enter his father's occupation and adopts religious and political views utterly different from those of his father.

The feminine equivalent , where a daughter has excessive love for her father and resentment of her mother is called the Electra complex.

oesophagus. The muscular tube, often known as the gullet, which conveys food from the mouth and pharynx to the stomach. It lies in front of the spinal column, behind the windpipe in the neck and behind the upper part of the heart in the chest. Food is propelled down the tube by muscular movements called PERISTALSIS.

It is the narrowest part of the whole digestive tube and swallowed foreign bodies tend to become lodged in it. The oesophagus may also become obstructed for other reasons: the commonest causes are: (1) scarring due to the swallowing of hot or corrosive fluids, (2) malignant disease arising in the oesophagus itself, and (3) external pressure especially from aneurysm of the aorta or malignant disease of lungs, bronchi, or mediastinum.

The gullet can be examined by an oesophagoscope, a tube with a light at the end and working in the same way as a periscope.

oestrogen. The two groups of hormones secreted by the ovary are known by the general names, oestrogen and progesterone. The oestrogens are the substances responsible for the development and maintenance of a woman's sexual organs and breasts, and in preparation for pregnancy they cause a thickening of the inside lining of the uterus.

Several synthetic oestrogens such as STILBOESTROL are available for therapy, e.g., for treatment of painful menstruation and for alleviation of symptoms at the menopause.

Most oral contraceptives contain small amounts of an oestrogen and a progesterone, the relative quantities and the particular synthetic oestrogen varying with the brand of contraceptive.

old age. See AGEING.

oliguria. Diminished secretion of urine. It occurs in some diseases of the kidney and in diseases of the heart and liver associated with OEDEMA. It may also occur temporarily in healthy people who have perspired excessively under conditions of abnormal warmth.

omentum. The omenta are double folds of peritoneum which contain fat and blood vessels and which separate abdominal organs from each other. The great omentum is attached to the lower border of the stomach and hangs like an apron in front of the intestines. The lesser omentum separates the liver from the stomach.

oncology. The study of tumours.

one-parent families. Families consisting of one or more children and only one available parent. Common causes of this situation include: (1) the death of one partner, leaving the other a widow or widower; (2) divorce; (3) desertion by one partner; (4) chronic illness or insanity of one partner; (5) cases of illegitimacy unaccompanied by any stable union.

The varying causes lead to considerable differences in financial circumstances, mental outlook and attitudes of relations. Thus the widow is in some, though by no means all, cases materially comfortable through inheriting life insurance or obtaining compensation for the accident or injury that killed her husband; the divorced person may have considerable alimony; but the unmarried mother or the woman whose husband has simply disappeared is often in dire financial straits. The widow and her children, if old enough, may look back to years of normal family life; the divorced or separated person may recall unhappy years of discord and bickering and may even have a permanent hostility to the opposite sex; and the unmarried mother has no personal experience of married life. The widower, though he may have to face the cost of employing a housekeeper, will in general receive the sympathy and practical help of his relatives, whereas in some cultures the unmarried mother is the subject of a stigma which may even make it difficult for her to secure employment. Again the widow and the unmarried mother can contemplate marriage but the divorced or deserted person in some cases finds the idea of re-marriage in conflict with long-existing religious tenets.

In most cases the solitary parent has to be the bread-winner for the household, involving placing young children in a day nursery or in the daily care of a child-minder (unless there is an available grandmother or aunt), and involving constant worry about children's illnesses. In any such illness there is a conflict between the needs of the children and the requirements of the bread-winner's job. It is easy to say on humanitarian grounds that the children must always take precedence, but the absence of one person in a highly responsible or highly specialized post may seriously impede the work of sixty other people.

Not least, the one parent has to try to

fulfil the role of both father and mother. It might be thought that, with a woman as sole parent, the absence of a father's authority might lead to excessive licence and 'spoiling'; but in many cases the effect is the reverse, the woman over-compensating for the absence of a husband by being over-strict, with harmful effects on the children's later ability to make decisions and exercise initiative.

In most western countries the problems of the one-parent household were largely ignored until recent decades. However, Sweden led the way by providing for such households special flats with adjacent nurseries, several developed countries now offer additional financial allowances in such cases, and helpful associations (such as, in Britain, the Society for the Single Parent and her Dependants) have come into existence. Also the spread of contraceptive measures (reducing the number of unmarried mothers) and improved facilities for the prevention and treatment of illness (reducing the number of deaths of parents) have between them considerably lessened the total number of one-parent families.

Nevertheless the situation of the solitary parent and her (or more rarely his) dependants is difficult; but it is worth remembering that even three generations ago the difficulties could be overcome, e.g., one child brought up in a one-parent family (Ramsay MacDonald) became prime minister of Britain and another (Charlie Chaplin) became perhaps the world's most famous cinema actor. See also DIVORCE.

onychia. Infection of the bed of a nail. Mild cases may clear up spontaneously, moderate cases respond well to antibiotics, and in severe cases removal of the nail may be required. If the nail is removed and the infection cleared, the nail will re-grow; but if the infection remains it may destroy the growing tissue, so that ultimately the nail comes off and does not re-grow. Hence deliberate removal of the nail to facilitate treatment of the infection may well save permanent loss of the nail.

operation, need for. The question of operative treatment arises under two different sets of circumstances.

Firstly, in acute illness the matter may be one of urgency and indeed of life or death. In acute appendicitis, for instance, or in a perforated ulcer of the stomach or duodenum, every hour of delay materially increases the risk to life. A death from an unnecessary operation is extremely rare, but every year hundreds of people die because operation was not performed or was performed too late. In any acute illness where the attending doctor desires a surgeon's opinion and where an experienced surgeon advises operation, neither patient nor relatives should hesitate.

Secondly, operation may be considered for the relief of a long-lasting condition. Examples are infected tonsils and adenoids, prolapse of the uterus, incurable arthritic joint, and ingrowing toenail. Here there is ample time for consideration of the advantages and disadvantages of operation as opposed to other available methods of treatment. Clearly decision will depend on many factors, including the patient's general health, but it is worth remembering that, with modern anaesthesia and modern surgical techniques, many operations involve little danger and little post-operative pain or discomfort.

ophthalmia. Inflammation of the eye or the membranes lining the eyelid. Conjunctivitis, iritis and trachoma are varieties of ophthalmia. Ophthalmia neonatorum, formerly common in new-born infants, was due to gonococcal infection during the journey through the mother's birth passage. In most developed countries the condition has disappeared, partly because of more efficient diagnosis and treatment of maternal gonorrhoea, but mainly because of routine treatment of the eyes of all newly born infants to prevent it.

Sympathetic ophthalmia is a curious condition in which, after an injury to one eye, the other eye becomes inflamed. Not only does the sympathetic inflammation need treatment, but the inflammation is long-lasting and hard to cure. Indeed, where both eyes were previously normal, it is not unknown for the injured eye to make a greater recovery of sight than the sympathetically inflamed eye. As a preventive measure many eye specialists, when treating an injured eye, use atropine or an antibiotic or both for the uninjured eye.

ophthalmologist. A doctor who specializes in treatment of diseases of the eye. A frequently used alternative name is ophthalmic surgeon, but not all doctors who have specialized on the eye undertake surgical work.

These terms should be differentiated from optician, a qualified, non-medical worker. An optician tests eyesight and prescribes spectacles but, if he discovers evidence of disease of the eye, refers the patient to an ophthalmologist.

ophthalmoscope. An instrument for examining the interior of the eye and especially the retina and its blood vessels.

opium. The dried juice of the seed capsules of the white poppy which is extensively grown in Asia. Opium contains several alkaloids, the most important being morphine and codeine. In the past the drug was normally given as a crude powder or as an alcoholic solution, laudanum, but nowadays the purified active ingredients are preferred for greater accuracy of dosage.

Opium has been used to relieve pain since the dawn of history. It reduces pain, slows respiration, constricts the pupils and produces a dreamy state with pleasant imagery or, if the dose is large, a deep sleep. Opium and its main alkaloid, morphine, are of the highest value for relief of pain, but their use has to be carefully controlled because of the danger of addiction. A craving for morphine can begin to appear after as few as three injections, and the drug habit, once established, is very hard to break.

In Britain dilute solutions of opium are readily available, e.g., a mixture of chalk and opium for the treatment of diarrhoea, but morphine and higher concentrations of opium are rigorously controlled under the Dangerous Drugs Act.

opium poisoning. Opium poisoning can occur by accident (especially in children), in attempted suicide, or through therapeutic misadventure. After a short initial period of euphoria and mental excitement, the condition manifests itself by increasing drowsiness going on to complete stupor, contracted 'pin-point' pupils which do not alter in size when light is shone on them, blueness and coldness of the skin, and stertorous or irregular breathing. The main danger is respiratory failure.

If the drug has been taken by mouth an emetic to cause vomiting may be useful. Irrespective of how the drug was taken, strong coffee helps if the patient can swallow, and most experts advise rousing the patient by movement. The most essential points in treatment, however, are the application of artificial respiration (aided by oxygen if available) if breathing becomes difficult, and (again if available) injection of 5 to 10 mg. of the specific antagonist, nalorphine. Given prompt treatment recovery from opium poisoning (as distinct from poisoning by its alkaloids) is highly probable, but in morphine poisoning the outcome is not so certain.

optic nerve. The bundle of nerve fibres forming the second cranial nerve which carry impulses from the retina to the back of the BRAIN.

optic neuritis and atrophy. Inflammation of the optic nerve is not a disease in itself but a symptom of such diseases as brain tumours, meningitis, chronic nephritis, gout and lead poisoning. It leads to failure of sight with blurring of vision, headache and pain in the back of the eye. Treatment varies with the cause.

Optic atrophy, i.e., degeneration of the nerve resulting in blindness, may follow uncured optic neuritis or may arise as a primary condition in organic nervous diseases.

orchitis. Inflammation of the testicles, characterized by swelling, pain and tenderness.

Orchitis occurs most frequently as a painful complication of mumps in adolescent boys and young men. Treatment consists of rest in bed with the scrotum supported by a pillow and pain relievers used as required. The inflammation disappears in a week or so but in some cases the disease leaves the victim sterile.

Less common causes of orchitis include gonorrhoea and enteric fever (in both of which antibiotics are useful), and injury.

organ transplant. See TRANSPLANT.

orgasm. The climax of the sexual act. In the male it is produced mainly by stimulation of the penis and results in the ejaculation of semen. In the female it is produced principally by stimulation of the clitoris. In both sexes orgasm is followed by relaxation of sexual tension and departure of blood from the previously engorged genital organs.

oriental sore. Also termed Delhi or Baghdad boil. A lesion, or more usually a number of lesions, of the skin and the tissues immediately below the skin caused by a protozoon (*Leishmania tropica*) normally transmitted by the bite of a sandfly. The sore begins as an itchy papule, enlarges over many weeks and becomes ulcerated, forming a boil which may take months to heal. Preventive measures are as yet almost non-existent in the countries in which the condition is common. There is no particularly effective treatment, although the injection of a 10 per cent solution of mepacrine hydrochloride is said to accelerate healing. If the sore becomes infected, usually as a result of scratching, antibiotics may be needed for the organisms causing the infection.

ornithosis. A feverish illness with symptoms resembling both pneumonia and typhoid fever, and caused by a virus transmitted by birds, especially from their dried excreta. It is sometimes divided into two varieties: (1) PSITTACOSIS, transmitted mainly by parrots, and (2) ornithosis proper, caused by a much smaller virus transmitted by pigeons, hens and other birds. In both varieties the mortality was very high until the advent of the tetracyclines, and even with early treatment with these recovery is by no means certain. Chlorotetracycline, 4 g. daily for two days and thereafter smaller dosage, is probably the drug of choice.

orthodontics. The branch of dentistry concerned with prevention and correction of faulty position of the teeth, usually by gradually moving teeth to better positions by the sustained slight pressure of a brace.

orthomolecular psychiatry. A school of medical thought, largely founded by Linus Pauling, which maintains that many mental diseases are caused by a twisting of molecules and which, in particular, emphasizes the importance of large intake of certain vitamins both for prevention and for cure. The adherents of the ortho-molecular school point out especially that 94 per cent of schizophrenics excrete abnormally low quantities of ascorbic acid, niacinamide or pyridoxine, and claim that the disease is benefited or cured by massive doses of these vitamins.

As so often happens with pioneers, the founders of this school of thought appear to overstate their case. There exists a good deal of evidence that many psychotic diseases (including at least a goodly number of cases of schizophrenia) are due to genetic abnormalities which, even if identifiable in advance, could hardly be prevented by massive doses of the water-soluble vitamins; and it is difficult to understand how such massive doses could remedy a genetic abnormality. Again, such human experiences as prolonged stress, insecurity, rejection and alienation play a large part in the causation of mental disorders (certainly including some cases of schizophrenia) but are disregarded by Pauling and his associates. In other words, the orthomolecular psychiatrists have not established the only cause or even the main cause of mental disorders and have not provided the sole method of treatment.

Nevertheless their published results are impressive, and they have certainly made out a case for trying massive doses of the B and c vitamins on schizophrenics. At the worst the treatment would do no harm and would not be excessively costly, and even if it improved or cured only a relatively small percentage of schizophrenics the benefit to the persons and to the community would be enormous.

orthopaedics. The branch of surgery that deals with the correction of deformities. The deformities in question include both congenital and acquired conditions, and forms of treatment used include massage, electricity, exercises, the breaking and resetting of bones, and a vast number of appliances.

orthoptics. A method of exercising the eyes, e.g., to correct squint.

osmosis. The diffusion of fluids through a semipermeable membrane into a solution where the concentration of the fluids is lower, thus equalizing the conditions on either side of the membrane. A semipermeable membrane is one of such nature that it acts like a sieve, holding back large molecules but permitting small ones to pass through. The walls of capillary blood vessels, for instance, are such membranes. They permit water, salts, and sugars and amino acids to pass through but prevent the passage of larger molecules. At the end of a capillary nearer to the heart (and receiving in weakened form the pressure of the cardiac contraction) the concentration in the capillary is greater than in the adjacent cells, so the traffic is from capillary to cell; at the far end of the capillary the concentration is greater in the cell than in the capillary, so the traffic is in the reverse direction.

ossification. Hardening of cartilage into bone, either as part of normal growth or in disease. The term is also used to indicate attitudes or beliefs becoming rigid and unalterable.

osteitis. Inflammation of bone. It may be acute or chronic and is the result of bacterial invasion, either from an external wound or from a local focus of infection e.g., in the mouth, throat or alimentary tract.

Osteitis deformans (Paget's disease) is a disease of later life in which certain bones, especially the long bones, lose some of their calcium and hence their rigidity, and then become deformed through weight-bearing. The first symptom is pain, and diagnosis is facilitated by radiological examination. Corticosteroids and sodium fluoride are used in treatment of the condition.

Osteitis fibrosa is a thinning of bones through over-activity of the parathyroid glands.

osteoarthritis. Gradual degeneration of one or more joints, with some loss of cartilage (the smooth tissue which lines the joint) and the formation of rough deposits of bone. It is a very common disease from 40 years onwards and is characterized by pain (generally worse at night), increasing stiffness of the affected joints, limitation of movement and in some cases deformed appearance with 'knobbly' joints.

There are three main types which may exist together. The mono-articular type affects the hip or shoulder mostly and is commoner in men; the polyarticular type affects many joints and is more frequent in women; and the spinal type creates a rigid 'poker' back and causes considerable pain.

Faulty posture, injury and excessive weight are predisposing factors, and prevention consists largely of their reduction or avoidance. There is probably also a hereditary factor, and certainly the disease appears to run in families.

In most cases deterioration is very slow and only three forms of treatment are needed: (1) movements and exercises to maintain the mobility of the joint as far as is practicable; (2) mild analgesics to control the pain; and (3) radiant heat, which not only lessens pain but also appears to have a positive beneficial influence.

In advanced cases surgical treatment may be needed to create a painless, immobile joint: a fixed knee or hip joint is often preferable to one with limited movement and causing considerable pain. A modern advance of striking value is the replacement of a badly damaged joint by an artificial joint. In successful cases, which are already numerous, the mobility and happiness of the subject are vastly improved.

osteoma. A benign (i.e., non-cancerous) tumour of bone, found most often in the skull or jaw. The tumour grows very slowly. If it presses on a nerve, hinders joint action or causes unpleasant deformity it can be removed by surgery. If it does none of these things it is probably best left in position.

Osteoma should be sharply differentiated from osteosarcoma, a highly malignant tumour liable to give rise to secondary growths, e.g., in the lungs. Where its situation makes its removal possible, an osteosarcoma should be excised as early as possible.

osteomalacia. A disease, mainly occurring in women, characterized by loss of calcium from the bones so that they become soft and yielding, with consequent bending and deformity.

The main cause is deficiency of vitamin D in pregnancy. The deficiency prevents the adequate absorption of calcium and phosphorus from the intestine, and the foetus gains its quota of these minerals at the expense of the mother. Essentially osteomalacia in an adult corresponds to rickets in a child.

Prevention consists of providing enough supplies of foods containing vitamin D (e.g. milk, butter, cheese and eggs), with artificial supplementation by vitamin pills or cod liver oil if necessary; but it should be remembered that there is also such a thing as over-dosage with vitamin D. Where the condition has occurred, termination of pregnancy is desirable with thereafter a diet rich in calcium, phosphorus and vitamin D.

osteomyelitis. Inflammation of the bone marrow through infection by pus-forming germs. The main symptoms are severe pain, tenderness in the affected part and high temperature. Antibiotic treatment has revolutionized the outlook in this formerly very dangerous disease, but surgical removal of the infected bone may still be required if antibiotic treatment is delayed.

osteopathy. A system of medical practice, founded in 1874 by A. T. Still (1828-1917). As outlined by Still, osteopathy is based on the self-sufficiency of the human body. It disbelieves in all drugs, vaccines and sera; it places little or no reliance on electricity or radiology; and it accepts surgical treatment in certain cases only as a last resort. Its main tenet is that 'disease is the result of anatomical abnormalities followed by physiological discord', from which it follows that natural healing will occur if the abnormalities are corrected. In other words osteopathy as originally understood holds that diseases are caused by displacements (especially of bones) and are curable by manipulation.

Since on one hand prevention and cure of deficiency diseases by vitamins and of various infections by vaccines and antibiotics respectively are now beyond dispute, and since on the other hand the development of radiology renders virtually all displacements visible, some of the basic tenets of osteopathy are manifestly in doubt. Nowadays most practising osteopaths accept that by no means all diseases respond to manipulation of bones and joints. While most osteopaths have departed from Still's view that osteopathy 'can be applied to all conditions of disease', some orthodox medical practitioners have accepted that osteopathy has had successes not explicable on purely psychological grounds, and that reduction of displacement by manipulation may have a valid place in the treatment of some diseases.

In orthodox medicine manipulative surgeons have undoubtedly learned something from osteopaths, just as osteopaths learned something from the bone-setters of the past. But the medical contention is that to consult an osteopath in the first instance is dangerous because the osteopath, trained only in the manipulative art, may diagnose incorrectly a condition – such as diabetes, anaemia or an acute infection – which will not respond to manipulation and urgently needs appropriate treatment of an entirely different kind.

osteoporosis. A thinning and weakening of bones, common in old people, especially those whose diet is deficient in calcium. The condition is commoner in women than in men, and cessation of ovarian function at the menopause is thought to be a factor in some cases. Excess of adrenal hormones is another possible factor and the condition sometimes occurs after prolonged treatment with corticosteroids. Where the spine is affected the main feature is episodes of backache, with inability to stoop or bend, and sometimes inability to move from the position at the time of onset, but with considerable periods of remission in which there is no pain or only a mild backache. Where a long bone, e.g., the femur, is mainly affected there may be no symptoms until there is a sudden fracture.

Apart from treatment of the fracture in the latter case, treatment involves rest during acute bouts, analgesics for the pain, adequate calcium and vitamin D, and gentle reintroduction of movement as the pain ends. Since, irrespective of the particular cause, loss of calcium from bones plays an important part, an obvious preventive measure is to ensure that elderly people have diets rich in calcium. Milk is an excellent source of calcium and is easily absorbed and digested.

osteosarcoma. See OSTEOMA.

osteosclerosis fragilis. A rare hereditary abnormality of bone growth, in which bones are unusually weak and brittle.

otitis media. See EAR.

otorrhoea. Discharge of pus from the ear. See EAR, otitis media.

otosclerosis. A hereditary condition in which the bones of the middle EAR become thickened and hardened, resulting in increasing difficulty in the transmission of sound impulses from the ear drum to the brain, and sometimes ultimately causing complete deafness. Treatment is either by fenestration, i.e., an operation whereby a new opening is made to the inner ear, or by removal of the affected bone and its replacement by a synthetic substitute. With either treatment the complete restoration of hearing occurs in most cases.

ovary. The female sex gland, and thus part of the female REPRODUCTIVE SYSTEM. The two ovaries are oval bodies nearly 4 cm. (about 1½ in.) long, situated on each side of the uterus. They contain ova (or eggcells) and they produce hormones,

The development of the ovum in the ovary

including oestrogen and progesterone, which give the adult woman her typical physical characteristics and largely regulate the menstrual cycle. During each menstrual cycle one (or occasionally more) of the ova ripens, comes to the surface of the ovary in a little follicle or blister and passes along a uterine tube to the uterus where it may be fertilized by a sperm.

Diseases. 1. Inflammation of an ovary may arise from the passage of infection along the relevant uterine tube. The condition is characterized by abdominal pain and tenderness, with rise in temperature. Treatment is with sulphonamides or antibiotics. Inflammation of the right ovary is liable to be confused with appendicitis.

2. Ovarian cysts are bladder-like growths which sometimes become remarkably large; they are mostly painless but may cause pain if they become twisted. Treatment is by surgical removal of the cyst.

3. Cancer of the ovary is difficult to differentiate from benign solid tumours until after removal, when laboratory tests can be performed on the tissue which has been removed. In most cases it is painless. In view of the diagnostic difficulty and the danger of spread of cancer, all ovarian tumours should be treated by surgical removal or by radiotherapy.

4. Displacement of the ovary can result from stretching or twisting of the ovarian ligaments. There is pain and tenderness, and surgical treatment may be necessary.

5. Insufficient production of ovarian hormones may cause delayed puberty or menstrual irregularity. Hormone treatment is usually effective.

overcrowding. Every person requires adequate air space, good ventilation without draughts and a modicum of privacy. Overcrowding increases the risk of air-borne (droplet) infections and also of contact infections. Hence respiratory infections and most specific fevers reach their peak incidence in winter when people are crowded together indoors and with windows closed for warmth. Overcrowding lowers general standards of health and of resistance to disease; and when a single room has to serve as the living, sleeping, eating and washing accommodation of a family, the resulting irritation, frustration and deterioration of morale is obvious.

Many developed countries prescribe minimum standards for living accommodation. In Britain it is laid down that, disregarding babies under 12 months and counting a child of under 10 years as a half, a house is overcrowded if two rooms contain more than 3 persons or three rooms more than 5 persons; and that to accommodate two adults a room must have a floor-space of at least 110 square feet.

Overcrowding in factories is also prohibited in some countries. In Britain the specified minimum is 40 square feet per person in a room at least 10 feet high, and the same minimum is now required for offices in which people normally work. Standards are also specified for schools and hospitals.

ovum. See OVARY.

oxalic acid. An irritant poison which looks like epsom salts and thus may be swallowed accidentally. If so taken, it corrodes the lining of the mouth, throat and stomach. Calcium compounds - such as chalk or whiting mixed with water - are the best antidote, and the patient should be kept warm and treated for shock. Since vomiting would return the corroding acid to the throat and mouth, emetics should never be given.

oxygen. A colourless, odourless, tasteless gas which constitutes one-fifth of our atmosphere and is essential to human and animal life. In respiration oxygen is taken into the lungs and carried in the haemoglobin of the red blood corpuscles to every part of the body.

Oxygen is valuable in any disease in which the lungs have difficulty in taking up air and in any condition in which there is insufficiency of oxygen in the arterial blood. For example, it eases breathing in pneumonia and severe bronchitis, and it is useful in congestive heart failure and coronary thrombosis.

Oxygen is normally supplied in compressed form in steel cylinders and is administered to the patient through a mask fitted over the nose and mouth, or through a tube passed through a nostril, or occasionally by a 'tent' covering the patient's head and shoulders.

In major operations the anaesthetist routinely has a cylinder of oxygen available and ready for use in the event of breathing difficulties developing.

Oxyuris vermicularis. See THREAD WORM.

ozaena. A chronic inflammation of the nose with crusting and partial wasting of the nasal membrane. It is probably the result of long-continuing untreated infection. Although NOSE DOUCHING (despite its possible dangers) and attention to diet and exercise may be tried, in many cases surgical treatment is necessary.

ozone. An unusual form of oxygen with three atoms to the molecule instead of two. It has a penetrating odour and is produced by the passage of electrical discharges through the air. In high concentration it is poisonous.

A little ozone is sometimes present in the seaside air, but the odour generally described as ozone comes primarily from seaweed; the health-giving powers of seaside air have never been scientifically demonstrated.

P

pacemaker. The part of the heart, the sino-atrial node, from which starts each wave of contraction of heart muscle. The tiny electrical impulse that originates in the node is conducted to all parts of the heart and causes the muscular contraction, with expulsion of blood down the arteries, that we call the heart beat.

If the natural pacemaker temporarily fails to work, as in certain forms of heart attack, an external artificial pacemaker, if available within a few minutes, can produce similar electrical impulses, thus re-starting the heart and maintaining the beat until the pacemaker recovers.

Where the pacemaker is permanently incapacitated or the conducting mechanism from it is seriously damaged, a battery-driven artificial pacemaker can be inserted under the skin of the chest.

paediatrics. The branch of medical science concerned with the prevention, diagnosis and treatment of diseases of children, and with the physical, emotional and mental growth and development of children.

There is no fixed age at which paediatrics ends and adult medicine begins. In the clinical field, separate curative facilities for children usually cease at about 12 or 13 years. In the preventive field the age of leaving school is an obvious border.

pain. Nature's primary indication that all is not well with the human machine.

The hurt or injury occurs in some part of the body, the message of distress is picked up by specific nerve-endings and carried by two types of sensory nerve fibres, and the brain interprets the message as pain, localizes it to the particular area and initiates necessary action. Biologically pain is very valuable in that it enables us to remove the endangered part from injurious influences, to decide consciously to avoid harmful stimuli and to seek medical aid for an injury or illness that might be disregarded if it were painless. Indeed, one of the unfortunate facts of life is that a few serious diseases (e.g., cancer and tuberculosis) tend to be painless in their early stages.

The sensory nerve-endings called pain receptors are more plentiful in some areas than in others. The cornea is particularly rich in them, so that eye injury causes immediate and severe pain. The teeth have very efficient pain receptors. The genitals have abundant pain receptors, so that injury produces intense pain and shock. The finger tips are well supplied, thus the tearing off of nails is an ancient form of torture. The buttocks are quite well supplied, so that, without adjacent vital structures that could be injured, they are a traditional site of chastisement. On the other hand, some internal organs lack pain receptors: for example, diseases of bone which do not affect its outer membrane are painless, as are many diseases of the brain.

Transfer of the message is impossible unless the relevant sensory nerves are intact. Hence in certain diseases of nerves a cut or burn fails to produce any sensation of pain; and in syringomyelia the sense of pain disappears but that of touch remains, indicating that the nerve fibres for these sensations are different. Once pain has served its purpose in calling attention to the area and helping diagnosis, it can be stopped by blocking the nerves, e.g., by injecting an appropriate drug.

Sensitivity to pain varies. Firstly, it varies with cerebral development: mammals and birds feel pain much more acutely than fishes and reptiles, and it is doubtful whether a worm can experience pain. Secondly, it varies with the degree of injury. Thirdly, it varies with the portion of the body affected, being less in parts poorly supplied with pain receptors. Fourthly, it varies with the individual: some people feel pain very acutely and even faint when subjected to what in others would be only moderate amounts of pain; and at the other end of the scale some people appear to have an unusually high tolerance of pain.

Pain is sometimes differentiated into 'burning', 'stabbing', 'gripping', 'gnawing', 'boring' and 'aching'. In addition there is the psychological anguish that is termed 'mental pain'.

The brain may sometimes ignore the message owing to preoccupation, as when in the excitement of battle a soldier receives a painful injury but remains unaware of it until later. Occasionally, too, the brain can be at fault in localizing pain, e.g., a person whose leg has recently been amputated may 'feel' pain in the absent toes; this is a phenomenon closely resembling referred pain.

Referred pain is that which is felt in a part of the body remote from the site of the actual injury or disease. This happens because the spinal cord is developed in segments, each with its own pair of spinal nerves. In the early embryo these segments are closely related to a similar segmental arrangement of the other developing tissue. Initially, each spinal nerve is thus related to the nearby skin, deep tissues, and viscera.

As growth and development proceed this close relationship is disturbed, with the result that the deeper structures and the skin may become widely separated although they continue to share a common nerve-supply. Pain impulses from the deep structures therefore reach the same point in the spinal cord as pain impulses from a remote skin receptor before they ascend the cord to be appreciated in the brain.

Since the brain is much more used to receiving stimuli from end-organs on the skin than from elsewhere, and because the cortex of the brain has a well-developed sensory 'map' of the body-surface and only rudimentary representation of visceral structures, it misinterprets the site of the pain. The actual pain is 'referred' to the segmentally-associated area of skin even although this may be some distance away.

Referred pain also occurs when nerve-trunks are damaged in their course by injury or disease. Pain is then experienced, not at the site of the damage but at the periphery of the nerve-distribution.

Common examples of referred pain are numerous. The heart condition angina pectoris may produce pain radiating down the left arm; abdominal conditions irritating the diaphragm may be felt as pain in either shoulder; the pain of renal colic is felt in the groin and upper thigh; hip disease may be referred to the knee; spinal caries, according to the level affected, may produce pains in the arms, 'girdle-pains' in the chest, lower abdominal symptoms, and pains in the buttocks and legs; and a blow on the inner side of the elbow may cause a tingling pain in the little finger.

To the physician pain is of great importance as an aid to diagnosis, and he may have to allow pain to continue until he has determined its cause. Thereafter, removal of the cause of pain and relief of the actual pain are the doctor's two primary objectives. Removal of pain is essential – as soon as possible after diagnosis of the cause – not only for reasons of humanity but also because continued severe pain creates shock and can even kill.

palate. The roof of the mouth, consisting of a bony front part, the hard palate, and a fibro-muscular hind part, the soft palate.

In the unborn child the right and left sides of the palate develop separately and normally fuse together. Failure to fuse results in cleft palate, a fairly common congenital defect, often associated with HARE LIP, a failure of the halves of the upper lip to fuse. The voice has a harsh nasal sound and pronunciation of the palatal consonants is indistinct. A repair operation is required and should normally be undertaken during the early months of life.

palliative. A medicine which relieves symptoms rather than curing the underlying disease. The term is often used in a derogatory sense, and certainly simply to relieve pain without ascertaining the cause is bad practice; but many conditions – such

as the common cold, shingles and tension headache – are temporary, so that palliation is all that is required. Aspirin (although of specific curative value in certain rheumatic conditions) is the palliative in commonest use, and other palliatives frequently employed are codeine and paracetamol.

pallor. Paleness of the skin, mainly due to constriction of the surface blood vessels. There are many causes, of which the four which follow are probably the most common. (1) Natural or habitual pallor occurs where, although the person is in good health, his skin is a shade thicker or his capillaries lie a shade deeper than in most people. (2) Prolonged pallor is in most cases a result of severe anaemia. It also arises from other causes such as chronic kidney disease and long confinement indoors. (3) Temporary pallor is a common consequence of fatigue. (4) Immediate pallor occurs in shock, fainting and sometimes in severe emotional disturbance.

In immediate and temporary pallor the cause is generally obvious, as is any necessary treatment. Prolonged pallor necessitates investigation unless the explanation is known. Natural pallor needs no treatment but adequate sunshine or a course of ultra-violet rays may improve the appearance.

palpitation. Awareness of the strength, rapidity or irregularity of the heart beat.

Excited action of the heart, creating this awareness, may occur as a result of indigestion, over-smoking, excess of alcohol, excess of tea or coffee, toxic goitre, anaemia or various diseases of the heart. The excited action may continue for a few minutes or for many hours.

Investigation is desirable because palpitation may indicate a condition needing treatment. Even more important, however, is reassurance, because the patient nearly always attributes the symptom to serious disease of the heart.

palsy. Until this century palsy was simply another term for PARALYSIS. In modern usage, however, palsy is generally reserved for conditions characterized not only by loss of power but by quivering of the affected part of the body. Nevertheless, facial neuralgia – a neuritis causing temporary paralysis of the muscles of one side of the face – is still sometimes called Bell's palsy.

pancreas. An elongated glandular structure lying on the back wall of the upper abdomen. Its rounded head is encircled by the curve of the duodenum and its body and tail extend to the left crossing the left kidney and reaching the spleen.

It consists of two distinct types of tissue. The main secretory cells produce digestive ferments which pass by small ducts to the main pancreatic duct and thence into the duodenum to assist in the breakdown and digestion of food. Embedded in the glandular tissue are enclosures of another

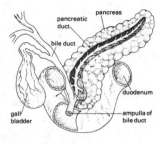

The pancreas

type of cells, known as the Islets of Langerhans. These produce the hormone insulin required for the metabolism of carbohydrate. They have no collecting ducts and insulin is absorbed directly into the blood stream, so that the Islets of Langerhans can be classed as ENDOCRINE GLANDS.

Animal pancreas is used as a foodstuff under the name 'sweetbread'.

Diseases. Deficiency of the pancreatic hormone insulin produces DIABETES. Absence or insufficiency of pancreatic enzymes which help digestion in the bowel cause intestinal disturbance and abnormal stools. In the congenital disease cystic fibrosis both lungs and pancreas show fibrosis and cyst formation and the affected child develops poorly and often has respiratory complications.

Apart from these special conditions acute pancreatitis is common, usually in association with inflammation of the gall bladder and gall-stones. Attacks tend to occur suddenly and constitute an abdominal emergency. Sub-acute pancreatitis is sometimes a complication of hypothermia in the aged owing to the effect of cold on the blood vessels and intestines.

The pancreas is a common site for malignant disease. Cancer of the head of the pancreas interferes with secretion of bile, producing jaundice.

pandemic. An outbreak of infectious disease not limited to one community or country but occurring on a wider scale.

papilloma. A tumour which appears as a raised area on the surface of the skin or the mucous membranes lining internal organs, glands and ducts. Skin papillomata are familiar as warts. Those which arise from mucous membrane are most commonly found in the bladder, larynx, stomach and intestine. Although initially benign, some types of internal papilloma have a tendency to become malignant and should be dealt with promptly.

papule. A pimple or small projection raised above the surface of the surrounding skin.

paracentesis. A minor surgical procedure in which a body cavity is punctured by a hollow needle to allow fluid to escape. This form of 'tapping' is most commonly employed in the relief of ascites (abdominal dropsy) but other applications are in the treatment of pericarditis, pleurisy, otitis media, and hydrocele.

paracetamol. A mild analgesic, a little stronger than aspirin, used to relieve pain, either alone or in combination with aspirin.

paraesthesia. Any unusual sensation (e.g., pain, heat, itching or tingling) experienced without any external cause. Paraesthesia is a common symptom in some diseases in which a nerve is compressed or irritated.

paralysis. Complete loss of the power of movement in any part of the body, produced by some damage to the nervous system or the muscular mechanism. Damage which causes loss of sensory reception is sometimes called sensory paralysis.

Various terms indicate the extent of any paralysis. Thus monoplegia means paralysis of one limb; diplegia, paralysis of both corresponding limbs; quadriplegia, paralysis of all four limbs; paraplegia, paralysis of both legs and the lower part of the body, seen particularly in spinal injury; hemiplegia, paralysis of leg, arm, and face of one side, as seen in the ordinary type of apoplectic stroke; crossed paralysis, affecting leg and arm of one side and the other side of the face, indicative of nerve tract lesions within the brain stem.

Paralysis may be spastic or flaccid. In spasticity there is loss of control of movement, muscle rigidity, exaggerated tendon reflexes, no alteration in electrical excitability, and only minimal wasting of muscle tissue through disuse. In flaccidity there is loss of all muscular power, complete limpness, absent tendon-reflexes, 'reaction of degeneration' to electrical excitation, and ultimately complete wasting away of muscle tissue. Strokes, spinal injuries, spinal tumours and multiple sclerosis are causes of spastic paralysis. Poliomyelitis causes flaccid paralysis.

paralysis agitans. See PARKINSON'S DISEASE.

paranoia. Originally paranoia was regarded as a separate mental illness characterized by a permanent pattern of delusions, generally of persecution, but with complete preservation of clear thought and action, and complete absence of hallucinations.

Paranoia is now regarded as a mild or early form of schizophrenia. Its particular symptoms are relatively rare, and although it may be separately identifiable it has to be assessed and re-assessed in the light of the later trend of the illness.

Most cases ultimately prove to be schizophrenia. However, it is possible to indicate a condition conveniently described as paranoia. Pronounced mental symptoms do not usually begin until middle life but a careful study of the earlier history will often reveal personality changes from adolescence onwards. In the developed disease the predominant feature is a completely consistent and systematized set of delusions, usually related to persecution, grandeur, personality, or status, which are maintained and supported with such persuasive detail and such unassailable logic as to be extremely convincing and likely to deceive many people. Paranoiacs thus tend to become leaders of religious and political movements, to swell the ranks of terrorist organizations, and to become tireless litigants and general trouble-makers.

It is precisely because they are so plausible that they are so dangerous. In the present state of knowledge there is no real cure for paranoia and it is often only after many years that increasingly antisocial behaviour or the development of increasing patterns of delusion make the condition recognizable and leave no alternative but to protect society by committing such cases to a mental hospital.

paraplegia. Paralysis of the legs and lower part of the body due to injury or disease of the spinal cord. Both voluntary movement and sensation are affected. In injury the PARALYSIS is of spastic type, but in other cases progression of disease may lead to a flaccid paralysis. The extent of the paralysis resulting from injury is determined by the level at which the spinal cord is damaged.

An important aspect of paraplegia is loss of control over bowel and bladder function, with incontinence and liability to ascending infection of the urinary tract.

parasites. Organisms which live on, or in, the body of another animal or plant and derive their sustenance therefrom. Although this definition could logically include the bacteria their presence is conventionally called infection rather than parasitism. If the association between host and invader is of mutual benefit this is recognized by using the term symbiosis.

Parasites of man may conveniently be divided into those living on the skin, ectoparasites, and those existing internally, endoparasites. Ectoparasites include fleas, lice, itch-mites and fungi such as ringworm. Endoparasites range from single-celled protozoans such as those of amoebic dysentery and malaria to the more highly organized flukes (trematodes), flat-worms (cestodes) and round-worms (nematodes) which exist in great variety, especially in tropical countries. Internally fungi also cause conditions like 'farmer's-lung' and actinomycosis.

Parasites vary in their potentialities for producing disease. Ectoparasites are mainly a source of irritation (although lice and fleas spread typhus and plague during epidemics), but biting insects transmit many tropical diseases. Some endoparasites like intestinal tape-worms are relatively harmless at that stage of

their life history, but many others produce serious injury particularly in such tropical diseases as schistomiasis and filariasis.

parasympathetic nervous system. One of the two divisions of the autonomic NERVOUS SYSTEM.

parathyroid glands. These ENDOCRINE GLANDS produce parathyroid hormone which controls calcium metabolism. They lie close to the thyroid gland in the neck.

paratyphoid fever. A specific infectious disease due to *Salmonella paratyphi*. The symptoms are mainly of gastro-intestinal disturbance with continued fever and sometimes a measles-like rash. It resembles classical TYPHOID FEVER and is difficult to differentiate clinically but the incubation period is shorter, the onset more abrupt, the duration of illness less prolonged, and toxaemia less severe. As in typhoid fever there is a risk of serious complications – haemorrhage, intestinal perforation, or myocardial toxaemia – but they are relatively rare and generally the fatality rate is low except in the elderly or debilitated. Often there may be little more than fever, malaise and transient diarrhoea.

While typhoid is spread by water, or occasionally food contaminated by a carrier or a missed case, paratyphoid is spread by food (especially milk and uncooked foods) similarly contaminated. The disease requires isolation and hospital treatment.

General measures of prevention are as for typhoid. Vaccine protection is available, often combined with protection against typhoid, and is a sensible precaution for persons travelling to any country in which the disease is still common.

paresis. Incomplete paralysis of voluntary muscles. If on testing a muscle or group of muscles feeble contractions can still be elicited the muscles are said to be in a state of paresis, as opposed to the state of paralysis.

Paresis tends to occur in the early stages of progressive diseases of the nervous system. On the other hand a paretic response after the total paralysis which has resulted from a stroke indicates some recovery of function and is to be regarded as a hopeful sign.

Parkinson's disease. A relatively common chronic nervous disease of later life, chiefly affecting males, characterized by muscular tremors, weakness and rigidity, and by a typical stooped posture, 'shuffling' gait and a mask-like immobile facial appearance. Alternative names for the condition are paralysis agitans or 'shaking palsy'.

The exact cause is unknown but the symptoms suggest that there is a disorder in the cerebral hemispheres of the brain, and within recent years it has been shown that patients have an abnormally low concentration of a substance dopamine in their brain tissue. Dopamine itself does not pass from the blood to the brain but a related substance, levodopa, overcomes this difficulty and cases of Parkinsonism have been substantially improved by the administration of this drug. Levodopa can cause serious side-effects such as nausea, vomiting, and disturbances of blood pressure and heart action, and a search continues for safer preparations. Systematic physiotherapy is also of service.

paronychia. Whitlow. See HAND (diseases).

parotid. The parotid glands, left and right, are the largest of the SALIVARY GLANDS.

parotitis. Inflammation of the parotid gland. Acute parotitis is usually due to infection reaching the gland from septic conditions in the mouth, and a salivary calculus may dilate or damage the duct making infection easier. Most cases recover spontaneously but local warmth and mouth washes may help.

Suppurative parotitis can occur as a sequel to acute parotitis, and also by spread from local sepsis in the jaw and adjacent structures or by blood-borne infection in septicaemia and other diseases. Abscess formation results and may be a serious complication since pus may reach the base of the skull or the deeper structures of neck and thorax. Surgical intervention will be required.

Epidemic or infectious parotitis is a specific infectious disease due to a virus and more usually called MUMPS.

passive movement. The movement of a joint by manipulation when, because of paralysis or some other cause, the patient is unable to perform the movement unaided.

Pasteur. Louis Pasteur (1822-95), French chemist. He showed that micro-organisms in the air are responsible for many diseases, and produced vaccines against rabies and anthrax.

pasteurization. A process for ensuring the hygienic safety of milk and for improving its keeping qualities by heating it to a moderate temperature for a prescribed time. Pathogenic bacteria are killed and other bacterial development considerably delayed.

Efficient pasteurization destroys the enzyme phosphatase in milk and this is used as a basis for the phosphatase test to check that the process is operating satisfactorily.

Pasteurization is also used in treating some other foodstuffs for similar reasons: cream and fruit juices are examples.

patella. The kneecap, an isolated bony structure flattened in profile and roughly triangular in shape, situated in front of the knee joint and incorporated in the tendon of the muscle which brings the thigh forwards. Its back surface, in contact with the lower joint surface of the thigh bone, is covered by articular cartilage.

Fractured patella is a common injury usually produced by sudden violent muscular action as in attempting to

recover balance. Successful repair generally requires open operation to wire the fragments in position.

The patella may also become dislocated, particularly in a leg misaligned through knock-knee deformity. Recurrent cases require operation.

pathogenic. Capable of producing disease.

pathognomonic. Signs or symptoms absolutely characteristic of a particular disease and sufficient to establish the diagnosis.

pathology. The scientific study of bodily changes produced by disease. Disease is manifested either by visible signs of structural change or by symptoms of disturbed function. Since function depends on structure any disease must basically be due to underlying changes either in structure or in chemical composition.

The methods employed in pathology are those of the anatomist, physiologist, physicist, biochemist and bacteriologist. Changes in physical structure may be recognizable with the naked eye (pathological anatomy) or by the ordinary microscope (pathological histology). Chemical changes may be detectable by ordinary qualitative or quantitative tests or by micro-chemical methods combining some form of chemical reaction with subsequent microscopic examination.

It is important, however, to appreciate that there may be changes which are not detected by any of these methods. The electron microscope now permits further exploration of the details of cell and molecular structure (cytology) while functional responses to infection and tissue interaction require the use of biological reactions classified generally as immunology. Enzyme reactions and the micro-chemistry of the cell also call for increasingly sophisticated chemical procedures.

Pathological investigation is thus two-fold in nature. The first step is to identify a structural difference and trace its evolution and the next is to discover its cause, making use as required of progressively more searching methods of examination until a satisfactory solution is achieved.

pediculosis. Infestation with LICE.

pellagra. A vitamin deficiency disease found mainly in regions such as the southern states of U.S.A., the Mediterranean shores and the Far East where maize is a staple article of diet. The symptoms are: wasting; inflammation of the mouth (stomatitis) and tongue (glossitis) with other indications of gastro-intestinal disturbance; a symmetrical scaly skin condition often with pigmentation; nervous manifestations such as numbness, tremors or paralysis; and mental deterioration. It is caused by lack of VITAMINS of the B_2 complex particularly nicotinic acid and riboflavin. It is readily cured by an adequate diet and the administration of appropriate vitamin supplements, although the scaly skin condition is slow to resolve.

Pellagra-like symptoms may also occur in patients on antibiotic drugs which tend to kill off intestinal bacteria that normally assist in the synthesization of vitamin B from foodstuffs.

pelvis. The massive bony ring at the lower end of the trunk which supports the vertebral column above and is itself supported by the legs. The main bone of the pelvic girdle is the ILIUM. The size and conformation of the female pelvis is of importance in relation to childbirth.

The name is also applied to the hollow interior of the kidney of which the ureter is the outlet.

pemphigus. A name for several diseases of the skin characterized by the formation of blisters.

(1) Pemphigus neonatorum: a form of impetigo seen in new-born infants usually due to staphylococcal infection. The delicate, soft skin readily separates to form blisters. There is often quite severe general upset but antibiotic treatment is effective. (2) Acute pemphigus: small skin blisters occurring in association with signs of blood poisoning. It is generally treated by sulphonamides or antibiotics. (3) Chronic pemphigus (pemphigus vulgaris): recurrent crops of watery blisters occurring on both the skin and the mucous membranes with deterioration of the general health. The exact cause is unknown. The condition, which is probably one of the collagen diseases, usually heals on treatment with corticosteroids.

penicillin. An antibiotic substance produced by a mould of the genus *Penicillium*. It was discovered by Sir Alexander Fleming in 1928, but its therapeutic effectiveness against many serious infections was not demonstrated until the 1940s.

Penicillin is now available in several forms. (1) Benzyl-penicillin or penicillin G, the original form. (2) Acid-resistant phenoxymethyl-penicillin or penicillin V, resistant to gastric juice and effective when taken by mouth. (3) Procaine-benzyl penicillin and benzathine penicillin which are longer acting. (4) Synthetic penicillins such as methicillin and cloxacillin. (5) Broad-spectrum penicillins which are active against a wider range of organisms, e.g., ampicillin. The use of penicillin has been a landmark in the treatment of bacterial diseases. It is essentially non-toxic except that some persons may develop allergic symptoms of asthma, skin eruptions or anaphylaxis.

penis. The male organ of copulation and the external organ of the REPRODUCTIVE SYSTEM. It consists of three elongated sections made up of spongy tissue, the spaces of which are occupied by blood sinuses. The middle section is traversed by the urethra, for the passage of urine and semen, and its outer end is expanded to form a bulbous extremity called the glans penis. The skin of the penis is thin and loose and, at the tip,

is folded upon itself partially to cover the glans as the foreskin, or prepuce; this is the skin which is removed in the operation of CIRCUMCISION.

Diseases. Congenitally, the penis may be diminutive with the urethra opening on its upper or lower surface instead of at the extremity. These abnormalities are epispadias and hypospadias respectively. When extreme they may give rise to difficulty in deciding the sex of an infant. In phimosis, another congenital condition, the foreskin is lengthened to extend beyond the end of the penis and so narrowed as to obstruct the urinary flow and be non-retractile. A narrow foreskin if forcibly retracted may cause paraphimosis, a partial strangulation of the glans. Both conditions require circumcision.

In the adult, venereal infections are the commonest causes of disease. The penis is a common site for syphilitic chancres. Gonorrhoea and other forms of sepsis produce balanitis or inflammation of the glans, and gonorrhoeal infection may extend up the urethra to produce a purulent discharge and later a urethral stricture. Warts are usually a complication of gonorrhoea. In elderly men the glans may develop papillomatous tumours which have a tendency towards malignant change, and cancer also occurs, commonly beginning as an ulcerated area in the groove behind the glans.

All the conditions mentioned require professional treatment but the correction of phimosis, sexual continence, cleanliness and hygiene are important preventive measures.

peptic ulcer. An ulcer occurring in the stomach or duodenum, or occasionally at the lower end of the oesophagus. See DUODENAL ULCER and GASTRIC ULCER.

perforating ulcer. A complication of chronic gastric or duodenal ulcer. The ulcerative process ultimately extends through the whole thickness of the wall of the organ concerned to produce a hole which allows gastric or duodenal contents to enter the peritoneal cavity and cause peritonitis.

Acute perforation produces sudden and intensely violent pain in the whole region accompanied by vomiting and signs of shock. It constitutes an emergency requiring immediate operative treatment.

Sub-acute and chronic perforations occur in similar but less dramatic fashion when there is a small leak which the body defences succeed in temporarily containing. An abscess eventually results which will also require surgical measures for its relief.

pericardium. The membranous sac containing the heart. It has two layers, an external one composed of tough and dense fibrous tissue, and an inner serous coat (the parietal pericardium) continuous with a similar layer covering the heart itself as the visceral pericardium. The space between the visceral and parietal serous coats is the pericardial cavity. Serous means 'exuding serum' and the opposed layers are thus kept smoothly lubricated to facilitate the heart movements.

Inflammation of the pericardium is pericarditis. It most commonly occurs in the course of acute and sub-acute attacks of rheumatic fever and also as a complication of septicaemia, pneumonia, empyema, pulmonary tuberculosis, cardiac infarction and penetrating wounds. It may also arise as a terminal incident in chronic diseases such as nephritis.

The symptoms are generally pain in the front of the chest, cough and breathlessness, with raised temperature, and rapid pulse rate. Fluids may collect, distending the pericardial sac, which seriously interferes with the heart's action. Acute pericarditis may be followed by chronic adhesive pericarditis where the two layers of the pericardium become adherent to each other and this also reduces the efficiency of the heart.

The treatment of pericarditis is that of the underlying disease, and the accumulated fluid may have to be drawn off by tapping (aspiration).

perineum. The area of skin with its underlying structures at the base of the trunk which surround the outlet of the pelvis. It forms a diamond-shaped region between the pubis in front, the buttocks behind and the thighs laterally. Through it pass the urethra and anus and in the female it also contains the external genitalia with the opening of the vagina.

The perineum is liable to be torn during childbirth and unless carefully repaired this may later on lead to incontinence or prolapse. Infected haemorrhoids may give rise to an abscess in the perineum.

period, menstrual. See MENSTRUATION.

periosteum. A fibrous membrane covering and closely adherent to all the surfaces of bones except in areas where there is articular cartilage, which gives a smooth surface at the joints.

In young bones the periosteum is thick and vascular and its deeper layers contain cells known as osteoblasts which form new bone during growth. In adult life its thickness is reduced but it still contains blood vessels which enter and nourish the bone. Hence the tendency of bone to die if the periosteum is stripped off by injury or disease.

Muscles and tendons are attached to bone through their incorporation with the periosteum.

peripheral neuritis. General inflammation of the peripheral nerves. The early symptoms are numbness, tingling, and tenderness over the nerve-trunks. This is followed by weakness and paralysis, loss of tendon reflexes, and muscle wasting. The condition is caused by a poisoning of the blood by (1) chemical poisons such as alcohol or arsenic, (2) bacterial toxins, or

(3) metabolic diseases particularly diabetes and beriberi.

A special feature of diphtheritic polyneuritis is its tendency to affect also the cranial nerves to cause disturbances in focusing the eyes, swallowing, and speech. The conditions which cause polyneuritis also damage the heart-muscle and there is a recognized risk of sudden heart failure particularly in diphtheria and beriberi.

The treatment in all cases is to remove or treat the cause of the poisoning of the blood, to stimulate the passing of urine and to aid perspiration (in both cases to help get rid of the poisons), to ensure adequate diet and to enforce rest until recovery. Beriberi requires specific treatment with vitamin B_1.

Peristalsis

peristalsis. The rhythmical movements of the small and large intestines by which their contents are gradually impelled downwards during the digestion of food and the subsequent elimination of waste material. Successive ring-like contractions pass slowly along the bowel sweeping forward any intestinal contents.

Similar peristaltic movements occur in the oesophagus and at the pyloric end of the stomach, and they are also seen in the secretory and excretory ducts of other organs.

Anti-peristalsis is peristalsis occurring in reverse of the normal direction of movement and mainly affects the oesophagus during vomiting.

peritonitis. Inflammation of the peritoneum, i.e., the membrane lining the abdominal cavity and covering the abdominal organs. The condition may arise from a ruptured appendix following failure to diagnose appendicitis, from infection of the uterus after childbirth, from a perforated ulcer of the stomach or intestine, or from various less common causes. Symptoms include severe abdominal pain, signs of shock and rigid ('boarded') abdominal muscles. Immediate medical treatment is essential. It includes intravenous feeding and administration of antibiotics, and may include removal of the accumulated fluid by drainage.

pernicious anaemia. A particular form of severe progressive anaemia. The name is obsolescent and the condition is now better described as megalocytic or megaloblastic anaemia because of the presence of large immature red cells in the blood stream. The disease usually commences in middle life and formerly had a uniformly fatal outcome within a few years; there is also a juvenile form, which is hereditary in origin.

Characteristics of the untreated condition are the insidious onset of great weakness, an appearance of typical yellowish pallor, sore tongue (glossitis), dyspepsia from lack of gastric acid, and nervous symptoms from spinal cord degeneration. Death results from debility and heart failure.

The blood shows a great reduction in red blood cells to as few as one-fifth of normal with a high proportion of immature forms which correlate with abnormal bone-marrow activity. Haemoglobin is not reduced proportionately so that the red cells are well-coloured compared with other forms of anaemia (high colour index).

Treatment was to no avail until, in 1926, it was discovered that the disease could be controlled by giving raw liver. Further work suggested that the liver normally produces substances essential for red-cell formation in the bone marrow and that these result from the interaction of an 'intrinsic factor' derived from the stomach lining and an 'extrinsic factor' from food. These essential substances were ultimately identified as cyanocobalamin (vitamin B_{12}) and folic acid, and their administration now completely restores normal function to the bone marrow.

Fortnightly or monthly intra-muscular injections of appropriate preparations are usually prescribed with periodic blood tests to check the position. Treatment needs to be continued for life.

personality. It is a matter of everyday observation that people differ individually in their attitudes to life and in their inter-reactions with their fellows. The impression which they make on others and their impact on the community as a whole can be summarized as their personality, which has been defined as 'that quality or assemblage of qualities which makes a person what he is and distinguishes him from other persons'.

To a great extent individual personality represents a summation of past experience and the modifications of behaviour which have resulted therefrom, but underlying this are certain basic attributes derived from inheritance. Many workers have attempted to correlate disposition with physical characteristics. Their observations have sought to identify three types of body build defined as (1) endomorphic: broad, muscular and athletic

with large body cavities and viscera and an active endocrine system; (2) mesomorphic: soft, rounded and fleshy; (3) ectomorphic: tall, narrow and spindly, poorly-muscled, and with small organs and a relatively stable endocrine system.

At one extreme, endomorphy tends to be associated with a pyknic type of personality; ectomorphs on the other hand display a leptic behaviour pattern. Pyknics have an extroverted and out-going attitude to life. They are sociable, active and energetic, 'hail-fellow-well-met', fluent conversationalists with strong, but not lasting, emotional reactions, and they show an ability to take positive decisions, to act on them promptly and generally to get things done.

In contrast, leptics are introverted and unsociable, inactive, ill-at-ease in society, and handicapped by shyness, diffidence, and reserve. Their immediate emotional reactions appear shallow and difficult to arouse but they may sometimes react strongly, and apparently irrationally, to trivial incidents as the result of a sudden release of accumulated resentment. Despite the superficial impression which they make of being misfits in society they may nevertheless be possessed of valuable attributes because their mental vision tends to be of longer range, with abilities to foresee and plan. Introverts have made many valuable contributions to knowledge and to the betterment of humanity.

In the development of personality there is thus a fundamental factor based on physical characteristics, but experience of life superimposes layer upon layer of modifications derived from upbringing (see CHILDHOOD, PSYCHOLOGY OF) and from education and emotional experiences; from the acquisition of enthusiasms, prejudices, intolerances, and bias; from habits and hobbies; and from vocational and non-vocational pursuits. Moreover personality does not remain fixed throughout life. It may alter with age and experience, and through physical, endocrine, and emotional factors. The demure, shy and retiring young girl may become in turn the brisk and competent wife and mother, and later still the frustrated, complaining, nagging spouse. The thrusting ambitious executive may become, through lack of material success, the soured and querulous bane of his colleagues. Physical defects may also profoundly alter personality. Illness, disability, disfigurement, or loss of sight or hearing may completely alter a person's attitude to life.

One of the most interesting features of personality is the difference which exists between the nationals of different countries and there is at least some evidence that this is related to the cultural patterns of the upbringing of children and to the influences of climate. It surely cannot be purely accidental that the residents of cold and temperate regions tend to show passivity and reserve compared with the spontaneity and ebullience found in those who live in a warm or tropical environment. It has been maintained, for example, that the clue to the Russian national character lies in the custom of 'swaddling' their babies. Long periods of immobilization alternating with joyous intervals of play are mirrored in their traditional adult attitudes of stolid, patient self-restraint, interrupted by episodes of explosive emotional release.

Personality tests. An appreciation of the fact that people possess different types of personality has aroused much interest in procedures for assessing their individual attributes, and such tests are now available in great variety. Many are based on structured questionnaires or on situations calling for interpretation by the examinee. One of the latter which has gained a good deal of acceptance is the Rorschach ink-blot test. The difficulty in devising such tests is to ensure that they really measure what they purport to do, that they are properly validated, and that they do not allow of cheating. It is often easy for an examinee to give socially acceptable answers to a questionnaire in the hope of gaining good marks rather than truthfully record his own attitudes. However, such tests are being increasingly used in research, in vocational counselling, and in personnel selection.

The personal attitudes for success are a good basic intelligence and a well-organized memory but other qualities are less easy to measure. Also required are self-assurance and willingness to listen, a pragmatic cast of mind, a taste for hard work, and the courage to take risks. There is no real substitute for intelligence but it is not enough in itself. Many who are intelligent lack the moral courage to act. On the other hand moral courage insufficiently modified by intelligence produces fanaticism. The task of education in the formation of personality is both to build on native intelligence and to foster desirable moral qualities.

personality, multiple. A disordered state of mind usually occurring in psycho-neurotic illness of hysterical type in which a patient appears to lead several different lives without being aware, at any one time, of the memories and experiences of his or (more commonly) her other identities. Hysterics adopt this type of behaviour in order to fulfil subconscious wishes or to evade difficulties, and multiple personality is only an extension of DOUBLE PERSONALITY caused by a further fragmentation of memory so that different sets of recollection and experience influence immediate behaviour.

personality, psychopathic. A behavioural pattern or relationship between an individual and his environment, characterized by markedly antisocial or asocial tendencies.

The psychopath is egocentric and largely incapable of displaying concern, sympathy or affection for others. His attitude to life is governed by his present needs without reference to the past or future. For him to want something is to take it and he feels neither guilt nor remorse at the consequences of his actions. Psychopaths form an important section of the criminal or delinquent members of society. Their developmental histories may show evidence of severe rejection in childhood and absence of conditions for forming secure personal relationships, but there are often genetic influences as well. As delinquents they are recognized to be most difficult to reform.

areas where sweat glands are most numerous

Perspiration

perspiration. The term signifies both sweat and the act of sweating. Sweat is secreted by sweat glands present in large numbers in the skin or subcutaneous tissue throughout the body although in some parts, such as armpit and groin, they are particularly numerous. Each gland is a simple tube coiled within the tissues and opening on the skin-surface by a funnel shaped duct. Sweat production contributes to heat regulation since its evaporation from the body-surface produces a cooling effect. If the surrounding temperature is at, or above, body temperature it is clear that heat cannot be lost by convection or radiation, and sweating compensates for this. If evaporation is poor because of high air humidity, this mechanism will also be ineffective and heat-stroke is threatened.

Sweating is mainly stimulated by the effect of body-heat on the temperature-regulating centre of the mid-brain and resultant impulses conveyed by the parasympathetic nervous system to activate the glands.

'Cold sweats' occur in fear or other emotional stress due to nervous influences disturbing the adrenalin-acetylcholine balance.

Excessive perspiration. Obese persons perspire readily and profusely. This is because the ratio of body bulk to skin surface is greater than in a thin person and so the capacity of the skin to lose heat by radiation and convection is relatively less.

This effect is physiological as it is in the sweating of febrile illness, but excessive sweating also occurs in nervous states, in conditions of toxaemia, anaemia and debility, and in certain diseases of the endocrine system such as diabetes and thyrotoxicosis. The sweat glands are inhibited by the sympathetic nervous system (adrenergic) and activated by the parasympathetic system (cholinergic) and in these pathological conditions the adrenalin-acetylcholine balance is disturbed.

Excessive perspiration is called hyperidrosis. If it remains on moist skin sites it may become invaded by bacteria to produce odours.

perspiring feet. Sweat-glands are very numerous on the palms and soles and some individuals perspire excessively from these sites, perhaps because of relative deficiency elsewhere. Just as some persons have a 'clammy' hand-shake, so others have sweaty feet.

It is a personal idiosyncrasy but one which calls for special attention to foot-hygiene because moist skin there predisposes to fungoid infections, 'soft-corns', and offensive odours. The feet should be washed daily and treated with an astringent lotion and dusting powder. Salicylic acid lotion followed by zinc, starch and talc dusting powder is a suitable régime. Socks should be changed daily and thoroughly washed. In warm weather and under suitable circumstances the wearing of sandals is helpful.

pertussis. See WHOOPING COUGH.

perversion or **sexual deviance.** A condition in which the person obtains sexual gratification otherwise than by ordinary intercourse with a partner of the opposite sex. Since 'perversion' implies obstinacy or wickedness, the older term – sexual perversion – is in the process of being replaced by the modern term, sexual deviance.

As Freud demonstrated, a child goes through stages of interest in the mouth (oral eroticism) through which tastes are felt and food enters the body, the anus (anal eroticism) from which emerge the excreta that appear to give such concern to parents, the genitalia, and later the genitalia of the other sex; and through a phase of great attachment to the parent of the opposite sex with some jealousy of the parent of the same sex, a phase of interest primarily in playmates of the same sex, and a heterosexual phase which gradually develops into adult love which is, of course, partly physical and partly idealistic, tender, romantic and protective. At any stage the emotional development may undergo arrest.

The deviation in which love is reserved for persons of the same sex is known as HOMOSEXUALITY in males or LESBIANISM in females. It may arise in part from strained relations with the parent of the same sex, so that, for instance, the boy with a cold and remote father may feel great need for acceptance by a man; or from over-possessiveness by the parent of the other sex, resulting in too close identification with that parent.

Essentially there are two types of homosexuality or lesbianism: in one the effeminate man or masculine woman identifies with, and often acts like, a member of the other sex; in the other type the person exhibits the normal characteristics of his or her sex but is strongly attracted to individuals of the same sex. In either case the homosexuality may remain latent and reveal itself only in a difficulty in forming heterosexual relationships, or it may lead to actual physical relations – usually anal intercourse in males or mutual masturbation in females.

Most adolescents pass through a stage of latent homosexuality and in adults there are many gradations, e.g., the completely heterosexual 'normal' person, the normally heterosexual person who has homosexual desires during prolonged separation from the other sex, the person who oscillates between heterosexuality and homosexuality, the latent homosexual who cannot obtain sexual gratification from either sex, and so on.

Sodomy, common in Ancient Greece and fairly common in Elizabethan England, has for centuries been illegal in many countries and its practice has been a common source of blackmail, but the modern tendency is to regard relations between consenting adults as permissible and that there is no justification for legal intervention.

The term SADISM is used where sexual excitement is obtained by inflicting physical or mental suffering on another person, usually, but not always, a member of the opposite sex, while MASOCHISM is the condition in which sexual gratification arises from undergoing actual beating or mental humiliation, again usually by a member of the opposite sex. There is often only a specific portion of the body involved, e.g., a particular sadist may gain satisfaction only from hurting the breast or the genitals, or a particular masochist may be stimulated only by flagellation of the buttocks. Masochistic tendencies may start with early severe punishment for sex play, with excitement and punishment linked, the origin of sadistic tendencies is still somewhat controversial.

In both conditions there are many variations. Examples are the apparently normal teacher or parent who nevertheless gets some pleasure from punishing children, or the apparently normal person who courts humiliation or even (in certain strata of society) blows, the person who beats or is beaten by a willing partner as an exciting prelude to intercourse, and the person for whom the whipping of another or of himself or herself serves as a complete substitute for intercourse.

Clearly a mild sadist and a moderate masochist can form a mutually satisfactory combination. Masochism by itself is not dangerous, since the pain is borne by the person who desires it and will cease when it exceeds the resulting pleasure; but sadism can be dangerous since the infliction of pain is by the sadist and the suffering is by the victim who may be powerless to resist.

There are elements both of sadism and of masochism in all of us. Why, but for sadistic impulses, would we laugh at knock-about comedy or avidly read newspaper reports of murder trials? Why, but for masochistic sensations, would we watch and sympathize with the sufferings of the hero or heroine of a tragedy? Yet in most people the sadistic and masochistic elements are relatively small, with one or other predominating but subordinate to normal sexual desires, and with pain-inflicting or pain-desiring components of the personality restrained by a mass of developmental, cultural and social forces.

NYMPHOMANIA, or inordinate sexual desire for a whole series of partners, is another deviation, as is FETISHISM, where an article of clothing creates erotic impulses, and VOYEURISM, the 'Peeping Tom' condition.

pessary. Any appliance worn inside the vagina. The term is used mostly for devices that support the uterus when it has been displaced downwards (prolapsed) as a consequence of childbirth. These devices are normally first inserted by a doctor or nurse, but many women quickly learn how to remove a pessary, clean it and re-insert it.

Diaphragms or rubber caps inserted as contraceptive devices, and medicated suppositories inserted into the vagina for the treatment of inflammation are also called pessaries.

Other forms of pessary are those employed to support the rectum.

petit mal. A minor form of EPILEPSY.

phagocyte. A cell able to engulf and digest invading bacteria and dead cells. Certain types of white blood corpuscle are phagocytes and can be considered as both the street cleaners and the policemen of the BLOOD: the former because they remove the remains of cells that die in the course of the ordinary wear and tear of the body, and the latter because they constitute the body's first line of defence, surrounding, sealing off, and dealing with invading bacteria.

phalanx. A segment of a finger or the bone of such a segment. The thumb and the great toe each have two phalanges, while all other fingers and toes have three.

phantom limb. The illusion that an amputated limb is still present. In the early days after amputation, sensations of distress in nerve fibres that were cut during the operation are commonly interpreted by the brain as pain in the part that has been removed.

pharmacist. A person qualified in preparing medicines and making up prescriptions. In most countries a person is not entitled to compound and dispense medicines prescribed by a doctor until he has passed necessary examinations. In Britain the appropriate qualification is Member of the Pharmaceutical Society, commonly contracted to MPS. A pharmacist is therefore a professionally qualified person but he is not qualified to practise medicine.

pharmacology. The branch of medicine that deals with the systematic study of medicinal substances, their actions on the body, their chemistry, their appropriate dosage, and the effects of over-dosage.

Pharmacology should be differentiated from pharmacy which is a narrower but related subject, namely the preparation and storage of drugs.

pharmacopoeia. An official list of approved drugs, their composition, chemical properties, preparation and dosage.

pharynx. The cavity of the throat, lying behind the mouth and separated from it by the soft palate and uvula above and on each side by the pillars of the fauces enclosing the tonsils. It extends upwards to the rear part of the nasal passages, while below it is continuous with the oesophagus. The trachea (windpipe) passes in front of the oesophagus and communicates with the pharynx by way of the larynx, which is protected by an overhanging lid, the epiglottis. The tonsils (commonly quite large in children and shrivelled in adults) are almond-shaped masses of lymphoid tissue which form part of the protective lymphoid tissue in this region.

Diseases. Acute pharyngitis, inflammation of the throat, is among the commonest of infections. It is caused by bacterial invasion and most frequently occurs after exposure to cold or to irritating vapours. Symptoms include dryness of the throat, pain on swallowing, and often aching of the back and limbs. The condition usually clears up within a few days, and severe cases respond well to antibiotics.

Chronic pharyngitis or 'clergyman's throat', results from excessive voice strain, or immoderate use of tobacco or alcohol. The main symptoms are a dry, tickling cough, hoarseness (largely from inflammation of the larynx), and a feeling of dryness in the throat. Avoidance of irritants and rest for the voice are the basis of treatment.

Inflammation of the tonsils, or TONSILLITIS, is frequent in children in both an acute and a chronic form but is rare in adults.

phenacetin. A synthetic drug used, alone or in combination with aspirin, to reduce fever and to relieve pain.

phenobarbitone. The most commonly used drug of the BARBITURATES. It is prescribed as a mildly sedative drug to reduce nervous tension or anxiety or to relieve insomnia. Like all barbiturates it is mildly addictive; and it should in no circumstances be taken simultaneously with alcohol, since two substances interact and each increases the effect of the other.

phenylketonuria. A hereditary disease in which the body lacks the enzyme necessary for the use of phenylalanine, a normal constituent of protein, so that toxic products from the abnormal breakdown of this amino-acid enter the blood stream and damage the brain and the nervous system.

Detection is by a simple urine test, normally employed for all babies as a matter of routine. Where the condition is ascertained early in infancy a special diet can prevent mental retardation, and sometimes the diet can be discontinued later in life.

The disease is inherited as a recessive, i.e., it appears only if both parents carry the abnormal gene; see GENETICS.

phimosis. A condition, in most cases inherited, in which the foreskin (prepuce) of the PENIS is abnormally tight and cannot be pulled back over the glans. In severe cases phimosis may interfere with urination, and quite often it is a cause of bed-wetting. Mild forms tend to disappear spontaneously, but in severe cases the operation of circumcision may be needed.

phlebitis. Inflammation of a vein. The area around the vein becomes red, painful, and tender, and the swollen vein may be felt as a hard cord.

Phlebitis occurs most commonly in the veins of the leg after childbirth, following a surgical operation, or after a prolonged period in bed. It also occurs in association with varicose veins.

ANTICOAGULANT DRUGS (i.e., those which slow down the clotting of blood) such as heparin are advisable because the condition is often associated with THROMBOSIS of the vein, and a clot, once it has formed, may become detached and cause damage elsewhere. Antibiotics and rest are the essentials for treatment, and warm fomentations (see POULTICES) help to relieve the pain.

phlegmasia alba dolens. White leg. A form of PHLEBITIS or thrombophlebitis occurring as a complication of childbirth and involving painful swelling and pallor of the whole leg. Skilled medical treatment is essential, not only because of the pain and swelling but also because of the THROMBOSIS, with the associated danger from detachment of fragments of the clot.

phobia. Irrational and baseless fear. Examples are AGORAPHOBIA, fear of open spaces; bacteriophobia, terror of germs;

CLAUSTROPHOBIA, fear of closed spaces; cynophobia, dread of dogs; and ailurophobia, fear of cats. In a typical case of fear of dirt the victim may feel obliged to wash his or her hands fifty times in the day, is unhappy whenever he does not yield to the compulsion to wash but can give no reason for being more exposed to dirt or more susceptible to its effects than are other people.

These pathological disorders are forms of NEUROSIS and are usually related to repressed impulses or to submerged guilt feelings. FREUD cast much light on their origin and made the successful treatment of serious cases possible.

In mild cases the victim should be advised to avoid the situations which create or exaggerate the fear: to attempt to 'fight' the fear is useless, and wherever possible the victim should continue his normal daily activities. Where the phobia seriously interferes with work or leisure activities, psychiatric treatment is needed.

phosphorus. A non-metallic element contained along with calcium in bone and also in the sheaths of nerves. Phosphates, i.e., organic compounds of phosphorus, are important MINERAL SALTS in body chemistry, energy being released by their breakdown and stored by their formation.

The element itself is a dangerous poison. Chronic phosphorus poisoning (phossy jaw) was formerly common in match factories but is now unknown. Acute phosphorus poisoning, e.g., from accidental swallowing of certain pesticides, is characterized by vomiting, abdominal cramp, diarrhoea, intense pallor, and signs of collapse. Atropine sulphate in doses of 1 to 2 mg. sometimes helps but the condition is often fatal. Prevention entails (1) the observation of strict precautions to prevent absorption by persons manufacturing or using phosphorus compounds (e.g., the use of protective clothing and wearing face masks), and (2) care that none of these compounds contaminates any form of food or drink.

photophobia. Intolerance of bright light by the eyes. This is commonly found in inflammatory conditions of the eyes and also occurs in migraine and in meningitis.

phthisis. Wasting of tissues, consumption. The term, now almost obsolete, was formerly used as a synonym for pulmonary TUBERCULOSIS.

physiology. The study of the working or functioning of normal cells, tissues and organs. Physiology can be contrasted with – but shades into – ANATOMY, the study of structure, and PATHOLOGY, the study of changes causing or caused by disease.

physiotherapy. Treatment of illness by physical measures, such as massage, heat, electricity, and exercises. Probably its most important contributions are towards restoration of function of joints and muscles after an injury or a stroke. Physiotherapy is a recognized profession, separate from medicine, nursing, and dentistry, but included in the group of professions supplementary to medicine.

pigeon chest. A deformity in which the breastbone (sternum) juts forward, creating a characteristic appearance, and in severe cases causing some limitation of movement of the heart and lungs. The condition is sometimes congenital but is usually a result of deficiency of calcium or vitamin D in the diet during the early years. See RICKETS.

pigment. The cells of the skin contain a pigment called melanin. The amount varies in different races, and in those of fair skin it is increased by the action of sunlight. The function of melanin is to protect the skin and underlying tissues against the sun's rays. Absence of pigment occurs in the hereditary condition of ALBINISM. Increased pigmentation is found in Addison's disease and sometimes in diabetes and exophthalmic goitre. In leucoderma there are patches of unpigmented skin surrounded by over-pigmented skin.

The blood pigment, haemoglobin, is responsible for the colour of a bruise or a black eye which follows bleeding below the surface of the skin. In jaundice the yellow pigmentation is due to bile pigments.

piles. A dilated and often inflamed condition of veins at the lower end of the rectum and anal canal alternatively called haemorrhoids. External piles originate in the part of the anal canal that is lined by skin, and in many cases they cause no symptoms except an occasional burning sensation when a constipated motion is passed. Internal piles originate in the part of the bowel and anal canal covered with mucous membrane. They may remain within the anal orifice and only occasion slight and intermittent bleeding, or they may form distinct fleshy masses which are protruded when faeces are passed and cause considerable pain, bleeding and itching.

Most cases are due to constipation and straining at stool, but they are common in pregnancy due to raised intra-abdominal pressure and they may be a symptom of more serious disease causing obstruction to the portal circulation. Extreme pain is usually due to the dilated vein becoming thrombosed and inflamed.

If the bowels are kept open with appropriate diet and bland laxatives, small haemorrhoids often subside with use of suppositories to reduce congestion. For more serious cases injection of an irritant fluid into the haemorrhoid may be required, causing scarring and obstruction of the distended vein. Surgical closure of the veins is seldom necessary.

Avoidance of constipation is an important preventive measure.

'Pill', the. A colloquial expression for oral contraceptive pills. See BIRTH CONTROL.

pimple. A small raised inflammatory spot on the skin, due to infection in a hair follicle or a sweat gland, and in many cases

(a)   anus

(b)   anus

Section through the end of the anal canal showing (a) an external pile, and (b) an internal pile

forming pus before healing. A pimple should in no circumstances be squeezed, both because squeezing spreads the infection and because the squeezing of a pimple may result in a permanent scar. Pimples are commonest in adolescence. See also ACNE.

pineal gland. A small, red, oval gland, about the size of a pea, situated at the base of the brain. It is probably a vestigial ENDOCRINE GLAND which in our primitive ancestors controlled the darkening of the skin on exposure to bright light. Despite various theories, e.g., that it is associated with sexual development, it has no proved existing function. Descartes regarded it as the place of residence of the soul.

pink eye. See CONJUNCTIVITIS.

pins and needles. The unpleasant sensation which arises in the course of a nerve after irritation, such as is caused by pressure from a limb being kept for a time in an awkward position. If the cause is not obvious and if the symptom recurs, the condition warrants medical attention.

pituitary gland. A small, pea-like body

situated in a depression of the sphenoid bone at the base of the skull, the pituitary is the most complex of the ENDOCRINE GLANDS.

pityriasis. A rather vague term used for any bran-like or scaly appearance of the skin.

Pityriasis rosea is a disease characterized by the development of pink spot-like marks which begin to scale in about ten days. The disease ends spontaneously in about six weeks, and the only treatment needed is reassurance and calamine lotion.

Pityriasis alba is a form of impetigo with scaly, whitish discs, mainly on the face.

placebo. A medicine without direct action on a disease, such as water with a harmless colouring agent added or a pill composed entirely of flour. It may be used simply to give the patient the feeling that some treatment is being employed, e.g., to retain his confidence and give him some comfort during an investigation that takes time but is essential before curative treatment can be started; or to reinforce medical advice where the advice alone would be less likely to be followed; or in alternate members of a series of patients to test the effects of a new drug. In respect of the latter use, the procedure is that only one person knows which patients have been given the new drug, and which the placebo; this prevents patients from feeling aggrieved at not being given the new drug, and also allows the doctors and nurses to judge progress objectively. However, if the placebo is given with apparent confidence, more than half of the patients receiving it feel the better for it, a fact which renders difficult the evaluation of a new drug.

maternal blood vessels

maternal blood bathing foetal blood vessels

umbilical vein

umbilical artery

placenta

umbilical cord

The placenta

placenta. The disc-shaped organ by which an unborn child gains nourishment from its mother. One surface of the placenta is connected to the baby by the umbilical cord, while the other surface is firmly attached to an upper part of the wall of the uterus, so that oxygen and nutrients can pass from the uterine blood vessels to the placenta while carbon dioxide and other waste materials from the baby can travel in the opposite direction.

Shortly after the child is born the placenta separates from the uterus and is expelled as the after-birth.

Placenta praevia. An unusual situation of the placenta where, instead of being attached to the uterine wall high up, it is attached low down and tends to lie across the opening of the uterus. In such a situation, as the birth process starts, there is danger to the mother from bleeding and danger to the child from lack of oxygen because of premature detachment of the placenta. Treatment is usually by CAE-SAREAN SECTION.

plague. A severe and highly fatal infectious disease, caused by a bacterium (Pasteurella pestis) and transmitted by rat-fleas. Rats are infected as a result of the bites of the fleas, and as rats die from the disease the fleas seek other hosts, including man, and, by biting, pass the infection to them.

The disease occurs in three main forms. (1) Bubonic plague, transmitted only by bites of fleas and therefore not directly transmissible from person to person, shows itself by painful swellings (buboes) in the armpits, groin and neck, extreme weakness, and high fever, often followed by dark blotches from bleeding into the skin. These blotches account for the mediaeval name, the Black Death. Until the era of antibiotics more than 50 per cent of sufferers from bubonic plague died and even now the chance of death is high. (2) Pneumonic plague, transmitted both by bites of fleas and by droplet infection, is a virulent pneumonia which is usually fatal. (3) Septicaemic plague, the rarest form, has no local signs of infection and almost always ends in death within three days.

Treatment of all types involves strict isolation, with attendants wearing gowns, masks, gloves, protective boots, and clothing impregnated with DDT, together with good nursing and high dosage with chloramphenicol (starting with 500 mg. every four hours) or streptomycin, both of which are strong antibiotics.

Preventive measures include periodic surveys in all areas where plague exists to determine the prevalence both of rats and of rat-fleas, measures for the destruction of rats and of fleas, especially those on ships arriving from infected ports, elimination of breeding places, rat-proofing of buildings and ships, periodic examination of rats for evidence of infection, isolation of patients and of contacts of pneumonic cases, and disinfection of the persons and clothing of all immediate contacts. An anti-plague serum, if available in time, confers a passive immunity for about a month, and a vaccine gives at least some immunity for several months.

During the fourteenth and fifteenth centuries successive waves of plague killed approximately half the population of Europe, but the last widespread epidemic was in 1665. Since then there have been only local outbreaks but these have originated in many parts of the world.

plasma. The fluid part of the blood in which the corpuscles are suspended.

plastic surgery. The branch of surgery which deals with the repair of disfigurements and the reconstruction of deformed parts of the body, mostly either by the use of tissue grafts or by the employment of artificial materials. An example of the former is a skin graft, where after an extensive burn of the cheek a flap of skin is partially detached from the arm and placed on the cheek, with the other end of the flap left attached to the arm. It is detached completely from the arm when blood vessels have begun to grow into it from the cheek so that it can live. An example of the use of artificial materials is the insertion of a glass eye.

platelets. Alternately known as thrombocytes, these are small spherical discs present in blood in a density of between 250,000 to 450,000 per ml. They are probably produced in the bone marrow, play an important part in the stopping of bleeding, and are necessary for the clotting of blood. If platelets are insufficient, as in the various types of purpura, multiple haemorrhages occur in the skin and mucous membranes. If platelets are abnormally plentiful, as tends to occur for some days after an operation or childbirth there is a possibility of the occurrence of thrombosis.

plethora. An excess of blood, generally showing itself by a fullness of the blood vessels of the face, and sometimes by nose bleeding and by a sensation of fullness in the head. It occurs mainly in middle-aged persons who over-eat and over-drink, and it is often associated with high blood pressure.

pleura. The double layer of membrane lining the outer surfaces of the lungs.

pleurisy. Inflammation of the pleura, i.e., the double layer of membrane lining the outer surfaces of the lungs. The inflammation is caused by bacterial or virus infection.

Dry pleurisy, where the inflamed membranes rub together, is characterized by sharp, stabbing pain on breathing and coughing, cough and high temperature. The condition occurs alone or may be a result of pneumonia, tuberculosis, or cancer of the lung.

Pleurisy with effusion, where the inflamed membranes are separated by fluid, commonly follows the dry variety. The pain disappears because the membranes are no longer rubbing, but breathing may be difficult and on inspection the affected side is seen to have reduced movement or to be completely immobile, while sounding the chest produces a note of dullness.

Treatment includes strapping the affected side to reduce lung movement, application of local warmth (e.g., poultices), the giving of analgesics to relieve pain and, if the fluid is present in large quantity, 'tapping' to drain it. The bacterial forms respond well to antibiotics, while virus pleurisy (Bornholm disease) usually subsides spontaneously within a few days. An x-ray examination is desirable after recovery, to eliminate the possibility of the pleurisy having been secondary to tuberculosis or cancer.

pneumoconiosis. A general name for diseases of the lung caused by inhaled DUST.

pneumonia. Inflammation of the lung as a result of infection by bacteria or viruses. The affected air pockets (alveoli), which normally hold oxygen for transmission to the blood and carbon dioxide received from the blood, become water-logged with inflammatory exudate and so incapable of performing their normal function.

Lobar pneumonia. In this condition the whole of a lobe of a lung is affected. The onset is sudden with pain in the side, short distressing cough, rapid shallow breathing, and raised temperature. Without specific treatment the temperature remains high for four to twelve days and then falls abruptly to normal within a few hours, the so-called crisis which is marked by profuse perspiration. Before the era of antibiotics fully 25 per cent of patients died, and pneumonia was particularly fatal in the elderly. Even in the antibiotic era the disease has quite a high death rate. The organisms most commonly responsible for pneumonia are the pneumococcus and the streptococcus. The germ is identified from the sputum and an appropriate antibiotic employed, but good nursing is as important as the right antibiotic.

Bronchopneumonia. Groups of alveoli near larger air-passages are affected in this type of pneumonia, so that there are small patches of inflammation or consolidation throughout the lungs. There are symptoms of severe BRONCHITIS, with increasing shortness of breath, discomfort in breathing, and often pain on both sides of the chest. While bronchopneumonia may occur alone, especially in the elderly, it often arises as a complication of measles, whooping cough, or bronchitis. Antibiotic treatment is important; the room should be kept moist with a steam kettle; and heart stimulants (e.g., brandy or coramine or strychnine) may be needed. As is the case in lobar pneumonia, skilled nursing is essential and for this reason it is generally desirable that the patient be treated in hospital.

Post-operative pneumonia. Formerly common, this third type is becoming a rarity. It arose partly from irritation of the lungs from the older anaesthetics (now replaced by anaesthetics less liable to irritate) and partly from prolonged and complete immobilization in bed (now replaced by minimal bed-rest after most operations).

pneumothorax. Air in the cavity between the two layers of pleura. It may occur from rupture of a tuberculous patch on the surface of the lung or as a result of a penetrating wound of the chest. Artificial pneumothorax is the deliberate introduction through a hollow needle of a measured amount of air into the pleural cavity to make it impossible for a diseased lung to expand and so rest it and facilitate healing.

While the occurrence of a large spontaneous pneumothorax is accompanied by pain, breathing difficulty and often signs of shock, the graded introduction of air into the pleural cavity should produce no symptoms either immediately or later. Patients are often at first afraid of having one lung temporarily put out of action, but most ordinary activities can be carried out perfectly well with only one functioning lung.

poisons. There is no arbitrary division between poisonous and non-poisonous substances. Many drugs which are life-saving in tiny doses (e.g., strychnine) kill in larger quantities; medicines that adults regard as harmless (e.g., aspirin) can poison young children; and substances essential to life (e.g., vitamin D, common salt, and even water) can destroy life or impair health if consumed in sufficient quantities.

Excluding the toxins of bacteria and the venom of snakes and insects, harmful substances can be roughly classified into four groups. (1) Corrosive irritants which irritate and inflame the alimentary canal and produce immediate symptoms, e.g., strong acids and alkalis. (2) Non-corrosive irritants which do not produce symptoms for half an hour or longer, e.g., arsenic. (3) Poisons affecting specific tissues, e.g., sodium cyanide, which prevents the transfer of oxygen in living cells. (4) Narcotics which act on the nervous system, e.g., morphia and prussic acid.

Evidences of poisoning. Symptoms appear suddenly in a previously healthy person. Depending on the type of poison they may appear immediately or some little time after the taking of the affected food, drink, or medicine. If the poison is derived from food several people may be ill simultaneously. Apart from these points the evidences vary with the actual poison.

Treatment of suspected poisoning. Summon medical aid immediately. If the poison is known, give the appropriate antidote, e.g., a solution of baking soda for an acid or of vinegar for an alkali, or if the poison is unknown a drink of milk, which will at least dilute it. Retain all food, drink, and vomited material since these may permit the identification of the poison and

of its source. If the patient is conscious ask him what he has swallowed: he may lose consciousness later. If he is unconscious, place him on his stomach with the head turned sideways to prevent suffocation if he vomits. If breathing stops, apply artificial respiration. Combat shock by application of warmth (e.g., hot water bottles) and, if he is conscious, stimulants (e.g., brandy or whisky). Emetics, such as a tablespoonful of mustard in a tumbler of warm water, are dangerous if the poison is corrosive – a circumstance often revealed by staining or burning of the mouth – and are again dangerous if the poison can form a vapour, as in poisoning by cleaning fluids. With these exceptions an emetic may be useful provided that the patient is conscious.

poliomyelitis. An acute infection of the central nervous system, causing no clinical symptoms in the majority of infected persons, fever and headache with some stiffness of the neck or spine in a sizeable minority, and temporary or permanent paralysis in about 2 per cent of cases. The condition was formerly called infantile paralysis, but it affects young adults and the middle-aged as well as children. The condition is caused by a virus which is transmitted mostly by droplet spray from the nose and throat of an infected person, and also to some extent by flies.

Although there are approximately twelve thousand people in Britain suffering from the persisting effects of poliomyelitis in the form of paralysis of one or more of the limbs, paralytic poliomyelitis is essentially a rare complication of a disease that is usually either symptomless or with symptoms resembling those of influenza. Hence both the diagnosis of a non-paralytic case and the tracing of the source of infection are difficult.

Paralytic cases require skilled nursing, preferably in hospital, with special equipment available during the acute phase, e.g., a respirator for use if respiratory paralysis threatens.

Vaccination. In country after country the introduction of poliomyelitis vaccination and the education of the public about its desirability and efficiency have virtually eradicated the disease. To take two years at random and using figures for England and Wales: in 1950 before vaccination had begun there were 5,565 cases of paralytic poliomyelitis; in 1965 there were 55 cases.

There are two types of anti-poliomyelitis vaccine.

1. The Salk vaccine consists of killed viruses which retain the capacity to stimulate the body to manufacture antibodies. Two intramuscular injections of 1 ml. are advised at intervals of four to six weeks, followed by a reinforcing injection about a year later and subsequent reinforcing doses at intervals of a few years. The desirable frequency of the reinforcing injections is still a little

uncertain, because when vaccination started the poliomyelitis virus was so widespread that persons with immunity conferred by vaccination might have their immunity strengthened by inhaling the virus, thus increasing their production of antibodies; as the virus becomes rare that stimulation of immunity is ceasing, so that we have to rely on reinforcing injections.

2. The Sabin vaccine consists of weakened strains of the virus and is given by mouth: three drops on a lump of sugar. Three doses are advised at intervals of about six weeks, with reinforcing doses later.

Both the injectable Salk vaccine and the oral Sabin vaccine produce a high immunity to the disease. While there is still argument about which is the better – with expert opinion in Britain tending to favour Sabin vaccine – it is highly important that all children and all previously unimmunized young adults should receive one or the other.

pollution. Defiling of the atmosphere, the land, the sea, or rivers by waste materials.

With increasing world population, rising industrialization, aggregation of people in towns, more and more cars and internal combustion engines, and steady increase in waste products and waste materials, pollution is becoming one of mankind's greatest problems, and indeed a problem critical for its survival. On the one hand it is vital that humanity appreciates and tries to counteract the health damage, financial cost, and ultimate results of air pollution by harmful gases, smoke, dust, and grit, the damage done to marine life by pollution of rivers, lakes, and seas, the harm to animal life resulting from widespread use of insecticides, and even the aesthetic damage created by slag-heaps and piles of disused cars, to say nothing of the continuous diminution of arable land by building of houses, factories, schools, and hospitals. On the other hand it has to be realized that urban life depends on a healthy industrial economy, that industry inevitably creates waste materials and waste products, and that to cripple industry by excessive regulations would lead to massive unemployment.

Air pollution. This is caused by smoke, gases, dust, and grit from domestic and industrial chimneys, railway trains, motor vehicles, and pollutants from industrial processes. It is estimated that fully 50 per cent of atmospheric pollution comes from domestic sources, with industry and transport also serious offenders. Some effects of the various pollutants are: (1) Interference with natural light, thereby reducing the manufacture of vitamin D and generally impairing health. (2) Increasing tendency to fog formation, with consequent increase in industrial, traffic, and domestic accidents. (3) Damage to paint work, building structures, etc., and increased rusting of iron. (4) Increased incidence of bronchitis,

pneumonia, lung cancer and emphysema. It is notorious that the death-rate in towns is almost everywhere higher than in the country despite rural areas having less variety of available food, more danger from winter storms, and often poorer medical and nursing care. The effects of air pollution on the respiratory system are best seen when a combination of cold, fog, and atmospheric contamination create the condition of smog – as in the 1952 London smog which killed four thousand people.

To some extent the smoke menace is being countered in heavily populated, developed countries by clean air legislation; but petrol-driven engines are beginning to give out more carbon dioxide than can be re-converted to oxygen and carbon by plant life, and are also giving out highly poisonous carbon monoxide – to such an extent that traffic policemen in Tokyo are now supplied with oxygen equipment for their personal use.

Land pollution. An example of land pollution is excessive use of insecticides: various countries, including Britain, have now banned the widespread use of DDT because of its long-term harmful effects on animals and man. Another example is pollution by radioactive materials: for instance strontium-90 passes to the soil, from it to the grass, thence to cows and their milk, and can in due course interfere with blood cell formation in the human bone marrow. Yet another example is the dumping of obsolete cars and other machinery – not only converting beautiful countryside into an eyesore but also using land that could otherwise be agriculturally productive.

Water pollution. The waste materials from factories, such as mercury compounds from paper mills, have enormously damaged fish life and in some areas have rendered the fish that survive dangerous for human consumption. For instance, in Japan people have died from eating tuna fish with high concentrations of mercury, and similar dangers have been identified in the Great Lakes of America and in Britain in the Bristol Channel. Another growing hazard is oil pollution from leaks from tankers and from accidental collisions. Yet another arises from the discharge of untreated sewage into the sea – very common in coastal towns.

Noise pollution. A form of pollution of which society is only in the process of becoming aware is noise – increasing rapidly through accumulation of population, universal use of the internal combustion engine, and increased use of materials that readily transmit sound.

The case for control of all forms of pollution is strong, but industrialists want their profits and their employees want their wage-packets, while householders like to keep their open fires and their cars. In general, therefore, there is a hostility to anti-pollution measures unless they can be achieved cheaply and preferably by the actions of persons other than ourselves. Yet increasingly air, water and land pollution are coming to constitute one of the world's two most fundamental problems, the other being the related problem of steadily rising population. Legislation alone is not the sole answer. The vast problem of pollution will be solved only by a combination of three things: education, to make people aware of the danger and of the need to accept and even demand control; research, to find measures which can reduce pollution with least damage to industrial efficiency and to personal comfort; and legislation, both to bring into line those who are too selfish to comply unless compelled to do so and to provide financial aid for those who could not otherwise afford to take effective steps for the reduction of pollution.

polycythaemia. Presence of red blood corpuscles in abnormally high quantity. The normal figure is about 5 million per cubic millimetre of BLOOD, and anything above 6.5 million is termed polycythaemia.

Apparent polycythaemia occurs in dehydration, where all bodily fluids including blood are reduced, and therefore the red blood corpuscles are more numerous in any measured quantity of blood. Genuine increase in corpuscles occurs in circumstances of any prolonged deficiency of oxygen, such as is occasioned by living at high altitudes or created by various diseases of the heart and circulation: the body manufactures extra corpuscles to cope with the harder work of carrying sufficient oxygen to the tissues.

Polycythaemia vera is an uncommon condition in which an excess of red cells and a thickening of the blood occur from causes as yet unknown. The disease is found mostly in the second half of life, and often creates headaches, dizziness, lack of concentration, purpling of the face, and enlargement of the spleen. True polycythaemia is one of the very few diseases for which bleeding (the blood-letting so extensively used in the seventeenth and eighteenth centuries) is still employed as treatment, although of course the modern method is insertion of a wide-bore needle into a vein, not vein cutting or application of leeches.

polypus. A tumour attached to a mucous membrane by a stalk. Such tumours occur in the nose, bladder, intestine, and uterus. They are benign (non-cancerous) but may cause trouble by obstruction (e.g., of breathing through the nose) and may very occasionally become cancerous if left. In general they are best surgically removed.

polyuria. The state in which an excessive amount of urine is passed. The normal quantity in an adult is about 1.5 litres (2.5 pints) daily, but varies with the amount of liquid drunk and the amount of sweat excreted by the skin. Broadly, patients suffering from polyuria may pass anything from 2 litres (4 pints) daily to the 23 to 27

litres (40 to 50 pints) excreted in some cases of diabetes insipidus.

Polyuria with albumin present in the urine suggests disease of the kidneys. Some of the causes of polyuria without presence of albumin are excessive fluid intake (e.g., the person who drinks a great quantity of beer or a large amount of tea or coffee inevitably passes much urine), nervousness, diabetes mellitus (in which the urine contains sugar), and diabetes insipidus. Since polyuria is essentially a symptom, treatment is to remove the underlying cause.

popliteal fossa. A lozenge-shaped hollow at the back of the knee, bounded by the hamstring muscles above and the calf muscles below.

liver

stomach

spleen

pancreas

large intestine

The portal circulation

portal circulation. The passage of blood from the stomach, pancreas, spleen and intestines to the liver by the hepatic portal vein. At the liver glycogen is extracted for storage before the CIRCULATION OF THE BLOOD continues through the hepatic vein.

port and airport services. Services designed to protect countries from the importation of communicable disease whether conveyed by passengers, crews or cargo. Apart from the general duty of preventing the entrance of infection, port health authorities are responsible for the inspection of imported food, the inspection of ships both for defects of hygiene and for evidence of rat infestation, and the medical inspection of aliens. Authorities responsible for airports have similar duties but also have to be aware of particular risks, such as the arrival of passengers who are incubating an infectious disease but owing to the speed of air travel do not yet show any signs of it, or the inadvertent transport in aircraft of insects harbouring the germs of a particular disease.

post-maturity. The condition of an infant whose birth is delayed beyond the normal time for the ending of pregnancy. In such delay there are dangers to the child since the nutriment passing through the placenta may be insufficient, and dangers to the mother especially if the child's bones begin to harden. It is therefore normal practice to induce labour artificially if it does not start within a few days of the expected date.

posture. The position of the body and limbs as a whole. Man's adoption of the erect position has had repercussions which are not wholly to his advantage. While use of the ancestral hind legs for standing and walking has enabled the front legs to be developed for climbing, grasping and throwing, a high incidence of hernia, varicose veins and flat foot is part of the price paid for an upright position.

Correct posture is very important for growth and health but unfortunately bad posture is often initially comfortable, although in due course it does harm by placing stresses and strains on parts of the body that were not intended to bear these burdens.

During the early development of postural defects much can be done by remedial exercises, but a child is apt to be bored by dull repetitive exercises and much better results can be obtained if the exercises are given as a form of interesting recreation and amusement.

Attention should particularly be paid to the posture of the scholarly, unathletic child who ignores the Roman maxim of 'a healthy mind in a healthy body', the abnormally tall boy or girl who so easily develops a stoop, and the short-sighted person whose round shoulders are essentially the result of peering forwards.

potassium. A silvery-white metal, of low density and unusual softness, that oxidizes rapidly in contact with air. The metal does not occur in nature in an uncombined form but potassium compounds are essential MINERAL SALTS for both animal and plant life. One of the things on which the maintenance of human life depends is the correct balance between potassium salts inside cells and sodium salts in the surrounding fluids.

With a normal diet the intake and excretion of potassium are equal at about 2.5 g. per day. Potassium depletion can occur in extensive diarrhoea and vomiting, and causes thirst, giddiness and confusion.

Pott's disease. See SPINAL COLUMN, TUBERCULOSIS OF.

Pott's fracture. See ANKLE.

poultices. Warm, pulpy masses applied to parts of the body to transfer heat in order to reduce inflammation, relieve pain or 'draw' pus from a boil. Nowadays it is customary to use kaolin preparations, such as antiphlogistine, available in tins and ready for application after heating. However, the older bread, mustard and linseed poultices are quite effective.

The mustard poultice is selected here for mention. Take one measure of mustard

and five of linseed; mix the mustard into a smooth paste with lukewarm water; pour the linseed, previously kept in a closed tin, into sufficient boiling water to make a smooth paste on stirring; stir the mustard paste smoothly into the linseed paste; spread on linen; apply to the affected part of the body for fifteen minutes; after removing the poultice dry the skin very gently with cotton-wool, dust with powder and cover with wool.

Fomentations. These are applications of cloths which have been heated by being wrung out with hot water (with or without drugs, such as turpentine or laudanum, added to the water). They serve essentially the same purpose as poultices.

pregnancy. The period from conception to labour, lasting for about 39 weeks in the human and for different lengths in animals, up to the 27 months of an elephant. Pregnancy is a natural and physiological state, not a period of invalidism. Despite the occurrence of occasional morning sickness in half the women during the second month, pregnancy is a time when a woman should feel at her best.

Duration of pregnancy. This is usually taken as 273 days, but variations from 240 to 320 days have been recorded. Since the exact date of fertile coitus is seldom known, the expected date of delivery is generally calculated as 280 days from the beginning of the last menstruation. Such calculation explains some of the variations in duration, since conception, arbitrarily assumed to occur seven days after the start of menstruation, may actually take place up to ten days earlier (just too late to stop the succeeding menstrual flow) or several days later.

Signs of pregnancy. The commonest presumptive sign is suppression of menstruation, but this is occasionally the result of disease or of fear of pregnancy, and very occasionally menstruation continues during the first month of pregnancy. Other presumptive signs include morning sickness (common but far from invariable in the second month); changes in the breast (sensation, fullness, enlargement and pigmentation successively); changes in the abdomen (in particular progressive enlargement); and quickening (the perception by the mother about the fifth month of the movements of the foetus). Absolute diagnosis depends on the feeling and counting of the foetal heart with a special stethoscope, the feeling of the foetal movements, or x-ray findings. Since none of these are really practicable before the fourth month, biological tests are much used. The Aschheim-Zondek test, for instance, consists of injecting the patient's urine into an immature female mouse: if the urine contains hormones produced in pregnancy, the ovaries of the mouse become swollen and congested in about four or five days.

Growth of the baby. An ovum fertilized

by a spermatozoon is called a zygote. The zygote repeatedly subdivides to form a globular mass of cells which then arrange themselves into an outer layer and an inner cell-mass, separated by fluid. The inner cell-mass develops into the future embryo and the outer wall ultimately becomes the chorion which unites with another sac, to form the amniotic cavity in which the embryo becomes suspended by the body-stalk or future umbilical cord.

Meantime the mucous membrane of the body of the uterus has become thicker and more vascular under hormonal influence and in this the developing ovum becomes embedded. The blood vessels of the chorion are thus brought into relationship with the maternal circulation. At a slightly later stage the blood vessels of the chorion are concentrated at one site opposite the body-stalk to form the placenta, which is supplied with blood from the embryonic circulation. The placenta provides an interchange system between the embryonic and maternal circulation. This stage is reached by about the end of the second month of pregnancy. Simultaneously the inner cell-mass has developed into a recognizable embryo, two inches long, and with all its tissues, organs and limbs differentiated. Conventionally it is then referred to as a foetus instead of an embryo.

It should be noted that the placenta also allows infective agents and drugs to cross to the foetal circulation, and so the embryo can be affected by certain diseases such as syphilis or rubella or by toxic agents which can damage its development particularly in the earlier months. X-rays can also have adverse effects.

During the next seven months further intra-uterine growth consists largely of a gradual increase in size and weight. The foetus by its fourth month is about five inches long, ten inches long at five months and about twenty inches long at full term.

All the materials needed for growth must come from the maternal circulation. A mother therefore needs extra food although quality is more important than quantity. By the end of pregnancy the additional requirement is some 500 Calories per day, and the developing foetus also makes increased demands on her iron and calcium intake which should be supplied by supplements of iron and folic acid and by additional milk.

Health in pregnancy. As already indicated, pregnancy is a physiological state, not a pathological state, and is a time when a woman should be at her best, with every faculty alert and her whole body full of life and energy. Nevertheless it is a very testing time.

During the nine months of pregnancy the woman's body has to adapt to hormonal changes, to the steady growth of the baby and to an average weight increase (including the weight of the baby) of about 1 kg. (24 lb.). In the second and

Pregnancy

third months of pregnancy she may well have bouts of nausea and sometimes slight actual sickness in the mornings, and may also develop frequency and urgency of urination because of pressure of the enlarging uterus on the bladder: later in pregnancy abdominal pressure may lead to indigestion, constipation, varicose veins, and occasionally piles. Mistaken attempts to 'eat for two' may also lead to indigestion and flatulence. In addition, specific diseases of pregnancy may occur, e.g., hyperemesis gravidarum.

While both excessive physical and excessive mental fatigue are undesirable and even dangerous, and while extreme emotional upset in the later months can lead to premature labour, health in pregnancy is best maintained by a continuation of normal activities, coupled with a philosophy of reasonable moderation. Exercise such as walking is useful although the more violent forms of exercise should be avoided. Food should be adequate and nourishing but not excessive: even at the very end of pregnancy a woman needs only about 25 per cent more Calories than before pregnancy. Fresh fruit, green vegetables, milk, butter, cheese and eggs should be plentifully included in the diet; an extra pint of milk daily is a useful source of calcium and provides most of the extra Calories needed. Too much meat is alleged to place a strain on the kidneys. Constipation should be avoided, with mild laxatives used as required. Clothing should not be constricting: belts and garters are not suitable. Adequate rest should be taken and the woman should have plenty of fresh air. Bathing is perfectly permissible but cold baths and very hot baths are undesirable. Sexual intercourse is undesirable during the later months.

Good antenatal care is important and the expectant mother is well advised to attend an antenatal clinic, discussion classes for prospective parents, and classes in psychoprophylaxis (a method of psychological and physical training for childbirth, particularly involving explanation and relaxation); but it cannot be sufficiently emphasized that pregnancy is normally a healthy period, not a time of illness and invalidism.

For false or spurious pregnancy, see PSEUDOCYESIS.

prejudice. An unfavourable opinion formed and maintained without knowledge, justification or adequate reason. Racial, religious and political prejudice is common, e.g., irrational dislike of persons with dark skin, Jews, Roman Catholics or Communists. Sex prejudice is far from rare: in some universities it is almost unknown for a woman to secure a senior post, and in women's professions in the process of being opened to men (e.g., health visiting and nursing) it is sometimes alleged that a good male student tends to receive a lower mark in examinations than a female student of equal merit. Prejudice may even extend to accents and colour of hair.

In health education where the educator is seeking to alter habits and attitudes awareness of the prejudices of the person being taught is vital. Anything that is in danger of running counter to a prejudice has to be tackled subtly and obliquely: it is hopeless to try to alter a person's prejudiced attitude by telling him bluntly that he is wrong. It is, of course, also important that the educator should try to become aware of his own prejudices.

premature ejaculation. See EJACULATIO PRAECOX.

prematurity. Birth occurring appreciably before full term. Since it is generally impossible to ascertain the exact date of conception the convention has been adopted of regarding a baby as premature

if its birth weight is less than 2.5 kg. (5.5 lb.). This rough and ready standard is reasonably accurate in cases where the infant at full term would have been expected to weigh between 3 and 3.5 kg. (7 and 8 lb.). Clearly, however, there are many cases in which the arbitrary standard is inaccurate. An infant born to well-built parents from families of above average size might well be premature even though its birth weight was about 3 kg. (7 lb.), whereas if the parents are small by reason of hereditary factors (as opposed to being stunted through poor nutrition or other environmental factors in childhood) the baby might be fully developed although weighing a little less than 2.5 kg. (5.5 lb.).

In some cases the delivery has to be brought on early because of maternal illness, and in other cases premature birth occurs spontaneously. The chance of spontaneous premature birth and the likelihood of early induction of labour becoming necessary are both greatly reduced by good antenatal care.

A premature infant suffers from three main disadvantages. Firstly, a mature infant can do without oxygen for a couple of minutes but the less well equipped premature baby cannot. Hence at the moment of birth, with change from oxygen exchange through the placenta to ordinary respiration, there is increased danger of brain damage. Secondly, protective fat develops only in the last weeks of a normal pregnancy. So a premature baby, lacking this fat, has difficulty in maintaining body heat. The baby should be kept in an incubator at about 24 °C. (75 °F.) or, failing that, in a specially warmed cot protected from all draughts. The baby should not at first be bathed but merely smeared with warm olive oil. Thirdly, since the stomach is small and the infant may be too weak to suck, feeding requires considerable care and patience.

During the first few weeks a premature infant is very vulnerable. Indeed fully one-third of all infant deaths are nowadays ascribed to prematurity. After it has survived the dangerous early weeks, however, it is not at materially greater risk than is a younger mature baby of the same weight or stage of development.

During the first two years or so the prematurity should be remembered in any assessment of the child's intellectual or physical development, e.g., a baby that was a couple of months premature is really only 10 months old at its first birthday. By about three years, however, the fact of prematurity can be forgotten, because the differences between a child of 40 months and another of 38 months (or of 40 months but born two months prematurely) are trivial.

premedication. The use of drugs in preparation for anaesthesia, e.g., atropine to reduce secretion in the lungs and morphia to allay anxiety.

prenatal diagnosis. Ascertainment during pregnancy of whether an unborn child suffers from certain hereditary disorders, with the aim of terminating the pregnancy if the child is abnormal but allowing the pregnancy to continue if the child is healthy. It is alternatively known as amniocentesis.

The method may be used for (1) certain chromosomal disorders (e.g., mongolism, where a mother over the age of 40 years has roughly a one-in-forty chance of giving birth to a handicapped child); (2) certain defects of the spinal cord (e.g., spina bifida, where the mother of a defective child has at least a one-in-ten chance of producing another handicapped child); (3) several diagnosable metabolic disorders; and (4) some severe sex-linked disorders (e.g., haemophilia).

Potential parents at risk may prefer to accept GENETIC GUIDANCE and family avoidance but if anxious to have a healthy child if possible, can be offered analysis of the amniotic fluid at about the sixteenth week of pregnancy on the understanding that they will accept termination of pregnancy if the examination of the fluid shows that the child is defective.

The procedure (called amniocentesis) is to withdraw about 10 ml. of amniotic fluid under a local anaesthetic, and then culture cells from the fluid to study the chromosomes (e.g., for the extra chromosome of mongolism) or examine the fluid for the presence of particular proteins (e.g., the alpha-foetoprotein of spina bifida). Diagnosis is not normally practicable before fifteen weeks, and is not yet possible at all for some genetic conditions, such as cystic fibrosis and phenylketonuria. The withdrawal of the fluid normally causes little discomfort, but very rarely quite serious complications ensue such as maternal haemorrhage, septicaemia and premature labour.

A major advance in 1974 in respect of spina bifida was the finding of alpha-foetoprotein in the maternal blood serum. There are occasional 'false positives', so a mother with the protein in her serum should be offered amniocentesis before the pregnancy is actually terminated.

The procedure is quite expensive in staff time – discussion with a health visitor or general practitioner, discussion with a geneticist, half an hour of the time of an obstetrician and a nurse (for the withdrawal of the fluid), considerable laboratory work, etc.; but the cost in time and money is trivial compared, for instance, with that of caring for many years for a partially paralysed, incontinent, mentally retarded victim of spina bifida.

prepuce. See FORESKIN.

presbyacusis. Diminution of hearing as age advances. The process starts in adolescence; persons of 17 or 18 years are too old to hear very high-pitched sounds that were perfectly audible to them several years earlier. As age increases more and more high-pitched sounds are unheard and in later life there may be difficulty in distinguishing some consonants, although vowels are still well heard. See DEAFNESS.

presbyopia. Decreased ability to focus the eyes as age advances. From the age of about 40 or 45 the lens becomes less elastic and it is more and more difficult for the person to obtain a clear view of near objects. Distance vision remains good but spectacles are required for reading and sewing.

preventable diseases. Apart from the degenerations of later life, most diseases are preventable, e.g., by genetic guidance, antenatal care, attention to emotional and physical health of children, immunization against infections, good diet but avoidance of obesity, adequate exercise, suitable recreations, avoidance of cigarette smoking and moderation in all things.

Preventable diseases are so numerous that only a few groups can here be selected for mention.

Infections. Until the middle of the twentieth century these were by far the greatest killers of mankind. Plague had several times destroyed a quarter of the population of Europe; malaria was unquestionably the biggest killing disease in the world; typhoid was the commonest fever of the developed countries in the nineteenth century; and as late as 1941 Scotland – a relatively small country – had over ten thousand cases of diphtheria and 517 deaths from that disease.

Some of the preventive measures introduced in recent decades have been: (1) eradication of food-borne infections by provision of pure water and uncontaminated food, with the result that typhoid and cholera have virtually disappeared from developed countries; (2) destruction of the breeding grounds of insects carrying infections such as yellow fever and malaria; (3) production of vaccines and education of the public about their desirability, with subsequent enormous reductions in smallpox, diphtheria, poliomyelitis and many other infections; and (4) virtual eradication of tuberculosis by a combination of better nutrition, better housing, follow-up of contacts, BCG vaccination and mass radiography.

To mention two other examples, ophthalmia neonatorum, a formerly common cause of blindness, has responded to routine instillation of drops in the eyes of babies, and rubella (German measles) – which when occurring in expectant mothers caused a high proportion of congenital defects in their offspring – is in the process of being eradicated by vaccination and public education about the need for vaccination. A few infections are not yet preventable. Gonorrhoea (unless we can prevent it by sex education and moral education) and the common cold are examples, but most infections are now deemed preventable, although it has to be remembered that health education about immunization and about food hygiene becomes more difficult as the particular preventable diseases become more rare.

Diseases of nutrition. It is essentially in the last fifty years that improved knowledge of nutritional needs, better available food supplies, identification of vitamins and other trace substances, education of the public about diet and budgeting, and the addition of minerals and vitamins to certain foodstuffs have combined virtually to eliminate from highly developed countries such diseases as rickets, scurvy, iron deficiency anaemia and simple goitre. We still find nutritional disorders in the very old, especially if living alone, and in immigrants still using a diet suitable only for a climate with greater sunshine and more warmth; and in the underdeveloped countries many deficiency diseases (e.g., kwashiorkor) are still very common. However, given a proper balance between population and food production so that enough food is quantitatively and qualitatively available per head of population, and given adequate health education of the public about dietetic needs at different ages, virtually all nutritional diseases can now be prevented.

Most diseases of pregnancy, labour and the puerperal state. Antenatal care, better nutrition, health visiting and midwifery services, and better obstetrics together reduced maternal mortality (on figures for England and Wales) from about 6 per thousand births a hundred years ago to less than 3 in 1941 (before the advent of antibiotics) and to 0.2 in 1971; and simultaneously infant deaths fell from 158 per thousand births in 1871 to 60 in 1941 and 18 in 1971. In terms of lives saved these reductions rival the savings from infections and utterly outstrip the saving of lives from any forms of medical or surgical treatment.

Home accidents. These were formerly the commonest cause of death from 1 year to 21 years and a very common cause of death and of disability in the elderly. Recent work has demonstrated that by studying the causal factors operating in different social groups and age groups and then educating persons at risk or persons responsible for children or veterans at risk, the incidence of home accidents serious enough to need medical treatment can be reduced by more than one-third. Particular value is placed upon home visits and one-to-one discussions by the health visitor. There is some evidence that the same techniques can be successfully applied to the reduction of traffic accidents and industrial accidents.

Hereditary diseases. It is becoming possible to identify many carriers of serious genetic defects (such as Huntington's chorea, spina bifida, deaf-mutism, the main variety of mongolism, and the main type of schizophrenia) and to

reduce their transmission by a combination of genetic counselling, health education, and contraceptive facilities.

Of the five groups so far mentioned it should be noted that the first two could be virtually eliminated and the last three very greatly reduced, although some home accidents would still occur and some developmental abnormalities would still take place.

Problems in the process of being solved. The psychoneuroses, aggressive behaviour and crimes of violence are very common today, and their treatment is unsatisfactory. For example, Eysenck produced evidence purporting to show that neurotics receiving treatment by psychotherapy responded very little better than neurotics not receiving such treatment, and Brown demonstrated that multiproblem families 'helped' by intensive social case-work were only marginally better than parallel families not receiving such aid. However, simultaneously with evidence of the limitations of clinical and social treatment there have appeared strong indications of the value of prevention. There are indications, for example, that aggressive behaviour and violence are often a response to arbitrary frustration and attacks on a child's self-esteem, and can be prevented by a warm, affectionate relationship with parents and associates. Delinquency on the whole appears to be caused by parental rejection, harsh or inconsistent discipline or broken homes, so that it can be reduced by campaigns to make every child a wanted child, by education of parents and prospective parents about child management, and by measures for the prevention of marital breakdown. It begins to seem quite likely that education of children, prospective parents and parents of young children may very substantially reduce the psychoneuroses, aggression, violence, delinquency and maladjustment.

Again, although man is mortal and diseases of old age can be postponed rather than avoided, there are enormous possibilities for the reduction of diseases at present associated with middle-life and the earlier portion of old age. We are beginning to understand, for example, that coronary thrombosis is in large measure caused by excessive stress, over-eating, heavy smoking and lack of exercise, and that all four factors are largely under human control. Again, we are in the process of realizing that chronic bronchitis – the 'English disease' – can in most cases be prevented by a combination of positive and negative factors: good nutrition, avoidance of obesity (both in the middle-aged who might develop bronchitis this year and in the child whose bronchitis may be half a century ahead), clean air, avoidance of cigarette smoking, warm and well-ventilated houses, immunization against diseases liable to produce effects on the respiratory system, and use of clothing that affords adequate protection against the elements.

The limitations of prevention. Although a few conditions so far afford scant possibilities of either prevention or treatment – with the common cold perhaps the disease for which there is least justifiable hope – it seems likely that the next half century will be the era in which disease as a whole, mental and physical, becomes recognized as preventable; that admission to hospital before the age of 75 or 80 will become increasingly infrequent; and that, within the next seventy years the occurrence of death in a person under the age of 75 years may well be so unusual as to warrant a special enquiry when it occurs. If this last suggestion at first seems fantastic, it may be noted that our grandparents would have thought the idea of a special enquiry into all deaths associated with pregnancy and childbirth utterly impracticable, and yet we already have it. It is also worth noting that long-term prevention of disease (e.g., reduction of senile psychosis sixty years later by fostering a child's capacity to form friends and develop fresh interests) is a science only still in its infancy.

Yet perhaps we need some moderation even in the application of measures designed to prevent mental and physical disorders. Perhaps the continued progress of mankind demands that some youngsters with personal unhappiness should challenge the beliefs and standards of their elders; that some adolescents should endanger life and limb, whether by attempting to climb an unscalable cliff or by experimenting with a new drug; and that some middle-aged people should continue to be regarded as eccentrics. PREVENTIVE MEDICINE has enormous potentialities for human health and happiness, but human progress may require that some people should not fully share in that health and happiness but should feel what Shelley called 'divine discontent'. Every health worker rightly aims at decreasing illness and improving well-being, but to some extent it is the unhappy, dissatisfied people – the people on the verge of neuroticism – who make scientific discoveries, produce works of art or change the patterns of human life.

preventive medicine. The science that seeks to reduce disease by identifying, removing or altering the causes or by modifying the response of the person on whom these causes operate. Preventive medicine is gradually evolving its own techniques and methods but was originally a combination of applied physiology, psychology, biology, sociology and medicine, with the persuasive methods taken at first from education and commerce.

'Preventive medicine' is an unsatisfactory term for two reasons. Firstly 'preventive' is far too narrow.

Improving, fostering and maintaining emotional, social and physical health are quite as important as the preventive aspects, though strict separation of 'promotion of health' from 'prevention of disease ' is not easy: we provide a good diet for a child to foster its growth and development, but incidentally the adequacy of calcium and vitamin D in the diet prevents rickets; and we give the same child plenty of warm, demonstrated affection, security and reasonable freedom to explore and make decisions in order to improve mental and emotional development, and we incidentally do much to prevent maladjustment, delinquency and sexual deviance. Secondly, 'medicine' seems to imply that the work is mainly that of doctors, whereas perhaps the biggest contributions can be made – and in part have already been made – by workers other than doctors, e.g., health visitors, health education officers, school teachers, personnel officers, and so on. Yet the alternative terms 'social medicine' and 'community medicine' are even less satisfactory. See also PREVENTABLE DISEASES and HEALTH EDUCATION.

priapism. Persistent and painful erection of the penis unaccompanied by sexual stimulation. The condition is sometimes due to a blood clot in the veins of the erectile tissue of the penis; sometimes it is a symptom accompanying stone in the bladder or urethra; it is occasionally a result of gonorrhoea, and has been known to occur, without other apparent cause, after prolonged sexual activity. Whatever the cause, the organ becomes woodenly hard, painful and extremely sensitive, and there may be difficulty in passing urine. Treatment varies with the cause, ranging from sedative drugs to anticoagulants.

prickly heat. An itchy rash of small watery blisters and red pimples, due to blocking of sweat glands, occurring through excessive perspiration in humid, tropical conditions, and affecting particularly the neck, face, chest, back, armpits and thighs. The rash usually disappears slowly after the body cools, but bathing – without soap – may help, as may the application of a dusting powder. In climatic conditions conducive to prickly heat alcohol and heavy meals should be avoided, especially by a newcomer in his first month or so, clothing should be light and porous, and the person at risk should endeavour to keep cool, e.g., by avoiding needless exertion and moving at a slow pace.

primary. There are two uses of this term. (1) The initial defect or disease from which may arise 'secondary' or subsequent trouble, e.g., the primary focus of cancer is in one part of the body but it may lead to secondaries elsewhere. (2) The main disease from which a person is suffering or the main factor in his treatment, with the implication that other diseases or factors are subsidiary and less important.

primipara. A woman who has given birth to

a child for the first time, in contrast to a multipara, the mother of more than one child. In recent years, however, some medical writers have tended to employ the term for a woman who is bearing her first child. Strictly such a woman is a primigravida and does not become a primipara until after the birth.

private practice. Medical, dental or other treatment provided outside any National Health Service and for which the patient pays directly.

problem children. A rather outmoded term to describe 'difficult' or 'maladjusted' or 'highly strung' children. See BEHAVIOUR (disorders), and CHILD GUIDANCE.

proctitis. Inflammation of the rectum. It usually occurs along with itching of the anus and may be due to threadworms, fungal infections, louse infestation or allergy. It may also occur in association with diabetes or with inflammation of the colon. Treatment varies with the cause, but the application of a towel soaked in warm water often relieves the symptoms and the avoidance of constipation usually helps.

progesterone. A female sex hormone secreted by the corpus luteum which develops each month in the ovary at the site from which an ovum has been released. The hormone stimulates the development of the uterus and prepares it for the implantation of the fertilized ovum. If pregnancy occurs progesterone prevents further menstruation and the release of more ova. If pregnancy does not occur the secretion of the hormone stops in a few days.

Because of its action in preventing the release of ova, progesterone is one of the basic elements in oral contraceptive pills. The hormone is also useful in the treatment of threatened or habitual miscarriage.

prognosis. A prediction of the probable future course and outcome of a disease. The prediction is based partly on the history of the disease in other people, partly on the previous health and constitution of the patient, partly on the drugs available and partly on the patient's response to these drugs.

progressive muscular atrophy. A disease characterized by progressive wasting of the muscles, most frequently the muscles of the arms, associated with degenerative changes in the central nervous system. The condition, commonest at 30 to 50 years, often causes paralysis within a few months, but in quite a number of cases there are long stationary periods each followed by a further deterioration. The cause is as yet unknown, no effective treatment or method of prevention has been devised, and so far all that can be done is to maintain the general health of the patient, e.g., by massage and passive movements.

projection. Unconscious reading into the minds of others of feelings, opinions and desires which we ourselves experience, e.g., blaming others for our own guilt or failure, or attributing to others our own stinginess or untidiness. Essentially projection is a defence mechanism which helps us to maintain our conception of our own dignity and merit, but it can lead to considerable bias in our judgment of others.

prolapse. Any protrusion or downward displacement of an organ. The term is most frequently used for downward displacement of the rectum or the uterus.

Prolapse of the rectum, with protrusion of a piece of bowel through the anus, is not uncommon in children and sometimes occurs in adults in association with haemorrhoids. In most cases replacement is possible without surgical operation.

Prolapse of the uterus, common in women who have given birth to several children, is usually a delayed result of injury during childbirth, e.g., stretching or tearing of the supporting muscles or ligaments. Possible lines of treatment include the fitting and wearing of a ring pessary, surgical reconstruction, and removal of the uterus.

Prolapse of an intervertebral disc is usually called SLIPPED DISC.

prontosil. Prontosil was the first drug found to have a specific effect on acute bacterial infections when administered by mouth. The sulphonamides have been developed from it and have taken its place.

prophylaxis. The medical term for prevention of disease. While prophylaxis may be anything from a vitamin tablet to a course of exercises or a complete reorganization of a person's way of life, the term is often used specifically for three types of preventive measures: (1) immunization and vaccination (specific prophylaxis of various infections); (2) the wearing of a condom and subsequent douching (prophylaxis of venereal disease and also of conception); and (3) teeth cleaning (dental prophylaxis). See also PSYCHOPROPHYLAXIS.

proprietary medicines. Patent medicines, with undivulged constituents and often claiming remarkable curative or preventive powers, were formerly very common in virtually all countries. They were intensely disliked by doctors because (1) if they were valueless they not only defrauded the patient but delayed his attempt to secure proper treatment; (2) if they had a value they were employed largely as a result of a self-diagnosis by the patient and therefore liable to be used for conditions in which they would not help; (3) if they had value and were selected for disease in which they would help they were in competition with the physician and liable to affect his income; (4) if a patient used a patent medicine and subsequently consulted a doctor, the doctor had no easy means of ascertaining whether the drug that he desired to prescribe was compatible with the drug already in the patient's system; and (5) it was basic to medical ethics that a doctor, having found a particular drug useful in a particular disease, should make the fact known to his colleagues so that patients in general could benefit from his discovery.

However, the position is now much improved. The Pharmacy and Medicines Act, 1941, made it an offence to advocate a proprietary medicine for the treatment of certain serious diseases, required disclosure of the ingredients of each patent medicine in precise terms and to some extent restricted the sale of these medicines; and the Food and Drugs Act, 1955, made it an offence to sell any food or drug which is not of the nature, substance or quality demanded by the buyer, and also made it an offence to use false or misleading labels. In addition, a trade association of manufacturers of proprietary medicines – The Proprietary Association of Great Britain – has devised a code of advertising standards.

Medicines in Britain are divided into those advertised solely to the medical profession and those advertised also to the general public, but the purchaser is fairly adequately protected, although occasionally an unscrupulous manufacturer can find a loophole in the law.

proprioception. Sensations coming from the muscles, ligaments, tendons and joints and from the labyrinths of each ear. These impulses – often never reaching the realm of consciousness – give information about the position of various parts of the body, so that posture is adjusted as required.

prostaglandins. Substances, produced in the body, which affect the nervous system and the blood flow in the kidneys, and also stimulate the contraction of uterine muscle. Because of this latter property it is possible that they may be developed as a contraceptive for use after sexual intercourse – a 'morning after' pill. Trials of synthetic prostaglandins are, however, still at only an early stage.

prostate. A glandular structure, normally about the size of a chestnut, lying at the neck of the bladder in males and surrounding the outlet of the urethra. The prostate secretes a clear, viscous fluid which lubricates the urethra and mixes with the sperm cells to form semen.

Diseases. By far the commonest disease of the prostate is enlargement, characterized at first by frequency of desire to pass urine, and later by partial obstruction of the flow of urine and sometimes by incontinence as a result of the bladder never being completely emptied. In most cases surgical removal of the gland is required, although a course of antibiotics should first be tried, because there may well be some inflammation which makes a relatively slight enlargement appear worse than it really is. As yet little is known about the cause of enlargement, so prevention is not practicable.

Acute prostatitis, inflammation of the gland, is an occasional complication of infection elsewhere in the urinary system. The condition is characterized by high temperature, pain in the lower part of the back and frequency of urination. Treatment is that of the original infection.

Chronic prostatitis, with similar symptoms but less fever, is often associated with cystitis. Both acute and chronic inflammation of the gland respond well to antibiotics.

Cancer of the gland occurs most frequently at 50 to 70 years. It is characterized by symptoms of enlargement (see above) but often exhibits more pain and leads to traces of blood in the urine. Rectal examination reveals a hard, irregular swelling. Until a few years ago surgical removal was recommended as the only effective treatment, but in recent years it has been found that treatment with stilboestrol in many cases results in complete cure.

prosthesis. The replacement of an absent or amputated part by an artificial one. Dentures, glass eyes and artificial limbs are examples of prosthetic devices.

In general artificial limbs are moved by the muscles of the remaining stump, but nowadays some are powered by electric batteries.

prostration. Complete physical or mental exhaustion.

protein. The complex FOOD substances containing nitrogen, and essential constituents of protoplasm of which all animal cells are composed.

On average the human body consists of approximately 70 per cent water, about 15 per cent fat and 12 per cent protein, with the muscles composed almost entirely of water and protein. Hence protein is constantly required for the building and maintenance of the body tissues.

Each protein molecule in the body is itself composed of a chain of amino-acids of which some twenty-two have been identified, including eight which the body cannot manufacture and which are therefore essential requirements in diet.

Foods containing protein can be divided into two types: those containing first class protein (i.e., protein with all the essential amino-acids) such as meat, fish, cheese, eggs and milk; and those containing second class protein (i.e., protein which is useful but lacks some of the essential amino-acids) such as peas, beans and lentils. During digestion the complex proteins of the foods eaten are broken down to their constituent amino-acids and then rebuilt to constitute the proteins of the bodily tissues. Surplus of protein can be used as bodily fuel and in conditions of starvation, protein will be used for fuel to the detriment of maintenance of tissues.

In communities where there is no shortage of food it should be remembered that excess protein in the diet is simply used as fuel which could just as well be supplied by the far more plentiful (and, incidentally, much cheaper) carbohydrate. Under these circumstances the nitrogenous portion is converted to urea and excreted in the urine. Indeed for energy purposes protein is an uneconomical food because considerable energy is used in its digestion, which is the basis of its employment in 'slimming' diets.

In developed countries many affluent people eat more protein than necessary, whereas in underdeveloped countries where MALNUTRITION is common, insufficient protein is usual. Severe protein deficiency leads to general weakness, swelling of the abdomen and lowered resistance to disease.

protozoa. Single-celled organisms, the smallest creatures that can be called animals. An example is the amoeba, found in most ponds, just visible to the naked eye and slightly smaller than the dot at the end of this sentence. They are usually regarded as the lowest form of animal life, just as fungi are regarded as the lowest form of plant life, with bacteria and viruses regarded neither as animals nor as plants. In general they do not reproduce sexually (most protozoa do not have male and female members of the species) but merely swell and then split into two, a process technically called multiplication by simple fission. Thus the amoeba that we see today is immortal in the sense that it has never lost an ancestor by death.

The vast majority of protozoa are harmless, but malaria, sleeping sickness and a form of dysentery are carried by parasitic protozoa.

prurigo. A vague term for a group of intensely itchy conditions in which the main physical signs are pimples with the tops scratched off and thickening of the skin. While the precipitating cause may be a trivial local irritant, the condition is in most cases fundamentally emotional in origin – a sort of direction of anger, thwarted elsewhere, against the self. Antiitching ointments, steroid hormones and tranquillizers may all help, but the essential treatment, and equally the essential means of prevention, is relief of the underlying emotional tension and therefore investigation of its causes.

pruritis. The medical term for ITCHING.

prussic acid. An intense and rapidly acting poison of the narcotic group occurring naturally in the oil of bitter almonds and identifiable from its characteristic almond-like smell. It is alternatively called hydrocyanic acid.

When taken internally the acid and certain of its salts (cyanides and isocyanides) cause a momentary sensation of burning in the mouth and are absorbed with extraordinary rapidity. Breathing becomes spasmodic, there are a few convulsive movements, unconsciousness supervenes and – usually within a couple of minutes – death results from paralysis of the respiratory and central nervous

systems. On post mortem examination the blood is a curiously bright red.

The poison, in addition to being very rapidly absorbed, is quickly destroyed by the tissues, so that, if the patient is still alive, artificial respiration should be tried, and continued until he has recovered or definitely died. If an oxidizing agent (such as hydrogen permanganate or potassium permanganate) is available it can be given in the hope of converting the prussic acid to a harmless oxamide. Intravenous injection of methylene blue (50 cc. of a one per cent solution) has proved effective in some cases.

pseudocyesis. Spurious or false pregnancy. This curious condition occurs in neurotic women, in women near the menopause who are very anxious to have a child, and in some eastern countries in women whose husbands could divorce them for barrenness. It is primarily emotional but the emotion affects the formation of hormones by the pituitary and other glands.

All the symptoms of pregnancy appear and many of the physical signs, e.g., the breasts and abdomen enlarge and menstruation may cease. Often the condition is so like a genuine pregnancy that examination under a general anaesthetic is necessary to establish the diagnosis. Under anaesthesia the hysterical fixation of the abdominal muscles collapses and vaginal examination reveals that the uterus is of only normal size. Treatment is essentially psychological and is far from easy.

The condition is not confined to human beings, but is sometimes seen, for instance, in female dogs.

psittacosis. A severe infectious disease with the general symptoms of pneumonia, but also with extreme weakness, slow pulse and often delirium, so that it may be mistaken for typhoid. The disease is caused by a virus, transmitted by parrots, parakeets, canaries and some other birds, and infection occurs through close contact with the birds or with their recent excreta. In most cases infection arises from sick birds, but occasionally an apparently healthy bird can act as a carrier.

Treatment consists of isolation of the patient and prompt and adequate administration of tetracyclines or other appropriate antibiotics. Although patient to patient transmission is rare, nurses handling a patient should wear thick gauze masks and all discharges from the patient should be disinfected. Infected birds and their carcases and cages should be destroyed.

There is as yet no method of immunization, but the condition is preventable by strict regulation of the import of, and traffic in, birds of the parrot family, with both a period of quarantine and a laboratory examination before any such bird is offered for sale.

psoriasis. A fairly common skin disease

characterized by the formation of red patches which are covered by fine silvery scales. The disease often runs in families and is not infectious, but its cause is still uncertain. The most widely accepted theory is that the condition is due to an inherited defect in the formation of the cells of the skin.

The guttate variety, which occurs in children, often follows an infectious disease which seems to trigger off the condition. Application of oily calamine lotion and administration of vitamin supplements often effect a cure within a few months.

Psoriasis of extensor surfaces (e.g., knees or elbows) may occur at any period of life. There is usually no itching and the patient should be encouraged to accept the patches as harmless and non-infectious. Many treatments have been advocated without much success, e.g., ointments containing coal tar and local application of steroid drugs. Exposure to sunlight may be useful.

Psoriasis of the flexures (e.g., armpits, genital area and below the breasts) is commonest in the obese, and treatment of the obesity may help.

The disease also occurs in the nails, palms and soles.

psyche. The human spirit or mind, including all its emotions, perceptions and activities. The term is used by psychologists and psychiatrists mainly because 'soul' has become restricted to spiritual or religious connotations and 'mind' is overwhelmingly associated with reasoning and remembering.

psychedelic drugs. Drugs which produce hallucinations. See HALLUCINOGEN.

psychiatry. The branch of medicine concerned with the diagnosis and treatment (and in some cases prevention) of emotional and mental disorders. See PSYCHOSIS, NEUROSIS, PSYCHOSO-MATIC DISEASES and MENTAL DEFICIENCY.

Perhaps a fair summary of the present state of psychiatry is this: emotional and behavioural disorders of children are preventable and also treatable; similar disorders in adults are in large measure preventable at long range but very hard to treat when fully developed; psychoneurotic diseases are in the main preventable at long range and are also in most cases curable; the reduction of mental handicap is fundamentally a matter of genetic counselling and in most cases existing mental handicap is incurable; the organic psychoses (e.g., those arising from brain damage through accidents) can be prevented; and there are some hopeful signs for the future prevention or cure of the other psychotic diseases.

psychoanalysis. A special method of exploring the unconscious mind, originated by Freud. It aims at bringing to the surface forgotten memories and hidden fears and conflicts. By so doing it often precipitates an emotional crisis, after which the patient is in a position to understand and cope with his problems.

After the analyst has taken a careful history and carefully noted any gaps in the patient's narrative, the usual method is 'free association'. Here the analyst may occasionally direct the patient's thoughts by a word or a phrase, but in general the analyst merely listens while the patient says anything that comes into his mind, however foolish or objectionable it may seem. Gradually his words begin to reveal the repressed matter lying in his unconscious, and so help to indicate the origins of his psychoneurotic or psychosomatic illness. The process is inevitably slow, perhaps taking two hours a week for a year.

Under hypnosis the procedure can be quickened, but the success rate is reduced, because in this case it is really the analyst who does the uncovering, whereas part of the value of the free association method lies in the patient uncovering hidden memories for himself.

A psychoanalyst is a doctor (or occasionally a non-medical psychologist) who has undertaken special training and has himself been analysed, so as to become aware, for instance, of his own prejudices.

Although disliked by some non-analytical psychiatrists and although very slow and therefore costly, psychoanalysis is of proved value in the treatment of the psychoneuroses (e.g., hysterias and obsessions), and some of its practitioners have claimed a measure of success in paranoia. It has limitations, however: firstly, it is useless unless the patient is willing; secondly, it tends to fail if the patient is too uneducated or too unintelligent to communicate well; and thirdly, it becomes difficult after the age of 45 to 50 years because of the patient's increasing mass of experiences.

psychology. The study of mental life, of behaviour and of all the activities of the individual, not only at one point in time but throughout his life span. Probably the science, which has developed enormously in the last sixty years, is best indicated by enumeration of a few of the problems with which it is concerned. Some examples are: how a child becomes 'socialized', acquiring the language, values and culture of the group in which it is brought up; how and why a child plays; how a child or an adult learns, and what things facilitate or impede the learning process; how and why we remember or forget; how people are influenced by instincts or innate drives; how we are motivated, both consciously and unconsciously; how we can measure intelligence; how we think; what factors stimulate our imaginations; what kinds of sensation contribute to feeling; what circumstances or factors create personality disorders in which the individual in effect turns against himself; and what circumstances or factors create behaviour disorders in which the individual turns against society.

Psychology is investigated both subjectively (by reasoned analysis, the usual method last century) and objectively (by observation and planned experiment).

An appreciation of psychological principles is essential to the understanding of all human relationships, from salesmanship to marital relations, and from personnel management to the education of children. Just as a knowledge of physiology is necessary to understand the functioning or malfunctioning of the body in physical disease, so a knowledge of normal psychology is essential to understand mental diseases and the many diseases in which body and mind interact.

Psychology is a vast subject, perhaps indeed the widest of all the sciences. There is certainly such a science as general psychology – just as there is such a thing as general medicine – but, like medicine, psychology is becoming increasingly divided into specialties.

Thus educational psychology is particularly concerned with teaching and learning. A practical example of its interests might be to investigate whether the traditional forty-five minute teaching periods in secondary schools and the traditional fifty to fifty-five minute lectures in universities and polytechnics are best, or whether more shorter periods or fewer but longer periods would facilitate learning and the retention of learning material.

Child psychology includes some of the matter of educational psychology but is also concerned with assessing children's personalities (as well as their intelligence) and helping children with emotional or behaviour problems.

Abnormal psychology deals, as the name implies, with the actions and behaviour of persons who are mentally ill or sexual deviants or otherwise removed from the average behaviour and values that we all call 'normal'.

Social psychology is concerned with the interaction of groups, the influence of the group on the individual and the influence of the individual on the group. It clearly comes near to sociology, just as clinical psychology (including the work of non-medical psychologists in mental hospitals and clinics) approaches psychiatry, and just as industrial psychology impinges on personnel management.

psychoneurosis. A general term covering anxiety states, obsessions, compulsions and causeless fears. See NEUROSIS.

psychopath. A rather vague term describing a person whose behaviour is habitually or repeatedly antisocial. In Britain the Mental Health Act of 1959 defines the term as a persistent disability of mind which results in abnormally aggressive or seriously irresponsible conduct, and needs medical treatment. See PERSONALITY, PSYCHOPATHIC.

psychoprophylaxis. Strictly the term simply means prevention or reduction of illness or pain by affecting the mind, but usually it is reserved for the psychological measures employed to prevent or diminish the pains of childbirth.

The pregnant woman loses much of her fear through being taught that childbirth is a natural and not particularly unpleasant process. Also she is encouraged to perform certain exercises again and again until she does them as routinely as a soldier stands to attention or shoulders arms. When the uterine contractions start she begins to perform these exercises and, apart from any actual help that they give, has her attention directed more to the exercises than to the 'labour pains'.

With adequate psychoprophylaxis some women voluntarily undertake childbirth without any analgesic or anaesthetic, while many others find that the anaesthetic can be given later and in smaller dosage than would otherwise be the case.

psychosis. Mental disorder involving sufficient loss of touch with reality to render a person 'insane', i.e., incapable of functioning independently in society. In descriptive terms the main types of psychosis are: (1) Manic-depression, in which the patient is either excited or depressed or alternates between these two states of mind. In this group there can also be included involutional melancholia where there are marked symptoms of depression associated with ageing. (2) Schizophrenia, in which there is a retreat from reality, an emotional nihilism, and often bizarre and incongruous behaviour combined with silliness, mannerisms, mental inertia, personality deterioration and often purposeless activity. (3) Paranoia which is characterized by suspicion and delusions of persecution, often well-constructed and systematized, maintained with apparent intelligence, and giving rise to appropriate emotional responses. (4) Dementia, in which there is a general decline of mental capacity and memory.

These purely clinical types of mental illness can develop in a variety of ways and a classification based on the cause may be described as follows: (1) organic psychosis, in which there is some demonstrable structural pathology of brain tissue or its vessels; (2) toxic psychosis, in which there is some exogenous or endogenous intoxication (i.e., intoxication originating from outside or from within); and (3) functional psychosis, in which no sufficient toxic or organic cause can yet be demonstrated in the present state of knowledge.

To these can usefully be added the 'defect reactions' in which there are constitutional absences or deficits rather than an acquired disease. These include patients with mental deficiency or with constitutional psychopathic inferiority as manifested by various types of unstable personality, the alcoholics and drug addicts, the kleptomaniacs and pyromaniacs, and those who exhibit other forms of antisocial behaviour.

Because of the growing appreciation that much mental illness arises from demonstrable causes it is absolutely necessary that practising psychiatrists must also be good general physicians, competent to track down the bodily conditions which are affecting the mind. Conversely, the general physician must be equally aware of the psychiatric effects of organic brain disease.

A clear distinction has to be drawn between psychosis and mental handicap. In the latter conditions the brain has been defective from birth or early childhood and the person can at no time reason like an ordinary individual. In the case of the psychotic the intelligence is normal and may indeed be very high.

psychosomatic diseases. Diseases in which mental events or disturbances cause physical effects.

No definition is wholly satisfactory because in all diseases and injuries there is an inter-action of mind and body, e.g., the soldier in the excitement of battle may not even realize that he has received a serious wound, the person with toothache often finds the pain decreasing as he enters the dentist's surgery, and the recovery of a seriously ill person depends considerably on whether he actually desires to recover. Broadly, however, a disease is termed psychosomatic when its main causal factors are in the mind.

In any normal person conscious emotion produces physical results, such as blushing from embarrassment, feeling a sinking sensation in the pit of the stomach from dismay, or having a quickened pulse rate during anger. These physical results are caused partly by action of the nervous system (including the sympathetic and parasympathetic nerves) and partly by release of hormones from the endocrine system.

Perhaps the easiest disease in which to indicate a mental element is duodenal ulcer. Prolonged emotional stress causes increased acidity of the gastric juice, with gradual erosion of the mucous membrane by the highly acid juice, so producing an ulcer. Moreover, a study of patients suffering from duodenal ulcer shows that they are on average more conscientious, more prone to worry, more rigid in attitude and keener to strive for success than are most people. In other words, although there are some physical factors predisposing to duodenal ulcer (e.g., faulty diet) the disease occurs mainly in persons of a particular type of personality and the mechanism is known.

In most organic diseases of mental origin the connection is not quite so clear-cut. Much emotion occurs at an unconscious level. This hidden and unfelt emotion nevertheless stimulates the sympathetic nervous system (altering, for instance, the rate of the flow of blood) and changes the rate of production of hormones (e.g., by the pituitary). Many – but perhaps not all – cases of asthma are produced by unconscious emotional factors. Thus a patient who has no conscious dislike of cats develops asthmatic attacks whenever he is in the presence of a cat and is thought to be allergic to the animal; but on being asked to study a picture of a cat he develops an attack, demonstrating that the condition in his case is psychosomatic, not allergic.

Apart from duodenal ulcer and asthma, diseases in which emotion can play a large part include migraine, colitis, hypertension, many skin diseases, and perhaps coronary thrombosis.

There is considerable argument about the number and prevalence of psychosomatic diseases. Some doctors maintain that about one-half of all physical illnesses fall into that category, while others would restrict the figure to nearer one-tenth. In a sense both are right. For perhaps 10 to 15 per cent of all persons consulting doctors because of physical symptoms, stress, fear or anxiety (conscious or unconscious) is the dominant causal factor; in perhaps another 10 to 15 per cent the mind plays an important part; and in yet another 10 to 15 per cent it contributes appreciably to the disease. Even a disease as physical and as clearly bacteriologically caused as tuberculosis has its main causal factors: in any particular age-group living under similar social and environmental circumstances there are relatively more cases of tuberculosis in persons who have recently been bereaved or jilted or lost their jobs than in persons in whom these factors have not operated.

It should be clearly understood that there is no question, in a psychosomatic disease, of the condition being imaginary. The man with a duodenal ulcer has a definite ulceration; the woman with asthma has a definite constriction of the smaller bronchioles and consequent difficulty in breathing out; the individual suffering from a psychosomatic disorder may die from it, in which case the pathological findings are demonstrable on post mortem examination.

If a disease is wholly or largely psychosomatic it may well need physical methods of treatment (e.g., drugs) to reduce or remove the symptoms; but for complete cure and avoidance of recurrence it will manifestly also need investigation and treatment of the underlying emotional problems, which – as already mentioned – are sometimes below the level of consciousness.

The best hope for the prevention of diseases of emotional origin would appear to lie in the fostering of strong and stable personalities in the early formative years, always remembering in such fostering the need for demonstrated affection (without 'smothering with love'), consistency, security, freedom to explore and investigate, and sufficient kindly authority to enable the child to learn without too much trauma that the needs and wishes of others have to be considered in addition to his own needs and demands.

psychotherapy. Treatment of emotional and mental disorders by verbal means, as opposed to drugs and physical measures. Essentially psychotherapy began with Freud's techniques of psychoanalysis but it nowadays also includes many less elaborate measures, such as simple counselling (by psychiatrist, doctor, health visitor or even social worker), group therapy (where a number of patients discuss their problems under the chairmanship of psychiatrist or psychologist, who in most cases keeps the discussion going but deliberately makes little personal contribution), and play therapy (in which children indicate, and sometimes solve, their conflicts in play).

ptomaine poisoning. An outmoded and inaccurate name for food poisoning. Decomposing proteins such as game hung for an unduly prolonged period produce alkaloid substances called ptomaines, and it used to be thought that these were the main cause of food poisoning. Certainly ptomaines are mildly poisonous (and one rather rare variety of shellfish poisoning is caused by a ptomaine), but they are produced when the food is in such a state of decomposition that it would be rejected by the palate. The real cause of food poisoning is specific bacterial contamination of food.

ptosis. See EYELIDS, DISEASES OF.

ptyalin. An enzyme present in saliva which converts starch into sugar and thus plays an essential part in DIGESTION.

ptyalism. Abnormal secretion of saliva. Common causes include oral sepsis, decaying teeth and trigeminal neuralgia. The condition also occurs in overacidity of the stomach, is sometimes caused simply by excessive smoking, and frequently occurs in the early months of pregnancy. Since saliva when swallowed carries air with it, there are usually symptoms of flatulence as well as excessive salivation. Treatment depends on discovery and removal of the primary cause, but 0.3 ml. of tincture of belladonna thrice daily, half an hour before meals, is often helpful in reducing the inconvenience of the symptoms, although it does not affect the cause.

puberty. The period of onset of sexual maturity. For consideration of the mental and physical changes in detail see ADOLESCENCE.

pubis. The front portion of the innominate or pelvic bone. It consists of a roughly square body and two branches, one passing backwards and upwards towards the acetabulum, and the other backwards and downwards to join a similar branch of the ischium. In the middle line of the body the two pubic bones join together to form the symphysis pubis.

public health. The science that studies individuals and families in their domestic, social and occupational groupings and in their working and living conditions, and seeks to promote mental and physical health, to reduce disease and to create the conditions for healthy living.

Essentially public health has passed through several overlapping stages.

1. The legislative stage – persuasion of legislators to spend money on water supplies, sewerage systems, reduction of overcrowding, food hygiene, and reduction of air and noise pollution; the era of the original medical officers of health and sanitary inspectors (now called environmental health officers).

2. The stage of interest in the physical health of mothers and children, seeking reduction of maternal and infant mortality, and improvement (e.g., by better nutrition and by immunization) of the health of pre-school and school children; the era of persuasion by public health doctors, health visitors and midwives.

3. The stage of interest in the well-being of the family, ranging from family planning and prevention of maladjustment to concern with the medical and physical health of the elderly; the era of modern health visitors, health education officers and social workers.

4. The stage of attempted integration of services that promote health and prevent disease with those that cure disease and care for the sick and disabled; the era in which environmental services were passed to the environmental health officers of local authorities, while purely social services were passed to social workers in these authorities; the era also in which the medical officer of health was replaced by the community physician with interest in both treatment and preventive services, and in which the health visitor (as an expert in prevention) began to work in collaboration with the general practitioner (an expert in treatment).

See HEALTH SERVICES, MEDICAL OFFICER OF HEALTH, and HEALTH VISITOR.

puerperal fever. Any condition producing after childbirth a rise of temperature to 38 °C. (100.4 °F.) maintained for twenty-four hours or recorded on two consecutive occasions. The term is generally applied to the septicaemia that was formerly common after labour. A synonym in the Victorian era was childbed fever.

In the process of childbirth the linings of the uterus and vagina are bruised by the passage of the child's head, and the separation of the placenta leaves a raw area. So the whole area is eminently suitable for the reception and multiplication of germs if they enter, e.g., from the hands or throat of the doctor or midwife.

During most of the nineteenth century hospital confinement was extremely dangerous because infection passed from patient to patient. In some hospitals as many as one mother in every four died from childbed fever. The arrival of antiseptics, with routine disinfection of the hands of doctors and midwives and of all instruments, brought the death rate from the condition down from one in four to nearer one in a hundred; and by 1900 the maternal death rate from all causes had fallen to about five per thousand total births. Antiseptic techniques, aseptic methods, better understanding of how bacteria spread, better maternal care and better obstetrics together made puerperal fever an extreme rarity, and with the advent of the sulphonamides and the antibiotics that rarity, when it does occur, is usually curable.

puerperium. The period immediately following labour during which the uterus and other organs return to approximately their previous sizes and positions. In normal circumstances the period lasts for six weeks.

The uterus is about 15 cm. (6 in.) long at the close of labour and can be felt quite distinctly in the abdomen; it dwindles by about a finger's breadth a day during the first seven or eight days and thereafter decreases more slowly. The bloodstained discharge from the uterus, the lochia, becomes paler and less copious after the first week. Bit by bit the organs return to normal, although lines remain on the abdomen and the vulva stays a little stretched.

Although childbirth is a normal process it is a strenuous one, and the puerperium is essentially a period of rest and recovery of strength. Apart from the husband and the patient's mother, visitors should normally be excluded for the first three days, and during the next few days the nurse should use her discretion, limiting visitors to such persons and numbers as will not tire the woman. Adequate rest, preferably including an afternoon nap, is important. The resumption of household tasks should be gradual.

After the stress of pregnancy and childbirth transient mild depression is not uncommon in the puerperium, and in a very small number of cases there develops a form of manic-depressive psychosis known as puerperal insanity. This requires skilled treatment, but the outlook is hopeful.

pulsation. The throbbing caused by the beating of the heart. Pulsation of the apex of the heart can usually be seen – as well as felt – between the fourth and fifth ribs. Abnormal pulsation of an artery may be due to an ANEURYSM, and capillary pulsation may occur in some cases of heart disease.

pulse. The pressure wave in an artery corresponding with each contraction of the heart. As these contractions push blood onwards into the arteries the increased pressure (systolic pressure) can easily be felt in any artery that can be compressed against a bone. Between each contraction less blood is pushed along the arteries and

Taking the pulse

the considerably lower pressure (diastolic pressure) can again be felt.

The pulse is generally most conveniently felt on the thumb side of the wrist in the radial artery. Each pressure wave reaches the wrist about one-tenth of a second after the particular beat of the heart. A doctor or nurse feeling the pulse seeks to ascertain several things: the rate, the regularity or irregularity, the force of the systolic contraction, the strength of the diastolic relaxation or rebound, and the condition of the arterial wall.

The normal pulse rate in people who have been at rest for some minutes varies between sixty and eighty per minute. The pulse accelerates with exercise (but in a healthy person rapidly returns to normal after the exertion is over), fear and excitement, and most fevers, with typhoid and diphtheria notorious exceptions. Irregularity of the pulse may be due to various diseases of the heart, some digestive disorders, overindulgence in alcohol, excessive smoking or excessive consumption of coffee. While the systolic and diastolic blood pressure can be more accurately measured by a sphygmomanometer, an experienced person can obtain a good approximate estimate from the pulse. In normal persons the arterial wall cannot be felt unless the patient is very thin, but in disease thickening, hardening and twisting may be noted.

pupil. The rounded aperture in the centre of the iris of the eye. Through this aperture light reaches the back of the eye. In dim light the pupil dilates to allow more light to impinge on the retina, and dilatation is also caused by action of the sympathetic nerves on the iris, by secretion of adrenalin (as in fear and excitement) and by drugs which temporarily block off the sympathetic nerves (e.g., belladonna and atropine). In bright light the pupil contracts to protect the sensitive retina, the contraction being initiated by action of the parasympathetic nerves. The pupil also contracts as the eyes are brought to focus on an object near to the face, and certain drugs, such as morphine, constrict the pupil.

In health the pupils are regular in shape and equal in size, and should contract briskly when exposed to bright light. The size, regularity and contracting power of the pupils are altered in certain diseases of the nervous system.

purgatives. See LAXATIVES.

purpura. A general name for a group of diseases in which blood leaks from capillary blood vessels causing purple spots under the skin or in mucous membranes.

Idiopathic thrombocytopenic purpura, occurring mostly in children and old people, is caused by an inadequate number of blood platelets. Salient features are multiple haemorrhages in the skin, and on blood examination a reduced platelet count and an abnormal fragility of red blood corpuscles. For the acute form of the disease transfusions of fresh blood or of suspensions of platelets are useful and ACTH often helps. For the more chronic form surgical removal of the spleen is usually necessary.

Purpura simplex, sometimes called 'rheumatic purpura' but really unrelated to rheumatism, occurs mostly in pre-school children and appears to be due to a deficiency of the capillary walls, not to a shortage of platelets. Corticosteroids and ACTH sometimes help, but there is really no specific treatment and relapses are common.

Heavy dosage of aspirin occasionally causes another form of purpura; and the small haemorrhages found in association with scurvy were originally thought to be due to deficiency of vitamin C but are now sometimes attributed to inadequacy of an alleged vitamin P with lack of C causing the scurvy but lack of P responsible for the purpuric spots.

purulent. Containing or discharging pus.

pus. A thick, yellowish fluid consisting of blood serum, broken-down blood cells and tissue cells, and killed bacteria. When bacteria invade any part of the body a process of inflammation begins: additional blood is rushed to the part bringing large numbers of white blood corpuscles whose function is to engulf and destroy the bacteria. The pus that is formed essentially consists of the 'corpses' from the battle.

The process of pus formation is called suppuration. When pus has formed and is under pressure it tends to track to the exterior of the body or to a hollow organ, and there form an abscess. The introduction of antibiotics has greatly decreased suppuration, because in many cases the antibiotic successfully kills the invading bacteria; but the old maxim, 'Where there is pus let it out' still holds, i.e., where there is any substantial amount of pus, incision and drainage are needed.

pustule. A tiny blister containing pus. Typical pustules are seen in acne vulgaris. The characteristic blister of anthrax is termed a malignant pustule.

pyaemia. A form of blood poisoning with formation of multiple abscesses throughout the body, and due to septic emboli – usually containing either staphylococci or streptococci – travelling from one point of infection. Symptoms include shivering, high temperature, rapid pulse, exhaustion and sometimes delirium, together with symptoms from the local abscesses. Treatment involves identification and usually surgical removal of the original focus of infection, the use of an appropriate antibiotic and the provision of ample fluids both to dilute toxins and to prevent dehydration.

pyelitis. Inflammation of the central part (the pelvis) of the kidney. It results from infection which can progress upwards from the urinary tract or downwards from any part of the body. Stone in the kidney and inflammation of the bladder are common causes, and the condition is not infrequent in pregnancy.

Characteristics include raised temperature, pain and tenderness in the loins, and frequency of passing urine; but in many cases there is merely a vague malaise, so that the condition is identified only by examination of the urine for bacteria.

The sulphonamide drugs are generally effective.

pyelography. An x-ray examination of the kidneys after they have been temporarily rendered opaque by injection of an iodine compound which concentrates in the kidneys. If the kidney that is to be examined is functioning well the compound may be injected into a vein and reaches the kidney via the blood-stream. If the kidney is not adequately filtering material from the blood, the compound has to be introduced into the bladder using a cystoscope.

pyelonephritis. Inflammation of the kidney and the renal pelvis. Treatment is by sulphonamides or antibiotics.

pyloric stenosis. Narrowing of the outlet of the stomach, the pylorus, through which food normally passes to the duodenum on its way through the DIGESTIVE SYSTEM. The common form occurs in young babies in the first few weeks of life, with cases in boy babies thrice as numerous as in girl babies. The affected infants suffer from projectile vomiting (i.e., true vomiting rather than the customary dribbling of feeds), steadily lose weight, and die if untreated. Some cases respond to atropine and similar antispasmodic drugs which relax the muscle of the pylorus. Other cases require a surgical operation which, while quite serious, is life saving. The condition is known to be of genetic origin.

A rather similar condition arises occasionally in adults as a result of scarring after a duodenal ulcer.

pylorus. The opening at the lower end of the stomach through which the stomach contents pass to the duodenum. The opening is controlled by a band of circular muscle fibres known as the pyloric sphincter. In PYLORIC STENOSIS the pylorus is narrowed and the passage of stomach contents becomes obstructed.

pyogenic. Pus-forming.

pyorrhoea. The term means simply a discharge of pus but as commonly used it usually refers to pyorrhoea of the sockets of teeth. In this condition there is chronic infection and ulceration of the gum margins which may extend into the tooth-sockets, destroying the lining of the teeth, invading the bone, and loosening the teeth.

In its earliest stages it commences as inflammation of the gums usually caused by poor dental hygiene but sometimes aggravated by other local factors such as mouth breathing and irregularity of the teeth, or by general diseases which lower tissue resistance. Once pyorrhoea has become established its ill-effects are irreversible because destroyed tissue cannot be replaced, but its further progress can be retarded by measures taken by a dental surgeon such as removing tartar and cutting away redundant gum-margin which forms pus-retaining pockets. The co-operation of the patient in carrying out gum-massage and maintaining satisfactory care of the teeth is also very important.

pyrexia. A synonym for FEVER.

pyrosis. HEARTBURN.

pyuria. The presence of pus in the urine. This always indicates some inflammatory condition in the urinary tract: nephritis, pyelitis or cystitis. Pus is detected in the urine by laboratory tests and the treatment is that of the underlying condition.

Q

Q fever. An infectious disease caused by a rickettsia-like organism, called *Coxiella burneti*, with an incubation period of two or three weeks and characterized by fever, headache, and usually chest pain, cough and scanty expectoration, indicating some lung involvement. The name 'Q' stands for Queensland, where the condition was first identified.

Ticks, wild animals, cattle, sheep and goats are natural reservoirs of infection, and the condition mostly occurs in persons working with animals or animal products; it is caught from air-borne spread of infected discharges or from direct contact with infected material. Patients suffering from Q fever are therefore found among veterinary surgeons, farmers, and employees of dairies, stock-yards, meat-packing plants and wool-processing factories.

Exact diagnosis depends on blood-tests. The duration of the disease is variable and relapses are frequent, but it very seldom kills and treatment by antibiotics is effective. Pasteurization of milk destroys the organism. A satisfactory protective vaccine is available and should be used for persons at risk; where the disease occurs there is a need for investigation and hygienic control of sources of infection.

quadriceps. The large muscle at the front of the thigh. Its function is to extend the leg.

quarantine. The period during which persons who have been in contact with an infectious disease have to be isolated to make sure that they themselves are not going to develop the disease and so become a fresh source of infection. The duration of quarantine varies with different diseases but for any one disease must cover its longest incubation period.

Nowadays quarantine is increasingly being replaced by SURVEILLANCE.

quickening. The stage of pregnancy at which the mother first becomes conscious of the movements of the developing child within her womb. Usually this awareness begins about the sixteenth to eighteenth week, which is approximately mid-term. By this time the uterus has enlarged and risen sufficiently to be in contact with the abdominal wall, and it is the transmission of impulses to the latter which enables the mother to sense them. The movements are initially quite feeble and have been picturesquely likened to 'the fluttering of a bird in the closed hand'.

quinine. A bitter-tasting alkaloid derived from the bark of the cinchona tree, originally from South America but subsequently grown in many warm countries. From 1638 it was used in Western Europe for both the prevention and the treatment of malaria. Essentially it renders the blood unsuitable for the multiplication of malarial parasites, so regular dosage in a mosquito-infested district will usually prevent malaria, and larger dosage will generally cure the disease. In recent years, however, quinine has been largely replaced for prevention and treatment of malaria by synthetic substitutes which are even more effective and have fewer toxic effects. Nevertheless quinine is a drug that has saved millions of lives.

Apart from its specific effect on malaria, quinine helps to reduce any high temperature and is a favourite preparation in colds and other febrile illnesses, e.g., as the liquid ammoniated tincture of quinine or as quinine sulphate tablets. Large doses may produce ringing in the ears, temporary deafness, headache and giddiness; and extremely large doses may cause death by paralysing the brain and the respiratory centre.

quinsy. A complication of severe tonsillitis resulting when infection causes pus to form within the tonsillar capsule, creating an abscess. Inflammation and accumulation of pus leads to severe pain and difficulty in swallowing. The fauces are swollen and discoloured and the affected tonsil is displaced towards the mid-line.

Early cases may sometimes be treated successfully by antibiotics, but a developed case will usually require the opening of the abscess and evacuation of pus, followed by antiseptic gargling. Immediate treatment should be followed later by removal of the tonsils since otherwise recurrence is common.

quotidian fever. A form of MALARIA with bouts of fever almost every day.

R

rabies. A virus disease mainly affecting carnivorous animals (dog, cat, fox, wolf, jackal, skunk, opossum, mongoose, stoat, weasel, etc.) and also common in bats. It is widely prevalent throughout the world except in Australia. In Europe only Britain, Scandinavia, Iceland, Spain, Portugal and Cyprus are free from it, because of quarantine regulations and constant surveillance. Elsewhere the disease is a real or potential hazard of serious importance.

Affected animals show restlessness, snapping, difficulty in swallowing (hence the alternative name 'hydrophobia' – fear of water), excessive salivation, fury, or lethargy, followed by paralysis, coma and death. In man infection results from being bitten by a rabid animal and causes severe inflammatory reaction in the central nervous system (encephalomyelitis).

The incubation period is very variable (three weeks to six months or more) depending on the site or severity of the bite. Symptoms in man are similar to those in animals with sudden onset of fever, headache, restlessness, muscular spasm (specially of the muscles used in swallowing and breathing), and in due course paralysis of these muscles, coma, and death, usually within a week. Once the condition has developed far enough for the symptoms to appear, the outcome is invariably fatal. Early treatment of suspected cases by anti-rabies vaccine provides the only hope.

Precautions. If there are special risks of contact with animals, vaccination to develop immunity should be advised. Otherwise the ordinary traveller abroad should regard any animal with circumspection and seek immediate competent advice if bitten. If this happens the animal should if possible be caught and kept under observation to see if it develops rabies. In many countries vaccination of dogs is compulsory so it is also helpful to identify the owner and find out if the dog has been recently vaccinated, since such a dog is unlikely to be developing rabies.

If there is any doubt whatever a course of anti-rabies inoculation should be started immediately. The success of treatment depends entirely on its initiation as soon as possible.

If rabies is imported to a country previously free it can easily become endemic. Its eradication would involve massive destruction of wild creatures and vaccination of domestic animals. So rigorous control of the importation of dogs and cats is very important.

radiant heat treatment. Treatment with INFRA-RED RAYS. Conditions in which such treatment is prescribed are neuritis, neuralgia, arthritis, fibrositis, inflammation caused by injury, cellulitis and superficial sepsis; it is also used as a preliminary to massage and movement in injuries and paralysis, and occasionally in nephritis.

radioactive drugs. Medicines which exercise their effect through the RADIOACTIVITY of their constituents. Radiotherapy, mainly employed for treating malignant disease, has until recently utilized radiation given by x-rays from outside or applied internally by implanted radium needles. These methods are rather imprecise and also tend to damage skin or other tissue within the field of radiation.

Various elements that are needed by particular cells or organs pass directly to them, e.g., iodine passes to the thyroid gland. So, if artificial radioactive isotopes of these elements are given as drugs they can convey radiation exactly to the diseased organ. Moreover, because they are later eliminated or have known short periods of decay, their effects can be predicted or controlled.

The most successful example of this technique is in the treatment of persons suffering from hyperthyroidism or from cancer in the thyroid. A carefully calculated dose is given of a draught containing radioactive iodine (iodine 131) and the thyroid gland, performing its normal function, concentrates this radioactive substance within itself and so destroys its over-active or abnormal cells. Similarly radioactive phosphorus can be used for the treatment of certain blood diseases such as chronic leukaemia and polycythaemia. Other radioactive drugs are also used in diagnosis as 'tracers' to study how certain elements are being absorbed or altered and to localize tumours.

Patients undergoing such treatment need careful supervision because their waste-products may be radioactive and require special measures for disposal. Incontinence raises additional problems.

radioactivity. All matter consists of atoms of various elements. Each atom has a central nucleus, providing almost all its mass, and made up of positively-charged protons and uncharged neutrons. Around it are negatively charged electrons and, since the atom is held together by electrical forces, the electrons are equal in number to the protons. The atomic weight of an element depends on the total of protons plus neutrons (M) but its atomic number (z), which determines its chemical identity, depends only on the number of protons. Some identical chemical elements exist as isotopes always with the same z number but with different numbers of neutrons and hence a different atomic weight or M number. Most of the common elements are stable isotopes and undergo no change because any unstable variants in their geological past have long since broken down to stable residues with protons and neutrons bound together by nuclear forces so strong that no particle ever escapes.

In general, nuclei are stable if the total number of particles is not too great and if the proportions of protons and neutrons are about the same. In certain naturally occurring elements, such as uranium, with unstable isotopes, these requirements are not met, and the atom breaks down liberating particles and energy. This is radioactive disintegration and it results in radioactivity characterized by the emission of alpha, beta, or gamma 'rays', although it is now known that the first two consist of particles, being helium nuclei (two protons plus two neutrons) and electrons respectively. Radioactive decay decreases with time, and each radioactive isotope remains active for a period which varies enormously, from centuries to a fraction of a second.

Many new radioactive isotopes can now be made artificially by bombarding stable nuclei with atomic particles in an atomic reactor. This alters the z or M numbers, or both, to values incompatible with stability. These isotopes are important in medicine both for diagnosis and for treatment because radioactivity affects cell function. They also have research uses as 'labelled atoms' which facilitate studies in physiology, chemistry, genetics and many other subjects since the behaviour of an otherwise indistinguishable sample of a particular chemical element can be traced by its radioactivity.

Dangers. After the discharge of an atomic bomb or after a major accident at a nuclear power station there can be three effects. (1) The blast wave, causing in the case of a megaton bomb total obliteration within a radius of one mile and severe damage for up to five miles. (2) Thermal effects, causing anything combustible within ten miles to burst into flames. (3) Radiation effects, essentially (a) a bone-marrow form, with nausea, vomiting, apparent recovery and then death in several weeks through aplastic anaemia, and (b) a latent form, in which either leukaemia develops in a couple of years or so, or there is apparently healthy survival but with the occurrence of genetic mutations in any offspring.

radiography. The production of images by means of radiation, especially x-rays.

radiology. The use of x-rays and radioactive substances in the diagnosis and treatment of disease. See RADIOTHERAPY.

radiotherapy. Treatment by x-rays or by the use of RADIOACTIVE substances. Radiation has the effect of damaging any tissue by ionization but cells are particularly susceptible when they are undergoing rapid growth and multiplication. Radiotherapy therefore has particular application in the treatment of malignant disease. The dose is adjusted so as to destroy the active cancerous cells without permanently harming the less active normal tissue.

The methods employed rely on conventional x-rays or on radium or the release of radium (radon). Deep x-ray therapy is applied by placing the patient under a beam of x-rays directed, usually from several different directions, to the site of tumour growth. With radium or radon, hollow needles containing the radioactive material are imbedded in the tumour. Now that it is possible to make radioactive isotopes, variants of this basic treatment have become possible. For general irradiation radioactive cobalt (cobalt 60) may be employed in a positioning device like a large x-ray machine (cobalt bomb).

Sometimes x-rays are also employed for the treatment of superficial skin diseases, especially those like ringworm which are due to fungi, but safer methods using new effective drugs are now more generally preferred. A complication of deep x-ray therapy is radiation sickness which usually manifests itself as a feeling of intense lassitude, sometimes accompanied by vomiting and diarrhoea, and by fever, a burning sensation in the mouth, and loss of hair. It may be necessary to stop the treatment temporarily or to reduce the frequency and intensity of applications. Radio-isotopes are also now used in the form of RADIOACTIVE DRUGS, to be taken internally for certain specific purposes.

radium. A radioactive element used in medicine for the treatment of malignant disease in RADIOTHERAPY.

radius. One of the two long bones of the forearm, situated on the outer side of the limb. Its upper end is small and forms a small part of the elbow joint but the lower end is enlarged to articulate with the wrist bones and forms most of the wrist joint. When indirect violence is applied to the forearm it is usually the radius which suffers damage so that a fracture of its lower end just above the wrist joint (Colles' fracture) is a very common type of injury in falls upon the hand.

rash. Any temporary eruption on the skin is known as a rash or exanthem. Similar effects on mucous membranes are called an enanthem. Rashes are produced by the action of toxins on the elements of the skin and particularly on its small blood vessels. They may be produced by external causes such as bacterial and viral infections, parasitic or chemical irritation and drugs, or internally by metabolic abnormalities and allergies.

They vary very much in type, and their appearance and distribution are often highly characteristic of a particular disease or condition. The following terms are used in describing the features of a rash:

Erythema: a uniform redness of the skin.

Urticaria: irregular firm raised patches or weals.

Macules: discoloured spots not elevated above the surface.

Papules: small, solid, round, pimple-like elevations.

Vesicles: small fluid-containing blisters.

Bullae: large irregular fluid-containing blisters.

Pustules: papules, vesicles, or bullae which have become infected and filled with pus.

Petechiae: small pin point haemorrhages into the skin.

Purpuric spots: discoloured areas due to haemorrhages into the skin.

Ecchymosis: a large isolated patch of haemorrhage beneath the skin, usually due to external violence.

A prodromal rash is one which occurs in the early stages of an infectious disease and does not have the full-blown characteristics of the typical exanthem.

Any rash is only a symptom, and treatment must be directed towards identifying and removing the precise cause. Where a rash causes itching calamine lotion or talcum powder sometimes relieves the symptom.

ratbite fever. This general term includes two very similar diseases which can only be differentiated bacteriologically. Each disease results from being bitten by an infected rat and the organisms responsible are *Streptobacillus moniliformis* and *Spirillum minus*. Most cases occur in India and the Far East, and in these countries are predominantly due to *Sp. minus*. In Europe and America the disease is relatively rare.

The disease has an incubation period of three to ten days. Characteristic features are an unhealed, septic and swollen rat-bite, enlargement of the related lymph-glands, a high, swinging temperature, a measly or haemorrhagic rash, and severe joint pains. The death rate in untreated cases is about 10 per cent, but antibiotic treatment (especially with the tetracyclines) is usually effective. Apart from rat-bites local outbreaks have occurred through consumption of contaminated milk. Preventive measures should include rat-control and pasteurization of milk.

rats. Rats are by far the most injurious domestic and commercial pests. They persist as an ever-present menace always ready to increase their depredations when defensive and offensive measures against them are relaxed. They destroy great quantities of stored food and spoil even more; they damage property by burrowing and gnawing; and they are carriers of several important diseases.

Two species are found in Britain: the black rat *(Rattus rattus)* and the brown rat *(Rattus norvegicus)*. Rats are very prolific: an unchecked rat population with access to adequate food supplies can double every two months.

Diseases. Bubonic plague is a disease carried by rats and transmitted to man by fleas. Although it is rare in developed countries there is always a risk of plague reaching a country by ship-borne rats. The worm disease trichinosis is transmitted by rats to pigs and may then infect man. Rats also transmit tape worms, spirochaetal jaundice (leptospirosis), and rat-bite fever. Apart from these specific diseases rats contaminate food by their excreta which may contain the organisms of food-poisoning (salmonellosis).

Control. In Britain the Rats and Mice (Destruction) Act 1919 requires the 'occupier' of land to take all necessary steps to destroy rats and mice thereon and to prevent infestation. However, eradication of rats requires expert knowledge and help is best obtained from local authority pest officers or from a commercial specialist. The measures required are the rat-proofing of buildings and systematic extermination by poison-baiting, gassing or trapping. There are also other legal powers to enforce the 'de-ratization' of ships.

Raynaud's disease. An unpleasant condition characterized by spasm of the arteries supplying the fingers and toes, usually affecting both hands and both feet and occurring particularly in cold weather. Young women are the principal sufferers and there is often a considerable psychological element involved. Three stages in the condition of the fingers and toes are described: (1) contraction of blood vessels – the affected parts are pale and numb; (2) asphyxia, i.e., lack of oxygen in the tissues so that they are blue, congested, and painful; (3) gangrene, so that parts become black and may separate, although not many cases proceed to this extreme.

Preventive measures should aim at avoidance of cold and the use of warm clothing. Drugs that dilate blood vessels are also helpful. Severe cases may require surgical measures to divide the sympathetic nerve fibres accompanying the limb arteries.

recessive. As applied to a gene, see GENETICS.

rectal douche. A douche is a stream of fluid directed against a part of the body or into any cavity for the relief or treatment of disease.

Instillation into the rectum of liquid intended to be retained and absorbed – such as a solution of glucose and salt where feeding by mouth is impracticable – is normally called injection; and a substance inserted to relieve constipation is termed an enema. Both are douches, but the term is more commonly applied to instillations for the treatment of worms (e.g., threadworms) and to the use of astringent, antiseptic or sedative lotions in inflammatory or ulcerative conditions, such as may arise from haemorrhoids, severe dysentery or malignant disease. The choice of a particular lotion depends on the exact condition.

rectal feeding. The rectal route may be used to supply liquid food when for any reason the normal route is not available or it is desired to afford the stomach complete rest. Rectal feeding is not very effective because the only foods absorbed from the rectum are glucose and salt.

rectum. The terminal part of the large intestine, in the DIGESTIVE SYSTEM, it is continuous above with the descending colon and below with the anal canal. It lies entirely within the lower pelvis. Faecal matter entering the rectum from above collects there until distension produces a desire to defaecate. Contraction of the rectum then expels the motion through the anal canal and the anal opening.

Diseases. Imperfect development of the lower opening of the rectum (imperforate anus) is a relatively common congenital defect noted at birth and requiring immediate surgical treatment.

Chronic inflammation ('proctitis') may be a downward extension of mucous colitis or due to dysentery, threadworms, or hookworms (bilharziasis). Less common causes are gonorrhoea, tuberculosis and syphilis. Ulceration may follow, and when it involves the anal canal is known as fissure-in-ano which gives rise to severe pain on defaecation. Sepsis tracking from ulcerated areas causes abscesses around the anus (peri-anal abscess or ischio-rectal abscess). This may ultimately produce a false passage to the exterior (fistula-in-ano).

Cancer is the commonest tumour, usually occurring after the age of 60.

PILES or haemorrhoids are varicose veins lying in the wall of the lower rectum and anal canal. Although very common and usually only the result of chronic constipation, their sudden late appearance in a person over 40 raises suspicion of more serious disease and calls for investigation.

reduce. To restore to the natural position, often referring to dislocated joints or factured bones.

referred pain. See PAIN.

reflex action. A rapid involuntary muscular response to some sensory stimulus. It is the result of an 'emergency short cut' through the NERVOUS SYSTEM to create an immediate response to a crisis before the signal reaches the brain. This is achieved by using the 'reflex arc' in the spinal cord. Reflex actions are classified as (1) superficial, (2) deep or tendon, (3) visceral. In superficial reflexes muscular action results from skin stimulation. An example is the plantar reflex in which stroking the

sole of the foot causes bending of the toes. The knee-jerk is a deep or tendon reflex, a tap on the knee-cap ligament causing straightening of the leg. Most involuntary physiological actions depend on visceral reflexes: food stimulating the pharynx is automatically swallowed and the need to pass urine or faeces is a response to distension of the bladder or rectum.

Investigation of reflex activity is an important part of clinical examination in disease of the nervous system and provides clues to the nature and site of any injury.

3. impulse passes up spinal cord reporting on sensation of pain and reflex action taken

2. instruction at spinal cord level to muscle to take action

1. nerve carries sensation of pain to spinal cord

Reflex action

refraction. Deflection of a ray of light from its path when it passes through a transparent substance, e.g., glass or water. It is this phenomenon which enables the eye to focus light onto the retina, and if the eye is so formed that the focus is not perfect, there is said to be a refractive error; see EYESIGHT.

registrar. A term with two specific meanings:
1. An official charged with keeping certain records. An example is the local authority registrar who maintains formal records of births, marriages and deaths in his district.
2. In the U.K. a doctor who has passed through the junior post-registration grades of house officer (house physician or house surgeon) and senior house officer and is aspiring to become a consultant in a particular specialty. A senior registrar in his third or fourth year normally holds all relevant higher qualifications and is of consultant calibre, but has not yet secured an appointment as a full consultant.

regression. In psychoanalytical theory regression is a defence mechanism: in anxiety a person may retreat to an earlier developmental stage of greater security. This is particularly seen in orphaned or neglected infants who regress into stupor and require stimulation before they will suck or otherwise respond. This suggests that there is a return to a pre-natal pattern of life when breathing and circulation were maternal responsibilities. Poor breathing and circulation impair nervous development and this leads to profound and persisting physiological and psychological consequences. Nowadays the usual prescription is a daily dose of TLC - tender loving care - combined with massage and sensory stimulation.

Adults may show similar regression especially in chronic alcoholism and involutional psychosis, and in schizophrenia where stupor and a curled-up position are seen as symbolic of an unconscious attempt to re-attain the secure and undemanding protection of the womb.

rehabilitation. Systematic measures that aim at restoring a person's physical, mental, social and occupational fitness after illness, injury or prolonged strain. Clearly there is a certain overlap with treatment, but essentially treatment is the curing of the particular condition or its improvement as far as is practicable, while rehabilitation seeks to cope with the weakness produced by the condition or by its treatment. The following examples illustrate the difference.

1. A coal-miner sustained a serious injury to an arm and a leg. Treatment involved many weeks in plaster. The fractures have now healed and from the aspect of treatment he is cured; but the unused muscles have become weak, so that he needs a course of exercises - rehabilitation - before being fit to resume work.

2. A man whose tuberculosis was diagnosed late has spent a year in hospital but is now regarded as cured. No further treatment is required (though as a safeguard he may be asked to attend occasionally for examination). During that year all his personal needs have been catered for, his decisions have been taken for him, and he has gradually become more and more dependent. He is in no condition to re-enter a community in which personal effort and initiative are demanded. He needs considerable re-education towards energetic independence and the acceptance of full social responsibility. For rehabilitation he may need a period of organized and graded occupational therapy, or intellectual stimulation through prescribed reading, lectures and group discussion, or planned social activites.

3. A bus driver of 21 years whose recreation was football had a serious accident; a leg had to be amputated and he has been fitted with an artificial limb. Treatment is completed and he can walk well with the artificial leg. As part of his rehabilitation he needs to be fitted for a different type of employment, convinced that he can enjoy recreations other than football, and helped to realize that his

former associates will not regard him as a cripple.

4. Through shortage of jobs a man has been unemployed for three years but jobs suitable for him are now likely to become available. There was no illness and therefore no treatment; but in these three years of increasing discouragement about posts he has become physically weaker and mentally demoralized. Manifestly he needs a period of mental and physical 'toning up' before becoming fit to undertake the particular form of work for which he is qualified.

In the past the term 'rehabilitation' was mainly understood as the application of physical measures such as physiotherapy, e.g., to improve the muscular action of a person whose arm had been temporarily paralysed as the result of a stroke. These physical measures remain highly important but nowadays constitute only one part of rehabilitation. As will be apparent from the examples given above, various educational, social, psychological and vocational factors may also be involved.

In most countries rehabilitation is still very inadequately and patchily developed. There are various reasons for this. In the first place, doctors, especially doctors working wholly or mainly in hospital, are primarily interested in diagnosis and treatment; and in most cases they know little about the requirements of the post to which the patient hopes to return or the social climate in which he will live after the discharge from hospital. Clearly a team approach is needed involving various combinations of the following specialists: the hospital nurse, the health visitor, the social worker, the physiotherapist, the occupational therapist, the speech therapist, the orthoptist (a specialist in the training of the eye-muscles), the remedial gymnast, the chiropodist, and in some cases the psychologist and the personnel manager.

In the second place, several countries already have a considerable shortage of qualified nurses, and such workers as health visitors, physiotherapists and occupational therapists are often in very short supply.

Thirdly, there is a tendency in many countries for physiotherapists, remedial gymnasts, occupational therapists and so on to be based in hospitals; but doctors, faced with a shortage of beds often dependent on a shortage of nurses, naturally seek to discharge patients as soon as clinical cure is complete or has advanced as far as is reasonably practicable; and many of the most important portions of rehabilitation are related to the stage after treatment has ended.

Nevertheless, there are advances in progress, such as the provision of day hospitals where the recovering patient spends the evenings and nights at home but has any necessary treatment and occupational therapy during the day. As a further example of advance the setting up in the U.K. of industrial rehabilitation units and government training centres may be mentioned. Additionally, progressive psychiatric hospitals are developing units for industrial therapy where work can be organized to resemble an industrial situation but can also be carefully regulated to the capacity of the individual patient.

Apart from shortages of skilled personnel, there are many difficulties. For instance, if a financially supported unit begins to produce and sell goods in a time of considerable unemployment, the ordinary (undisabled) producers of these goods begin to question whether it is beneficial or harmful to restore a disabled person to full capacity at the cost of making another person unemployed.

A very practical aspect of rehabilitation is the development and use of aids for the disabled. These range from obvious items like artificial limbs and purpose-built cars which can be driven by a person with the use of only one leg or one arm to many ingenious gadgets to deal with the recurrent difficulties of everyday domestic life. Many such devices have been produced by voluntary organizations (e.g., in the U.K. the British Red Cross Society and the National Fund for Crippling Diseases), but in general advice is available from the health visitor, community nurse or social worker.

rejuvenation. Ageing appears to be an inescapable outcome of the activities of any biological organism, and rejuvenation in the sense of any real renewal of youth remains a mere dream. In extreme old age there is an inevitable deterioration in the efficiency of physical and mental functions.

The main theories advanced to explain this are that ageing is caused by loss of (or injury to) cells that the body has lost the capacity to replace; that cells produced late in life are not as good as the same type of cells developed during youth; and that the changes are not so much in the cells as in structureless components of the body, for instance the walls of blood vessels. These theories may all be true.

Since cell-function in a complex organism is influenced by chemical messengers or hormones, and since ageing of reproductive cells precedes ageing of other tissues, it was only a short step to the hypothesis that if production of sex-hormones could be maintained the ageing of other tissues could be delayed or reversed. This led to the development of an operation for transplanting to man the testes of anthropoid apes. At that time (1930) this 'monkey gland' form of rejuvenation gained some notoriety, but the claims made for it were not fulfilled. From what we now know of tissue-matching and tissue-rejection (see

TRANSPLANT) it is clear that the procedure was foredoomed to failure. It may be that there are still unexploited possibilities using human tissue but there would be enormous practical difficulties. Experience in the use of sex hormones such as testosterone in the treatment of testicular inadequacy or of the male climacteric has not produced any convincing results.

The most effective practical hopes of delaying the ill-effects of old age lie in the extension of two fields of medical work: (1) efforts to maintain and improve the physical and emotional health of persons around the age of retirement, e.g., attention to diet, excercise, eyesight and hearing, and the fostering of leisure interests; and (2) identification and treatment of diseases of later life at an early stage, where they can be cured or at least ameliorated.

relapsing fever. A specific infectious disease due to generalized infection by a spirochaete, *Borrelia recurrentis*. Man acquires the disease from infected lice or ticks. Louse-borne relapsing fever may become epidemic and is mainly found in Africa, Asia, and South America. The tick-borne variety is more usually endemic and occurs principally in tropical Africa.

The incubation period of the disease is three to twelve days (usually eight) and it shows itself as an intermittent fever in which feverish episodes of two or three days alternate with non-feverish periods of two to four days in up to ten or more 'relapses'. In untreated cases, especially in the epidemic form, as many as half may die, but the infection responds well to antibiotic treatment.

Prevention depends on the control of lice and ticks by insecticides and repellents, and on precautions against tick-infestation by clearing land, reducing small mammal populations, controlling stray dogs, and dipping livestock.

relaxation therapy. Treatment by resting the activity of both body and mind has long been employed in both mental and physical diseases.

1. Anxiety and emotional tension are symptomatic of life in advanced societies. Noise, the pressures of modern life, materialism, and disregard for the individual and of his emotional needs and capacities have all led to an increasing prevalence of psychosomatic disease, depressive, obsessional or anxiety states, phobias, hysteria and hypochondriasis.

Relaxation therapy as now understood and practised in the treatment of such disorders depends on the use of new psycho-active drugs which are used simultaneously with psychotherapy. The drugs employed vary in strength. Powerful ones are used in acute mental illness and have revolutionized the work of mental hospitals. Minor tranquillizers or anti-anxiety agents are nowadays prescribed and taken on an ever-increasing scale.

2. On the physical side muscle spasm is a

feature of injuries and various acute and chronic inflammatory conditions. Although it is a protective response it can be a major cause of pain and discomfort; and relaxation by rest, correct posture, massage and infra-red radiation can do much to help. Return to mobility is encouraged by passive movements controlled by the masseur or by active movements performed in a relaxed fashion with the weight of limbs or body supported by slings or by floating in the physiotherapy pool.

3. Systematic training in relaxation is also the basis of a regime developed to encourage painless and NATURAL CHILD-BIRTH.

renal. Of the kidneys.

renal colic. Stones may form in any part of the urinary tract through the deposition of urinary salts. The presence of a stone (or CALCULUS) in the kidney causes pain in the loin and blood in the urine. At intervals there may be attacks of more agonizing spasmodic pain starting in the loin, and radiating downwards to the groin. There may be frequency of passing urine and evidence of fresh haemorrhage with vomiting, abdominal rigidity, and all the symptoms of shock and general collapse.

Such an attack of renal colic is due to intermittent contractions of the pelvis, of the kidney and of the ureter in attempting to drive the stone downwards along the ureter. Similar pain may be produced by the passing of a blood clot or of urinary crystals (gravel). Immediate treatment employs sedatives, rest, and local application of heat, but the condition requires full genito-urinary investigation to determine what further measures are needed. Operation may be called for if the stone has not been passed.

renal dialysis. See KIDNEY MACHINE.

reproduction. The fundamental difference between living and non-living things is that only the former possess the ability to grow by assimilation of food and to multiply by reproducing new organisms like themselves.

Reproduction may be either asexual or sexual. The asexual pattern is seen in simple single-celled organisms where the cell and its nucleus become elongated and shaped like dumb-bells and then split into two new individuals, a process known as binary fission. A further development of this is a splitting into several new individuals simultaneously; this is multiple fission. The multiplication in the blood stream of the parasite which causes malaria is an example.

Sexual reproduction on the other hand is preceded by a linking of male and female sex-cells spermatozoon and ovum respectively. These sex-cells or gametes unite to form a zygote by the process of fertilization. The zygote then undergoes repeated sub-division and gradually grows into a new individual.

Fertilization: the head of the sperm enters the ovum, creating a single cell

Some simple animals and many plants possess both male and female reproductive organs in one individual and are capable of self-fertilization. They are said to be hermaphrodites. In other instances the ovum is capable of development without fertilization and this type of reproduction is known as parthenogenesis. See REPRODUCTIVE SYSTEM, HEREDITY and GENETICS.

reproductive system. Reproduction in the vertebrates, including man, is sexual, i.e., fertilization requires union between an ovum from the female and a spermatozoon from the male. The result is a zygote or embryo which is then protected and nourished within the female for a period of gestation, varying with the species, until growth by cell-division and differentiation produces a miniature replica sufficiently developed to be born and to survive. The reproductive system therefore provides for the production of ova by the female and spermatozoa by the male, for arrangements to secure their union, and for the accommodation of the embryo until it reaches a required stage of development.

The female reproductive system

The female pelvis contains the uterus or

- vas deferens
- bladder
- seminal vesicles
- prostate gland
- rectum
- epididymis
- scrotum
- penis
- urethra
- testis

The male reproductive system

womb, a pear-shaped, hollow, muscular organ designed to accommodate and nourish a growing embryo and to expel it when mature. From its upper border arise two narrow ducts (one on each side) known as the Fallopian tubes; these terminate as trumpet-shaped, fringed extremities close to the ovaries.

An ovum is liberated each month from an ovary and conveyed by the Fallopian tube to the uterus. If it encounters a spermatozoon it may become fertilized and the resultant zygote embeds itself in the lining of the uterus and develops as an embryo. The lining undergoes a regular monthly cycle of change designed to make sure that it is suitable for implantation; this is known as MENSTRUATION.

The lower end of the uterus is the cervix which links these internal organs to the vagina, a muscular tube opening externally at the vulva. This is a cleft bounded in front by the mons veneris, a fatty pad, overlying the pubic bone and carrying the pubic hair; at the sides by two thick folds of skin, the labia; and behind by the perineum. The forward ends of the labia are joined to enclose the clitoris, a small, sensitive organ corresponding to the male penis. In the virgin state the lower vaginal opening is partially closed by the membranous hymen ruptured at first intercourse (defloration).

The male organs basically consist of the sex-glands or testes for the production of spermatozoa and, in addition, other structures to ensure that the spermatozoa

can subsequently be deposited within the female genital tract. The spermatozoa are conveyed from the seminal tubules of the testes inside the scrotum towards the base of the bladder by the vas deferens of the spermatic cord. Also at the base of the bladder are the prostate gland and two sack-like pouches, the seminal vesicles. The gland and vesicles produce a fluid which mixes with spermatozoa from the vas to become the seminal fluid or semen.

From here the liquid passes along the urethra, a duct extending down the centre of the penis, the external male organ of copulation. The end of the penis has a sheath called the prepuce or foreskin. (This is removed in the operation of circumcision; where it is not so removed it should be pulled back during bathing and the underlying part, in which debris can accumulate, kept clean.) Part of the structure of the penis is a spongy layer, the spaces of which are occupied by blood vessels. Under sexual stimulation the spongy tissue becomes distended with blood so that the whole organ becomes enlarged, stiffened, and erect, preparatory to copulation. During sexual intercourse (see COITUS) the erect penis enters the female vagina and contractions of the vas deferens and seminal vesicles force seminal fluid into the penis from which it is forcibly and rhythmically expelled into the vagina as an ejaculation.

It should be noted that in the female the urinary tract is quite separate from the genital tract, but that in the male the urethra carries both urine and semen.

resolution. A term describing the successful repair of tissue damage by inflammation without the formation of pus, ulcers or gangrene.

respiration. Apart from some insignificant exceptions, like some types of bacteria, all living organisms require oxygen to maintain life. In the chemical changes undergone by living cells oxygen is combined with carbon and hydrogen derived from food materials. This process, known as oxidation, produces carbon dioxide (CO_2) and water (H_2O), and at the same time liberates the energy required for heat production and muscular activity. Oxidation of hydrogen is an important source of body water, but the carbon dioxide is simply waste matter. The whole process in which an organism exchanges oxygen and carbon dioxide between itself and its environment is known as respiration.

In general, single-celled organisms and simple multi-cellular plants and animals live in a fluid, so that this respiration takes place directly between the cells and their surroundings. In larger and more complex organisms that is no longer possible because the area of external surface becomes relatively smaller as bulk increases and the surface itself changes on account of the need for support and protection so that a more complex arrangement needs to be developed. This is provided in all the higher animals by the circulation of the blood. The essentials of such a system are a network of capillary vessels carrying blood to all the cells; lungs or gills to allow the blood to take up oxygen from the environment and get rid of carbon dioxide; and a blood-pump or heart to move the blood from the lungs to the cells and back again.

The process of respiration can be divided into internal respiration, which is the exchange of gases between cells and blood, and external respiration which is the gaseous interchange in the lungs between the blood and the air. Respiration has another important function because the level of CO_2 in the blood helps to determine the pH or acid-alkali balance of the bloodstream, and this is delicately adjusted by the rate and depth of breathing. See METABOLISM and RESPIRATORY SYSTEM.

respiratory system. The elements of the respiratory system are the lungs and the respiratory tract, which comprises the nose, pharynx, larynx, trachea, bronchi and bronchioles and provides a route for air to enter and leave the lungs. Within the nose are the two nasal passages. They open externally at the nostrils and are separated internally by the midline nasal septum. They are designed to humidify and warm air which is breathed in by contact with moist mucous membrane; the area of the mucous membrane is increased by the turbinate bones which are three thin, curved, shelf-like projections into each nasal passage.

Behind the nose is the pharynx, a tubular cavity communicating above with the mouth and nasal passages and below with the larynx. At the upper end of the larynx is a flap of cartilage, the epiglottis, which folds over during swallowing to close the upper opening of the larynx and so prevents the entry of food or fluid.

The larynx, voicebox, or Adam's apple is a hollow piece of cartilage containing the vocal cords which can be drawn together so as to vibrate in the air-stream and produce sounds for the purpose of VOICE and SPEECH. The channel through the larynx is continued downwards in the neck and chest as the trachea or windpipe. In mid-chest it divides into smaller tubes called bronchi. These branch to the right and left lungs and then by further subdivision to the main lobes of each lung – three on the right and two on the left. These main branches again divide and redivide as the bronchial tree or bronchioles and so reach every part of both lungs. They end as very fine tubes less than 1 mm. in diameter, each lying close to a small segment or lobule of the lung consisting of a group of alveoli or air-sacs. The trachea, bronchi and bronchioles are lined by cells with fine hair-like projections, called cilia, the purpose of which is to move secretions outwards with a whip-like action. The alveoli are lined by flattened cells so that within them is separated from the capillary blood vessels of the lungs by a microscopically thin layer in order to facilitate the movement of oxygen from the air to the blood in the capillaries and of carbon dioxide in the opposite direction.

The lungs themselves appear spongy and are inherently elastic, so that they shrink and contract when not distended by air. In life they completely fill the chest cavity. During the act of breathing in, the size of the CHEST is increased by the muscles of respiration; the diaphragm moves down and the ribs are lifted upwards and forwards. This produces a partial vacuum and air enters the lungs along the respiratory tract; this process is known as inspiration. On expiration the muscles of respiration relax and air is expelled by the natural elasticity of the lungs and by return of the chest wall and diaphragm to the resting position.

Control of respiration is effected by nerve impulses from the respiratory centre in the mid brain. When the centre is stimulated the rate and depth of breathing are increased to meet the demands for greater respiratory interchange of oxygen and carbon dioxide. The most important stimulus is a rising concentration of carbon dioxide in the blood stream. This normally occurs after exercise or in asphyxia. Other factors also may either inhibit or stimulate the centre: examples are gasping from sudden immersion in cold water, 'winding' by abdominal blows, coughing induced by partial obstruction, sneezing produced by irritation of the mucous membrane, and the rapid respiration which may accompany fear or anger. These are involuntary reactions but the brain also exercises voluntary control to meet the need for a controlled air-flow during speech and singing.

nose
pharynx
larynx
trachea

bronchus
bronchiole
diaphragm

bronchiole

alveoli

The respiratory system

Diseases. Diseases of the lungs and respiratory tract are very common, ranging in severity from the relative triviality of the common cold to conditions of the utmost gravity. In a survey in Britain, National Health Insurance statistics show that they are responsible for more than one-quarter of the total days of work-absence.

The main causes are infection, allergy, tumour and damage by dust, the first-named being by far the most frequent. They may be classified as follows:

1. Infections: these may occur in the upper respiratory tract or the bronchial tree and lungs. Examples of the former include the common cold, sinusitis, pharyngitis, tonsillitis, laryngitis and tracheitis. The infecting organisms are either viruses, as in colds and influenza, or various harmful bacteria, most frequently streptococci. Bronchial-tree and lung infections include acute and chronic bronchitis, bronchopneumonia, lobar pneumonia, pulmonary tuberculosis, pleurisy and fungus infections. These are due respectively to the pneumococcus, *M. tuberculosis*, and various types of moulds. Bronchiectasis, emphysema, and abscess

of the lung may occur as later complications.

2. Allergy: responsible for hay-fever and for many cases of asthma.

3. Tumours: these may be simple or malignant. Nasal polypi are common and papillomata occur on the vocal cords, the so-called 'singers' nodes'. Except for these, simple tumours are rare, but the larynx, trachea and bronchi are frequent sites for cancer, particularly in smokers. Although the lungs themselves and their related lymph-nodes may occasionally give rise to primary malignant tumours, tumours of the lungs are usually secondary to malignant disease elsewhere.

4. Dust-diseases: these are occupational in origin, due mainly to the inhalation of particles of silica or of other kinds of inorganic or organic dust. They produce chronic fibrosis of lung tissue.

rest. Cessation from motion or disturbance. A fundamental need of all living organisms is that their activity should be interrupted or reduced at appropriate intervals in order to allow recovery of strength by the elimination of waste products and the replenishment of energy resources. In addition, more prolonged periods of freedom from disturbance may be required for repair of tissue.

All this is a matter of common knowledge and experience. The whole body needs a nightly period of repose which we recognize as sleep. Muscles become fatigued by excessive exercise, and recover when rested; the mind becomes tired by long-continued mental effort; the special senses become blunted by over-use. The heart secures its necessary respite not only from diminished activity during sleep but also in small amounts between each heart-beat.

The above are examples of the need for rest as a normal physiological provision, but in disease rest becomes an essential aid to any form of treatment in order to secure reduced activity, either of a particular tissue or organ, or of the body as a whole. In many conditions, particularly those associated with fever and toxaemia, there is wasting and tissue destruction. These impose strain on the circulatory and excretory systems and this strain must be reduced as far as possible. Healing of diseased organs depends on tissue repair; unnecessary movement extends the area of infection, increases damage, and discourages or delays attempts at restoration.

In certain circumstances rest can be secured by mechanical or therapeutic means. Fractured limbs can be splinted; a lung can be immobilized by temporarily collapsing it; iritis can be treated by paralysing the ciliary muscle with appropriate drugs; and rest of the mind, important in many illnesses, can be secured by psychotherapy or by the use of tranquillizing drugs. The degree of rest which should be imposed depends on the particular condition. It may range from the absolute bed-rest necessary for the patient with a heart-attack to the holiday which is recommended to complete a period of convalescence. Professional advice must be the guide.

A person seeking to organize his own rest should note various points. Physical rest should include adequate time in bed each night and at least an hour of complete relaxation at some time during each day. Mental rest is often the most difficult to achieve: it involves the deliberate fostering of a determination not to think at night about the worries of today or the problems of tomorrow; it also involves a certain reorientation of attitudes – a conscious creation of degrees of priority and a firm decision to omit or postpone tasks or engagements for which there is not adequate time available.

The subject of rest is inseparable from that of sleep, which if inadequate will not only delay the cure of disease but will also undermine previously good health. The causes and treatment of sleeplessness are more fully discussed under INSOMNIA.

restlessness. Excessive or relentless activity occurs most often at night and in association with sleeplessness (INSOMNIA), which is itself a feature of many illnesses and largely a problem of good nursing. Over-activity by day, with or without sleeplessness at night, is an important feature of certain diseases, e.g., hyper-thyroidism, the manic phase of manic-depressive psychosis, and a form of brain damage that leads to constant jerky movements. It may also occur in adults and children who are physically uncomfortable, over-tired or over-anxious.

It is sensible to look for simple causes first. For instance the person who is restless in bed – especially if he is a young child or an invalid unable to remove causes of discomfort – may be hungry or thirsty, his feet may be cold, or he may be too hot or too cold generally. His bed may have an uncomfortably hard mattress, wrinkled sheets, unremoved crumbs or badly placed pillows. He may need to pass urine or empty his bowels. If he is a patient his bandages or splints may be too tight. If such causes are eliminated, the restlessness may be a result of fears, persisting anxiety, or over-fatigue.

Restlessness may be more specifically related to his disease. The patient may be fevered, with a hot dry skin or, conversely, excessive perspiration. He may have pain, headache, breathlessness, palpitation, flatulence or abominal discomfort. If he has had an operation restlessness is an important warning of internal haemorrhage.

It is essential to identify the cause of the distress and take steps to afford relief. Drugs should be a last resort. By depressing vital functions they delay the elimination of toxins and are no substitute for the beneficial effects of normal sleep and rest if they can be secured by simpler methods.

resuscitation. Emergency restorative measures applied to a person who is unconscious or apparently dead as a result of respiratory or cardiac failure.

The need for resuscitation as a first-aid procedure usually arises from some accidental or unexpected cause as in drowning, choking, gas or narcotic poisoning, electrocution, or a heart attack. In these circumstances ARTIFICIAL RESPIRATION should be started immediately; mouth-to-mouth breathing is effective and simpler to carry out than the older standard methods. Where the heart has stopped external cardiac massage may be of use but requires care and experience. See First Aid section at the end of the book.

Resuscitation may also be needed for new-born infants, and in the course of anaesthesia for surgical operations, but in these circumstances specialized equipment and resources are provided as a precaution.

retention. In retention of urine there is a stoppage of voiding of urine through a defect in the urinary apparatus. As urine accumulates, the bladder becomes distended and painful. If hot hip baths or hot fomentations applied to the abdomen do not give relief, it may be necessary to pass a catheter into the bladder.

retina. The light-sensitive inner lining of the EYE.

retirement. It is now a generally accepted pattern of British life that men should give up work at 65 and women at 60. This is a development quite uncharacteristic of less advanced societies and even of our own recent past. By adjusting pace to age and physical capacity, men used to work for as long as they were reasonably effective. Although their output might diminish they retained respect as sources of knowledge and skill, as local oracles, and as peacemakers in disputes. In the domestic field much the same was true of the older woman who often maintained or increased her sway.

Various factors have operated to change all this. Social legislation has introduced retirement pensions at a fixed chrono-logical age and technological advances have also had their effect. The older worker may be steadier, more accurate, and more conscientious, but he is also slower, less strong, and less adaptable. His skills and knowledge soon become outmoded by progress. We live in a world where machines rapidly become obsolete or disposable and there is perhaps a tendency to view men in a similar light.

The position of women has also changed radically with their increasing employment outside the home, not only before marriage, but also after their main family responsibilities have been fulfilled. They too find themselves with problems of retirement unknown to their mothers and grandmothers. Changes in society have undermined the status of the older woman as a respected figure in home or village. The younger generation tends to move away to new housing areas and grandparents are left alone in a world with which they are out of sympathy and which they cannot influence.

In the past an elderly person was more of a rarity and to that extent more likely to be accorded respect. In 1900 only 6 per cent of the population was over pensionable age. In 1980 the figure was almost 17 per cent and still increasing: the average man who reaches the age of 65 can look forward, on British statistics, to fourteen years of rich, zestful life, and the average woman to seventeen such years. This change has been due not to any spectacular increase in longevity but simply to there being fewer deaths in infancy, childhood and young adult life.

The average expectation of life at birth is now 69 years for men and 76 years for women. This is a remarkable difference between the sexes and in large measure appears to be accounted for by the fact that attainment of retiral age generally forces on men a much more dramatic change than on women who have to remain active and interested in domestic tasks which to some extent they have done all their lives whether or not they also had paid employment. For men, however, retirement means that their feelings of usefulness and importance are suddenly taken away. This may be a shattering and demoralizing experience with rapid onset of boredom and loss of interest in life. Lack of mental stimulus soon has repercussions on physical well-being. Most parents try to prepare children for the first big change in life, from home to school; and the bulk of formal education should be a preparation for the change from dependent child to self-supporting adult, spouse and parent. Yet curiously little attention is paid to preparation for the equally big change from worker to pensioner. Full discussion of preparation for a healthy old age is beyond the scope of this article but six very important points are here selected for mention.

1. Attention to physical health. In particular the person around retirement age may find his hobbies and interests becoming limited by deteriorating vision, often easily corrected by suitable spectacles and good lighting. His communication with others may be lessened by poorer hearing, sometimes improved by removal of wax from the ears and in other cases helped by an appropriate hearing aid. He may begin to suffer from corns or bunions, requiring the attention of a chiropodist.

2. Decisions about food, drink and exercise. The overweight person and the person who is retiring from a physically strenuous job should cut down their intake of starches and sugars. The person who is

facing a serious reduction of income should become aware of the need for adequate protein (with milk, eggs and fish often cheaper than meat) and for sufficient vitamins (with the possibility of much of the fruit and vegetables being supplied from his own garden). He may have a tendency to constipation through insufficient roughage in the diet or inadequate exercise. As he ages his dentures may cease to fit his shrinking gums and need renewal, since chewing difficulties can discourage him from maintaining a healthy diet. An occasional drink does no harm but alcohol may have to be reduced because of its cost to a retired person. Regular but moderate exercise is important: non-strenuous activities like walking and bowls are best.

3. Need for creative activity. Considerably before retirement he should begin to consider how he is going to occupy his vastly increased leisure time. Interests that appeal to different types include studying a subject for which time was not available earlier, painting, gardening, piano playing and sewing. Bowling is an excellent recreation and helps to create social contacts. Walking is good exercise but is more solitary.

4. Maintenance of social contacts. If he contemplates moving house, e.g., to be near his children, he should do so while still active enough to make new friends, and he should in any case consider how he is going to find substitutes for the many contacts that he had in the course of his work. Whether he moves house or not he should try to join some form of congenial social organization. One way in which he can very usefully make new contacts is by joining one of the many organizations that seek to help persons who are older or more handicapped than himself.

5. Financial matters. Monetary preparation for retirement should begin about ten years earlier, since some savings can make the difference between physical comfort and bare existence. It may also be possible to work out other economies for the future period of lessened income. For instance, the house may be too large, and transfer to a smaller house may reduce housework and save money. The heating system may be wasteful of fuel, and the cost of installing a more economical system could perhaps be met during full employment but not after retirement. Not least, skilled advice should be sought regarding the best way of investing any savings.

6. Finding people and organizations that can help. Before retirement a person is wise to familiarize himself with agencies that can help him. In the U.K. the family HEALTH VISITOR can do much to suggest methods of maintaining physical and mental health, preventing accidents and injuries, and rearranging the domestic budget; the local office of the Department of Health and Social Security can give

information about pension and possible supplementary allowances; and the local education department may organize pre-retirement courses.

In retirement the person should continue to follow the lines indicated in the six points above, to lead a reasonably active life, and to realize that he is entitled to call on the services available – whether on his general practitioner (who in Britain receives a larger annual payment for an old person than for an ordinary member of his list), or on his health visitor, or on the social work department. In looking ahead he has to face the fact that all men are mortal, but he should also appreciate that advances in modern medicine should make the suffering of severe pain unnecessary.

Two further points may be noted. Firstly, age tends to accentuate the traits of earlier life. Hence the person of advancing years may need a self-assessment. If, for example, he tended earlier to give vent to rages, raising his blood pressure, he may now have to cultivate self-discipline lest he creates the circumstances for a stroke. If he over-smoked, he may now grossly over-smoke and create a danger of chronic bronchitis; or if he was careless over his clothing and appearance, he may have to take pains lest he become an unshaven, unwashed, disreputable-looking old man.

Secondly, if he lives with a younger relative, he should remember that the relative needs a private life and adequate time to enjoy it. At least some old people change their image from that of beloved parents to that of hated tyrants by seeking to have a younger relative available for twenty-four hours in each day.

Measures are therefore necessary to ensure that retiral from work is not followed by the tragedy of physical and mental deterioration. Industry should seek to make retirement more flexible and abandon the rigidity of a set chronological age. Re-training for non-manual jobs, the provision of sheltered or part-time work and the organization of outwork for the housebound are possibilities which might be studied so that pensioners could be meaningfully employed. Training for leisure is as important as training for work and can diminish many of the problems and ill-effects of enforced idleness.

There is immense scope too for organized effort by social agencies. Adequate retiral allowances linked to cost of living indices are of course a first essential but equally important are all the measures now being developed, all too slowly, to ensure that elderly people are integrated with the community and do not become prey to loneliness and isolation. The significance of the whole question of retirement becomes very clear when it is remembered that about half the people who reach pensionable age can expect to have more than a quarter of their lives ahead of them.

retrograde amnesia. See AMNESIA.

retrolental fibroplasia. Around 1940, the use of incubators with an oxygen-rich atmosphere was introduced for the resuscitation and care of premature infants. Unfortunately some surviving infants were found to be blind because of increase in fibrous tissue behind the lens of the eye. Most surprisingly, it was discovered that this effect was caused by high concentrations of oxygen which nobody had even suspected might be harmful.

Since then the practice has been to limit oxygen-concentration, or to give it intermittently, and the condition of retrolental fibroplasia has virtually disappeared.

retroversion. A backward displacement of the UTERUS out of its normal position.

rhesus factor. A substance present by inheritance in the blood of most people but not of all.

In 1940 it was discovered that red cells from rhesus monkeys when injected into laboratory animals produced agglutinins which in turn would react with red cells from 83 per cent of human blood samples. Persons with such cells were designated rhesus-positive (Rh+ve); the other 17 per cent were rhesus-negative (Rh-ve). These proportions vary with race.

Demonstration of this rhesus factor next led to an appreciation of the cause of haemolytic disease of the new-born. If a Rh-ve woman is bearing the child of a Rh+ve man, the unborn child may inherit the Rh factor from the father. Normally foetal and maternal bloodstreams remain quite separate so that no difficulty need arise if their Rh grouping is different. However, if the placenta is damaged even minimally (e.g., by toxaemia, accidental haemorrhage, or obstetrical operations or manipulations), Rh+ve foetal red cells gain access to the Rh-ve maternal circulation and cause an antibody to form. This antibody then diffuses back into the foetal circulation and destroys foetal red cells so that the infant is either still-born or shows signs of severe anaemia at birth, with jaundice and other symptoms which may cause death or disability.

This does not happen in the first pregnancy. Several stimuli are required to produce significant amounts of antibody, so it is the second and succeeding infants who are likely to be affected. For good antenatal care it is important to identify the Rh-ve mother and assess the formation of antibodies so that steps may be taken in good time to treat the infant by exchange transfusion, replacing its damaged blood. This can now be done even before birth. Another procedure that aims to prevent the development is active Rh immunization in Rh-ve mothers by giving injections of appropriate immuno-globulin shortly after delivery. The object of this is to neutralize the antigenic effects of any Rh+ve foetal red cells which may have crossed the placenta.

rheumatic fever. An alternative name is acute articular rheumatism. Streptococci cause various diseases: upper respiratory tract infections, tonsillitis, scarlet fever, erysipelas, and puerperal fever are specific examples, but the germs are also a common cause of impetigo, wound infections, cellulitis, osteomyelitis, otitis and septicaemia.

Rheumatic fever may occur as a sequel to streptococcal infection, usually of the upper respiratory tract. Although the actual infection may be insignificant or may have gone unrecognized, the fact that it did occur can be demonstrated by laboratory blood-tests.

So rheumatic fever differs from conventional infection by being a reaction brought about by toxin from previous or present streptococcal conditions. Its main clinical features are fever and arthritis of many joints, very often heart involvement shown by rapid pulse, chest pain and breathlessness, usually anaemia and loss of weight, and sometimes twitching movements, nodules below the surface of the skin, and rashes. Mild and unrecognized attacks may occur and definite and even severe heart disease may develop in the absence of obvious rheumatic fever.

The acute stage is usually treated with salicylates and sometimes with cortisone to reduce inflammation in the joints, but prevention is all-important. Any initial or predisposing infections should be promptly and adequately treated by antibiotics. Since acute rheumatism is particularly prone to recur, the long-term use of prophylactic penicillin is now standard practice with the object of minimizing the risk of heart complications.

rheumatism. A general term for a group of disorders that cause pain in the joints, muscles and bones. RHEUMATIC FEVER, which is a specific infection though sometimes called rheumatism, is considered elsewhere, as is RHEUMATOID ARTHRITIS. The present article deals essentially with muscular rheumatism and so-called chronic rheumatism in adults, and with rheumatism in children.

Muscular rheumatism. An ill-defined term which may be regarded as synonymous with fibrositis, a condition of acute or chronic inflammatory change affecting the fibrous tissues of the body, and in particular those which form the muscular sheaths and tendons, and the joint capsules and ligaments. The symptoms are predominantly pain and muscle spasm. Lumbago is perhaps the most familiar example of the condition but any group of muscles may be affected.

An exact cause is often difficult to identify, but sepsis, diet, metabolic defects, trauma, occupation, fatigue and climate may all play a part. The condition is common in cold countries and especially in persons whose occupations involve exposure to damp, cold, and excessive strain. Damp and cold act by depressing the circulation, so encouraging the accumulation in the tissues of the end-products of metabolism.

Treatment depends on accurate assessment of the causes but principles to be observed are: removal or correction of any predisposing factors, treatment of any identifiable general disease, local treatment relying mainly on rest, warmth and physiotherapy, and analgesics.

Chronic rheumatism. To such extent as it can be differentiated from muscular rheumatism, chronic rheumatism is usually taken to mean subcutaneous fibrositis or panniculitis. This is characterized by painful and tender hard nodules under the skin at various sites, but commonly over the inner aspects of knees, the back of the neck, and the outer aspects of arms and thighs. These are particularly frequent in over-weight persons and may also be associated with menopausal changes and hypothyroidism.

To secure relief the nodules should be dealt with locally by massage. This must be as vigorous as the patient will tolerate and may be assisted by the application of local heat. Treatment must be persistent and prolonged in order to break up and disperse the condensations of fibrous tissue.

Rheumatism in children. When children are alleged to be suffering from 'rheumatism' (with swollen, painful joints and a raised temperature) the condition is generally RHEUMATIC FEVER, a disease liable to damage the heart unless promptly treated. There is, however, a less acute condition in children characterized by recurrent pains in limbs and joints, fatigue, pallor and loss of weight. In general this should be regarded - and treated - as a mild form of rheumatic fever, and not dismissed as 'merely growing pains'.

Predisposing heredity or environment? Many workers have suggested for adult rheumatism and for rheumatism in children that certain people have an inherited tendency to develop the disease. In particular it has been claimed that where rheumatism - whether true rheumatism or rheumatic fever - occurs in childhood one or other parent often has rheumatism, and that two types of children are particularly susceptible - the red or sandy-haired youngster with freckled complexion, and the child with lank dark hair, long eyelashes, a pale complexion, bluish sclera of the eyes, massive teeth, and a nervous disposition.

Rheumatism, however, is a disease with a well-defined 'social pathology'. Statistics related to social class show a greatly increased incidence in the lower socio-economic groups. Poverty is associated with bad housing, dampness, inadequate heating, deficient light and ventilation, over-crowding and poor nutritional standards.

Much research has been done on the relative importance of these factors and it is clear that over-crowding is the most potent. The fact that outbreaks of 'acute rheumatism' occur in residential schools, barracks, and training-ships where general hygiene, nutrition, and medical supervision are usually good, supports this view. Limitation of cubic space is not perhaps the sole factor because infrequent air-changes, lack of daylight, and dust accumulation all help to maintain a harmful concentration of bacteria. Disturbed sleep, and lack of opportunity for open-air exercise may also impair resistance to infection. In short, contact is probably more important than constitution in the bacterial form; and in the common muscular rheumatism or chronic rheumatism of adults climate, occupation and environment undoubtedly play the main part.

rheumatoid arthritis. A particular form of arthritis of many joints affecting chiefly the smaller joints of the hands and feet and generally showing a symmetrical distribution. All the structures within the joints may be involved. Women are chief sufferers (five to one) and the age-incidence is mainly from 20 to 50 years, although there is a variety which affects children known as STILL'S DISEASE.

In the acute stage painful joint symptoms may be accompanied by a low or variable fever and by fatigue, loss of weight and anaemia. Later on there is severe muscle-wasting with deformity and loss of movement resulting from contractures, fusing together of joint cartilages, or partial dislocations.

The exact cause is still unknown but indications point to the influence of infection or toxaemia, possibly streptococcal. In many cases there is some obvious point of infection such as decayed teeth or diseased tonsils which can be dealt with. A large proportion of patients have absence of gastric hydrochloric acid which would favour chronic intestinal infection.

It is a formidable disease because of its serious crippling potentialities. The acute stage requires treatment by rest, analgesics to relieve pain, and immobilization of affected joints, with daily passive movement. A wide range of more specific therapy has been employed at various times with varying degrees of success and failure. Salicylates, vaccines, and injections of gold salts have all had their advocates. Gold salts are to some extent back in favour but most current treatment largely relies on the new anti-inflammatory drugs based on phenylbutazone, with or without the help of steroid compounds.

rhythm method. A non-contraceptive method of birth control in which intercourse is restricted to the time of physiological sterility ('safe period') in each menstrual cycle. Generally, the ovary expels only one ovum per cycle, approximately fourteen days before the start of the next menstrual period, and the ovum is only available for fertilization for twenty-four to forty-eight hours. Spermatozoa only remain viable in the female genital tract for three to five days. There is thus a maximum period of seven days during which conception is theoretically possible, but in practice this may be longer because of menstrual irregularity.

In applying the rhythm principle by the calendar method a woman must first keep a prior record of her menstrual history for six to twelve months. From this she determines her shortest and longest cycles. In a regular twenty-eight-day cycle the period from the tenth to the eighteenth days, counting from the first day of the period, is unsafe. With irregular cycles the following example will show how to calculate the unsafe period. Shortest cycle, say 25 days: subtract 18=7; longest cycle, say 31 days: subtract 10=21: unsafe period between seventh and twenty-first day from the start of last period.

The rhythm method

The alternative temperature method depends on the fact that the body temperature rises slightly immediately after ovulation and remains up for three days until the ovum starts to disintegrate. A record of morning temperatures is kept and the safe period can then be determined as extending from the fourth day after the initial temperature rise until the next cycle commences. An obvious weakness is that many factors other than ovulation can cause a slight rise in temperature.

The rhythm method has the approval of the Roman Catholic Church but is troublesome to apply and mistakes occur more often than with any other form of contraception. It should not be relied on if menstruation is very irregular, after childbirth, near the menopause, or during illness, dieting or medication.

riboflavin. One of the VITAMINS of the B-complex, also known as vitamin B_2.

ribonucleic acid. See RNA.

ribs. The twelve pairs of curved bones which enclose the chest-cavity. The upper seven pairs are the true ribs which articulate behind with vertebrae of the spinal column and join the sternum or breast-bone in front. In addition to forming the thoracic cage of the chest, the ribs move upwards and forwards ('bucket-handle action') by muscular action when breathing in, so increasing the size of the chest and sucking in air from the exterior. The reverse takes place when breathing out.

The lower five pairs are the false ribs and three of these, instead of reaching the sternum, have their front ends attached by cartilage to the rib immediately above. The last two pairs have no attachment in front and are therefore known as floating ribs.

A fractured rib is a common type of injury, and ribs may also be malformed or deformed by disease, especially in rickets, diseases of the lung or spine, and in some kinds of paralysis. In the so-called 'rickety rosary' the front ends of the ribs become enlarged and bulbous to form a bead-like row of projections along each margin of the sternum. This also occurs in infantile scurvy.

rickets. A deficiency disease in which lack of vitamin D upsets calcium and phosphorus metabolism. This vitamin is obtained from a suitable diet, and is also produced by the body itself through the action of sunlight on precursors in the skin (photosynthesis).

Rickets occurs in infancy and early childhood. In the initial stages there is mainly retarded physical development and failure to thrive. The infant tends to be either lethargic or fretful, his muscle development is weak and he is reluctant to sit, crawl, or walk, the appearance of teeth is delayed, the abdomen may appear distended, and there is often excessive sweating. Later on, bony changes appear: bulging of the forehead; delayed closure of the skull fontanelles, enlargement of ends of long bones; curvature or deformity of limbs; and deformity of chest or spine.

Both breast-milk and cow's-milk tend to be deficient in vitamin D, especially in the winter months. Artificial milk powders are usually fortified to some extent but all infants should be given a vitamin concentrate in addition.

Rickety infants are prone to develop complications due to other infections, but otherwise early cases, adequately treated, make complete recovery. If neglected, any bony deformities are likely to persist.

rickettsia. A specific group of micro-organisms, intermediate between the bacteria and the viruses. Many different species have been identified and incriminated as the causal agents of such diseases as Rocky Mountain spotted fever, boutonneuse fever, Siberian tick typhus, rickettsiapox, marine typhus, Tsutsugamu-shi disease, louseborne typhus fever, and trench fever. Q fever is caused by a rickettsia-like organism.

Rickettsia are widespread in wild and domestic animals and then become parasitic in various arthropods, such as ticks, lice, fleas, and mites. Infection spreads to man through bites by these insects, by contamination of his skin from their crushed bodies or their faeces, and by inhalation of infective dust. The various diseases are broadly similar, with a short incubation period, followed by an intermittent or remittent fever of some weeks' duration, and the appearance of some form of rash. Exact diagnosis often depends on blood tests.

Most of the infections clear up even without special treatment, but epidemic typhus may have a fatality rate of 40 per cent, and untreated cases of Rocky Mountain fever also produce a substantial number of deaths.

The use of antibiotics (chloramphenicol group) is very effective in cutting short the course of these diseases and has significantly reduced the former risks of mortality.

rigor. An ague, or severe shivering attack, produced by the effect which toxins in the blood-stream have on the temperature-regulating centre in the mid-brain. Rigors may occur during the early stage of any infection, or during the course of a disease associated with organisms circulating in the blood, as in septicaemia or malaria.

In the first or 'cold' stage of a rigor the patient appears pinched and blue, he shivers uncontrollably, and his teeth chatter. His temperature rises to perhaps 40 °C. (140 °F.) and he passes into the 'hot' stage, with restlessness, thirst, a hot dry skin, and further rise of temperature. There then follows the 'sweating' stage with profuse perspiration and gradual decline of temperature.

A rigor may also sometimes be produced by shock (e.g. following an accident involving breaking a limb) and is quite common after some surgical operations.

rigor mortis. A Latin phrase meaning 'rigidity of death'. It usually develops about six hours after death and gradually passes off within a day or so. It is due to chemical and enzyme reactions which cause the muscles to become fixed in a state of general contraction so that the corpse is absolutely stiff and inflexible.

ringworm. Fungus infection of the keratinized areas of the body – the hair, skin and nails. Various species of fungi are responsible and collectively they are called dermatophytes. The scientific name for ringworm is tinea.

Tinea capitis (ringworm of the scalp) is due to various species of *Microsporon* and *Trichophyton*. It begins as a small papule and spreads concentrically leaving scaly bald patches. Initial infection is usually from animals – cattle, cats, dogs – but person-to-person spread may follow.

Tinea corporis (ringworm of the body) is due to a species of *Epidermophyton*, *Microsporon* or *Trichophyton*, and appears as flat, scaly, spreading, ring-like lesions. Infection is by indirect or direct contact, especially in gymnasia and swimming-baths.

Tinea pedis (athlete's foot) is mainly due to *Epidermophyton floccosum*, and is characterized by scaling and cracking of the skin between the toes. Spread is by contact with contaminated floors in shower-stalls and swimming-baths.

Tinea unguium (ringworm of the nails) is usually seen as a spread from toes in which the nails thicken, become brittle, and disintegrate.

In the past ringworm was notoriously difficult to treat and potentially hazardous forms of therapy, using x-rays or thallium acetate were sometimes employed. However, standard treatment now uses a new antibiotic drug, griseofulvin. Prolonged courses may be required for more resistant types of the disease.

Prevention depends on hygienic measures of disinfection in swimming-baths and similar places, the avoidance of contact with affected animals, and the regular changing, disinfection, and washing of clothes and footwear.

Areas of fungal infection show fluorescence under ultra-violet light, and this can provide useful diagnostic help.

RNA. These initials stand for ribonucleic acid which forms part of the chromatin in every cell and is concerned with the process by which the inherited genes in the cell-nucleus control cellular growth, development, reproduction, and behaviour.

The cell-nucleus holds information about how the cell should behave, and this information is derived from its predecessors and passed on to its successors when the cell divides. Each item of information is a gene and collectively these genes form the chromosomes. The effect of a particular gene is to instruct the cell to manufacture a particular kind of protein.

Genes are composed of short lengths of deoxyribonucleic acid (DNA) which is a long chain-like molecule. The characteristics of each gene are determined by the arrangement of four chemical groups attached to the DNA chain. Taking these three at a time, sixty-four different arrangements are possible, and this number of 'triplets' is sufficient to specify and determine the particular arrangement of some twenty amino-acids of which every different protein is composed.

Within the cell, and separate from the nucleus, are other aggregations of chromatin material called ribosomes. They contain RNA and are the site of protein synthesis as the cell grows and develops.

The problem is to transfer instructions from the genes in the cell-nucleus to the ribosomes in its cytoplasm. This function is carried out by RNA 'messengers' which are molecules of ribonucleic acid carrying the pattern determined by the genes. Messenger RNA leaves the cell-nucleus and attaches itself to the ribosomes.

Amino-acids then find their appropriate 'triplets' and arrange themselves in a chain as specified by the RNA to form the particular protein required.

It has been discovered how to make synthetic pieces of RNA and these have proved capable of controlling the assembly of a predetermined protein. It is possible that in the future further developments will provide a direct means of controlling heredity, at least to some extent. This opens up the prospect of being able to breed individuals to pattern who might be monsters or geniuses or immune to disease. Even although this may never be practicable it is no longer mere science fiction.

Rocky Mountain spotted fever. A communicable disease caused by *Rickettsia rickettsii*, and transmitted by species of hard TICKS *(Ixodidae)*. It occurs during spring and summer in most of the United States and also in Canada, Mexico, Colombia and Brazil. It is the prototype of several similar conditions known generally as tick typhus occurring in Southern Europe, the Levant, Africa, India, Siberia and Queensland.

Onset is sudden with fever and headache, followed on the third day by a rash of elevated and non-elevated spots, appearing first on the extremities and then spreading to the whole body and forming tiny haemorrhages.

In untreated cases, 20 per cent of cases die, but the disease responds well to tetracyclines. Blood tests are helpful in the diagnosis.

Preventive measures aim at reduction of tick populations, avoidance of tick-infested areas, and the use of protective clothing to prevent tick-bites. A vaccine is available but annual reinforcement is required.

rodent ulcer. A relatively common type of malignant ulcer arising from proliferation of cells in the deeper layers of dermis or true skin. The condition is technically a carcinoma but it differs from other tumours of similar origin in being only locally malignant and it never spreads by metastasis to related lymph-glands.

It chiefly affects the skin of the upper face in elderly persons and starts as a flattened hard nodule which breaks down and ulcerates on the surface. Over a period of years, if untreated, it gradually invades and destroys the tissue beneath and may produce great disfigurement.

Early treatment by wide excision and subsequent skin-grafting affords good prospects of complete cure, while x-rays or radium are also successfully employed.

Rorschach test. A test for the assessment of emotional elements of personality, extensively employed in psychological investigation. The patient is shown a series of ten 'ink-blot' designs and asked to describe what the irregular patterns suggest to his mind. His responses are then studied and interpreted as clues to significant aspects of his personality. It is an example of a projective test, so-called because the patient is unconsciously forced to reveal his own personal attitudes.

rosacea. A condition of chronic congestion of the blood capillaries affecting particularly the skin of the nose and the surrounding central area of the face. It is usually related to persistent indigestion, and it is aggravated by alcohol, strong tea, and too hot or spicy foods.

Eventually it leads to thickening of the skin, giving a lumpy red appearance to the face, and to over-action of the sweat-glands whose follicles become distended with secretion and may become infected (acne rosacea). In late stages the overgrowth of skin and the tissue beneath it converts the nose into a bulbous swelling known as rhinophyma or, popularly, 'brandy-nose'.

Treatment requires investigation of gastric function and the correction of excess or deficient acidity, the avoidance of unsuitable food or drink, and applications to the nose of such preparations as calamine lotion. Rhinophyma can be treated surgically with expectations of a good appearance.

roughage. In addition to nutrients any normal diet also contains material which is not digested and not absorbed from the human intestine. Such material, derived mainly from cereals, fruit, and vegetables, is variously described as dietary fibre, residue, or roughage. Although everyone knows that 'an apple a day keeps the doctor away', professional opinion has varied about the value and importance of roughage, and distinguished gastro-enterologists have been prepared to maintain that the human gut is designed for a meat and not a vegetable diet.

However, fibre-containing diets are now in favour. Studies of primitive races have suggested that diverticulitis, appendicitis, and cancer of the colon are less frequent when there is a high intake of vegetable fibre. It is also known that fibre influences fat digestion, so that persons on high-fibre diets have lower levels of blood cholesterol and therefore might be expected to be at less risk of developing arteriosclerosis and subsequent heart disease. There are effects also on water retention and on the metabolism of bile.

Much research remains to be done, but evidence is accumulating that roughage is a valuable protective constituent, and that a good diet should include suitable sources such as whole-meal bread, vegetables, and fruit.

roundworms. A general name for worms of the class Nematoda. Many roundworms are parasitic in man and cause symptoms either from the presence of mature forms in the gut or tissues or by movement of larvae about the body.

In temperate countries, the genera of importance are: (1) *Trichinella* which causes TRICHINOSIS, generally acquired by eating infected pork. (2) *Ascaris* which usually develops in the intestine and may produce effects from pressure or blockage or cause pneumonia or nephritis as larvae move around. (3) *Enterobius*, the common THREADWORM, is a common intestinal parasite of children, especially in institutions.

In tropical countries the range is much wider and the effects are frequently disabling not only to individuals but to whole populations. *Ankylostoma* and *Necator* (HOOKWORM), *Filaria* (elephantiasis and 'Calabar swelling'), *Oncocerca* (lesion of deeper surface of skin and blindness), *Trichuris* (whipworm) and *Dracunculus* (Guinea-worm) are some examples.

Different species of round worms are spread in various ways: by direct eating of their eggs, by larval penetration of the skin, and by bites from insect-carriers. Control requires expert knowledge of some complicated life-cycles, but many effective drugs are now available. The vermicidal drugs actually kill the worms and the vermifugal ones expel them from the body.

rubella. See GERMAN MEASLES.

rupture. A popular term more or less synonymous with HERNIA, though the term is usually restricted to some form of abdominal hernia.

S

sacroiliac pain. Pain in the lower part of the back and occasionally spreading down the leg. It is generally caused by osteoarthritis.

sacrum. A large wedge-shaped bone at the lower end of the spinal column formed by the fusion of five sacral vertebrae.

As viewed from behind it is situated between the two hip-bones, and its concave front aspect forms part of the cavity of the lesser pelvis. It articulates above with the fifth lumbar vertebra and below with the coccyx or rudimentary tail. Its articulations with the hip-bone are the sacroiliac joints.

sadism. A manifestation of abnormal personality in which pleasure, and especially sexual pleasure, is derived from the infliction of cruelty upon another. As a sexual PERVERSION or deviation, sadism may involve the whipping, beating, or maltreatment of a sexual partner in order to achieve arousal, but the term is also used to describe an attitude of mind which derives satisfaction from contemplating or securing the discomfort of others. Treatment is by psychotherapy.

safe period. See RHYTHM METHOD.

St. Anthony's fire. See ERGOT, ERYSIPELAS.

St. Vitus's dance. An old-fashioned name for CHOREA.

salicylates. Salts of salicylic acid which reduce temperature in fevered conditions, lessen pain and promote sweating. Sodium salicylate, a white crystalline substance soluble in water, is employed in the treatment of rheumatic fever, but in large doses may cause dizziness and head noises. Methyl salicylate or oil of wintergreen is sometimes used externally as a liniment for inflammation and sprains. Acetylsalicylic acid, better known as aspirin, is one of the most widely used of all medicines.

saline. See NORMAL SALINE.

salivary glands. Saliva is secreted by three pairs of glands and passed to the mouth by ducts. The submaxillary glands are situated beneath the floor of the mouth, and close to the inner surface of the angle of the lower jaw. Each has a duct opening beneath the tongue. The sublingual glands lie beneath the tongue on each side of the mid-line and have a number of small ducts. The parotid glands lie below and in front of the ear, overlapping the vertical part of the lower jaw; each has a duct which reaches the mouth at a point on the inner surface of the cheek opposite the second upper molar tooth.

Secretion of saliva is a reflex phenomenon caused mainly by stimulation of taste-buds in the tongue and mouth, but

parotid gland

sublingual gland

submaxillary gland

Salivary glands

also by the anticipation or smell of food.

The functions of saliva are to keep the mouth moist, to assist in the swallowing of food and to start the process of digestion.

The chief disorders of the salivary glands are inflammation (PAROTITIS) produced by ascending duct-infection or by MUMPS, and the occurrence of calculi in the ducts.

salpingitis. Inflammation of a tube. Although sometimes referring to the Eustachian tubes, which pass from behind the eardrum to the back of the nose, the term normally relates to the Fallopian tubes which extend between the ovaries and the upper part of the uterus.

Most cases of salpingitis are due to infection ascending from the uterus, and caused either by gonococci or by pus-forming organisms associated with septic conditions of the uterus. Abortion and childbirth may be complicated by this condition. Tuberculous salpingitis is also not uncommon, either blood-borne from elsewhere in the body, or spreading from the membranes surrounding the abdominal contents.

The symptoms are deep-seated pelvic pain, vaginal discharge and menstrual irregularity, with tenderness on either side of the abdomen and hardness detectable on vaginal examination.

Treatment can be aimed at preservation or may eventually require surgery, but the availability of suitable antibiotics has revolutionized the management and outcome of the condition. In salpingitis the ovaries are usually involved as well, and there is always a substantial risk of subsequent sterility either from ovarian damage or because the Fallopian tubes have become blocked.

salt. In chemical terms, a salt is any compound of a base or inorganic radicle with an acid, but ordinarily 'salt' is taken to mean common salt or sodium chloride (NaCl). Sodium chloride is an essential constituent of the blood plasma and tissue-fluids because of its role in maintaining these at the correct osmotic tension to ensure that the water-content of cells remains stable. See OSMOSIS.

Normal saline is a solution of salt, having the same osmotic pressure as blood plasma, and containing 0.9 gm. of common salt per 100 ml. of water. It is used to raise the blood-volume, and hence the blood-pressure, in conditions of shock and collapse. It may be given by various routes, but is usually given rectally, or by injection into the skin or into a vein.

In ordinary circumstances any normal diet provides adequate amounts of sodium chloride, but bacon, milk, and milk-products are especially good sources.

Salt is excreted in the perspiration, and excessive sweating (as in hot climates or occupations) may so reduce the osmotic tension of the blood that muscular cramps result. Additional salt must be taken to restore the depletion.

A salt-free or salt-poor diet is sometimes ordered in kidney disease where the inability of the kidney to excrete salt leads to water-retention and oedema.

salts, mineral. See MINERAL SALTS.

sand-fly fever. A disease, resembling influenza, with fever lasting three or four days, headache, malaise, nausea, and limb pains. The virus which causes it is transmitted to man by the common sand-fly, *Phlebotomus papatassi*, a small, hairy, blood-sucking midge, which bites at night, and is found on the Mediterranean coast and also widely in sub-tropical and tropical parts of Africa, Asia, Central and South America.

The incubation period is three to four days; one attack confers a lasting immunity; there are no specific measures of immunization or treatment; the disease simply runs its course, causing no danger to life.

Preventive measures include insecticidal spraying of, and around, human habitations, with personal use of insect-repellents and mosquito-proof bed-nets.

sarcoma. A type of malignant tumour or CANCER resulting from the unregulated proliferation of connective-tissue cells such as those of ordinary fibrous tissue, bone, cartilage, muscle, and pigmented tissue. It is to be distinguished from carcinoma, which always arises from epithelial cells.

Sarcomata, as a rule, are very malignant, fast-growing, and vascular. They are apt to spread rapidly, either directly, or by blood-borne and lymph-borne metastases.

Various terms are used to describe special types according to their origins.

Osteosarcoma, chondrosarcoma, myosarcoma, and melanotic sarcoma arise from bone, cartilage, muscle, and pigmented tissue respectively.

satyriasis. A psychological abnormality in which a man has an abnormal desire for sexual relations. It is very similar in cause, effect and symptoms to the condition of NYMPHOMANIA in woman.

scabies. A skin infestation caused by a small spider-like parasite, the itch-mite or acarus (*Sarcoptes scabiei*). The female acarus is about 0.4 mm. in length and the male rather smaller; they are just visible to the naked eye as glistening white dots. The female burrows into the horny layer of the skin to lay her eggs and she prefers the thin parts such as the finger-webs, the fronts of the wrists, the armpits, and the breasts. At the affected sites small vesicles form and the burrows tend to fill up with dirt and so may be seen as fine twisting lines.

The main symptom is itching, and as the patient scratches he inflicts further skin-damage which usually becomes infected. The disease is very contagious and newly-hatched mites readily migrate from person to person and also contaminate bedding.

Treatment is relatively easy and effective, using lotions based usually on benzyl benzoate, but it must be thorough, and it is advisable to treat a whole family simultaneously. Clothing and bedding should be washed and disinfected to prevent recurrence.

scalds. Tissue damage or destruction caused by moist heat through contact with hot liquids or hot vapours such as steam. Scalds do not differ essentially from burns and their effects are classified in six degrees of severity in exactly the same way, although carbonization does not occur. See BURNS.

Most scalds are of first, second, or third degree, with reddening, blistering, and skin destruction respectively. They produce pain and inflammatory reaction, together with the general effects of shock, and these may be severe if large areas of skin are involved.

Minor scalds can be satisfactorily treated by the application of medicated tulle with a protective dressing and bandage. Extensive injuries require admission to hospital and first-aid treatment should be limited to the provision of a sterile dressing covering the whole area, either dry or moistened with normal saline or sodium bicarbonate, together with measures to relieve pain and combat SHOCK.

Severe scalds of third degree or worse cause serious skin damage and lead to subsequent scarring and contraction. Skin-grafting may be required to achieve a satisfactory functional result and to restore an acceptable appearance.

scapula. The shoulder-blade, a flat, triangular bone situated on the upper rear aspect of the thorax between the levels of the second and seventh ribs. It forms part of the shoulder-girdle, articulating at the point of the shoulder with the collar-bone. The upper end of its outer border is expanded to form the shallow glenoid cavity into which fits the head of the humerus, the long bone of the upper arm.

Fractures of the scapula are rare because it is mobile and well-surrounded by muscle layers. A congenital elevation of one or both scapulae is sometimes seen and is known as Sprengel's shoulder. In 'winged scapula' or scapula alata, which may occur in persons of feeble muscular development, or as a result of damage to nerves, the lower angle of the scapula projects unduly.

scar. A mark left on the skin or on other tissue after a wound or sore has healed. Cicatrix is an alternative name. If tissue has been destroyed the defect is made good by ingrowth of fibrous tissue instead, and it is characteristic of the latter that it contracts, thus producing the puckered and depressed appearance which scars usually have.

Extensive scarring, especially near joints, may cause disabling contractures. Occasionally there may be some overgrowth of scar tissue to produce an unsightly raised appearance known as keloid scar.

Troublesome or disfiguring scars can be treated by excision and skin-grafting.

scarlet fever. Haemolytic streptococci cause various infections differentiated by the method of infection, the tissue affected, and the presence or absence of a rash. Development of a rash depends on the balance between toxin-formation by the organism, and antitoxin immunity in the patient. Although bacteriological tests show the same infection as other cases of streptococcal sore throat, scarlet fever or scarlatina has very clearly recognizable characteristics.

Usually of sudden onset, its features are fever, constitutional disturbance, inflamed throat with exudate on tonsils and pharynx, tender, swollen neck-glands, a generalized rash (a general blush with fine darker points) which avoids the face (circumoral pallor), and the so-called 'strawberry tongue' – initially with white fur and red papillae and gradually peeling to appear generally reddened.

The incubation period is one to three days and it is mostly likely to occur in young children, although infants under one year are seldom affected. Severe cases are less often seen nowadays, and treatment with antibiotics cuts short the disease and lessens the risk of serious heart and kidney complications. Cases should be isolated for at least seven days from onset, or until symptoms disappear. Peeling of skin begins during the second week and may take some weeks to be complete, especially on the soles and palms. The dead fragments of skin flaked off do not convey infection.

In epidemic outbreaks search should be made for some common source of infection. It is often possible to trace it to contaminated milk or food, or a chronic CARRIER.

Schick test. A test of susceptibility to DIPHTHERIA.

schistomiasis. See BILHARZIASIS.

schizoid personality. Since sufferers from schizophrenia tend to be incapable of feeling or expressing emotion and to live in a dream world of their own, the term schizoid personality is sometimes used for persons mildly approximating to that condition, i.e., for persons who, although within the bounds of normality, are cold, unemotional, self-sufficient, aloof and withdrawn. In a small minority of cases the adolescent of this shy, retiring, introspective disposition develops into a schizophrenic, but in the great majority of cases he simply develops into a rather solitary, self-sufficient and unemotional adult.

schizophrenia. A type of mental illness. From derivation the term means a splitting of the personality. Schizophrenia is perhaps the commonest of the serious mental illnesses since it accounts for about one-quarter of all admissions to mental hospitals. Its significance for society, and for the individual, is even more important, because it principally affects young people on the threshold of their lives and careers. For this reason it is sometimes referred to as dementia praecox.

Most cases begin between the ages of 15 and 25 and onset after 40 is very rare (except in the paranoid type). It is slightly more common in males than in females.

Its exact cause is still unknown but there is undoubtedly a considerable hereditary factor. The inherited defect appears to be some inborn metabolic abnormality, and this hypothesis is strengthened by the similarity which exists between the disease and the effects of certain hallucinatory drugs such as mescaline and lysergic acid.

Although mental stress, in the form of overwork, a broken love-affair, or other tragic experience, may sometimes be regarded as a starting-point of breakdown it is usually possible to show from a detailed clinical history that this was only the latest of a series of disturbing events which fostered or accelerated a latent disposition. In retrospect, the schizoid personality may be indentifiable from an early age: the quiet, shy, solitary, model child, who is introspective, submissive, or sentimental, and the adolescent who is unusually touchy, suspicious, obstinate or resentful of advice are both suspect, though not all of these will later show signs of the disease.

The essential feature of schizophrenia is a retirement from reality into a world of fantasy. To the outside observer this change appears as a disorder of thought, emotion or lack of emotion unrelated to actual circumstances, and domination by hallucinations which lead to abnormal impulses and conduct. It is usual to describe four main types of the disease according to its principal manifestations.

1. Simple schizophrenia: deterioration of emotional reaction with apathy and with-drawal.

2. Hebephrenia: 'silly' behaviour, inap-propriate smiling and laughter, coining of words, and hallucinations.

3. Catatonia: stupor, negativism, suggest-ibility and impulsive conduct.

4. PARANOIA: preservation of thought and emotion to a late stage, but with delusions of persecution or grandeur.

The treatment of schizophrenia is rather unsatisfactory. Many methods have been tried. Shock therapy by insulin or electrical devices has enjoyed a vogue which is now being replaced by the use of new drugs and more intensive psychotherapy.

Although some cases do recover, at least to some extent, there is likelihood of permanent damage to personality. Acute cases and those which commence at later ages are rather more hopeful. There may, however, be some scope for prevention of the condition. If the schizoid type of child is identified, the child guidance service and child health services can help to foster his social integration and to safeguard him from situations of mental stress.

school health services. There are three main reasons why the provision of school health services should rank second only to antenatal and pre-school health services. (1) School children constitute about one-fifth of the population. (2) They are in the process of mental, physical and emotional development. (3) They are a group accessible to efforts to improve their attitudes to health maintenance.

The services seek to safeguard the health of school pupils, to secure early treatment of remediable defects, to minimize the physical and educational handicaps imposed by disability, to create attitudes and habits conducive to health maintenance, and to keep a watchful eye on the hygiene of buildings, meals and equipment.

The school doctor normally examines pupils after school entry, before they leave school, and at other times at the request of the school nurse, teacher or parent. He pays particular attention to posture, nutrition, orthopaedic defects, sight and hearing, and also arranges for any needed medical treatment or modification of the educational programme.

The school nurse may be a health visitor also visiting homes in the district (preserving continuity of care), or a health visitor full-time in the school, or a nurse without subsequent training. Her functions are to carry out checks of cleanliness and infestation, to investigate outbreaks of infection, to pay attention to immunization, and to keep unobtrusive watch on the health of the pupils. If a health visitor she will also be actively involved in health education.

The school dentist routinely inspects children's teeth and arranges – or provides – treatment when needed. He is often assisted by a dental hygienist, qualified to carry out such simple procedures as scaling.

Most authorities also provide minor ailments clinics, special clinics for sight testing and hearing testing, etc.

The sciatic nerve

sciatica. Neuralgic pain occurring in relation to the sciatic nerve. The roots of the nerve arise from the lower part of the spinal cord and emerge between the lumbar vertebrae and through openings on the inner surface of the sacrum. The composite nerve-trunk which they form then passes through the lesser pelvis and follows a course down the back of thigh and leg.

Sciatica is due either to inflammation of the fibrous tissue enclosing the nerve-fibres (neurofibrositis) or to pressure on the nerve-roots and nerve-trunk from various causes including 'slipped' inter-vertebral disc, osteo-arthritis, or disease within the pelvis.

Investigation is required to determine the exact cause. Cases due simply to neurofibrositis may respond to rest, warmth, counter-irritation, analgesics, and physiotherapy. Stretching of the nerve is sometimes advocated. A SLIPPED DISC and other physical causes of pressure may require an operation to relieve the pressure.

sclerosis. A hardening of any tissue. It arises as a sequel to tissue damage caused by inflammation, toxaemia, or restriction of blood-supply, and is characterized microscopically by proliferation and condensation of the supporting or interstitial tissue. Common examples are cerebral sclerosis in which diminished blood-supply leads to nerve damage and overgrowth of neuroglia, the connective tissue of the central nervous system; ARTERIOSCLEROSIS; and disseminated or MULTIPLE SCLEROSIS.

scrofula. An old-fashioned name for TUBERCULOSIS of the lymph-glands, usually in the neck, which become enlarged and then break down to cause chronic suppuration, with thickened, unhealthy overlying skin and discharging sinuses. The condition is rarely seen nowadays because it was due to bovine tuberculous infection derived from milk and has now been largely eradicated by control of herds and pasteurization of milk.

Another name for scrofula was 'king's evil' because of the irrational belief that it could be cured by the touch of a king.

scrotum. A pouch of skin, situated in the male crotch, and providing two separate compartments for the right and left testicles and the lower end of the corresponding spermatic cords. Its external appearance varies with circumstances. Under the influence of warmth, and with age and debility, it is roomy and flaccid; with cold, and in the young and robust, it is contracted, corrugated, and closely applied to the testes. This is due to the contraction of muscle-fibres in its wall. Apart from its normal contents the scrotum may be enlarged by the presence of the lower part of an inguinal HERNIA, by the fluid accumulation of a HYDROCELE, by a VARICOCELE due to varicose veins of the spermatic cord, or by disease of the testes and their appendages.

scurvy. A deficiency disease due to insufficiency or lack of vitamin c (ascorbic acid). The early symptoms resemble those of a severe anaemia with weakness, lassitude, dizziness, and a tendency to bruising from slight injuries. The most striking subsequent changes are in the mouth where the gums swell, bleed and ulcerate, with eventual loosening and loss of teeth. The effects are primarily due to interference with blood-formation in the bone-marrow, and to increased fragility of capillary blood vessels.

Adult cases mostly occur in elderly persons on an inadequate diet. Vitamin c is chiefly obtained from fresh fruit and vegetables, and it is easily destroyed by over-cooking.

Treatment is simple and rewarding: administration of ascorbic acid effects a dramatic cure within a few days. After that it should be ensured that the diet includes enough fresh fruit and green vegetables.

Infantile scurvy. Like adult scurvy, this is due to lack of vitamin c in the diet and it is particularly apt to occur in artificially-fed infants unless steps are taken to ensure an adequate supplementary intake. It is seldom seen in breast-fed infants unless the mother herself suffers from vitamin c deprivation.

The symptoms are those of anaemia with a tendency to bleeding. Haemorrhages into the skin occur, and sometimes also from the digestive and urinary tracts. In the absence of teeth, the mouth effects are less noticeable, but the ends of long-bones are usually painful and become swollen because of haemorrhage into them and derangement of bone-formation.

The condition responds rapidly to the administration of vitamin c. To prevent it occurring, all infants should receive 20 to 50 mg. ascorbic acid per day, and this applies to breast-fed infants too, since the vitamin content of breast-milk is quite variable. Fresh orange-juice contains nearly 1 mg. per ml. and commercial concentrates usually supply 2 mg. per ml.

sea-bathing. Cold baths have a tonic effect and induce a general feeling of well-being and exhilaration. In sea-bathing the salt makes little difference and the benefits are essentially those of a cold bath, although sun, wind, wave-movement and the usual presence of other participants all contribute to the degree of pleasure and mental stimulation which results.

Sea-temperature commonly varies from 4.5 ° to 21 °C. (40 ° to 70 °F.) and the first effects on entering the water are a contraction of skin blood vessels, a feeling of chilliness, and a tendency to gasp from reflex disturbance of respiration when water reaches chest-level. Reaction sets in on leaving the water. The skin 'glows' as its vessels dilate, pulse and respiration increase, and the individual feels active and stimulated. If immersion is over-prolonged, chilliness may persist, with shivering and a 'blue' skin, and activity may be depressed even to the stage of collapse.

Moderate bathing is thus bracing and beneficial to those who are healthy and robust, but it should be indulged in cautiously by the young, the old and the debilitated, and children in particular should be supervised to ensure that their enthusiasm does not lead them to stay in too long. It is also inadvisable to bathe soon after meals. The risk of cramp or collapse is increased because of blood being already diverted to internal organs for the purposes of digestion.

sea-sickness. See TRAVEL SICKNESS.

sebaceous glands. The sweat glands of the body, which are present all over the body surface but are most numerous on the palms and soles. They consist of coiled tubes in the deep layers of skin with corkscrew-like ducts running through the outer layer and ending in tiny cup-shaped depressions on the surface. These glands are one of the main excreting channels getting rid of body waste as SWEAT.

seborrhoea. Excessive secretion of sebum, the oil produced by sebaceous glands. The condition, commonest at and soon after puberty and often decreasing with advancing age, is partly hereditary, partly due to hormonal upset and partly the result of faulty diet. The skin becomes greasy, thickened, coarse and muddy-coloured, and acne is a common complication. The most effective treatment is to decrease the fats and carbohydrates in the diet, with corresponding increase in proteins, vitamins and minerals, and to wash frequently with soap and water.

secondary. Arising as a result of some other ('primary') defect or circumstance.

secretion. A term used both for a substance formed and released by a gland or organ and for the process by which the substance is formed and released. To mention some examples, endocrine glands secrete hormones, the liver secretes bile and the tear glands secrete tears, and each of these products of an internal manufacturing process is a secretion.

sedative. A drug, or less often another agency such as a warm bath, which reduces over-activity of the nervous system and therefore diminishes mental excitement and irritability. Moderate doses are often useful in emotional stress, while larger doses are prescribed to induce sleep or to reduce pain.

The borderlines between sedatives and HYPNOTICS and TRANQUILLIZERS are not very clear. Essentially a hypnotic aims to produce sleep (as does a large dose of a sedative) and a tranquillizer aims to calm excitement (as does a smaller dose of a sedative).

Sedatives, such as the various barbiturates and the bromides, are extremely useful drugs but are perhaps employed too frequently nowadays. In conditions of serious distress or excitement they are invaluable, but they are sometimes used in situations in which ten minutes of calm discussion between patient and doctor would be equally effective.

semen. A thick, whitish fluid containing spermatozoa (produced in the testicles) and also containing secretions from the seminal vesicles (situated beside the prostate). During the process of ejaculation semen is discharged from the penis.

semicircular canal. Part of the balancing mechanism of the inner EAR.

senescence. The process of AGEING.

sensation. Perception of stimuli, irrespective of whether these are of light, sound, smell, touch, pressure, pain, heat or cold. The mechanism of sensation starts in the relevant receptors, e.g., the rods and

cones of the retina of the eye or the nerve-endings in the skin. From the receptors electrical currents pass along nerve fibres to the brain, and the experiencing of the sensation actually occurs in the brain.

sentiment. In colloquial usage a sentiment is a thought, feeling or mental attitude influenced by emotion. In psychological writings the term is used rather more precisely for any complex emotional attitude towards a person, object or situation which has been built up in the course of experience. Thus a normal parent's sentiment towards his child usually combines tenderness, affection and at times sternness; and hatred of persons of different colour or different religion is a complex and often permanent attitude largely created by personal experience and by social surroundings. Many feelings and actions that we deem logical and rational are really inspired by our sentiments.

septicaemia. Blood poisoning caused by the entry of disease germs into the blood stream and their survival and multiplication there. The original infection may be in a wound of the skin (sometimes apparently trivial) or inflammation of a bone, joint, vein or heart-valve. The symptoms include high fever, shivering, sweating and pains in joints and muscles. The condition was very serious indeed before the era of sulphonamides and antibiotics and is still serious, but timely and adequate treatment with an antibiotic or sulphonamide to which the germ is sensitive usually effects a cure.

serum. The clear, yellowish fluid which separates from the blood corpuscles when a blood clot is formed. Serum contains several proteins, including gamma globulin which may contain antibodies against a particular infection.

Serum may be obtained from a person or animal convalescing from – or highly immunized against – a particular infectious disease (e.g., measles or diphtheria). It may be used for injection to prevent the disease in contacts or to reduce its severity in those who are actually suffering from the disease. In a small minority of cases there may be a SERUM REACTION to injection.

serum reactions. Allergic reactions to the injection of SERUM occur in a proportion of people. With the unconcentrated serum of the past, where large quantities had to be injected to provide the necessary amount of antibodies, the proportion was as high as one person in six, but with modern concentrated serum it is much lower. Reactions are of two main types.

1. *Serum sickness* occurs mainly in patients sensitized by a previous injection of the same protein. After a latent period of six to fourteen days following the injection, a rash appears, sometimes localized to the site of the injection but more often generalized or patchy. There is itching, rise of temperature, sometimes joint pains and occasionally nausea and

vomiting. The condition, if untreated, seldom lasts for more than twenty-four hours; application of calamine lotion relieves the itching and a hypodermic injection of adrenalin usually relieves the condition completely.

2. *Serum shock* occurs within two hours of the injection of serum and is characterized by shivering, chilliness and signs of collapse. An extreme form of this reaction is called anaphylaxis, with breathing difficulty and sudden collapse, usually within minutes of the injection. Adrenalin can be life-saving here, and the general treatment is that of SHOCK. The best preventive measure is attempted desensitization before injection of persons known to be sensitized or known to suffer from allergic conditions. For desensitization a small injection of the particular serum is given under the skin about half an hour before the main injection.

sex education. Sex is an inescapable part of life and a happy and well-balanced sex life is essential for the health of both body and mind.

The Victorians tried to conceal sex under a mass of dogma, convention and secrecy, so that some men and many women embarked on matrimony with little awareness of sexual matters. Frigidity, marital unhappiness, extra-marital relations, high illegitimacy rates and high incidence of venereal diseases were one result, while over-large, unspaced and often unwanted families with exhausted mothers were another.

Today sex is freely discussed, and books and films on sexual matters are freely available, but every study of adolescents reveals gaps and misconceptions in their knowledge even of the physical aspects. Clearly, therefore, we need substantially more sex education. In particular, we can no more rely solely on parents – some of them ignorant even of anatomical terms and ignorant also of aesthetic and moral aspects – to teach children about sex than to teach them about geometry or physics.

It seems essential for a start that every child should be taught the anatomy and physiology of sex with full realization of how the male and female organs complement each other for the achievement of nature's primary purpose, the perpetuation of the species. It seems desirable that such instruction should be given in some detail before hormonal changes arouse sexual desire. The instruction should obviously include consideration of menstruation and its hygiene, explanation of nocturnal emissions and their harmlessness and full discussion of masturbation.

This physiological approach is, however, only a beginning. On sexual relations are built marital love, home and family, and many of the finest things of life. The aesthetic aspects have to be taught and fully discussed. The world is already overpopulated and over-large families are common: the importance of family postponement, family spacing and family limitation has to be considered, with due discussion of contraceptive techniques and their advantages and limitations. Heavy petting has to be considered from the aspect that it is normally a prelude to sexual intercourse and that arousal of passions without their normal release may be physically and emotionally harmful and may also lead to exaggeration of the physical responses in sexual relations and under-valuing of the intellectual, emotional, temperamental and aesthetic sides of relationships between the sexes.

Promiscuity has to be discussed with due attention both to the religious and moral arguments in favour of chastity, and to the claims by advocates of 'freedom', i.e., that the sexual instincts should not be unnaturally dammed up by continence and that repression and inhibition may produce neurosis and maladjustment. The dangers of venereal diseases, abortion and emotional disorders have to be considered in respect of pre-marital and extra-marital relations.

Marriage has to be considered as the general foundation of society, with discussion not only of sexual adjustment in marriage but of wider aspects of mutual consideration.

Perhaps not least, sex education should include an introduction to parentcraft and a consideration of the emotional and physical needs of young children.

Parents can do a great deal in children's early years by answering questions honestly and with brevity of detail appropriate to the child's age and mental development, and by realizing that – since sexual matters do not appear important to the child – he may well forget the information and later ask the same questions. As the child grows older, parents who have devoted some thought to the points mentioned earlier in this article can clearly regard their continuing sex education of the child as part of the general process of helping him to progress to physical, emotional and intellectual maturity, and indeed as part of good family relationships.

It is a common mistake, however, to assume that a thoughtful and well-informed parent can undertake the whole of the child's sex education and that sex education outside the home is needed only for children whose parents are ignorant or embarrassed. There are times when discussion between the child and an emotionally detached adult can be more fruitful than discussion with a parent, and times when an adolescent is more prepared to accept the statements of an 'outsider' with some claim to expertise than to accept those of mother or father. Also, since full sex education extends into many different fields (physiology, ethics, population problems, marital adjustment and child psychology are examples) very few parents would feel competent to do justice to all aspects.

Ideally sex education in the home and outside the home should supplement and reinforce each other; but in some homes sex education is virtually non-existent; and some parents who would never assume that they alone and unaided should give their child his total knowledge of religion or music or citizenship, resent the participation of professional workers in the sex education of the child.

Not every secondary school teacher, perhaps not every health visitor and certainly not every school doctor is competent to tackle the vast subject of sex education, including for example the elements of counselling for children with suspected genetic defects, discussion of the relative merits of oral and other contraceptives, and dispassionate consideration of the arguments for and against pre-marital intercourse. Yet these three individuals - teacher, health visitor and doctor - reinforced by the health education staff of the local health board and themselves reinforcing and supplementing intelligent parents can vastly improve future marital happiness, can reduce premarital conceptions, can decrease the births both of unwanted and of illegitimate children and can curtail the incidence of venereal disease.

sex hormones. A person's sex is determined by the sex chromosome from the father at conception (see GENETICS). The mother's sex chromosomes, normally designated x and x, are both female, while the father's are an x chromosome and a rather smaller Y chromosome. If the child gains an x from both parents it becomes a female with ovaries. If it gains a Y from the father it becomes a male with testes.

All the other sex characteristics are determined by hormones which are chemical secretions from the glands of the ENDOCRINE SYSTEM; the sex hormones are formed in the ovaries or testes but influenced by hormones of the pituitary. Both males and females produce two groups of sex hormones, androgens and oestrogens, but in different proportions. If androgens predominate, male characteristics appear, such as deepening of the voice at puberty and the appearance of facial hair; and these may appear in women in whom the hormones are out of balance. If oestrogens predominate, female characteristics appear, such as development of the breasts.

sex instinct. The inborn urge which impels animals of the opposite sex to approach each other at certain times and, by sexual intercourse, to effect the union of the male germ cell (sperm) and the female germ cell (ovum) so that the species may be reproduced and continue.

In human beings the operation of the instinct is modified by sentiments, ideals of conduct, social conventions and acquired codes of behaviour; and the instinct is generally regarded as including not merely 'lust' (as in the mating of some lower animals) but also certain protective impulses and tender emotions. The sex instinct, in short, falls into at least three separate categories - physical or sensual attraction between the sexes, mental or intellectual attraction, and the domestic complex concerning family and home. Any one of these three may be dominant and the three may be in conflict.

It was formerly thought that the sex instinct was dormant until puberty, but Freud and his followers showed that in some measure sexual life begins in infancy. It is at first concerned with gaining pleasure from the stimulation of the oral and then the anal regions of the body, the 'auto-erotic stage'. Next the child's interests are temporarily directed towards himself, the stage of narcissism. This is followed by a period of interest in persons of the same sex, the homosexual phase. From about 7 years until puberty there is a latent period under favourable conditions of environment and training, and at puberty there is a marked increase in strength of the sex interest with, in most cases, a change of interest from the same sex to the opposite sex. An over-development or exaggeration of one of the natural stages in sexual development tends to lead to sexual peculiarities in adult life.

The picture of childhood sexuality given above is, however, complicated by the fact that the child has two parents and tends to develop an affection for the parent of the opposite sex and a resentment, sometimes below the level of consciousness, of the parent of the same sex. In most cases this over-concentration on one parent and resentment of the other disappears without trace, but in some instances an excessive fixation of the son on the mother (or the daughter on the father) makes it difficult for the youngster to fall in love or makes the youngster seek an exact counterpart of the qualities of the loved parent. This is the cause of much marital unhappiness and lies at the root of many neurotic illnesses.

In puberty and the years of economic dependence that follow it there is often a conflict between the powerful sex instinct and the forces of tradition and social convention that oppose its gratification. ADOLESCENCE is a time of stress and conflict, and many adults, forgetting their own teenage difficulties, are unsympathetic in their attitudes and reactions.

In most societies gratification of the sexual instinct is secured by marriage, with subsequent procreation and protection of offspring, increasing bodily and mental harmony between man and woman and mutual expansion of personalities. Mutual adjustment of the sexual instinct in marriage is a primary factor in the creation of long years of trust and happiness. Failure of such adjustment may lead to prolonged unhappiness, psychoneurotic illnesses, infidelity and disease.

In women the sexual appetite tends to wane after the menopause although there is considerable individual variation. In men there is no definite period of decline of sexual desire and sexual potency but decrease between 50 and 60 years is fairly common, although some men of over 70 retain full sexual vigour.

sex-linked characteristics. See GENETICS.

sex perversion. See PERVERSION, SEXUAL.

sexual development. See DEVELOPMENT.

sexual deviance. See PERVERSION, SEXUAL.

sexual intercourse. See COITUS.

sexual relations. Sexual reproduction is the means whereby two individuals of opposite sex combine their genetic material to form new individuals who are not genetically identical with either parent. In complex animals, including man, the sexual act is influenced by hormonal cycles, instinctive drives, affection, the pleasure of touch and the relief of tension through orgasm. Reproduction is a natural process, essential for the preservation and perpetuation of the species, but it may quite often be detrimental to the immediate well-being of its practitioners – from the male mantis that is eaten by the female after he fertilizes her to the human couple faced with a young child's needs, implying less available money, less leisure and temporary inability of one of the couple to engage in remunerative employment.

In primitive communities the change from polygamy and polyandry to something approaching monogamy probably followed the establishment of settled homes, and was in part a recognition of woman in the role of home-maker and in part a response to the need to restrict the rate of growth of the population. In the earliest civilizations there was certainly nothing shameful about sexual relations, and woman was not devalued: goddesses were worshipped no less than gods, illegitimacy carried no stigma, female queens and priestesses were common enough and indeed matriarchy may have been the commonest form of rule.

Somewhere around the fourth century B.C. there began to develop new attitudes: politically, that the warrior was the only person fit to rule, with woman being bit by bit demoted to a chattel, without rights and even without a soul; and aesthetically and morally, a prudishness and guilt about matters of sex and a concept of virginity as the ideal state.

The early Christian church, while following both the Greeks and the Jews in supporting monogamy against polygamy for those who must marry, greatly devalued women, glorified virginity and continence, and deemed all pleasure in sexual intercourse wrong. Extra-marital relationships became associated with guilt and the fear of hell-fire, and even marital intercourse was considered something that should not be enjoyed but undertaken only with a view to the procreation of children.

The rehabilitation of woman came very slowly: the right to vote and the right to own property came within living memory, equal pay does not yet fully exist, traditionally female professions (such as nursing) are still paid less than comparable traditionally male professions, and it is only very recently that a woman's passport has ceased to indicate her marital status. Throughout this very slow process of rehabilitation enormous efforts were made to protect the 'innocence' of girls, to limit male company to well-chaperoned occasions, to teach self-denial and self-discipline, and to ensure that girls came to matrimony knowing little or nothing about sex and with a vague idea that sexual relations should be reluctantly tolerated rather than enjoyed – and inevitably a large amount of frigidity, marital unhappiness and psychosexual disorders resulted.

The Second World War probably did more than anything else to change attitudes: there were jobs for all, and the woman who became an unmarried mother no longer feared poverty; with death quite likely for the civilian as well as for the soldier there was a freer 'live for the present' atmosphere; and the preachers and moralists who had failed to prevent two wars lost status in the eyes of the young.

The allegedly permissive society of the last forty years, the spread of sex education and the availability of contraceptives have combined to produce a new attitude to sex – an enjoyment of a natural function, a reduction in prudery and a separation of sexual relationships from reproduction of the species. These changes occurring gradually over a century might have been purely healthy, a reversion in fact to the attitudes of ancient Greece and Egypt before the subjugation of women; but, occurring in a single generation, they have sometimes produced confusion and conflict.

sheath. A contraceptive or prophylactic condom made of fine rubber and worn over the penis during sexual intercourse.

It was widely used in many countries in the seventeenth and eighteenth centuries, and curiously became called in Britain a 'French letter' and in France 'le chapeau anglais'. Even today it is probably the most widely used contraceptive device in virtually all countries.

If filled with air (like a balloon) to check for leaks before being placed on the penis prior to intercourse it is a reasonably good contraceptive and also lessens the chance of transmission of syphilis or gonorrhoea. If additionally it is coated with a spermicidal cream its efficiency as a contraceptive rises to about 99 per cent, a figure outstripped only by the modern contraceptive pill. The use of a spermicidal cream also prevents vaginal discomfort from friction.

The best patterns have a teat-shaped end to collect the ejaculate and minimize risk of backward seepage to the free margin of the sheath. Sheaths must be of reliable quality, and since rubber perishes with age, they should also bear a date beyond which they should not be used.

The advantages of the sheath include the very small effort required, as contrasted for instance with the physical effort needed for insertion of an intra-uterine device or the mental effort needed to remember to take an oral contraceptive every day. A second advantage is the fact that no doctor is required, the sheaths being purchasable without prescription. A third advantage is that a sheath lessens the likelihood of transmission of venereal disease.

Although a few men and women maintain that even a very fine sheath on the man's penis reduces the pleasure of intercourse, the main disadvantage is of course that it is worn by – and normally purchased by – the man, whereas it is usually the woman who is the more anxious to avoid bearing a child.

shellfish poisoning. Essentially there are three types of shellfish poisoning.

1. *Bacterial.* Shellfish that grow near sewage outlets are liable to harbour infecting organisms from the sewage, e.g., the organisms of typhoid, dysentery and food poisoning. In Britain, local authorities have power to declare contaminated areas unsafe and to forbid the sale of shellfish from these sources. Where contamination is possible but less severe, authorities also have power to provide tanks in which shellfish may be cleansed by immersion for several days in water sterilized by chlorine. Where bacterial poisoning from shellfish occurs treatment is that of the particular disease.

2. *Toxic.* Mussel poisoning is sometimes caused by a ptomaine, mytilotoxin, produced by bacterial activity and not destroyed by cooking. Symptoms are those of collapse, with giddiness, coldness, lividity and often an itching nettle-rash. The stomach should be washed out with large quantities of water, the patient needs to be kept warm, and stimulants should be given freely.

3. *Allergic.* Some individuals have an idiosyncratic reaction to crabs, lobsters, mussels and oysters, developing within a few hours of eating them an irregular raised rash, diarrhoea and vomiting, and sometimes signs of collapse. The patient should be kept warm, anti-histamine drugs may be tried, and subsequently the person should avoid shellfish.

shell shock. An acute anxiety neurosis following exposure to extreme danger. There are usually underlying emotional factors but a traumatic experience is the final trigger in the production of the disorder. Common symptoms include headache, anxiety, depression, nightmares and fatigue.

The term was frequently used in the First World War but has subsequently been replaced by broader terms such as anxiety neurosis, traumatic neurosis and effort syndrome.

shingles. The colloquial name for herpes zoster, an acute infection of a nerve root causing very severe, stinging pain in the skin served by the particular nerve, and in due course a crop of blisters appears over the same area. Pain and raised temperature occur for three or four days before the appearance of the blisters and the latter tend to dry off and shrink during the next week or ten days, although in frail or elderly people the pain may persist for months.

A dusting powder of starch or zinc oxide is helpful, and pain may be relieved by aspirin or phenacetin, or if necessary by pethidine. Claims have been made that corticosteroids are helpful. When it affects the nerve supplying the upper face and eye, there is a danger of damage to vision and special care must be taken to reduce this risk.

The virus which causes shingles is identical with that of chickenpox. A person with shingles may infect children with chickenpox, but it is very rare for a child with chickenpox to cause shingles in an adult.

shivering. Uncontrollable trembling or quivering. It is a normal reaction to sudden intense cold and is beneficial in that it generates heat in the muscles. Shivering, or rigor, also occurs in the early stages of many feverish diseases, such as influenza and pneumonia, and bouts of shivering are particularly associated with malaria and glandular fever.

shock. A condition associated with failure or collapse of the circulatory system. Common causes include injuries (especially in the neighbourhood of the heart, lungs, intestines and genitalia), burns, failure of the pumping mechanism of the heart, severe haemorrhage and occasionally serious emotional upset. The symptoms vary with the degree of shock but typically include prostration and exhaustion; nausea and abdominal discomfort; headache and giddiness; and coldness and shivering. The patient is pale, his pulse is rapid and feeble, his breathing is shallow and his pupils are dilated.

Essential features of treatment are to lay the patient flat, preferably with the head a shade lower than the feet so as to increase the supply of blood to the brain, and to keep him comfortably warm; this is most easily done by placing warm (but not uncomfortably hot) water bottles at the feet, armpits and the inside of the thighs. Provided that he is able to swallow and provided also that the digestive organs are undamaged he should be given hot tea or coffee, and reassurance is even more useful. If the breathing becomes enfeebled,

ARTIFICIAL RESPIRATION may be needed.

The term 'shock' is used colloquially in Scotland to mean apoplexy or STROKE.

shock therapy. See ECT.

short sight. The common name for the defect of EYESIGHT known medically as myopia.

shoulder. The part of the body surrounding the ball-and-socket joint between the head of the humerus and the glenoid fossa of the scapula or shoulder-blade. Movement of the shoulder joint is usually good in all directions but mobility is paid for by lack of stability: dislocations of the head of the humerus, usually downwards and forwards, are commoner than dislocations of any other joint. Fractures are also not uncommon. Inflammation of the tendons of the joint leads to the painful condition known as frozen shoulder.

Siamese twins. See TWINS.

sickle cell disease. A hereditary condition in which the red blood corpuscles are sickle-shaped, fragile, and contain an abnormal type of haemoglobin. The disease is common in people of African and West Indian descent.

From childhood onwards the victim tends to display pallor, lassitude, weakness and other signs of anaemia, together with enlargement of the spleen. At intervals the victim suffers from infarctive crises, i.e., bouts of acute pain in muscles and joints.

Diagnosis (by blood test) is essential, both for correct management of the disease and because the giving of iron – useful in most anaemias – can do harm. Treatment of the crises consists of reassurance, warmth and analgesics. Treatment of the disease involves attention to general health, prompt attention to any infection, and special care before and after any operation.

The disease is transmitted as a Mendelian recessive, i.e., a child will suffer from it only if both parents are carriers. The condition is therefore preventable if carriers, known as persons with sickle cell trait, are identified (by blood test) and thereafter do not marry other carriers, though they can safely marry people who are not carriers.

side-effect. A secondary and usually undesirable result of a particular drug or other treatment, e.g., a sulphonamide may cure a particular infection but in a small number of patients produces a rash as a side-effect.

silicosis. A disease of the lungs caused by breathing dust from rocks containing silica for prolonged periods. The condition occurs in rock miners, quarriers and sandblasters. It develops gradually, with the sufferer becoming progressively shorter of breath and having a persistent dry cough.

The silica dust particles form silicic acid in the tissues of the lung and this results in scarring and thickening, with ultimately the signs and symptoms of chronic bronchitis and emphysema.

Treatment is essentially that of chronic bronchitis and emphysema. Prevention is largely a matter of providing special ventilation; where that is not practicable, breathing masks should be worn.

sinew. The tendon of a muscle, i.e., the fibrous tissue between the meaty part of the muscle and the bone into which the muscle is inserted. For example, the fleshy soleus and gastrocnemius muscles in the back of the calf combine to end in a bundle of tough fibres, called the tendon of Achilles, running down to the heel bone. This tendon, although it is occasionally torn, is probably the strongest sinew in the body.

Colloquially the term is often employed to describe muscular strength or vigour.

sinus. This term has two meanings.

1. In anatomy, a hollow space or cavity, usually in bone. The term is applied mainly to the cavities in the skull – the frontal sinuses in the forehead, the maxillary sinuses in the cheeks, the sphenoidal sinuses at the back of the nose and the ethmoidal sinuses behind and below the frontal sinuses. Inflammation of the mucous membrane lining a sinus is termed SINUSITIS.

2. In pathology, a burrowing, elongated ulcer, which starts at a blind end (e.g., in bone) and opens on the skin or on a mucous membrane. A sinus differs from a fistula in having one blind end.

sinusitis. Inflammation of the mucous membrane lining one of the SINUSES which connect with the nose. Such inflammation often occurs during a cold in the head or other upper respiratory tract infection but may also be caused by allergic reaction or by prolonged irritation by dry air. The nose feels stopped up and has a copious thick discharge, the face and head have a sensation of heaviness, and there may be headache or pain behind the eyes if the frontal or ethmoidal sinuses are involved and pain in the cheek if a maxillary sinus is affected. Treatment consists of rest in a reasonably even temperature, a nasal decongestant spray, and in severe cases an antibiotic. If the symptoms fail to clear after a week's treatment, it may be necessary to consider inserting a needle into the affected sinus (working under local anaesthesia) in order to wash and drain it.

skeleton. The rigid scaffolding to which the body owes its shape.

In the process of evolution two types of skeleton have developed. (1) The exoskeleton or hard outer shell, as in crustaceans: this provides an excellent passive defence but limits movement and has to be cast off at times as the animal grows, leaving it temporarily defenceless. (2) The endoskeleton or inner scaffolding of vertebrates: the endoskeleton of man and other vertebrates, while essentially a central framework, nevertheless provides very complete protection for the brain and considerable protection for the thoracic and pelvic organs.

skull
collar bone
scapula
sternum
ribs
humerus
spinal column
radius
wrist
pelvis
palm
ulna
fingers
femur
patella
tibia
fibula
ankle
foot
toes

The skeleton

The human skeleton can be considered as consisting of an 'axial' and an 'appendicular' part.

The axial portion includes: (1) the SKULL, i.e., the eight bones of the cranium and the fourteen bones of the face; (2) the thirty-three bones of the vertebral or SPINAL COLUMN; (3) twelve pairs of RIBS, each joined behind to the vertebral column and the upper ten joined in front to the sternum; and (4) the STERNUM, or breast bone.

The appendicular portion consists of (1) the pectoral girdle, consisting of SCAPULA (shoulder blade) and clavicle or COLLAR BONE, with the bones of two upper limbs attached; and (2) the PELVIS, or pelvic girdle of ilium, ischium and pubis, with the bones of two lower limbs attached. Each upper limb has one HUMERUS (arm-bone), two forearm bones the RADIUS and ULNA, eight WRIST bones, five bones of the palm and fourteen finger bones (three for each finger but only two for the thumb). Each lower limb has one FEMUR (thigh bone), one small PATELLA (knee-cap), two leg bones the TIBIA and FIBULA, seven ankle bones, five bones of the sole and fourteen bones of the toes.

Every movement of the body is brought about by contraction of muscles anchored to particular bones.

skin. The outer covering of the body consists of two main layers, the dermis or true skin and the outer layer of epidermis or cuticle. The dermis has a framework of tough fibrous and elastic tissue and contains loops of blood capillaries and nerve fibres with endings specialized for sensations of pain, touch, pressure and temperature. It also contains the sebaceous glands which excrete sweat. The epidermis is a protective outer layer without blood vessels. The deeper part of the epidermis contains growing cells but the surface consists of dead cells which are constantly shed and replaced from the growing cells. Hairs are epidermal growths which emerge from little pits called hair follicles. Nails of the fingers and toes are hardened and horny modifications of epidermis.

The skin is a tough, waterproof, elastic outer covering which protects the soft structures beneath from dehydration, soaking, minor injuries and bacterial invasion. It is an important sense organ, making us aware of such things as pain, heat, cold and touch. The sweat glands play an important part in the excretion of waste products. Both by dilating or contracting its blood vessels (so that more or less heat is given off by radiation) and by adjusting the amount of perspiration, the skin helps to regulate body temperature. In sunny climates it is the main source of manufacture of the body's vitamin D. Not least, it is the organ that is seen – the organ that attracts or repels other people by its beauty or ugliness, the organ that reveals emotions, and the organ that often provides indications of bodily health or disease.

Skin

An index of health. In many respects the skin is a useful guide to the body's well-being, constitutional changes being quickly reflected in the appearance and functioning of the organ that is most easily seen. Thus pallor occurs in the anaemias (although some people who are not anaemic have a natural pallor) with a curious lemon-yellow tint in severe cases of pernicious anaemia; yellowing of the skin and mucous membranes characterizes the various types of jaundice; bronzing is seen in Addison's disease; in cancer and advanced syphilis there is a characteristic earthy hue; and in chronic heart disease and chronic bronchitis there is a dusky, bluish tinge. Many acute infections are diagnosed mainly by their skin eruptions, e.g., the blotchy rash of measles, the rather finer rash of rubella, the fine reddening (except around the mouth) of scarlet fever, and the crops of papules and pustules of chickenpox. Again, the skin of a diabetic is often dry and inelastic; the perspiring forehead of rickets is almost proof of the diagnosis; and a thick, harsh skin suggests deficiency of the thyroid gland.

Diseases. As the most exposed organ of the body the skin is subject to so many disorders that classification is almost impossible. A few out of several hundreds are mentioned here:

1. Skin infections: bacterial, e.g., impetigo, boils, erysipelas; virus, e.g., warts; fungal, e.g., ringworm; and parasitic, e.g., scabies.

2. Rashes arising from acute infections, such as those of measles, German measles, chickenpox and scarlet fever, and the rose-spots sometimes seen in typhoid.

3. Increased sensitivity or pruritus (itching), sometimes occurring by itself in the elderly, and often appearing as a symptom of diabetes, gout, renal failure or cirrhosis of the liver.

4. Decreased sensitivity, as in

syringomyelia, leprosy and peripheral neuritis.

5. Changes of pigmentation, either an increase, as in pigmented moles (melanomata), which are birth marks, and freckles (ephelides) or a decrease, as in albinism.

6. Disorders of secretion: increased perspiration (hyperidrosis) in conditions of abnormal heat, exertion or fear, and also in association with hyperthyroidism and acromegaly; increased oiliness (seborrhoea), often due to hormonal influences; and abnormal dryness (xeroderma), often hereditary.

7. Disorders of skin circulation, e.g., chilblains and rosacea.

8. Dermatitis of various types, including contact dermatitis, the commonest of all occupational diseases.

9. Eruptions of large blisters, as in pemphigus.

10. Cancer of the skin, e.g., rodent ulcer.

11. Miscellaneous other conditions among which are psoriasis and acne vulgaris.

skin grafting. See GRAFTING.

skin writing. A curious condition, otherwise known as dermographia, in which the slightest scratching of the skin produces a red weal, so that it is possible to write on the skin with a finger, with the marks remaining visible for some minutes. The condition is allergic and is akin to urticaria or nettle-rash. Stimulation or injury of cells liberates histamine which causes a dilatation of skin blood vessels and localized reddening and swelling, and often occurs in persons with other allergic symptoms.

skull. A general name for the eight domed bones of the cranium that protect the brain and the fourteen bones of the face; the upper jaw is part of the skull while the lower jaw is hinged to it. In most animals the cranium is placed in the back part of the head and the face looks upwards as well as forwards. In man, because of the enormous development of the cerebral hemispheres of the brain, the cranium is above the face as well as behind it, and consequently the face looks straight forward.

Disorders. The commonest disorders of the skull are congenital malformations and fractures.

Since the bones of the skull develop round the brain and gaps for growth are present in the early years, congenital malformations are not caused by defects of the skull but result from disorders of the brain which in turn cause alterations of the skull. In microcephaly the brain is of abnormally small size and therefore a small skull develops to house it. In hydrocephaly there is excess fluid round the brain and so the skull enlarges to make room for it.

Fractures of the cranium are common, although slightly reduced by the wearing of crash helmets by motor-cyclists; such fractures are very important because of

Frontal view of the skull

Side view of the skull

their complications. Since there is no available space between the brain and the skull, relatively minor bleeding can create enough pressure to cause death. Hence operation may be essential to stop the bleeding or to allow excess fluid to escape.

Fractures of the bones of the face are also quite common, as is dislocation of the jaw.

sleep. The partial suspension of the activities of the nervous system which normally occurs at regular intervals and leads to restoration of the body's energy.

Although the transition from waking to sleeping may be abrupt, sleep is usually preceded by a feeling of languor, a heaviness of the eyelids, a relaxation of the muscles and a decreasing acuteness of the senses, with sight fading first and touch being the last to go.

An infant in the early weeks of life sleeps for over twenty hours out of each twenty-four; a child of 1 year sleeps for around fourteen hours daily; a child of 8 years needs at least ten hours; a child of 12 on average requires nine hours although individual differences are beginning to appear by this age; and most adults need about eight hours, although a few adults require substantially more or less and there are two or three cases on record of adults who appear able to exist without sleep. As a rule continued deprivation of sleep causes symptoms resembling those of drunkenness and is injurious to physical health as well as to mental health.

During sleep all the chemical processes of the body are slowed, but brain activity – as demonstrated by the electroencephalogram – undergoes a change but does not cease. Whereas electrical waves from the waking brain are rapid and irregular, in deep sleep they are slow and regular but with occasional periods of increased electrical activity associated with rapid movements of the eyes. Some workers suggest that these active periods are associated with dreaming but evidence is hard to obtain since most people do not remember their dreams or even whether they have been dreaming.

Slumber is encouraged by comfort, darkness and silence, in other words by an absence of strong sensations, but paradoxically it is sometimes aided by monotonous repetitive sensation, such as a sound occurring every thirty seconds. Most of all, sleep is influenced by physical and mental tiredness and by habit.

Inability to sleep is known as INSOMNIA.

sleeping sickness. An infectious disease of tropical Africa, caused by a minute parasite called a trypanosome and transmitted by the bite of an infected tsetse fly. The incubation period varies from one to three weeks. The early stages of the disease are characterized by irregular fever and rigors, intense frontal headache, areas of puffiness on the legs and face and enlargement of the lymph glands. After some months further symptoms appear: mental and physical inertia, shuffling gait and a tendency to fall asleep. Untreated cases usually die within a year. Various arsenical drugs are useful in treatment but the doses required for therapeutic effect come dangerously near to the poisonous level. The tsetse fly that carries the parasites usually acquires them by biting antelopes or other wild animals, or by biting infected persons.

Preventive measures include mass injections of the local population with one of the appropriate drugs (to prevent the tsetse fly from becoming infected when it bites); clearing of bush around villages and beside roads (to remove flies); and fly control by suitable insecticides. Tsetse flies mainly bite by day, so journeys across infested country should be made by night.

A rather similar disease – American trypanosomiasis or Chagas' disease – occurs in Central and South America. Here the organism is transmitted in the excreta of various bugs and the disease, although often fatal in children, is less deadly in adults.

The disease should not be confused with 'sleepy sickness', a colloquial name for ENCEPHALITIS LETHARGICA.

sleeplessness. See INSOMNIA.

sleep walking. The occurrence during sleep of certain muscular actions which imply activity of the portion of the brain controlling the relevant muscles. In the most marked form the person may rise from bed and perform a complicated series of actions. If the eyes participate in the activity the person may see and avoid objects in his path.

Minor forms of sleep walking – or somnambulism, to use the medical term – include talking during sleep and such actions as sitting up in bed while still asleep. As a rule there is on wakening no recollection of the nocturnal activities.

Sleep walking is sometimes regarded as allied to hysteria but in most cases it is probably an expression of deep emotional conflict. Where it occurs as a single episode it is worthwhile to try the effect of reducing cerebral activity for the last couple of hours before the time of going to bed and avoiding heavy meals in that period. Where somnambulism continues or recurs medical advice is desirable.

sleepy sickness. A colloquial name for ENCEPHALITIS LETHARGICA.

slimming. A deliberate and sustained attempt to lose weight. In underdeveloped communities where malnutrition is common and plumpness is a sign of affluence and power, slimming is virtually unknown. In the affluent societies of Western Europe and North America, and especially in the middle and upper classes in these countries, people are becoming increasingly aware of the dangers of obesity. Excessive weight puts a strain on the heart (which has to pump blood to a gradually enlarging territory), the kidneys (which have to remove waste products produced in that enlarging territory) and the joints and muscles (which have to bear more weight). Obesity raises the chance of such diseases as chronic bronchitis and diabetes, and it increases the severity of conditions like pneumonia. Furthermore, it diminishes prowess in sport and looks unsightly. Hence attempts to reduce weight are very common.

Persons seeking to lose weight should remember three basic points.

1. Excessive eating is often employed to camouflage life's problems. If a person eats as a form of compensation for bereavement or loneliness or sexual frustration or lack of work satisfaction, a reduction of food, however achieved, merely removes the compensation without tackling the basic cause. Attention to underlying factors may be far more important than attention to the diet, and slimming in the presence of sympathetic and encouraging associates is far easier than slimming without support and help.

slipped disc

2. Our weight depends essentially on our intake of Calories. If for our particular body size and amount of exercise we need 2,600 Calories daily and eat 2,300 we shall lose weight; if we need 2,600 and normally eat 2,800 we can expect to gain weight, unless we are the kind of person - lucky in a weight-conscious affluent society but in dire straits in famine conditions - who makes inefficient use of our food.

To lose weight the fundamental need is to consume fewer Calories. Certainly we can seek to increase our calorific needs by more exercise, but violent exercise can be dangerous for those not accustomed to it and even mild exercise, while increasing Calorie expenditure, also increases appetite. Again, we can temporarily remove some weight by getting rid of excess fluid, as by saunas or Turkish baths, but the fluid - being the amount that is normally needed for our bodily size - will in due course be replaced. For sustained weight reduction we need a Calorie intake less than our Calorie expenditure, with gradual increase to balance expenditure after the weight loss has been achieved.

For weight maintenance an average-sized, middle-aged man of fairly sedentary occupation needs about 2,600 Calories daily, and a similar woman, being rather smaller, needs about 2,300 Calories. Tables giving the Calorie values of different foods and drinks are available in many textbooks on nutrition and dietetics. In general a slow reduction of weight (through eating perhaps 200 Calories a day less than are expended) is desirable over a number of weeks, with ultimate return to a Calorie intake that will simply maintain the reduced weight without either increase or further reduction. Sudden dramatic reduction of food intake may cause illness or exhaustion and is in any case likely to be followed by increased eating and restoration of the overweight condition after the period of extreme dietetic effort. Broadly, an overweight person can seek unaided to cut his Calorie intake by about one-tenth, but for more drastic reduction he would be wise to enlist the help of a doctor, health visitor or dietitian.

3. In attempting to reduce food intake we cannot afford to reduce all food components equally. The adult DIET should contain about 75 g. (2.5 oz.) daily of protein, or - since no food is pure protein - about three times that weight in lean meat, white fish, cheese, eggs and legumes (i.e., peas, beans, etc.). Unless our intake of protein has been grossly excessive its reduction would be dangerous to health. Again, sharp curtailing of our intake of animal fat (e.g., butter and cheese) could create a deficiency of the fat-soluble vitamins A and D; reduction of bread consumption may lead to a shortage of the vitamin B complex; most of us get 40 per cent of our needed vitamin C from potatoes, so that omission of potatoes from the diet may lead to deficiency of vitamin C unless we

are eating plenty of lemons, oranges, tomatoes and green vegetables; and cutting down on milk and milk products may create a deficiency of calcium. Yet again, to prevent constipation we need a reasonable amount of ROUGHAGE - foods of low dietetic value but appreciable residue.

Having ensured that we have adequate protein, adequate vitamins (possibly by addition of vitamin supplements to the diet), adequate calcium from milk and milk products, and adequate roughage, we can reduce our Calorie intake by particular attention to the reduction of carbohydrates (e.g., sugar, sweets, cakes, scones, white bread, to a lesser extent brown bread and potatoes), secondarily to the reasonable reduction of fats (e.g., butter and fried foods), and thirdly to the reduction of proteins to such extent as they were previously excessive. In arranging such reduction we can very much please ourselves so long as the total reduction is adequate: for instance, we may need to curtail our combined Calorie intake from whisky, potatoes, bread and cakes, but there is no particular virtue in cutting out the two that we happen to enjoy and leaving the two that we could happily do without. What we should aim at is a palatable, personally satisfying diet that will gradually reduce our weight over a number of weeks and that thereafter, with slight additions, can be maintained permanently.

The many 'slimming diets' in current vogue are mostly based on maintenance of adequate protein supplies and adequate vitamins, and reduction of total Calories by diminution of carbohydrates and, to a lesser extent, of fats.

Appetite depressants can help at the beginning of a period of weight reduction but some are addictive and some produce side effects. If needed, they should be taken under medical supervision. Usually, however, psychological help is more important than the use of drugs. Such help includes attention to the underlying causes of the obesity, encouragement to persevere with the diet, sympathy with occasional dietetic indiscretions and relapses, and even pleasant conversation at meals to make a relatively small meal take longer to consume.

slipped disc. The vertebrae of the SPINAL COLUMN are separated by cartilaginous discs, and slipped disc is the painful condition that occurs when a disc cracks or becomes slightly displaced and so presses on a nerve. The dominant symptom is pain, occasionally felt near the site of the injury, as in lumbago, but more often experienced in the muscles which are supplied by the nerve concerned, e.g., displacement of the fourth or fifth lumbar disc is felt as sciatica, i.e., pain in the back of the thigh and the calf. Common causes include sudden, abrupt movement, for instance lifting a heavy case to the rack of a railway compartment may injure a lumbar disc, and the 'whiplash' injury when a stationary car is run into from behind, causing the head to jerk backwards and then quickly forwards with possible cracking of a cervical disc. Often, however, no cause is found and there is only a vague attribution to prolonged bad posture.

While heat, massage and analgesics all help the pain, they afford only temporary relief. These temporary measures are usually necessary, and most cases respond to rest, sometimes including the wearing of a supporting collar for a neck injury, and often including the use of a board under the mattress for a back injury and occasionally the wearing of a spinal brace. Where these measures are not followed by return of the disc to its normal position and shape, manipulation by an orthopaedic surgeon (or by an osteopath) sometimes helps.

Young or early middle-aged adults with long backs, the commonest victims of slipped disc, can to some extent console themselves with the knowledge that the ageing process renders recurrence of the injury less likely. On the other hand, where the condition occurs after the age of sixty and fails to respond to rest and measures to relieve pain, a surgical operation may be required.

Slipped disc

slough. A portion of dead tissue (e.g., the core of a boil) that is cast off from the living tissue. Sloughing is the falling away of such dead tissue.

smallpox. The most infectious of all diseases, caused by a virus and characterized by a rash of pimples which became filled with pus and finally dried with crusting and often left permanent pitting of the skin. From the time when it was first identified in the tenth century it was one of the major killing diseases. Spread was by droplet infection from persons sick with the disease or incubating it, by articles recently contaminated by discharges from such persons, and possibly by aerial transmission for very short distances.

There were two forms, a major variety which had (even in the 1960s) a death rate of about 30 per cent, and a minor variety with a death rate of about 1 per cent. Treatment consisted of very strict isolation, rest, good nursing, analgesics,

and attention to the eyes. No antibiotic, sulphonamide or other drug was effective.

Vaccination, however, gave an absolute immunity for several years, and in most cases an immunity for life. Vaccination of the public in country after country made the disease a rarity. Then general vaccination was no longer needed, and vaccination was confined to contacts of cases, including, of course, the doctors and nurses involved. Finally – perhaps the greatest triumph of health education and preventive medicine – in 1979 smallpox was declared to have been eradicated from the world.

smear. A preparation of blood, secretions, etc., smeared onto a glass slide for examination under a microscope.

In *cervical cytology*, the doctor or nurse takes a smear from the mucous membrane of the cervix of the uterus. The specimen so obtained is stained and then examined under a microscope to see whether there is any abnormality in the cells. If any abnormality is found, an operation is desirable before the cells actually become cancerous.

Smears are also used for a wide range of other tests.

smegma. A soapy-like mixture of dead skin cells and oil from the sweat glands that collects in folds of the skin, and especially around the clitoris and the foreskin of the penis. It is important that the genitals should be kept clean, because there would appear to be an association between the presence of smegma in a man and the occurrence of cancer of the cervix in a woman with whom he has frequent sexual relations.

smell, sense of. Smells are identified by delicate, hair-like endings of the olfactory nerves in the mucous membrane of the upper and back part of the nose. From these smell receptors impulses pass inwards to the olfactory tract, which is an outgrowth of the brain. In many animals the olfactory tract is hollow and of considerable size; but in man it is much smaller and more solid, so that man has a relatively poor sense of smell.

Nevertheless our perception of smell, weak as it is, accounts not only for our perception of odours but also for much of our taste. Certainly the taste receptors on the tongue identify the four basic taste sensations (sweet, sour, salt and bitter) but most of what we normally regard as taste is actually smell. Hence if the upper part of the nose is blocked with excessive mucus, as in a severe head cold, we have difficulty in differentiating by taste foods of the same consistency. Loss of the sense of smell is known as ANOSMIA.

Many attempts to classify smell have been made, the most recent being into burned, fragrant, rancid, sour and blends of these. Sensitivity to scents and odours increases when the atmosphere is moist (explaining why flowers smell more perceptibly after the dew has fallen) and when the temperature rises. For some smells there is differing sensitivity between the sexes, e.g., men can in general detect the odour of coffee more quickly than women. There are, however, considerable individual differences, and even in any one person there may well be some day to day variations of sensitivity to odours.

smoking. While many dried plants can be smoked (e.g., opium) the term normally means the drawing into the mouth of the smoke created by burning tobacco.

Although it was realized that over-indulgence in tobacco could lead to chronic inflammation of the throat, hoarseness, excessive secretion of mucus and an irritating cough, and that it could impair the appetite and make the complexion 'muddy', smoking was not significantly associated with the occurrence of serious diseases until after the middle of the present century.

Smoking is an expensive pastime but its devotees claim that the expenditure is well worthwhile. Smoking certainly facilitates social intercourse, and indeed one of its dangers is perhaps that all smokers tend to smoke more when in company. A pipe, and perhaps a cigarette or a cigar, is alleged to be emotionally calming, and smoking certainly gives a nervous person something with which to occupy his hands.

Undisputed physiological effects of smoking are that it raises the blood sugar (so that it is satisfying to a hungry person who is temporarily unable to obtain food), that it tends slightly to quicken the heart rate and to increase the blood pressure, and that it after a time raises the level of blood platelets and appears to increase their adhesiveness (a point which may explain the relation of heavy smoking to coronary thrombosis).

Over the last thirty years evidence has been accumulating about the relationship between smoking and various diseases, but widespread publication of the facts has produced singularly little change in smoking habits – perhaps because virulent anti-smokers have damaged their cause by exaggerating the dangers. It is probably fair to say that smoking is not the sole cause or even the main cause of any disease, but that smoking, especially heavy smoking and in particular heavy cigarette smoking, increases the likelihood of various diseases. Here are a few points.

1. Influence on duration of life. Heavy cigarette smokers have an appreciably greater chance of early death. The evidence may be summarized by expressing the percentage of men aged 35 who may expect to die before the age of 65 as – non-smokers, 15; smokers of 1 to 14 cigarettes per day, 22; smokers of 15 to 24 per day, 25; smokers of over 25 per day, 33. The American Framington study which followed up a cohort of men for eighteen years showed little difference in the life expectation of non-smokers, ex-smokers, pipe smokers and smokers of under 10 cigarettes per day but confirmed the reduced life expectation of heavy cigarette smokers.

2. Influence on coronary thrombosis, a very common disease of middle and later life. Various studies have shown that the ratio of coronary attacks in heavy cigarette smokers to that in non-smokers is approximately 14 to 10. Coronary thrombosis is common enough in non-smokers, so smoking is certainly not the main cause, but the ratio should certainly cause the heavy smoker to think.

3. Influence on lung cancer, still a relatively uncommon disease. Here the evidence is much more definite. Lung cancer is about thirty times as common in heavy cigarette smokers as in non-smokers, and tobacco has been proved to contain several substances liable to cause cancer (carcinogens).

4. Influence on other respiratory diseases. A smoker's cough (commoner in cigarette smokers than in pipe smokers) is indicative of irritation of the respiratory system, and chronic bronchitis is much more frequent in smokers than in non-smokers. Other respiratory diseases, such as asthma, appear to be no more common in smokers than in non-smokers.

In general it appears that cigarette smoking is much more associated with harmful effects than pipe or cigar smoking, possibly because a cigarette burns at a higher temperature, or because different portions of the tobacco leaf are used.

Some advocates of smoking have pointed out that comparison of smokers and non-smokers is not necessarily of like with like. Psychological studies have suggested that heavy smokers are more energetic, restless and extroverted than non-smokers, so that (irrespective of smoking) they might be more liable to coronary disease. That, however, hardly holds true for lung cancer which has been produced experimentally in animals by measures equivalent to heavy smoking.

Again, advocates of smoking have indicated that smoking depresses the appetite, that most people who stop smoking gain weight and that obesity may be more dangerous than continuation of smoking. Anti-smokers maintain that the death rate in ex-smokers (despite possibility of obesity) is less than in continuing smokers, but the question once more arises of whether we are comparing like with like.

Everything written about smoking is controversial. It has some proved and some probable associations with diseases, it is expensive, it gives personal pleasure and is an easily acquired addiction, and while about 80 per cent of people can discontinue it if they so desire, the other 20 per cent find discontinuation extremely difficult. Many doctors and other health workers have reached the position of saying: (1) that they unhesitatingly advise children not to start and adolescents and young adults who are light smokers to discontinue; (2) that they do not advise long-continuing smokers in older age-groups (say from 60 years upwards) to seek to discontinue unless they have diseases actually harmed by smoking; and (3) that they are in some doubt about how to advise persons between 30 and 60 years.

If the undesirability of smoking is accepted various measures need to be considered:

1. Fiscal measures that increase the tax until people hesitate to pay the amount demanded. Duty on tobacco, already very heavy in countries like Norway, Sweden and Britain, now amounts in Britain to nearly one-fifth of the Government's revenue, whereas the cost in Britain of diseases directly attributable to smoking is relatively small. It would be a very bold Chancellor of the Exchequer who would so vastly raise the tax as to deprive himself of a large slice of national income, and a very fervent anti-smoker who would advocate such action with a balancing steep increase in income tax. Moreover, sudden cessation of purchases of tobacco would have serious effects on the economy of tobacco-growing countries.

2. Restriction of advertising. This has been tried in Britain in respect of television advertising with very doubtful results. There was no marked drop in the sale of cigarettes. Also a study by a health visitor of children's smoking habits just before the ban of television advertising showed no relationship between the brands bought and the brands advertised. Equally, a formal warning on cigarette packets that smoking may damage health has proved ineffective. Just as a child will climb a particular tree if told that it is dangerous, so perhaps many of us respond to the challenge of taking a risk.

3. Health education of adults. The value of campaigns is a little questionable. (1) It is possible that the adult who increases weight by stopping may be at greater risk than before. (2) The person who gains real or imaginary consolation from tobacco may substitute more dangerous consolations, e.g., drugs. (3) Anti-smoking campaigns concentrating on mass media have in general failed. (4) Anti-smoking clinics have not really proved their value. Since smoking by expectant mothers has detrimental effects on babies and since most expectant mothers are still fairly young, an approach to them might be useful. Again a campaign to influence selected groups that in turn influence the community – e.g., doctors, nurses and teachers – might be worth trying.

4. Health education of those who are not yet confirmed addicts. Campaigns directed to school children and adolescents are probably the most useful line of approach. In such campaigns two things should be avoided: (1) health arguments – about disease thirty years later – make little impression on the young or merely worry them about the risks that their parents are taking; and (2) it is fatal to associate health education with a kill-joy attitude consisting of a series of negatives – a condemnation of cigarettes, alcohol, sweets, cannabis, promiscuous sex and so on. Perhaps the best hope lies in an appeal to the boy's athletic strength ('wind' for football and racing) and to the girl's beauty (stained teeth and tobacco-laden breath).

5. Production of a carcinogen-free cigarette. This would seem obviously desirable, but in countries like Britain every time that a firm announces the manufacture of a cigarette free of cancer-producing substances, the Treasury intimates that it will be subjected to exactly the same taxation as ordinary tobacco.

6. Encouragement of changing from cigarettes to a pipe or small cigars. This would seem clearly desirable but most of the exponents of the dangers of smoking appear to have an 'all or nothing' approach.

7. Encouragement of moderation in smoking. Some of the many published investigations show little if any differences between light smokers and non-smokers, and all published studies highlight the danger of heavy smoking. There might well be a far better response to appeals to keep cigarette consumption to under ten per day and not to inhale than to appeals to stop smoking altogether.

snake bite. Poisonous snakes occur in all tropical and sub-tropical countries and to some extent in more northern climates. Not all snakes are poisonous, but identification of the biting snake is important because a specific antidote, if available, is more effective than a general one for all snake bites. In general the poison is injected from hollow fangs which connect with poison glands, and identification involves study of the fangs.

The highly poisonous cobras and mambas have fangs fixed in the upper jaw with few or no other teeth in that jaw, and these snakes usually have heads covered with large scales. Vipers and pit vipers (such as the rattlesnake of North America) have erectile fangs which when relaxed lie in a sheath of mucous membrane, and most of them have heads covered with small scales; some are very poisonous but the adder of Europe is seldom fatal to adults. There are also several varieties of highly poisonous sea snakes.

In general snake bites are indicated by two clean puncture wounds, often about an inch apart. Immediate treatment consists of the application of a tourniquet between the bite and the body (to reduce circulation of venom) with subsequent loosening of the tourniquet for a few minutes every quarter of an hour. If practicable, the patient should be immediately transferred to hospital, with reassurance given meantime, together with any available measures for relief of pain. The affected part should be put at rest and the patient's breathing safeguarded during removal to hospital. Incision of the wound and sucking away of the venom is no longer considered useful, although it has a long history.

The symptoms vary according to the type of snake but after initial shock and pain usually include the development within twenty minutes of swelling and paralysis of the bitten part. Generalized effects include colic, pallor, vomiting and sometimes collapse with both respiratory and circulatory distress. Specific anti-venom (or failing that, polyvalent antivenom) can be life-saving; stimulants can help the flagging respiratory and circulatory systems; as much rest as is practicable is essential, and corticosteroids can also be of help. Antivenom, so useful for the bites of many tropical snakes, is of doubtful value for adder bites, because in almost all cases the victim recovers without serum treatment about as rapidly as with it, and in a few cases serum produces a violent allergic reaction.

In the absence of prompt skilled treatment the outlook varies from a 50 per cent chance of death from the bite of a black mamba to a 1 per cent chance from that of a European adder.

sneezing. Sudden expulsion of air through the nose, occurring as an involuntary reflex action to remove irritation. Sneezing may be caused by the presence of irritating particles (e.g., pepper, snuff, and the pollen of some flowers) or may be an early symptom of cold in the head, influenza, hay fever or certain infections (e.g., measles). When a person with an infection, such as a head cold, sneezes otherwise than into a handkerchief he is liable to spray infectious droplets around for as much as a couple of yards.

Repeated sneezing may imply that control of the relevant muscles has been lost and has to be regained, as in the case of continued hiccough. A cold sponge pressed against the face sometimes helps.

snoring. Noise due to vibration of the soft palate, generally occurring from sleeping with the mouth open, especially when lying on the back. Occasional snoring can often be stopped if the sleeper can be induced to turn on to his side. In children snoring is usually due to the presence of enlarged adenoids.

The term is normally reserved for noisy breathing during sleep. Similar noisy breathing, also due to flapping of the soft palate, occurring when a person is not asleep is called stertor and arises in apoplexy, drunkenness and morphine poisoning.

snuffles. Noisy breathing through the nose (in contrast to snoring where the breathing is through the mouth). The condition is associated with nasal catarrh.

social aspects of health. Nearly all illnesses involve social factors, just as nearly all

social problems involve health factors. Yet interest in the relationships between health and disease on the one hand and social factors and circumstances on the other spread gradually. In part it was due to the social awareness of some forward-looking public health medical officers and of a smaller number of general practitioners, in part to the rising professional status of health visitors (e.g., in the U.K.) and public health nurses (e.g., in Sweden) who from the nature of their work could not avoid becoming aware of the social circumstances and attitudes of their clients, and in part to the emergence of sociology as an independent science and to the slightly earlier emergence of modern psychology. By the middle 1950s the medical officer of health had been described as 'a sociologist with clinical insight' and the post-nursing training of student health visitors was beginning to include sociology.

Interested health workers began to realize that some diseases (e.g., coronary thrombosis) were associated with af-fluence and others with poverty, and that many less obvious factors played a part, e.g., susceptibility to tuberculosis is increased in persons suffering from serious bereavement. Health workers and social scientists in collaboration also established many points. To give two completely different examples, they showed that upbringing and life style from birth onwards had as strong an effect on an expectant mother as had the nine months of pregnancy, and they demonstrated that in industries handling asbestos safety precautions to reduce the intake of asbestos particles were not enough by themselves since workers often regarded masks and other devices as uncomfortable and as hindering productivity and so reducing income.

Physical and environmental factors affecting health are nowadays well recognized, e.g., the adverse effects of over-nutrition, under-nutrition, faulty diet in respect of individual constituents, overcrowding, excessive noise and inade-quate exercise. Mental and social factors are in the process of becoming recognized, e.g., it is now appreciated that during the comradeship and collaborative effort of the Second World War various mental and psychosomatic diseases became less common, and that these diseases are more frequent in conditions of obvious loneliness (such as a lighthouse keeper) or partially disguised loneliness (like a clergyman in a remote district with no other persons of good education near him) than in close-knit communities (such as a miner in a mining town).

Many difficulties still interfere with the full application of social knowledge to the improvement of health and the reduction of disease. A few may be mentioned here. Firstly, skilled medical treatment is inevitably given mainly in hospitals, where neither doctors nor nurses can know much about the social circumstances, values and cultural pressures affecting a short-stay patient, never having seen his home or place of work. Secondly, health workers, especially doctors, often unknowingly seek to force middle or upper class ideas and values on their patients. Again, health workers may not be consulted in illness: a woman with severe backache may decide against investigation and treatment because of the anticipated costs (in a country without a national health service) or because of the feared impact on her family if she is temporarily transferred to hospital. Yet again, some people - especially some social scientists - question whether the doctor should be the sole arbiter of what is or is not perceived as illness, e.g., deciding whether a person whose behaviour is at variance with that of the surrounding neighbourhood should be diagnosed as insane and removed to a closed institution, or deciding which of two equally ill patients should be admitted to the only available hospital bed.

Even in health education, the branch of the health and disease services to which sociology has made the largest contribution, there are still some educators who fail to change attitudes and habits because they unconsciously attribute their own beliefs and values to the people whom they are trying to teach.

Moreover, in the U.K. the rigid separation of health services and social services has certainly not contributed to increased awareness of the interaction of health factors and social factors.

sodium. A metallic element of remarkably low density and great softness and one of the essential MINERAL SALTS in the diet. The element does not exist in pure form in nature, and is best known in the form of some of its salts, e.g., sodium chloride (common salt). Sodium chloride is present in all bodily fluids and the maintenance of its level is essential to life. See SALT.

sodomy. Anal intercourse, i.e. intercourse in which the penis is inserted into the anus, commonly practised by active homosexuals, and sometimes between men and women.

soft sore. See CHANCROID.

somatic. Pertaining to the body as opposed to the mind. In medicine the term is used when differentiating physical ailments from mental or psychological illnesses, and psychosomatic is the word employed when mental or emotional causes produce physical effects.

somatotype. A term sometimes employed in attempts to classify physique. A big-boned, well-muscled person is described as being of mesomorphic somatotype and a small-boned, poorly-muscled person is of ectomorphic somatotype, while a third type is called endomorphic. Determination of somatotype involves a complicated series of measurements.

Undoubtedly we need some classifica-tion of physique: for instance the old idea of saying that a man of a particular height had a particular optimum weight was clearly faulty, since large-boned and small-boned persons of equal height would have appreciably different ideal weights. Nevertheless, many workers consider that the twenty separate measurements required for determination of somatotype are too elaborate for general use.

somnambulism. See SLEEP WALKING.

sore throat. Inflammation of the tonsils, pharynx, oesophagus or larynx, with pain and usually reddening. Common causes include excessive talking and shouting, excessive smoking, and bacterial and virus infection. Serious throat conditions include quinsy, Vincent's angina and cancer of the oesophagus.

The value of gargling and of various types of slowly dissolving lozenges is in some doubt, but they can be tried, along with avoidance of the causal factor, if known. In general the continuation of a sore throat for more than three days justifies the seeking of medical advice, and if there is any breathing difficulty associated with the sore throat the doctor should be consulted at once.

spa. An institution specializing in the regulated drinking of (and bathing in) natural water, usually with a high content of mineral salts. The aim of the treatment is the removal of the waste products of faulty metabolism through the kidneys, the bowels and the skin.

Spa treatment, e.g., for rheumatism, is a very old method of attempting to combat disease. In so far as any benefit accrues from spa treatment it is probably due not to the drinking of the water but to the ordered discipline of spa life, the complete change of diet and the mental peace resulting from the removal of ordinary daily cares and worries.

Spanish fly. See CANTHARIDES.

spare-part surgery. A term sometimes used for the replacement of damaged parts of the body by parts made of stainless steel alloys, silicones, plastics or other inert materials. False teeth are the oldest and best known example. Steel alloy replacements are already quite common for the hip joint and are occasionally used for the elbow joint and the knee. Plastic tubes are sometimes employed to replace diseased portions of blood-vessels. Silicones are used to repair damage to the ear, the chin bone and the testicle, and battery-run cardiac pacemakers coated with silicone can replace a defective natural pacemaker in the heart.

In many cases replacement of a damaged joint or organ by inert material is easier and simpler than TRANSPLANT surgery from a very recently deceased person, because transplant surgery (involving living tissue) often produces a rejection reaction, whereas inert materials do not produce such reactions and do not irritate neighbouring tissues.

spasm. A sudden involuntary contraction of a muscle or group of muscles. The muscle fibres in the walls of blood vessels and other tubes may also develop spasm to obstruct blood-flow or otherwise affect function; arterial claudication produced in this way occurs particularly in the heart and brain and in the limbs. Bronchial spasm produces asthma.

Spasm also occurs in epilepsy and other diseases of the central nervous system; it is a feature of such conditions as chorea, meningitis, tetanus and rabies; it is characteristic of strychnine poisoning; and spasm of the hands and feet is a symptom of infantile tetany. Various occupational cramps such as writer's or telegraphist's cramp are similarly the result of muscular spasm.

Spasms of psychogenic origin are described under TIC.

spastic. A form of paralysis in which the affected muscles are kept taut or in spasm. While a spastic paralysis can occur at any age (e.g., as a result of brain injury or of stroke) the term spastic is usually applied to a form originating before birth though not always recognizable in the first few months of life. In a typical spastic the legs are usually more seriously affected than the arms and the person walks with a curious stiff gait. Mental development is sometimes also retarded.

The causes of the condition include shortage of oxygen to the brain in the interval between the baby getting his oxygen from the mother's blood and starting to breathe for himself, jaundice of the new born, and birth injury, all in large measure preventable. Yet the condition is not uncommon, although the emphasis on it in developed countries nowadays implies not that it is increasing but that other forms of handicap in children (e.g., those due to rickets, tuberculosis and poliomyelitis) have decreased sharply. In general a severely affected child is best educated in a special school for spastics.

specialization. In the context of disease and its treatment, specialization means that particular knowledge and skills have come to be differentiated into increasingly narrow fields recognized as specialities and practised by individuals who concentrate on 'knowing more and more about less and less' and who follow careers as specialists.

The range of recognized specialities is now immense. In broad terms the nine 'families' within the whole range of the medical profession are: general medicine; general , surgery; obstetrics and gynaecology; general practice; psychiatry; community medicine; pathology; anaesthetics; radiology and radiotherapy. Many are still further subdivided. General medicine for instance includes sub-specialities in: internal medicine; cardio-vascular disease; clinical pharmacology; communicable diseases; dermatology; endocrinology; gastro-enterology; geriatrics; clinical haematology; neurology; renal disease; respiratory disease; rheumatology; and venereology.

Specialization now occurs also in other health professions. For instance the health visitor and the midwife are specialized nurses with extensive post-qualification trainings, and in each of these professions there is further specialization, e.g., the specialist health visitor concentrating on health education of groups or on the well-being of old people, or the midwife with specialized experience of premature babies.

On the whole, specialization improves and increases skills and is therefore beneficial to the patient; but a stage may be reached at which many people have expert knowledge of the various diseases from which members of a family suffer but nobody really understands the particular family and its problems and interactions.

spectacles. A set of two glass or plastic lenses in a frame, worn in front of the eyes to improve the clarity of the EYESIGHT.

Probably the commonest error of spectacle users is to forget to clean them frequently. Dust from the atmosphere easily settles on the lenses, as does grease. Yet people who would never dream of facing the day's activities without washing their faces will frequently put on spectacles that have lost half their effectiveness through being uncleaned.

speech. The power of articulating words intelligibly. Many animals possess some power of vocal communication. Yet the ability for exact and detailed communication in words – the ability to say 'A tall, white-haired man wearing spectacles is coming up the garden path' – is specifically human.

Words are formulated in a speech centre of the cerebral cortex, a centre which lies on the left-hand side of the brain in right-handed persons and on the right-hand side in left-handed persons. The sounds themselves, i.e., the VOICE, are produced by vibration of the vocal cords of the larynx; and essentially the vowel sounds are formed by the larynx but produced by the shape of the mouth, while the consonants depend mainly on the position of the palate, tongue, lips and teeth.

Some of the many causes of speech disorders are as follows.

1. Deafness. A person deaf from infancy will not learn to speak unless taught by special methods. A person who becomes deaf later in life may gradually undergo changes in his speech because he no longer hears himself pronouncing words.

2. Mental handicap. In extreme cases the person does not have the intelligence to understand what is said or to formulate answers. In less extreme cases his vocabulary will be small and his articulation poor.

3. Emotional disorders. These may

produce stammering or stuttering, or sometimes complete absence of speech.

4. Damage to the speech centre, e.g., from a stroke, a brain tumour or multiple sclerosis. Depending on the nature of the damage speech may be totally absent, or slurred, or unrecognizable gibberish.

5. Abnormalities of the larynx. Examples are the hoarseness or even temporary speechlessness of laryngitis, and the loss of voice following surgical removal of the larynx.

6. Abnormalities of the mouth, palate, tongue or teeth. Examples are the defective speech associated with hare lip and cleft palate, and the milder articulation difficulties associated with badly fitting dentures.

Treatment manifestly varies with the cause; but except in cases of serious brain damage it is likely that speech therapy, or psychological treatment, or any necessary dental or surgical attention will materially improve the speech.

spermatic cord. A bundle of fibrous tissue and rudimentary muscle fibres containing the duct of the testis and the blood vessels of the testis and epididymis and thus forming part of the male REPRODUCTIVE SYSTEM. The passage of the cord from the abdomen to the groin, through the subcutaneous inguinal ring, creates a weak spot at which a hernia sometimes develops.

spermatorrhoea. Involuntary discharge of seminal fluid occurring at times other than during copulation. Seminal emission is common during adolescence and young adult life and has no sinister significance. At these ages the testes are very active in sperm-production and the distended seminal vesicles periodically discharge excess secretion.

Spermatorrhoea is also sometimes a symptom in neurasthenia and becomes a matter of further needless anxiety to the patient.

spermatozoon. A mature male germ-cell. Spermatozoa develop in the testes and are the fertilizing element of male seminal fluid where they are present in great numbers. Each is a single modified cell with a flattened oval head, an elongated cylindrical neck and body, and a long filamentous tail. Their overall length is about six-hundredths of a millimetre.

Spermatozoa are actively mobile by using their tails and so are capable of ascending from vagina to uterus and Fallopian tubes of the female REPRODUCTIVE SYSTEM. Fertilization of a mature ovum generally occurs in the Fallopian tube; a single spermatozoon pierces the capsule of the ovum, achieves fusion with the female nucleus and so starts the development of a new individual.

sphincter. A ring-like band of muscle-fibres found at the entrances or exits of hollow organs and ducts. Muscle contraction reduces the diameter of the ring, narrows or closes the opening or passage and thus

Spermatozoa

controls the flow of any contained material.

The best known examples of sphincter muscles are the cardiac sphincter at the junction of oesophagus and stomach; the pyloric sphincter at the lower end of the stomach; the anal sphincter at the lower end of the anal canal; and the urethral sphincter at the outlet from the bladder. Sphincter oculi is a term sometimes used to describe the circular muscle fibres in the iris which constrict the pupil and so control the amount of light passing through to the retina.

Sphygmomanometer

sphygmomanometer. A clinical appliance for measuring arterial BLOOD PRESSURE. An inflatable cuff is wrapped around the patient's arm and air pumped into it until it constricts the arm sufficiently for the pulse-beat to be stopped. This air pressure is meantime also raising a column of mercury against a scale and the blood pressure is recorded according to the height of the column of mercury.

spider. A name applied to eight-legged, wingless, predacious arachnids, most of which spin webs in which to trap their prey.

Although most varieties, like the ordinary garden spider, are harmless to man, fear of spiders is remarkably common.

Dangerous varieties whose bite can sometimes kill include the American black widow, also found in some European countries; the Russian karakut spider; and the Australian night stinger. After initial local pain, swelling and reddening, bites from these insects are followed by a general reaction of muscle pains and spasms, sweating, fever and rapid pulse, and danger of circulatory collapse. If available, an injection of calcium gluconate into a vein helps the muscle pains and spasm; and antivenines have been prepared and are available in some countries.

The notorious tarantula, much utilized by writers of fiction, gives a very painful bite but is unlikely to prove fatal to any animal as large as man.

spina bifida. A congenital abnormality affecting the spinal cord and spinal column. During the early life of the embryo the outer layer of cells running down the back of the body curls over to form the neural groove and this closes right over, becoming a tube lying just below the surface skin. As development continues, this tube forms the spinal cord with the vertebrae of the SPINAL COLUMN protecting it. The cord lies within the vertebral canal, formed by the neural arches of the vertebrae. In spina bifida the primitive neural groove fails to close and the vertebral canal becomes deficient at the back because of the faulty development of the vertebral arches. These defects lead to anatomical and functional abnormalities of varying degree: in spina bifida occulta involvement of the cord and its membranes containing cerebrospinal fluid; in meningo-myelocele the protrusion also involves part of the spinal cord and associated nerves; in myelocele the unprotected and malformed nervous structures lie exposed in a central cleft.

About 2,000 new cases of spina bifida occur in Great Britain each year. The incidence varies from 1 in 500 to 1 in 250 births and it is a major handicapping condition of childhood. Its cause is largely genetic, although social class, birth order, nutritional state, maternal age, and infections during early pregnancy have also been shown to have significant effects.

Before the introduction of early surgical treatment in the 1950s most cases died in early life but now a long-term survival rate of 50 per cent may be expected.

Survival, however, raises great problems not only of clinical management but of educational, social, and emotional adjustment. Some 60 per cent of the survivors require special education because of physical and mental handicap

vertebral projections

body of vertebrae

spinal cord protruding through defective vertebrae structure

Spina bifida

since the effects of spina bifida include defects of movement due to paraplegia, urinary and faecal incontinence, sensory defects, skin ulceration, and brain damage resulting from hydrocephalus, often an associated condition. The care of a child with spina bifida is a team effort involving medical and nursing skills, together with guidance in relation to educational, social and employment difficulties. The parents also require help and social support. In view of the substantial hereditary element in the condition there is need for GENETIC GUIDANCE and family planning advice.

spinal column. The vertebral column or main axis of the body consists of a series of bones called vertebrae, united to one another by intervertebral fibro-cartilaginous discs and by ligaments. The vertebrae number thirty-three and, although conforming to a standard pattern, they have individual characteristics as the cervical (seven), thoracic (twelve), lumbar (five), sacral (five), and coccygeal (four) vertebrae. In the first three groups the twenty-four vertebrae are each separately mobile so that the column is flexible. It can bend in all directions and rotate to a limited extent, but the sacral and coccygeal vertebrae are fused to form the sacrum and coccyx respectively.

Each of the vertebrae has four projections, two upper and two lower, which form the joints with the corresponding parts of the adjoining vertebrae and, in the case of the lowest of the lumber vertebrae, with the sacrum below. Between these joints there are firmly attached pads of fibro-cartilaginous tissue known as the intervertebral discs.

The vertebrae each have an arch towards the back and these, lying as they do one above the other, form the vertebral canal in which lies the spinal cord, which ends at the level of the first of the lumbar vertebrae. The spinal nerves leave the cord and emerge pair by pair, from between the vertebrae and from openings on the inner surface of the sacrum.

The bones of the spinal column are supported and laced together by fibrous ligaments and attached to this composite structure are the muscles which provide the power for voluntary movement – bending forwards (flexion), backwards (extension), and sideways (lateral bending), and also some rotation.

Viewed from the side the column has certain natural curves, concave backwards in the cervical (i.e., neck) and lumbar (small of the back) regions and concave forwards in relation to the thorax (chest) and sacrum (low back). The size and massiveness of the vertebrae increase progressively from above downwards and the upper two cervical vertebrae – the atlas and axis – are particularly specialized in form to support the skull and to permit rotation of the head.

Injuries. The spinal column is very strong but indirect violence may produce fracture-dislocations with risk of injury to the spinal cord, which runs within the vertebral canal, but in lesser injuries the continuity of the column is preserved.

Such lesser injuries include sprains, twists, partial and complete dislocations of the joints between vertebrae, and fractures of the vertebral bodies, neural arches (the parts of the vertebrae which enclose the spinal canal), or of the articular, spinous or transverse processes (the projections from the neural arch which provide anchorage for the muscles of the back). Sprains are commonest in the more mobile cervical and lumbar regions and are produced by sudden and excessive stretching of ligaments as in 'whiplash' car accidents or over-lifting. There is pain and muscular spasm but no x-ray evidence of injury. Fractures result from direct blows, sudden excessive bending, or abnormal stresses. An x-ray will confirm bony injury and such cases require rest and orthopaedic measures to secure repair, followed by physiotherapy.

In complete lesions the column is broken and displaced (fracture-dislocation), a common result of falls or of riding and traffic accidents. The chief risk is to the spinal cord itself which gets crushed between the arch and body of the adjacent vertebrae, so that PARAPLEGIA results. Skilled and prolonged treatment is needed but prospects are poor. The cord ends at the level of the first lumbar vertebra and lesions below this involve only the leash of nerve-roots known as the cauda equina, and subsequent restoration of function is more possible.

Deformities and diseases. Deformities of the spinal column may result from congenital defects, from diseases of the bone, or from the effects of soft-tissue changes. Apart from SPINA BIFIDA congenital conditions are rare. There may

be absence of a part or whole of one or more vertebral bodies, fusion of adjacent vertebrae, or other defects. In disease there may be defective ossification, bony softening or bone destruction.

However, most of the postural defects are due to muscular or ligamentous changes; see CURVATURE OF THE SPINE.

The small joints of the spine are also prone to develop arthritic changes, especially in later life, producing SPONDYLITIS (inflammatory changes) or spondylosis (joint fixation); and damage to an intervertebral disc is a frequent cause of disability known as SLIPPED DISC.

spinal column, tuberculosis of. Tuberculous infection of the vertebrae is sometimes called Pott's disease. Bacilli reach the affected site through the blood stream from a pre-existing focus, usually in the lungs or in the lymphatic glands of the neck or abdomen. Such primary lesions are now rare in most developed countries because of better control of sources of bovine and human infection. Consequently the incidence of any type of bone or joint tuberculosis has dramatically declined.

Most cases occur in children below the age of puberty. The disease usually affects the vertebral bodies, especially in the thoracic and lumbar regions, and these become eroded, with symptoms of pain and rigidity, and then collapse to reduce the deformity of kyphosis. In the thoracic region this appears as the typical angulation commonly called 'hunch-back'. Lumbar involvement causes less obvious deformity but pus produced may track down within the sheath of the psoas muscle (the muscle attached to the front of the lumbar vertebrae and passing in front of the hip-joint to the femur) to appear at the pelvic brim as a psoas abscess.

The treatment of spinal tuberculosis requires prolonged rest, orthopaedic appliances to immobilize the affected area, and anti-tuberculous drugs. With an adequate regime most cases eventually make a good recovery.

spinal cord and nerves. The spinal cord is an elongated cylindrical part of the central nervous system occupying the canal in the spinal column from the base of the skull to the level of the first lumbar vertebra. In an average adult it is about 45 cm. long and 1.25 cm. in diameter, tapering towards its lower end, and is enclosed within three layers of membranes corresponding to the meninges of the BRAIN. It is composed almost entirely of nerve-tissue with a core of grey matter or nerve cells surrounded by white matter consisting of nerve fibres which are disposed as 'tracts' conveying impulses up or down its length.

At regular intervals there arise thirty-one pairs of spinal nerves each having an anterior and posterior root, the latter distinguished by an oval swelling or spinal ganglion containing nerve cells. These spinal nerves are bundles of both motor and sensory nerve fibres which respectively relay outward impulses to related muscles and carry incoming sensory stimuli. The motor fibres leave the cord by the anterior root and fibres carrying sensory impressions enter by the posterior root.

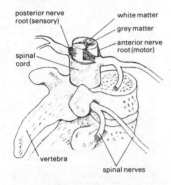

posterior nerve root (sensory)

white matter

grey matter

anterior nerve root (motor)

spinal cord

vertebra

spinal nerves

Anatomy of the spinal cord

Within its membranes the cord, like the brain, is also surrounded by cerebrospinal fluid acting as a water-cushion for support and protection. Since cerebrospinal fluid may show changes in certain diseases, a sample may be helpful for diagnosis. This is obtained by lumbar puncture, a hollow needle being inserted between the lumbar vertebrae. Similarly drugs may be injected for treatment or to produce spinal anaesthesia.

Diseases. The brain and spinal cord are continuous, lined by the same membranes and subject to the same diseases but with great differences in frequency. This article deals only with diseases of the cord, but see also BRAIN.

Haemorrhages and tumours (both common in the brain) are very rare. Such tumours as occur are seldom tumours of the cord itself but either meningiomas (growths in the lining membranes) or bony tumours which press on the cord. However, nerves which run from the spinal cord to the various parts of the body are often involved in certain general diseases, some of which (like poliomyelitis, locomotor ataxia and shingles) are due to specific infections.

For most of the other diseases of the spinal cord the causes are less clear.

Some, like Friedrich's ataxia, are familial or hereditary, some, such as syringomyelia, are due to congenital defect, and a particular type of hardening of the nerves at the side of the cord is associated with pernicious anaemia. Other common conditions include multiple (or disseminated) sclerosis and progressive

muscular atrophy, the causes of which are still uncertain.

Special mention must be made of spina bifida, since improved surgical techniques are now saving many children born with this congenital condition.

Injuries. Fracture-dislocations of the vertebral column are very likely to injure the spinal cord and because of its small size the damage usually severs the cord with complete paralysis below the site of injury. The spinal cord does not heal and the results are a permanent loss of movement and sensation (paraplegia).

spirochaete. A general name applied to any long, filamentous, spirally-coiled bacterium. Spirochaetales should be distinguished from the Spirillaceae, another family of curved and sinuous shape but which have other characteristics, and cause quite different diseases.

Spirochaetes cause relapsing fever, Vincent's angina, Weil's disease or spirochaetal jaundice, canicola fever, syphilis, and yaws.

spleen. A large organ situated in the left upper part of the abdomen and of an elongated flattened oblong shape. Its size and weight are very variable but in the adult it is about the size of two hands placed palm to palm and weighs some 200 g. (7 oz.). It is soft, and very well supplied with blood vessels.

Although not essential to life it has several important functions. It acts as a blood-reservoir to augment the blood-volume when the need arises; it breaks down and disposes of damaged or worn out red cells and sets free their haemoglobin which passes to the liver for conversion to bilirubin; it produces new white cells especially in intra-uterine life and in infancy; and it protects against infection by removing micro-organisms from circulation.

The spleen is well protected by its situation high up under the ribs but it is sometimes ruptured by direct or indirect violence. Because of its vascular nature haemorrhage is usually severe. The damage is difficult to repair surgically and it is often necessary to remove the whole organ.

Diseases. The spleen may undergo atrophy in old age or from debility and arterial degeneration, and it may suffer damage to its blood vessels from embolisms in endocarditis and septicaemia, but the usual sign of splenic disease is enlargement of the organ, often to a gross extent – it may reach a weight of 4.5 kg. (10 lbs.). Enlargement (splenomegaly) is easily detected clinically and always calls for further investigation. Its causes are complex because the spleen has several distinct functions.

Its role in bodily defence mechanisms involves the filtering out and destruction of bacteria, protozoan parasites and worn out blood corpuscles. This explains the enlargement seen in infective conditions such as typhoid fever, miliary tuberculosis, malaria, kala-agar, hookworm disease, haemolytic anaemias and polycythaemia.

In post-natal life, its foetal function in blood formation is normally assumed by the bone-marrow but there may be renewal of its primitive activities in diseases such as leukaemia and lymphadenoma. Other splenic cells play a part in the metabolism and storage of fat, haemoglobin and iron. Derangement of this mechanism is seen in Gaucher's splenomegaly and other similar diseases. There is also a condition known as splenic anaemia or Banti's disease characterized by splenomegaly, anaemia, fibrosis of liver and spleen, and jaundice, sometimes controlled completely by removal of the spleen.

Apart from these more individual diseases, the spleen may be affected by amyloid disease, a form of waxy degeneration occurring in chronic toxaemia. It may also be enlarged from the effects of cirrhosis of the liver.

splint. For the use of splints for fractures see First Aid section at the end of the book.

spondylitis. Inflammation of one or more of the vertebrae, often leading to permanent stiffness of the spine (spondylosis) and deformity (kyphosis), and characterized by recurrent severe episodes of backache or, less commonly, of referred pain in the leg. Spondylitis may be due to some infections, e.g., tuberculosis, but the majority of cases are of anchylosing spondylitis, a condition possibly allied to rheumatoid arthritis, thought to be genetic in origin, and affecting mostly young men of athletic habits.

The old treatment of immobilization and use of back supports and braces is now seldom advocated, and deep x-ray therapy is also largely discontinued, partly because of the high relapse rate and partly because of the danger of producing leukaemia. Aspirin and other analgesics are useful; a hard mattress is desirable; and the modern drugs phenylbutazone and oxyphenbutazone are valuable. In general, if the patient endeavours to maintain mobility in the long periods between spasms, the disease appears to burn itself out by about the age of 45 years.

sporadic. A term derived from the Greek word for 'scattered' and used mainly in relation to infectious disease to differentiate the isolated case or small local outbreak from the presence or occurrence of disease in endemic or epidemic prevalence.

spores. Certain bacteria (e.g., those causing anthrax, tetanus and gas gangrene) assume an inert form (spores) to resist adverse conditions. Spores can resist temperatures up to 100 °C and can survive for periods in dust or soil.

spotted fever. A colloquial term most commonly employed as a synonym for cerebrospinal fever (meningococcal meningitis), but Rocky Mountain fever and typhus may also be so described.

sprains. If excessive force or violent movement forces a joint beyond its normal range of action in any direction the supporting ligaments may be overstretched or torn and the result is a sprain. In a sprain-fracture fragments of bone may be simultaneously torn from the point at which the ligaments are attached. In most cases the synovial membrane surrounding the joint is also damaged with the effusion of blood and synovial fluid into the joint cavity. Muscles and tendons may also be torn. There is usually severe pain and some degree of shock shown by feelings of faintness and nausea.

Sprains should be x-rayed to see if there has been injury to the bone. Otherwise the principles of treatment are to put the affected joint in a position of ease and to limit effusion and provide support by a firm, well-padded bandage. Sometimes a splint will be required to ensure adequate fixation. Once effusion subsides (four to five days) passive movements are commenced, followed by gradual active use, avoiding the production of pain or muscular spasm. Other measures may also be required to protect injured structures until they are soundly healed. In general, sprains require to be treated efficiently to avoid persistent or recurrent disability.

sprue. A disease or group of similar diseases characterized by chronic diarrhoea due to unabsorbed fat, loss of weight (both from failure to absorb fats and from voluntary restriction of intake of food because of the diarrhoea), anaemia (from failure to absorb folic acid, vitamin B_{12} and iron), inflammation and soreness of the tongue, and sometimes bone pains and mental apathy.

1. Non-tropical sprue. Best treated initially with a gluten-free diet, i.e., exclusion from the diet of ordinary wheat flour and of all articles made from it. In about 60 per cent of cases the dietetic treatment effects a complete cure but the gluten-free diet has to be continued. In the 40 per cent that do not respond, a high protein, low fat diet is useful and a course of such antibiotics as tetracycline or neomycin should be tried.

2. Tropical sprue. Has similar manifestations but appears to respond better to adequate dosage of folic acid, although a diet containing high protein and low fat is also useful.

squint. For accurate binocular vision (i.e., using both eyes together) the visual axis of both eyes must be correctly aligned so as to converge and meet at the point on which vision is directed. If this does not occur one eye is in a faulty position. This condition is strabismus; the eye is said to 'squint' and its deviation is either obvious to the observer or, when slight, may be demonstrated by optical tests.

Strabismus produces double vision and because this is confusing the brain tends to suppress the image produced by the squinting eye, which gradually loses its visual acuteness. Squints may arise from actual paralysis of muscles controlling the eye movements but in the common squint of childhood there is no paralysis and the squinting eye moves with the sound one but maintains its deviation. Hypermetropia, or long sight, is often associated with the condition.

Squints require supervision by an ophthalmologist, and any persistent deviations observed should be attended to immediately. Various lines of treatment are employed according to circumstances. These include the wearing of spectacles, measures to enforce use of the squinting eye such as a patch or certain drugs that temporarily diminish the vision of the sound eye, exercises, and surgical procedures on the eye muscles.

stammering. Halting or hesitant speech due to spasm or incoordination of the muscles involved. Frequently the first consonant or syllable is repeated several times and this is STUTTERING. Speech is composed of words, and words are formed from vowels and consonants. Vowels are produced in the larynx by the vocal cords vibrating in a flow of air and their sounds are modified by changes in the shape of the mouth. Consonants are formed by interruptions of the air-flow at various 'stop' positions by the lips, teeth, tongue and soft palate. Speech thus depends on an air-flow provided by the respiratory muscles and muscularly controlled by other movements of the mouth, tongue, and adjacent structures. Consonants are interpolations in vocalized sounds; the stammerer adopts the correct 'stop' position for the one he intends to say but he maintains this too long and fails to allow the vowel to follow without delay.

Stammering affects about 1 per cent of children and is more frequent in boys. It is often associated with left-handedness, particularly if the child has been forced to use his right hand for schoolwork. It may appear either at speech-learning stage or later after some stressful experience. Occasionally it may be familial or imitative. Stammerers can usually sing or whisper without difficulty. In verse or song the metre demands orderly management of breath and attention is diverted from articulation to respiration. Other neurotic disorders may be associated indicating that it is a symptom of anxiety or repressed aggression.

Treatment requires much patience. The dominant hand should be determined and the child allowed to use it. Otherwise the emphasis is upon speech training and on child guidance methods. The speech therapist determines which of the 'stop' positions particularly give trouble and then concentrates on exercises and practice for breath-control, voice production, and correct 'stopping' until speech becomes automatic and not a conscious and laboured effort. Child guidance seeks to uncover hidden conflicts. These two activities complement each other. Conquest of speech difficulties gives confidence in other directions and vice versa.

staphylococci. Cocci are minute spherical micro-organisms about one-thousandth of a millimetre in diameter. Staphylococci occur as little compact groups, in contrast with the long chains formed by streptococci.

The two principal species of staphylococci are *Staph. albus* and *Staph. aureus* which develop in culture as white and golden-yellow colonies respectively. *Staph. albus* is ubiquitous and relatively harmless, and can almost always be found on the skin. Both types may however be found in superficial skin infections such as pustular acne, boils, carbuncles, styes, ear infections and so on. *Staph. aureus* is more invasive and is common in such conditions as osteomyelitis. It may subsequently reach the blood stream and cause septicaemia. Contamination of foodstuffs with these organisms and their toxins can also cause staphylococcal food poisoning.

starch. See CARBOHYDRATE.

starvation. The result of denying to the body nutriments adequate to provide its requirements for food and energy. Deprivation may be absolute as in voluntary fasting, hunger-strikes or severe famine; partial when food is scarce; or it may result from disease processes interfering with the intake, digestion, or assimilation of food.

In starvation the body initially secures its needs by drawing upon its own reserves of glycogen and fat. Metabolism of fat in the absence of carbohydrate causes acidosis. When these stores are exhausted tissue protein is then used and extreme wasting develops. Starvation associated with disease is known as cachexia.

Three weeks may be regarded as the average length of survival from starvation if water is available. Deprivation of water cannot be withstood more than a few days. In partial starvation (e.g., 600 Calories daily) people become apathetic, dazed and incapable of coherent thinking.

status lymphaticus. The thymus gland, consisting of lymphoid tissue, is situated in the lower neck and behind the upper part of the breast-bone. It is one of the ENDOCRINE GLANDS and is concerned with antibody formation and defence against infection. It increases in size until puberty and then gradually atrophies.

Some children who are fat, anaemic and lethargic have enlargement of the thymus with overgrowth of lymphoid tissue elsewhere and sometimes die unexpectedly, especially under anaesthesia. Such 'thymic deaths' were once ascribed to status lymphaticus (the lymphoid state) but this is no longer regarded as a satisfactory diagnosis. However, an enlarged thymus can cause respiratory difficulty by pressure on the air-passages, producing respiratory stridor or thymic asthma. Death may thus result in a mechanical way from acute respiratory failure, the likelihood of which is obviously enhanced by anaesthesia.

Thymus enlargement if demonstrably causing symptoms is treated by x-ray irradiation.

stenosis. A narrowing or restriction of any vessel, duct, tube, or canal in the body. The term is most commonly used in relation to disease of the valves in the heart which may result in aortic, pulmonary, mitral or tricuspid stenosis. Arteries may also be narrowed by degenerative disease of their walls and this is of particular importance for the blood supply to heart and brain.

Another frequent site for stenosis is the pylorus or lower outlet of the stomach. See PYLORIC STENOSIS.

sterility. Although also used medically to indicate a condition of being free from germs (e.g., in phrases like 'the sterility of the operating theatre') the word normally means inability to have children. In males sterility is essentially a failure to produce living spermatozoa, and should not be confused with impotence, i.e., the inability to achieve successful intercourse; and in females it is inability to give birth to a viable child.

In an infertile marriage both husband and wife need investigation since the cause of sterility may lie in either.

Female sterility. In primary sterility conception has never taken place; secondary sterility is infertility after one or more previous pregnancies, often as a result of infection following labour or damage to the uterus.

The general causes are complex because a woman has not simply to provide an ovum ripe for fertilization. Before conception her other organs must be able to receive spermatozoa from the male and facilitate their ascent in the genital tract; and after conception they have to provide for the nourishment and protection of the developing embryo during pregnancy.

The basic essential is ovulation or the production of mature ova by the ovaries. Normal menstruation is an indication that this is occurring and confirmation can be obtained by a laboratory test on a tiny portion of the womb-lining which shows the monthly series of changes related to hormone output by the ovary. Hormone disorders and chronic ill-health may affect ovulation.

A comprehensive gynaecological examination of the reproductive system should uncover causes likely to prevent access of spermatozoa. These may be malformed or underdeveloped states of the vulva, vagina, cervix or uterus; the nature of the vaginal secretion is also important.

Fertilization usually takes place in the Fallopian tubes and any factor which prevents descent of the ovum or ascent of the spermatozoa will prevent a union of these germ-cells. Salpingitis (inflammation of the Fallopian tubes) is much the commonest cause. Evidence of blockage or obstruction can be obtained by air-insufflation or by x-ray examination.

Finally, there is the problem of the uterus inadequate to the demands of a full-time pregnancy: conception occurs but pregnancies repeatedly abort. The uterus may be small and poorly developed, malformed or malpositioned, or the seat of some pathological process such as fibroids. Many such cases can be rectified by appropriate surgical treatment.

It will be clear that female sterility is a condition of very diverse causation and that decisions about possible treatment must rest primarily on a painstaking investigation of each individual case.

Male sterility. This not uncommon problem is usually due to some organic disease of the sexual organs. A primary cause is non-production of living spermatozoa by the testes. Testicular atrophy results from certain genetic conditions; from developmental faults as in undescended testes; and from fibrosis of the testes with destruction of the germinal tissue. The latter may occur as a sequel to mumps or other generalized infective conditions, or as a result of x-ray exposure, or in other local diseases affecting both testes.

Secondary causes are those which prevent spermatozoa reaching the exterior. These are practically always due to past inflammatory disease, usually gonococcal in origin, which causes blockage or obstruction. The sites of this may be in the vas deferens, the urethra, or the tubules between testis and epididymis.

Diagnosis of male sterility depends on microscopical examination of seminal fluid for actively mobile spermatozoa. Although some of the obstructive causes may prove to be temporary or intermittent and resolve with treatment or by spontaneous recanalization, there is little hope of any improvement in the cases of non-production of living spermatozoa.

sterilization. 1. In relation to reproduction. Any procedure whereby an individual is rendered sterile or incapable of fathering or bearing children. See BIRTH CONTROL.

2. In relation to surgery. The elimination of micro-organisms from instruments and dressings in contact with wounds and, in special circumstances, even from the air of operating theatres. See ASEPSIS.

sternum. The breastbone, a long flat bone extending from the neck to the abdomen and forming the centre of the front wall of the chest. It articulates at its upper end with the clavicles and its margins unite successively with the cartilaginous ends of the seven upper pairs of ribs.

Fracture of the sternum is uncommon but it is often distorted or displaced by disease, as in rickets, abnormalities of the spinal column, or disease of the respiratory tract. The junctions of ribs and sternum become enlarged in rickets and infantile scurvy to produce the characteristic 'rickety rosary' or 'scurvy-beading'.

stethoscope. An instrument employed to convey sounds, especially of the heart and lungs, to the ear of the examiner. A modern stethoscope consists of two ear pieces attached to flexible rubber tubes which in turn lead to a conical mouthpiece. The mouthpiece is placed against the appropriate part of the body and the sound is transmitted along the tubes to the ears.

stiff neck. The common variety of this condition is acute rheumatic torticollis. It is generally caused by exposure to damp, cold or draughts which precipitate or aggravate an attack of fibrositis involving the neck muscles and their fibrous sheaths. The onset is usually sudden with considerable pain on head-movement and the affected muscles can be felt to be rigid and tender. In chronic torticollis or wry-neck the head assumes an abnormal attitude, usually tilted to one side and slightly rotated to the other side.

Minor injuries to the neck muscles and intervertebral ligaments produce similar signs and symptoms. 'Whiplash' strains arising in traffic accidents are a common cause.

Another variety is reflex torticollis induced by inflammation of adjacent structures such as inflamed glands, cervical abscess, decaying teeth, or disease of the spine.

Rheumatic torticollis usually responds well to rest, local heat and analgesics. Injuries should be investigated to exclude fracture. Other causes require appropriate treatment based on the exact diagnosis.

stilboestrol. A synthetic compound with effects similar to OESTROGEN. It is used in the treatment of cancer of the prostate gland, for contraceptive purposes, for the suppression of lactation, for the treatment of menstrual disorders, in certain skin diseases, and in senile degeneration of the vulvar and vaginal mucous membrane.

still-birth. A child born after the twenty-eighth week of pregnancy and showing no signs of life. Twenty-eight weeks has been generally assumed to be the shortest period of gestation which can produce a viable child. However, there is a growing body of opinion that even younger foetuses can now be regarded as viable because of improved methods of resuscitation and post-natal care, and it has been suggested that twenty-four weeks should now be the criterion, though this is a matter of some controversy.

Since a still-born child has developed successfully until at least its twenty-eighth week, its death must have occurred either from pathological conditions within itself or from extrinsic factors affecting it during subsequent intra-uterine life or at birth. The possible causes within itself are comparatively rare and chiefly due to developmental abnormality.

In intra-uterine life and during labour the child's safety depends on the health of the mother; on the proper functioning and adequacy of the placental circulation; and on the absence of complications during labour which lead to insufficient oxygen reaching the baby or to birth injury. The causes of foetal death or of premature birth with its attendant risks can be summarized thus:

1. In the mother: malnutrition, pre-eclamptic or eclamptic toxaemia (an infection of the blood), high blood pressure, heart disease, diabetes, thyrotoxicosis (resulting from disorders of the thyroid gland), syphilis and sometimes other infections.

2. Affecting the efficiency of the placenta: several previous pregnancies, multiple pregnancy, haemorrhage before labour, and umbilical cord abnormalities.

3. During labour: prolonged and difficult labour; abnormal position of the foetus; some sedatives; injury to the brain either through the size of the head being disproportionate to that of the birth canal or through over-vigorous use of forceps to assist delivery.

The prevention of still-birth depends on several factors: (1) supervision of the expectant mother's physical and emotional health and education about diet, exercise, and so forth – all aspects in which the health visitor can play an important role; (2) skilled antenatal care to anticipate, uncover, and treat threatened departures from normal; (3) hospital resources to provide at need in-patient antenatal care and planned delivery; and (4) skilled help to ensure effective resuscitation of the baby if needed.

The reduction in the numbers of still-births in the third quarter of this century is in large measure an indication of the success of health services in such countries as Sweden, Norway and Britain; but in these countries the proportion of still-births remains higher among the poor than among the wealthy, higher in women over 35 years than in younger mothers and higher in women who have already had four or more children than in those having their first or second.

Still's disease. A type of rheumatoid arthritis occurring in children. It usually appears between the ages of 2 and 4 years; onset may be abrupt with high fever and painful swelling of many joints, or more insidious with gradually increasing stiffness and swelling of the small joints of fingers, hands and wrists. Other special characteristics are enlargement of lymph-glands and spleen and often heart complications, particularly pericarditis.

Wasting, anaemia, muscle contractures and deformities usually follow. Although remissions or arrest do occur the course of the disease tends to be progressive and may lead to complete invalidism. Rest is essential and other treatment is usually by salicylates, steroids and physiotherapy.

Surgery may be required to deal with contractures. Death from intercurrent infection or cardiac complications is not unknown.

stimulant. Any substance that temporarily quickens the rate of a mental or physical activity. If a stimulant is to be effective there clearly must be a certain amount of reserve power in the organ that is to be stimulated. To use a stimulant where there is no such reserve power is simply the equivalent of whipping an exhausted horse.

There are a vast number of drugs which stimulate various functions in the body, e.g., digitalis stimulates heart muscle, and diuretics stimulate the action of the kidneys. Since such stimulants act in a variety of different ways the word is seldom used in medicine.

In common parlance the term is generally employed for two types of substance. (1) It is used (correctly) for drugs which temporarily increase mental alertness, such as the amphetamines and to a smaller extent the caffeine contained in coffee and tea. They have after-effects of course, because the central nervous system cannot be overworked for some hours without cost, but are genuine stimulants. (2) The term is very commonly used for alcohol. Alcohol has many uses: it provides a very rapid source of energy in exhaustion, it creates bodily warmth after exposure to cold (although it should not be given while the person is still exposed to cold), and it removes inhibitions and decreases shyness; but it actually lowers reaction time and mental and physical activity, and is therefore really the reverse of a stimulant.

stings. See BITES AND STINGS.

stitch. A severe pain, usually experienced on one side of the abdomen just below the ribs, and commonly brought on by unaccustomed running or other excessive exertion. It is due to cramp of the abdominal muscles which are maintaining firm contraction in order to protect the abdominal organs from being jolted about. It rapidly recovers with rest and no special treatment is required.

The word 'stitch' is also synonymous with a surgical SUTURE, used in sewing up wounds.

stomach. A capacious musculo-membranous pouch forming part of the DIGESTIVE SYSTEM between the lower end of the gullet, or oesophagus, and the duodenum, or beginning of the small intestine. Situated in the upper abdomen, it is J-shaped with the vertical part expanded to form the fundus and the hook of the J narrowing to the pyloric antrum and sphincter. Food enters through the cardiac orifice just below the diaphragm and is retained for digestion for about four hours. Ferments and hydrochloric acid for this purpose are secreted by multiple glands in the mucous lining of the organ. Muscular movements of the stomach churn and mix its contents with the digestive secretions.

When gastric digestion is complete, the pyloric sphincter, or lower opening, relaxes to allow the prepared contents to pass to the small intestine for further treatment and subsequent absorption.

Diseases. Minor disorders of the stomach are very common.

Indigestion or dyspepsia may be due to acute or chronic gastritis caused primarily by stomach irritants which include dietary indiscretions, alcohol, and chemical and bacterial toxins. It is a symptom also of other diseases accompanied by infection, fever, or metabolic upset. Actual erosion of gastric mucous membrane occurs in GASTRIC ULCER, producing both pain and dyspepsia.

Disorders of secretion may produce either an excess or deficiency of hydrochloric acid. Excess (hyperchlorhydria) is usual in gastric ulcer; deficiency (hypochlorhydria) is common in anaemia, debility and malignant disease.

Gastric ulcers may bleed, causing either frank haematemesis (vomiting of blood), or detectable traces in the stools.

Pyloric stenosis is obstruction to the outlet from the stomach. A congenital form occurs in infants but in adults it results from chronic ulceration or malignant disease.

Cancer may arise from the cells lining the inner surface of the stomach. It is a common disease, with an incidence which is higher in males. Indeed it is the most frequent malignant disease in men. No adult age is exempt but it tends to occur in older persons, and while many cases are a sequel of chronic gastric ulceration, others arise without any history of previous gastric disease.

Early symptoms are often vague with indigestion, loss of appetite, anaemia, weakness and wasting. Such a history in a previously healthy person over 40 should arouse suspicion and suggest a need for x-ray investigation. Further effects depend greatly on the actual site of tumour growth. At the pyloric end of the stomach early obstruction produces vomiting. The vomit is often characteristic ('coffee-grounds' from altered blood). Other late features are absence of gastric hydrochloric acid and development of enlarged lymphatic glands at the root of the neck on the left side from direct spread along the thoracic lymph duct.

Treatment is surgical removal of the organ (gastrectomy), but success depends on early diagnosis.

stomatitis. See TONGUE.

stone. A stone-like mass, technically called a calculus, formed within the body, usually in hollow organs or secretory ducts.

Calculi commonly occur in the gallbladder, the kidney, the urinary bladder, and the ducts of the salivary glands.

Gall-stones are composed either of cholesterol or bile-salts; stones in the urinary tract are derived from the precipitation of salts normally held in solution in the urine and vary in composition – calcium oxalate, uric acid and urates are the most usual constituents. Salivary calculi are generally composed of calcium carbonate or phosphate or a mixture of these.

Gall-stones and urinary caculi often give rise to much pain and ill-health, and appropriate surgical treatment is required.

stools. The faeces, or material evacuated from the bowel. The characteristics of stools may provide important diagnostic clues. Normally a single stool of about 100 g. (3.5 oz.) is passed each day. It should be of semi-solid consistence, neither fluid nor hard, and roughly cylindrical; ribbon-shaped stools may indicate some constriction higher up; there should be no excess of mucus nor any other abnormal constituent; the colour, which tends to be darker on a predominantly meat diet, should range from light to dark brown. Inspection of the stools may show obvious blood, pus, bile, mucus, or parasites such as tape-worm segments. In addition attention should be paid to:

1. Colour: clay-coloured in obstructive jaundice; green in digestive disorders, especially of young children; black and tarry (melaena) from altered blood.

2. Consistency: resembling pea-soup in typhoid fever and intestinal infections; like rice-water in cholera; hard, rounded and separate (scybala) in chronic constipation.

3. Appearance: slimy with mucus in colitis; purulent in chronic dysentery; pale, bulky and oily from excess of fat which may be present as neutral fat in pancreatic insufficiency or as fatty acids and soaps if there is defective absorption, as in sprue or coeliac disease; frothy in carbohydrate fermentation which may follow intestinal infection.

Infants' stools present special features. For the first few days they are dark green and fluid from bile and mucus from the intestine. They then become soft and yellow and only gradually change as a mixed diet is introduced. By two years they should be formed and definitely faecal. During digestive upsets they are often green and may contain curds from undigested milk or froth from fermentation of excess dietary sugar.

Laboratory examination by micro-scopical, bacteriological or chemical methods will provide still more information, and a specimen of faeces is frequently requested for these purposes. It is usually collected in a special sterile glass container equipped with a scoop or spatula attached to the cap and should be transmitted to the laboratory with the minimum of delay.

strabismus. See SQUINT.

strain. The result of tearing or over-stretching muscle fibres, usually by a sudden or unusual movement. A strain manifests itself by sudden pain which increases on movement of the muscle, swelling, and sometimes bruising. Treatment includes rest of the part, cold compresses to reduce swelling, a firm bandage for a few days, and analgesics if the pain is severe: aspirin or paracetamol usually suffices. The essential difference from a SPRAIN is that the latter involves tearing of ligaments and is in general more severe.

strangulation. (1) Compression of the windpipe. (2) Compression of a part of the body so that its blood supply is cut off, e.g., strangulated hernia.

strangury. Painful and ineffectual effort to pass urine. By derivation the word means 'to squeeze out urine' and this describes the difficulties of the patient who makes frequent paroxysmal, painful and spasmodic attempts to urinate but each time only succeeds in voiding small quantities which are often mixed with blood or pus.

Strangury (or dysuria) is a common symptom of such conditions as renal colic, acute cystitis, urinary retention from prostatic obstruction, and especially of acute urethritis, usually of gonorrhoeal origin.

streptococci. BACTERIA are tiny, single-celled organisms which multiply by simply dividing into two. Cocci are varieties of bacteria roughly spherical in shape. Streptococci are cocci in which division occurs always on one axis, so that a single streptococcus after three successive divisions appears as a chain of eight.

Streptococci cause many diseases, from scarlet fever to septicaemia.

streptomycin. An antibiotic derived from the soil-fungus *Streptomyces griseus* and prepared for clinical use as the crystalline sulphate or chloride. It has to be given by injection into a muscle as it is absorbed from the digestive system.

Streptomycin has a wide range of anti-bacterial activity but its main use is for the treatment of tuberculosis in which it is very effective. Its chief drawback is a liability to induce severe deafness. Both it and its derivative, di-hydro-streptomycin, have a specific action on the auditory and vestibular nerves. Signs of toxicity such as a ringing in the ears, vertigo, nausea and nystagmus (involuntary rapid and jerky movements of the eyeball) may appear within a few days on high dosage (3 to 4 g.), but they are mostly seen in tuberculous patients under prolonged treatment. A decision to continue treatment despite such symptoms means acceptance of a risk of severe deafness but may be justified by the severity of the actual disease.

Another important feature is its tendency to encourage the emergence of strains of the infecting organism which are resistant to the drug, thus leading to the failure of the treatment. For this reason it is usual to give streptomycin in association with other anti-tuberculous drugs such as para-amino-salicylic acid.

stress. Anything which disturbs the natural balance of the body and its tissues. While the term usually means mental stress, it is perhaps useful first to consider physical stress.

Bodily health depends on the health of individual cells and they in turn need a constant internal environment provided by the tissue fluids in which they are continuously immersed. When the body is functionally over-taxed it is said to be under stress and the symptoms of such stress can be related to adverse changes in the internal environment induced by untoward or excessive physical or mental activity.

Physical over-exertion causes stress because muscular function requires adequate supplies of fuel and oxygen and rapid elimination of the resulting metabolic waste-products, e.g., carbon dioxide and water. If the elimination is insufficient for the needs of a particular situation the result is fatigue which persists until relieved by rest. To give a simple example, in running we consume more oxygen and build up carbon dioxide in the tissues faster than we can breathe it out; so immediately after running we still breathe fast to get rid of the carbon dioxide and our muscles feel tired because of the excess carbon dioxide. Within physiological limits no harm results.

Repeated physical stress tends to produce HYPERTROPHY so that a particular tissue becomes more capable of dealing with the loads imposed upon it: for instance, long distance runners tend to develop enlarged hearts by the end of their athletic careers. In some cases of prolonged and repeated physical stress there may also be trends towards accelerated degeneration and these can be compared to physiological ageing. There may also be other man-made and external factors which reinforce the effects of this accelerated degeneration. Amongst these are environmental pollution, the physical contacts which encourage infection, and sometimes new habits and new ways of life.

The influence of mental stress is more subtle. Society influences individuals just as the tissue-fluids influence individual cells. It provides a regulating mechanism to preserve its harmonious functioning, and each individual is subject to these regulatory pressures. It prescribes codes of acceptable behaviour and it tends to discipline, persecute, or ostracize those who will not or cannot conform; alternatively it grades its members by systems of value and prestige, based on race, religion, language, occupation, or wealth, from which escape is difficult. Those who conform avoid pressures and conflict; those who rebel and those who prove inadequate are equally liable to suffer unpleasant consequences.

External social or cultural pressures, e.g., attempts by parents and teachers to induce a non-academic boy to fit himself for entry to a profession, or intolerance of the person whose religious or political views differ strongly from those of his associates, or hostility to the incomer from a different background and with different traditions and customs, all evoke primitive responses and fundamentally these represent preparation either for flight or fight.

Under these emotional drives the body liberates hormones which stimulate its capacity either to escape or conquer. These hormones come chiefly from the pituitary and adrenal glands but also include other secretions with specific 'target organs' such as the skin, stomach, colon and cardio-vascular system. Unfortunately the problems which beset the individual in an organized community can seldom be satisfactorily resolved by direct action, and the hormonal stimuli, if repeated, eventually lead to a state of persistent reaction or over-reaction shown by symptoms of anxiety, fear, frustration, hate, anger, or rage.

Anxiety is perhaps the commonest manifestation of stress. It stems from conflict and conflict may arise from various causes: from the need to exercise a difficult choice; from unsatisfying personal relationships; from competitive standards of living which bring financial worries and may force husbands to accept promotion posts for which they are unfit or wives to undertake full-time work in addition to looking after children and house; from insecurity and dissatisfaction at work; from the isolation of young families and the loss of kinship networks in a mobile society; and from the many other complexities and perplexities of modern life.

Emotional upset of this kind may lead on to obvious disease. The end result of chronic anxiety may eventually be a neurosis, but more commonly it produces physical symptoms affecting various bodily systems. This is psychosomatic disease and a wide range of modern complaints are so determined. Headaches, insomnia, twitches, tics, skin-rashes, digestive upsets, peptic ulcers, colitis (inflammation of the colon), palpitation, high blood pressure, coronary thrombosis, dysmenorrhoea (menstrual pains) and infertility are common examples, but there are many other less well-defined conditions. Repeated absence from work for apparently trivial causes may itself be a sign of such illness and may represent an appeal for help in escaping from some intolerable work situation.

Skin diseases are of particular interest in a psychosomatic context because the effects of emotions on the skin are easily observed, as in blushing in shame, pallor in fright, sweating in fear, and hair-erection and goose-flesh in apprehension and horror. Exteriorization of such emotions when experienced in excess is reflected in such conditions as pruritus (itching), urticaria (nettle-rash) and rosacea (chronic congestion of the blood capillaries leading to a lumpy red appearance of the face.

It is sometimes said that stress is largely a result of modern civilization; that in the simpler cultures of the past the peasant or artisan could work at his own pace, seldom moved away from his relatives and early associates, and had his major decisions taken for him by a possibly benevolent feudal superior, landlord or priest; in short, that stress is in large measure a consequence of emancipation, education, greater opportunity and 'progress'. This is probably an over-simplification, since the peasant of the past was subject to the stresses occasioned by the sheer difficulty of survival in years of poor harvests, together with the strains caused by living in an overcrowded, insanitary dwelling, the physical stresses created by unremitting toil and the mental stresses of constantly trying to please an overlord of often uncertain temper and little benevolence. The stresses today are different, but not necessarily greater. Anyway, even if a return to nature could remove some of the stresses of a mobile, competitive, highly mechanized and highly specialized culture, very few people would be willing to abandon such 'luxuries' as modern heating, lighting, transport and methods of communication, and fewer still would be prepared to have major decisions taken for them by a military or ecclesiastical superior.

Yet, instead of merely treating stress diseases, and often treating them very ineffectively, perhaps we should as a society be directing our attention to the reduction of needless stress. It may be, for instance, that academic education has concentrated too much on fitting children for a career, and has produced on the one hand the 'drop-out' and on the other hand the over-ambitious, over-concentrated career worker without leisure interests or healthy recreation. Perhaps, since most people work for only one third of their waking life up to the age of retirement, education should be for leisure as well as for work. Perhaps again, as machinery increasingly takes over repetitive tasks, work can be made more enjoyable and more meaningful to the persons engaged in it. Yet again, having in large measure conquered death except in extreme old age, perhaps we can use family planning facilities to prevent the continued growth of population and to give the individual (even in cities) a modicum of privacy and reasonable access to green fields and woods. Not least, perhaps we can re-establish compassion, tolerance and unselfishness as desirable qualities to some extent lost in an era of material progress.

We have to realize, however, that some stress (and its accompanying diseases) is the penalty for human advance. Without some stress we would have fewer reformers, inventors or poets.

stricture. An abnormal narrowing of any duct or passage in the body. The usual causes are spasm, inflammation, scarring and tumour, and the commonest sites are in the oesophagus, ureters, urethra, and rectum.

Urethral stricture leads to retention of urine and is perhaps the condition most likely to occur suddenly with urgent symptoms. Cases due to spasm or inflammatory congestion can be treated by inserting a catheter to release urine from the bladder; partial stricture due to scar tissue after urethral infections such as gonorrhoea may be relieved by gradual dilation with appropriate instruments; other conditions may require surgical measures to relieve or remove obstruction.

Strictures elsewhere will generally need operative treatment eventually.

Some causes of stroke

stroke. Damage to the brain, mostly occasioned by (1) bleeding from a weakened artery (cerebral haemorrhage), (2) clotting of blood in a diseased artery (cerebral thrombosis), (3) blockage of an artery by a plug of fat or mass of bacteria or bubble of air (cerebral embolism), or (4) pressure on the vessel by a tumour. Associated underlying conditions include arteriosclerosis and high blood pressure.

The onset is usually sudden in embolism and gradual in thrombosis, while in haemorrhage it may be gradual or, if the bleeding is sudden and profuse, very rapid indeed. Manifestations vary according to the amount and situation of damage but often include unconsciousness and heavy breathing.

A stroke causing only minimal brain damage may create a few minutes of haziness and confusion, with no later symptoms, but a massive stroke may result in immediate death. Where the damage is serious but not fatal within the first week – the danger period in respect of death – some paralysis of the arm or leg is common; this is known as HEMIPLEGIA.

In any case of suspected stroke the patient should have restrictive clothing, such as the collar, loosened and should be placed on his side to remove the danger of his choking on his own saliva. Medical help should be summoned immediately. In serious stroke both skilled medical treatment and skilled nursing care are required and it is not possible in the early weeks to forecast how much paralysis of limbs and possible speech impairment will remain.

Prevention of stroke is largely the prevention of arteriosclerosis and high blood pressure, and essentially the same measures are desirable as are mentioned in the article on CORONARY THROMBOSIS. Additionally, since stroke often occurs during or just after violent exertion or strong emotion, persons with high blood pressure should seek to avoid these factors.

Alternative names for the condition are apoplexy and cerebrovascular incident.

stupor. A condition of extreme mental apathy in which the person does not respond at all to his surroundings. It may arise in such diseases as melancholia, schizophrenia and epilepsy, and also occasionally in hysteria. The stuporous patient makes no effort to take food or to attend to the calls of nature, so that measures like spoon-feeding may be necessary. The condition is usually transient, but where it persists for more than a few days, electro-convulsive treatment is worth considering.

stuttering. A condition, allied to STAMMERING, in which a person has difficulty with the initial word of a sentence or phrase and tends to repeat the word or the first syllable of it. The condition is sometimes caused by sudden fright or other emotional shock, and it occasionally occurs after debilitating diseases.

Stuttering in childhood is commoner in boys than girls, and in left-handed rather than right-handed people, and it is sometimes associated with homes with such disturbing factors as parental discord, jealousy or over-strictness. Probably the most important factor in treatment is the fostering of self-reliance and confidence, but in addition a good speech therapist can often help.

stye. See EYELIDS, DISEASES OF.

styptics. Preparations for applying to a wound to check bleeding from a skin surface either by constricting the capillary blood vessels or by inducing clotting of blood. Alum, perchloride of iron, tannin, copper sulphate and silver nitrate are common styptics. In the absence of an available styptic, applications of cold or very hot water will often check an oozing of blood.

subacute. A term used to describe a condition intermediate between acute (which describes an incident of a sudden nature) and chronic (which indicates a long-standing condition).

subarachnoid. The fluid-filled space between the middle of the three membranes lining the brain (the arachnoid) and the innermost membrane (the pia mater).

Subarachnoid haemorrhage. Bleeding into the subarachnoid space with consequent pressure on the brain; it may occur through rupture of an aneurysm on one of the small cerebral arteries or through collapse of the weakened wall of one of these arteries. There are two sharply demarcated types. The apoplectic type is characterized by intense headache followed by unconsciousness, and can in some cases be differentiated from stroke only by lumbar puncture (the taking of a sample of cerebrospinal fluid, in which blood is found if the condition is a subarachnoid haemorrhage). In this type about one-third of the patients die, mostly within forty-eight hours, and most of the others make a full although often slow recovery. Where the haemorrhage is less in quantity the meningitic type occurs, with symptoms and signs rather like those of meningitis. In both types surgery may be necessary to deal with the cause of the bleeding.

subconscious. The totality of mental experience and activity operating beneath or beyond consciousness and therefore without the awareness of the person. The term is sometimes employed to include activity under the control of the autonomic nervous system and of hormonal activity (e.g., involuntary acceleration or slowing of the heart rate or the respiratory rate), but it is generally used to cover deep-seated drives (especially sexual and aggressive) and ideas and memories that have been repressed because they are incompatible with the standards or beliefs in the conscious mind.

The deep-rooted tendencies in the subconscious often come into conflict with the standards of morality, ethics or aesthetics that an individual has acquired from his parents, teachers and associates. The repressed ideas and impulses are prevented by a psychological mechanism called the censor from reaching the conscious mind in direct form, but frequently reach it in distorted forms or by roundabout methods. Many (but not all) dreams and many mistakes in speech are explicable in terms of the emergence of items from the subconscious.

Behaviour, far from being completely rational, is to a considerable extent a compromise between acquired standards and values and impulses from the subconscious.

See also UNCONSCIOUS MIND.

subcutaneous. Under the skin. A subcutaneous injection is one given just under the skin as opposed to the more superficial intradermal injection, which raises a bleb in the skin, and the deeper intramuscular injection.

sublimation. The process whereby prohibited or repressed tendencies, especially sexual and other biological energies, are diverted into channels that are permissible, realizable and socially constructive or creative. For instance, the unmarried woman who has a strong maternal instinct may sublimate by diverting her desire to care for a child of her own into the acceptable channel of working in a children's nursery, or may lavish on a pet animal the affection really intended for a non-existent child. Similarly a man who has a very strong power-drive but cannot gain a top-ranking post in his profession or business may sublimate by becoming the dominant figure in a particular social, political or religious organization.

Sublimation is an important psychological mechanism and its successful employment prevents much misery. Like any other mechanism, however, it can be misused. The man who would badly like to hit his boss but instead beats his children for trivial misdemeanours is sublimating in an unfortunate way, as is the man who compensates for a feeling of inferiority by heavy consumption of alcohol. Conversely, the man with similar feelings of aggression who names a golf ball after his employer and then drives it round the golf course is getting rid of his impulse without harming anybody.

subliminal. A sensation too slight or transient to be consciously perceived. Such a sensation may enter the subconscious and so may subsequently affect behaviour.

subluxation. Partial dislocation of the bones of a joint without separation being complete. Probably the commonest example is subluxation of the head of the radius (one of the two long bones of the forearm); following a sudden wrench to the elbow, especially of a child; the head of the radius is pulled forward, and the elbow is very painful and the forearm useless until the bone has been restored to its natural position.

subphrenic. Below the diaphragm. A subphrenic abscess is an abscess in the space between the diaphragm and the upper part of the liver. It occurs most commonly as a complication of gastric ulcer or other disease of the stomach; it is characterized by pain and high temperature, and is both hard to diagnose and difficult to treat.

suckling. The term used for BREAST-FEEDING a baby.

sudden death. Where a person dies in Britain without having been treated by a doctor within the previous fourteen days, or where the doctor involved is not satisfied as to the cause of death, certain legal formalities are required and in circumstances of suspicion or uncertainty a post mortem may be demanded.

suffocation. Unconsciousness or death resulting from lack of air to breathe or blockage of the respiratory passages. See ASPHYXIA.

sugars. See CARBOHYDRATE.

suicide. The intentional taking of a person's own life. The recorded incidence of suicide, the methods used and the occupational and age groups mainly involved vary considerably from country to country and from year to year. Broadly, recorded suicides are commoner in highly developed countries (with Sweden particularly high) than in developing countries; in some advanced countries they account for something like one in every fifty deaths of adult males and one in every hundred deaths of adult females. They tend to be commonest at around 55 to 60 years of age, although not uncommon around the ages of 18 to 30. In general, recorded suicide is most frequent in people whose occupations involve strain, responsibility or overwork, or whose occupations make the persons accustomed to violence, or whose occupations provide ready access to easy means of suicide.

Figures for recorded suicides are probably not particularly accurate. In the first place, an unknown but perhaps considerable number of suicides, especially at the upper end of life, are certified as having died from natural causes: if a person has been suffering from an incurable and painful disease, and if the attending doctor finds that he has died earlier than had been expected and mildly wonders whether the patient has contrived to take an overdose of pain-killing drugs, there is clearly a likelihood that the doctor will simply certify the death as due to the disease, rather than distress the bereaved relatives by refusing to certify and demanding a post mortem examination. Secondly, an intelligent person can sometimes make a suicide appear like an accident: for instance, his gun appears to have gone off while he was cleaning it. Thirdly, there occur quite a number of unintentional suicides; e.g., in order to call attention to his distress and need for help in a dramatic way a person jumps into the sea with every intention of being rescued or, failing a rescuer, of regaining the shore by his own efforts, but no rescuer appears, the current is stronger than the apparently suicidal person had realized, and he drowns.

Some psychologists have attempted to link suicide with the extreme end of the spectrum of masochistic inclinations, and to talk of the turning of sadistic aggression upon the self.

While there may be some truth in these statements, it is perhaps wiser for the present to stick to the long-standing classification of deliberate self-destruction into altruistic, egotistic and anomic.

Altruistic suicide, where the person places a higher value on the maintenance of society than on the preservation of his own life, is rare in Europe and North America. Examples are the suicide of

Some causes of suicide

Japanese officers after defeat or capture, and the formerly common custom of suttee in which Hindu widows threw themselves on their husbands' funeral pyres.

Egotistical suicide, generally to punish relatives or associates for some real or imaginary injury, is probably commoner than is often appreciated. It clearly implies immaturity or defect of personality and is probably the form of self-destruction that has led to suicide being associated with the phrase 'being of unsound mind'.

Undoubtedly, however, the common variety of suicide is the anomic type, with anomie defined as a state of confusion of values and lack of social cohesion. It is because this type vastly outnumbers the other types that the proportion of suicides to the total population of a community is to some extent an indication of the degree of stress and the amount of social breakdown. To give two examples: despite the worries, fears and dangers of a war the number of suicides often falls during a war, when people tend to collaborate and experience a sense of common purpose; conversely, there are more suicides in periods of heavy unemployment and financial stringency.

Suicides of anomic type are proportionately commoner in single, divorced and widowed persons than in the married, in persons in solitary occupations than in those working closely with others, and in immigrants (whether from overseas or from distant parts of the same country) than in persons with firm roots in a neighbourhood.

The general pattern of anomic suicide is fairly clear - a decision to end things, fostered by loneliness, unwantedness and confused values, with often the moral and social standards of the suicide's upbringing clashing with those of the community in which he has been living. Many statements about suicides are, however, largely unproved. For instance, it is often alleged that there are more suicides among Protestants than among Catholics, but for Catholics certification of death as suicide raises problems of sanctified burial and these problems may well influence certifying doctors in cases that are not absolutely clear-cut. Similarly, statements about social class differences in suicide rates disregard the greater opportunities of the intelligent, the educated and the affluent of making a self-destruction appear a natural death.

Prevention of altruistic and egotistic suicide is clearly very difficult and involves long-term alteration of the whole attitudes and system of values of the person. Prevention of anomic suicide is not easy, although companionship and acceptance reduce its likelihood.

Unsuccessful attempts at suicide are many times commoner than successful attempts and are probably in many cases never intended to succeed but are essentially a desperate cry for help. Obviously any unsuccessful attempt at self-destruction warrants full investigation of the person's background and problems to ascertain whether there is any acceptable way of giving him the help that he needs.

While on general principles dangerous drugs should be kept under strict control, a great deal that is said about their use in suicidal attempts is of highly doubtful value. In the few cases where the attempt is sudden and unpremeditated it may be facilitated by the availability of a particular drug, but in most cases the attempt is not the result of sudden impulse. In general to lock away hypnotics and sedatives without tackling the basic problem leading to suicidal impulses is merely to compel the intending suicide to substitute drowning or cutting of his wrists for what might have been an easier form of death.

sulphonamides. A group of drugs that prevent the multiplication of bacteria and so enable the defence mechanisms of the body to destroy the invading organisms. The sulphonamides rendered curable many infections of former high fatality, and until the advent of penicillin and other antibiotics they dominated the treatment of infections caused by bacteria. Since some bacteria have now acquired a resistance to several antibiotics, the sulphonamides are still of the highest importance.

With sulphonamides as with antibiotics correct dosage is important. Excessive dosage is liable to produce toxic side-effects. Insufficient dosage or too early cessation may create organisms that have acquired a resistance or immunity to the particular medicament.

Sulphanilamide. Now used mainly as a dusting powder for wounds or burns, often in combination with penicillin powder.

Sulphapyridine. This drug reduced the mortality of cerebrospinal meningitis from 30 per cent to under 3 per cent; it is now little used because of its tendency to cause rashes and gastric disorders.

Sulphathiazole. At present usually deemed the drug of choice for most serious bacterial infections in which sulphonamides are for any reason considered preferable to antibiotics.

Sulphamezathine. An alternative with remarkably few toxic or side effects.

For most infections soluble sulphonamides are needed, as above, but for bacterial infections of the gastro-intestinal tract (such as bacterial dysentery) what is needed is a sulphonamide that is not easily absorbed. Here sulphaguanidine and sulphasuxidine are the sulphonamides of choice.

The sulphonamides are not effective in diseases caused by viruses.

sunbathing. Attempts to improve health or acquire bronzing by exposure to the sun's rays.

In any such efforts gradualness is the key to success, with initial exposures of only five or six minutes, with the eyes protected by dark glasses, and preferably with the exposures in the morning or evening when the rays are not at full intensity. Injudicious exposure can cause painful SUNBURN and even sunstroke. The danger is particularly acute where a person goes on holiday to a warmer and sunnier climate and, ignoring the change from his normal surroundings, exposes himself to the direct rays of the sun.

sunburn. The painful reddening and ultimate peeling of the skin that results from excessive exposure to bright sunshine. Very fair persons are abnormally sensitive to sunshine, as are victims of some diseases (e.g., porphyria) and persons taking some of the sulphonamide drugs.

Prevention of sunburn is essentially by avoidance of exposure, and this may include skin protection by long sleeves and a broad hat, the use of various creams and lotions, and caution in SUNBATHING. Where the skin is red and sore, cooling lotions such as calamine and witch hazel are useful. Where there is in addition weakness and giddiness, with feeble and rapid pulse and hot, dry skin, the patient requires treatment for HEAT STROKE.

In tropical climates repeated sunburn with peeling of the skin often leads to wrinkling and sometimes leads to skin cancer.

sunlight treatment. Since vitamin D is produced by activation of ergosterol in the skin by the ultra-violet rays of the sun, sunlight is obviously of value in preventing rickets in children whose diets are low in that vitamin. In general, a moderate amount of sunshine is certainly invigorating, has some general tonic effects and produces psychological benefits, although a graduated increase of exposure to sunshine is essential to avoid sunburn.

Many experts, however, are now a little sceptical about the value of sending a patient with such a condition as tuberculosis of the bones or joints to a sunny and dust-free atmosphere (such as the High Alps) and even more sceptical about the merits of sunlight lamps which produce ULTRA-VIOLET RADIATION in the privacy of the patient's home. Certainly both natural and artificial sunlight treatment (or heliotherapy) have their place in the prevention and treatment of some diseases, but their role was grossly exaggerated in the early decades of this century, and there is a salutary lesson in the saying, 'Mad dogs and Englishmen walk out in the midday sun'.

sunstroke. See HEAT STROKE.

superego. The portion of the unconscious mind which acts as a censor, preventing repressed ideas and impulses from rising from the unconscious (the id) into consciousness (the ego). There are clearly very close connections between what the psychoanalysts term the superego and what religious persons call conscience.

superinfection. A second infection by a different germ arising during the course of an initial infection.

In any severe infection the bodily resistance is weakened so that 'the soil is ripe' for invasion by another organism; and, while the particular antibiotic or sulphonamide employed for the first infection is presumably of known effectiveness against the initial germ, the second invader may well be resistant to it.

Where fever and other symptoms recur, after having begun to respond to treatment, it is often useful to check – by sending appropriate specimens for laboratory investigation – that there has not been a secondary infection requiring a different treatment.

suppository. A cone-shaped mass, usually made of cocoa-butter or gelatin or glycerine, which is used for the introduction of drugs into the rectum. A suppository is solid at room temperature but melts at body temperature, liberating the contained drug. A suppository may be used (1) to initiate action of the bowels in constipation, (2) to allay the inflammation and congestion of internal piles, (3) to reduce pain in any disease of the rectum, or (4) to get a drug into the circulation.

To introduce the suppository it is placed with the pointed end nearest the anus and gently propelled forwards with a screwing movement of the finger. It must be pushed inwards beyond the sphincter muscle, because otherwise it will not be retained.

suppuration. The formation of PUS.

suprarenal glands. Otherwise known as adrenal glands, and lying on the top of each kidney, these are very important members of the system of ENDOCRINE GLANDS.

surgery. The treatment of injuries, diseases or deformities by manual operation or instrumental appliances. Surgery is essentially the last medical resort, and an admission that both prevention and medical treatment have failed. See also OPERATION, NEED FOR.

surveillance. A watch kept over a person regarded as liable to develop a particular infection.

Under the formerly common system of quarantine, persons who had been in contact with a case of serious infection were required to remain isolated in their homes for slightly longer than the incubation period of the disease. That measure checked the spread of diseases transmitted from person to person, but where the contacts were numerous it could damage the entire life and productive work of a community. Furthermore, in the cases of diseases of long incubation periods it served little purpose in the earlier part of these periods since the contacts – whether in the process of developing the disease or not – would not yet be infective.

Quarantine is increasingly being replaced by surveillance. Under this system the persons regarded as contacts remain at work, or in the case of children remain at school, but are inspected daily by doctors or health visitors and are excluded from work or school if any symptoms or signs of the disease appear. Essentially surveillance depends for its success on the idea that a particular infection can be identified just before the person becomes infectious. There are inevitably some diseases for which surveillance is not applicable, and where applicable the system depends entirely on the expertise of the inspecting doctor or health visitor. The saving to the community is, however, enormous: under the quarantine system a hundred contacts might be kept off work for a fortnight (losing the community the equivalent of four years of a man's work) and then one might develop the disease; under the surveillance system the hundred remain at work and about the thirteenth day perhaps two are excluded – the man who is developing the disease and another who has symptoms warranting momentary suspicion.

suture. The drawing together of two sides of a wound by stitches or clamps. The term is also used for the stitches so employed. Cotton and linen stitches, used for centuries, have nowadays been largely replaced by silk thread, nylon thread, catgut and metal clamps. Catgut has the advantage that it is ultimately broken down in the tissues and absorbed, whereas other stitches have to be removed after the wound has healed sufficiently.

Suturing promotes rapid healing and helps to prevent the formation of unsightly or disfiguring scars. In general it is needed whenever a wound is too large to heal readily by itself.

swab. Essentially a solid stick with cotton wool, gauze or cloth wrapped round one end. Swabs are employed (1) to clean out natural cavities, such as the ear or nostril; (2) to clean wounds, e.g., to mop away blood or pus during an operation; and (3) to obtain samples for bacteriological examination, as in swabbing the throat of a person suspected of early diphtheria or tonsillitis. In major operations, especially on the abdomen, it is standard procedure that all swabs used are counted so as to ensure, before the wound is closed, that they have all been removed.

swallowing. The passage of food from the mouth to the stomach.

One cannot simultaneously breathe and swallow, because in the act of swallowing the epiglottis blocks off the respiratory channel to prevent food from entering the trachea. Thereafter involuntary contractions of the pharynx and oesophagus force the food downwards towards the stomach.

If the epiglottis fails to perform properly its function of sealing off the trachea, as can happen when a person tries to talk or breathe with food in his throat, there is danger of a particle of food passing into the respiratory tract and causing choking.

swallowing difficulty. Difficulty in swallowing may arise (1) in a baby as a result of congenital defects such as a cleft palate; (2) from any painful or inflammatory condition of the throat such as quinsy; (3) from paralysis of the muscles concerned in swallowing, as in certain organic nervous diseases; (4) from pressure of a tumour in the vicinity of the throat; and (5) in hysteria. Where the difficulty persists for more than a few hours medical investigation is desirable. Treatment varies with the cause.

sweat. See PERSPIRATION.

sycosis. See BARBER'S RASH.

sympathectomy. The operation of cutting over-active nerves of the sympathetic nervous system to prevent the effects of their activity, e.g., to avoid constriction of a particular artery.

In most cases it is possible to block the nerve temporarily with a local anaesthetic, and so to verify before the operation that surgery will be likely to have the anticipated effects.

sympathetic nervous system. One of the two branches of the autonomic or involuntary NERVOUS SYSTEM. Sympathetic drugs, such as tolazoline or propanolol, inhibit some or all of the activities of the sympathetic nervous system.

symptom. A manifestation of disease or disorder noticed by the patient or prospective patient, e.g., pain, swelling, cough, abnormal sweating, itching, backache, fatigue or irritability. Although the difference is a very fine one, the symptoms reported by the patient are normally differentiated from signs, i.e., things noted by the doctor or other health worker. The distinction is made because the patient according to his temperament may exaggerate or minimize his symptoms, or even fake them to secure an excuse for being off work or to gain compensation for a non-existent injury, whereas the signs are noted by an impartial and skilled observer. Yet many manifestations of illness can be both symptoms and signs.

Nose bleeding, high colour, pallor and breathlessness on exertion are examples.

A symptom, especially pain, is what usually induces a person to seek medical help. However, one of the tragedies of existence is that symptoms develop after - and in consequence of - pathological changes which may be irreversible. Thus the person in the early stage of pulmonary tuberculosis may look and feel healthy: the characteristic cough, night sweats and loss of weight do not appear until the disease is well-developed in the lung. The first symptoms of duodenal ulcer appear after the mucous membrane has been so eroded as to produce a definite patch of ulceration. Cancer in almost any part of the body may be symptomless until the tumour has not only grown to an appreciable size but has started to cause secondary growths elsewhere. The first evidence of disorder of the coronary arteries may be sudden death from coronary thrombosis.

There are hundreds of different symptoms. To mention a few examples, symptoms probably related to the head include the various types of headache, dizziness, fainting, sleep disturbances, skin disease of the scalp, various types of baldness, changes in the colour and texture of the hair, and so on. There is no simple classification, and a single symptom may be produced by any one of several disorders. Even the organ affected may not be directly indicated by the symptom, e.g., pain over the heart in a young person is more often than not caused by a disorder of the stomach, coughing may be evidence of wax in the ear, and pain in the leg may be a manifestation of a damaged intervertebral disc. So a doctor before attempting to make a diagnosis has usually to consider not merely the particular symptom of which the patient is complaining but also all the other symptoms and signs that are present.

Until the twentieth century the whole system of medical care was normally based on the appearance of symptoms which induced the sufferer to make a layman's diagnosis of illness and consult a doctor. Nowadays opinion in the health professions increasingly recognizes that intervention merely in a crisis is unsatisfactory, and favours paying substantially more attention to preventive measures. (1) Health education, in an effort to maintain and improve physical and emotional health, seeks to create habits and attitudes compatible with good health. (2) Prevention of disease may be achieved by several means, either specific prevention such as immunization against various infections or presumptive prevention such as avoiding the main causes of child maladjustment or of postural defects. (3) Health screening in advance of any symptoms, as in the periodical medical examination of pre-school and school children, is most rewarding. Attention to health education, disease prevention and health screening has already greatly improved the physical and mental health of persons in the first two decades of life, but most adults still have no contact with the health services until they themselves initiate that contact after symptoms have appeared.

syncope. Temporary loss of consciousness through deficient blood supply to the brain. The term is synonymous with FAINTING.

syndrome. A group of signs and symptoms which are together characteristic of a particular disease and have been given a specific name, generally that of the person who first described them. The recognition of a syndrome can be of great value for accurate early diagnosis.

synergy. Co-operative or reinforcing action, as when two or more nerves or muscles work together. An example is the movements of forefinger and thumb to grasp an object. The term is also used for two drugs that reinforce each other.

synovitis. Inflammation of the lining membrane of a joint cavity. Causes include infection following wounds or injuries and also transmission of germs from other parts of the body. Symptoms include pain, reddening and swelling, and the joint is usually kept bent. Rest and hot fomentations help, but sulphonamides or antibiotics are often required.

syphilis. A dangerous venereal disease of slow development, caused by a spirochaete, the thread-like *Treponema pallidum.*

Transmission occurs in four ways: (1) during sexual intercourse with an infected person - this accounts for 99 per cent of cases; (2) from mother to unborn child via the placenta (see congenital syphilis below); (3) very rarely from kissing a person with a syphilitic lesion on the mouth or by contact with very recent and still moist discharges from an infected person, as in the communal use of drinking cups; and (4) even more rarely from infection of an unnoticed scratch on the hand when treating a patient - an occupational hazard of doctors and nurses.

The incubation period is one to six weeks. Thereafter the disease may be conveniently divided into three stages.

The primary stage is characterized by the appearance of a hard, painless, red papule at the site of infection - usually the foreskin or glans penis in the male and the labia in the female. The papule enlarges to the size of a pea and then breaks down to form an ulcer with sharply cut edges and a hard base, while the adjacent lymph glands become enlarged and 'shotty'. At this stage diagnosis can usually be confirmed by the Wassermann test of blood, and the disease is fairly easily cured, but because of the absence of pain the victim may not seek treatment and may not even know that he has the disease.

The second stage, in six to twelve weeks, is characterized by general symptoms

The primary stage of syphilis

indicating the presence of spirochaetes in the blood-stream – mild feverishness, lassitude, headache and a non-itchy rash which can be mistaken for various skin diseases. Where the skin is moist, raised patches, called condylomata, may appear with a highly infective discharge. The Wassermann test, if made, is always positive and the disease is still easily curable, but the condition may be missed and the stage subsides without treatment although infection still lurks.

In untreated or inadequately treated cases the third stage may appear between five and twenty years later. It may take various forms – the appearance of a gumma, a chronic abscess which causes symptoms by compressing healthy tissue; an attack on the blood-vessels, causing, for instance, aortic aneurysm (a bulge in the wall of the main artery of the body) which may be fatal; and in particular two different diseases of the central nervous system. Of these, tabes dorsalis (or locomotor ataxia) is characterized by loss of the reflexes that co-ordinate voluntary movement, curious stamping gait, sudden intense stabbing pains in the legs, and impairment of bladder control. Anti-syphilitic treatment, analgesics and special exercises all help but the outlook is not very good. The other syphilitic disease of the nervous system, general paralysis of the insane, shows itself successively in gradual deterioration of the personality with increasing loss of emotional control and increasing lack of concentration, delusions of grandeur, and finally paralysis and complete absence of mental activity.

Heavy dosage of penicillin can arrest the disease but little or nothing can be done to remove such mental deterioration as has already occurred.

With adequate dosage of penicillin syphilis is definitely curable in the first and second stages; and in consequence of early diagnosis and efficient treatment tertiary syphilis has now become an extreme rarity.

Prevention of syphilis is inevitably linked with reduction of promiscuity. The non-promiscuous couple, whether married or unmarried, clearly run no risk of the disease; if one of that couple acquires the disease through an act of promiscuity – perhaps during a prolonged absence of the normal partner – only two people are likely to become infected, and if the disease is identified in one the treatment of both is a virtual certainty; but in casual promiscuity or prostitution one infected person may infect many partners. Preventive measures include health education (including sex education and education both about the avoidance of syphilis and about recognition of the primary sore); moral education (to reduce casual sexual relationships); advice about the use of condoms, which afford a partial protection, and about chemicals for use after intercourse; provision of facilities for healthy recreation (to reduce the likelihood of casual sexual encounters); efficient contact tracing (very difficult where the couple have met on the street or in a public house and do not even know each other's names); and registration and periodical medical examination of prostitutes.

Congenital syphilis. Where the mother has uncured secondary syphilis, transmission of infection to unborn children through the placenta is highly probable. In congenital syphilis the disease is found in many internal organs, and in many cases the child dies in the uterus. Indeed the classical picture in a syphilitic mother is a series of pregnancies resulting successively in early miscarriage, later miscarriage, still birth, a living child with syphilis and a healthy living child. Although that is an average picture the variation is great: there are even cases on record of one twin being born with typical syphilis and the other being born healthy.

In a surviving syphilitic child common manifestations include emaciation and sallow complexion, a syphilitic inflammation of the lining of the nose, 'saddle-nose' (from destruction of the nasal bones) and 'bossing' (a heaping up of spongy bone on parts of the skull).

Apart from prevention of infection of the mother by measures to reduce syphilis, prevention is by adequate and timely treatment of the mother. Where a child is found to have congenital syphilis, penicillin treatment is usually effective if given early.

syringe. An instrument, consisting of a hollow barrel, a plunger and a hollow needle, which is used for injecting fluid into a muscle, vein or body cavity, or for drawing off a sample of blood or cerebrospinal fluid. Formerly syringes were made of glass and required very careful sterilization, but nowadays disposable syringes are normally employed; these are used once and then discarded.

syringomyelia. A chronic disease in which cavities develop in the spinal cord and brain stem. The condition is almost certainly congenital but symptoms do not appear until late childhood or early adult life. The characteristic early feature is a loss of sensation, so that the hands often have several painless cuts or burns, and on examination portions of the body are found unable to detect pain or heat, although they can still appreciate touch and vibration. Later there is some atrophy of muscles, especially of the arms, and sometimes a thickening and brittleness of the bones.

Progress of the disease is very slow, with long periods in which the condition becomes no worse; but as yet no useful treatment or means of prevention has been discovered.

systole. The rhythmic contraction of the muscle of the heart which normally occurs about sixty to eighty times per minute and has the effect of pumping blood into the arteries. The converse phase of relaxation in which blood flows into the heart from the veins is termed diastole.

T

TAB. A combined vaccine used against typhoid and the two common types of paratyphoid, A and B. If given several weeks before the person is at risk, i.e., early enough to permit of the development of immunity, it gives a reasonable protection for at least a year. If given to persons at immediate risk, e.g., in an outbreak where they have consumed the same food or drink as the early cases and are therefore in the position either of incubating the disease or of having escaped, it is useless and indeed, by invalidating the Widal test, makes the diagnosis of cases appreciably more difficult.

In a highly developed country with good standards of hygiene TAB is rarely necessary, but in unhygienic conditions and particularly in the potential disruption caused by war it can be of enormous value.

tabes. Any disease involving wasting of tissue. The term, however, is nowadays virtually restricted to tabes dorsalis, a degenerative condition of the spinal cord that occurs in advanced stages of untreated or inadequately treated SYPHILIS.

tachycardia. Unduly rapid beating of the heart. It occurs as a normal event after considerable exertion and in emotional excitement, but may also be a sign of hyperthyroidism or of disease of the heart. To set a borderline is difficult because the normal heart rate at rest varies from about sixty to about eighty beats per minute, but broadly a rate in excess of eighty-eight, persisting more than five minutes after the end of exercise or the occurrence of emotional excitement, can be termed tachycardia.

Paroxysmal tachycardia, in which the heart suddenly starts to beat at perhaps twice its normal rate and equally suddenly reverts to its normal speed, is usually indicative either of hyperthyroidism or of heart disease (especially mitral stenosis). The state may, however, be precipitated by excessive exertion, strong emotion, heavy smoking or heavy consumption of tea, coffee or alcohol. Reassurance is essential because the patient, especially in a first attack, tends to be very anxious, but attacks nearly always end spontaneously without doing much harm. Drinking iced water sometimes ends an attack as does massage of the heart. If the attack continues, quinidine (300 mg.) and a sedative are useful.

taenia. Certain species of TAPEWORM. Care should be taken to distinguish *Taenia* from *Tinea*, which is the scientific name for RINGWORM.

talipes. See CLUB FOOT.

talus. Formerly called the astralagus. One of the seven bones of the foot. With the lower ends of the tibia and fibula it forms the ankle joint.

tapeworms. Intestinal parasitic worms, each consisting of a head, neck and many segments.

The common tapeworms are *Taenia saginata* (the beef tapeworm) and *Taenia solium* (the tapeworm of pork). In the former case the patient usually becomes aware of the infestation only by seeing segments of the worm in his faeces, although in time he begins to lose weight and to have vague ill health. The eggs are normally discharged in the faeces and form cysts in the tissues of animals that swallow the larvae but not as a rule in man. In the case of *Taenia solium* the larvae are liberated within the human body and cysts – cysterci – may form in any muscle or organ, causing symptoms which depend on the site.

Prevention is by adequate inspection of meat and pork and by proper cooking of these foods.

Less frequently encountered are the *Bothriocephalus latus* of Central Europe, which enters man through the eating of infested fish, and the *Echinococcus granulosis* or dog tapeworm, which causes hydatid cysts in man.

tarsus. The base of the foot. It consists of seven bones with a covering of compact tissue. Nearest the leg are the talus and the calcaneus; intermediate is the navicular; and nearest the toes are the three cuneiform bones and the cuboid. These seven bones support the weight of the body in standing and walking.

A taste-bud

When cleaning the teeth the brush should be swept down from the gums (a) so that the bristle-heads clean between the teeth (b). There are three movements required: on the outside (c), the inside (d), and the tops (e) of the teeth

taste. The sensation of taste depends on tiny elevations of skin in the tongue, palate and epiglottis, each containing a taste-bud; this is a cluster of spindle-shaped cells from which nerve fibres pass to the facial and glossopharyngeal nerves. The taste-buds detect only four tastes: sweet, perceived best by buds at the tip of the tongue; sour, appreciated best by buds at the sides of the tongue; bitter, identified by buds at the back of the tongue; and salt, for which the buds are more widespread but are largely near the tip and sides of the tongue. Solids are not tasted until at least partially dissolved by saliva.

The finer distinctions of taste are really dependent on the sense of smell. Hence the apparent blunting of taste when the sense of smell is impaired, as by a cold in the head.

tattooing. Pricking indelible pigments into the skin to form words or pictures. Tattooing is much favoured by older adolescents and young adult males, who are sometimes embarrassed later by, for example, an arm branded with the name of a girl who is now only vaguely recalled as the subject of a long past and only temporary infatuation. Removal of tattoo marks is difficult and usually requires minor surgery.

While not illegal in Britain, it is frowned on by doctors and other health workers because an inadequately sterilized needle can transmit serum hepatitis or occasionally syphilis. In this connection it should be remembered that qualified doctors found the sterilization of syringes and needles both difficult and time-consuming, and gladly began to use disposable ones when these became available. Moreover, the virus of serum hepatitis can be transmitted to the tattooing pigment from an infected person undergoing tattooing, so that, even if a fresh needle is used, the next person tattooed may be at risk.

Tay-Sachs disease. See AMAUROTIC FAMILY IDIOCY.

tears. See LACRIMAL.

teenager. A person whose age is over 12 and under 20 years. The term is seldom used for persons of 18 or 19 years but commonly employed for youngsters of 13 to 17 - the difficult phase in which they are in some respects regarded as responsible young adults and in other respects treated as dependent children. See ADOLESCENCE.

teeth. Every person develops two sets of teeth during life.

The twenty temporary, deciduous or milk teeth consist in each jaw of four central, chisel-shaped incisors for biting food, two conical canines on each side of the incisors for tearing food, and, further back, four cuspid-shaped molars for grinding. The temporary teeth begin to erupt at 6 to 9 months, a lower central incisor being usually the first to appear, and dentition is complete by about 2½ years.

The thirty-two permanent teeth consist of four incisors, two canines, four premolars and six molars. The first molars

labels:
incisors — 6 to 9
canine — 8 to 12
— 16 to 20
molars — 12 to 16
— 20 to 30

Milk teeth, showing the age, in months, when they usually appear

begin to emerge, further back than the temporary teeth, at about six years and thereafter the temporary teeth are gradually - and usually painlessly - pushed out by their successors. Dentition is usually completed by 14 to 15 years, except for the third molars (wisdom teeth) which appear around 17 to 25 years.

labels:
incisors — 6 to 8
canine — 7 to 9
— 9 to 13
pre-molars — 9 to 12
— 10 to 13
molars — 5 to 7
— 11 to 14
— 18 to 40

Permanent teeth, showing the age, in years, when they usually appear

A tooth consists primarily of the hollow interior or pulp, soft connective tissue containing a mass of blood vessels and nerves, and a thick outer shell of dentine (or ivory), a hard cellular substance. On the outside the dentine is lined with enamel, an even harder non-cellular material on the exposed surface or crown, and with bony cement at the root.

Tooth development is impaired by deficiency of any of the following: calcium, vitamin C, vitamin D, fluorine, and manganese and other trace elements. Since teeth begin to develop before birth, although not erupting till long afterwards,

these deficiencies are also important in the expectant mother.

Disorders of the teeth. Dental decay (caries) is the commonest cause of toothache. The bacteria normally present in the mouth produce enzymes which act on starches and sugars, both creating acid and forming a 'plaque' of debris on the surface of the tooth. The acid, kept in contact with the tooth by the plaque, gradually destroys the enamel and dentine of the tooth.

For the most part it can be prevented by careful dental hygiene. Where unprevented it leads to the formation of a cavity which provides access for the food products to the pulp. A small cavity may be closed by a filling but a large cavity may well necessitate extraction of the tooth.

Gingivitis and peridontitis (inflammation of the gum) are usually painless until an abscess begins to form, generally necessitating removal of the tooth after the abscess has passed the acute stage, although in a reasonably early stage the abscess may respond to treatment with antibiotics.

Malocclusion occurs when the teeth grow unevenly, largely through overcrowding; this happens because the human jaw has receded in the course of evolution. In a case of malocclusion the teeth are unsightly and also useless because they do not meet their opposite numbers. Orthodontic treatment at the age of 9 or 10 years can often remedy the defect.

Dental hygiene. Care of the teeth includes at least seven points:

1. Vigorous and thorough tooth brushing, preferably morning and evening, but particularly in the evening, with the entire front and back surfaces of the teeth vigorously brushed with a reasonably hard toothbrush containing many bristles - about fifteen forwards and backwards horizontal strokes, i.e., sixty double strokes in all. In this brushing tooth-pastes are quite useful, especially those that contain added fluoride, but the brushing is far more important than the paste.

2. Eating foods that require adequate chewing to clean the teeth. Examples of such foods are rye bread, Scandinavian flat bread, toast, and such raw vegetables as cucumber and carrots.

3. Eating plenty of fruits and green vegetables to ensure sufficiency of the water-soluble vitamins, especially vitamin C.

4. Taking a diet containing adequate amounts of calcium and vitamin D.

5. Normally drinking water in which any deficiency of fluoride has been corrected, to bring the fluoride content to approximately one part per million.

6. Limiting the consumption of sweets, cakes, sweet biscuits and sweet puddings, and ensuring that they are eaten before - and not after - tooth brushing.

7. Having a dental inspection, with

scaling of the teeth if necessary, twice every year.

In general the standard of dental hygiene in Britain is not high. As a nation we tend to eat far too much sugar and white flour, many of our water supplies are deficient in fluoride, too often tooth brushing is forgotten or undertaken in a very perfunctory manner, and visits to the dentist are postponed until pain indicates the presence of unprevented dental caries. As a whole, therefore, British adults and children have bad teeth. By the age of 2 years, half the children in Britain show signs of tooth decay, and by the age of 12, less than 4 per cent of children are free from decayed, filled, or missing teeth.

On the other hand, it is possible to carry insistence on dental hygiene to excess. Our teeth will not suddenly decay because we were so tired last night that we did not brush them properly, or because we succumbed to temptation and ate a couple of sticky sweet cakes. It is the general and habitual attention to dental hygiene that matters, not the occasional deviation from it.

teeth, artificial or **dentures.** Artificial or false teeth may be partial, replacing only a number of teeth, or complete, replacing all the teeth in a jaw. Their provision is essential to allow a person who has lost teeth to chew properly, and they also prevent the face of such a person from developing a sunk-in appearance.

After dentures have been inserted, soft foods may have to be eaten for a couple of days until the patient becomes used to the dentures. A return visit to the dentist is often necessary as false teeth may press at one or two places and require adjustment. It is important to wear the dentures on the day before visiting the dentist, so that he can see the reddened areas and thus identify the exact points of pressure. Speech may be slightly indistinct for the first two or three days after starting to wear dentures.

The care of artificial teeth includes rinsing or brushing them after meals and placing them overnight in water containing salt or denture cleaner.

teething. The stage of eruption of the teeth, starting at about 6 to 9 months in the case of the milk teeth and continuing until about 15 years for the permanent teeth, with the last of the permanent teeth (the wisdom teeth) erupting at between 17 and 25 years.

Many young children are fractious and irritable during teething, but it is a mistake to attribute all illnesses in such children to teething. The teething process can sometimes be hastened by giving the child a rusk or hard crust to try to chew, and the diet during teething should contain adequate quantities of vitamins A and D (e.g., from appropriate dosage of cod liver oil or halibut oil drops) and adequate calcium (e.g., from a pint of milk and an egg daily).

television and health. Many criticisms, mostly casual and unproved, are made of the effects of watching 'the box'. In excess it reduces access to fresh air, limits the taking of healthy exercise, converts people from active providers of their own entertainment to passive viewers, limits discussion and family conversation, damages the creative imagination by imposing pictures and scenes as visualized by someone else, and may harm the eyesight, although probably no more so than does intensive reading. On the other hand its supporters say that it brings to the viewer a much wider view of life, that it raises for consideration aspects of problems that a person in a narrow cultural atmosphere may never have encountered or imagined, and that it is a profound educational influence.

There is a modicum of sense in both attitudes. Clearly extreme viewing – like other extremes – can be harmful; but there is little if any concrete evidence that a moderate amount of viewing does any damage either to parents or to their children. The wise parent will, however, try to exercise unobtrusive censorship not only over quantity but also quality, ensuring, for example, that an excitable child does not see an alarming play shortly before going to bed.

temperament. Natural disposition. The tendency of a person – partially inherited and partially created by relationships with others in the formative years – to be easily angered or slow to anger, optimistic or pessimistic, extroverted or introverted, and cautious with strangers or 'hail-fellow-well-met'.

temperature. The normal temperature of the body varies with time of day (lowest in the early morning) and with the part of the body (lower in the armpit than in the mouth and higher in the rectum). The average mouth temperature of the human is 36 ° to 37.2 °C. (97 ° to 99 °F.). Some warm-blooded creatures, especially birds, have higher temperatures, although all mammals, including humans, fall into the warm-blooded class; and cold-blooded creatures, e.g., reptiles and fishes, have much lower temperatures.

Temperature is kept fairly even by maintenance of a balance between heat production (e.g., by muscular exercise) and heat loss (e.g., by sweating), with the amount of heat loss regulated by a centre in the brain.

In some diseases, such as most fevers, the mechanism for regulating heat loss is thrown out of control, so that the temperature rises. It may rise as high as 43 °C. (110 °F.) but there is risk to life after it reaches 41.6 °C. (107 °F.).

In extreme cold, starvation, severe loss of blood and some diseases the heat regulating mechanism cannot cope with the heat loss, and so the temperature falls.

°C   °F

Temperature conversions

It may sink to 32 °C. (90 °F.) but there is danger when it passes below 35 °C. (95 °F.).

Old people are peculiarly liable to suffer from a cold environment with which their heat regulating centre cannot cope. Their temperature falls gradually, often without them becoming aware that they are cold. The condition is called HYPOTHERMIA.

temper tantrums. Episodes of uncontrolled rage, usually in small children, but occasionally also occurring in old people. A tantrum may be sheer blackmail, or it may be an attempt to express a very genuine and urgent need, as in emotional starvation, or again it may be a reaction to a terrifying situation. In the last case the situation, which may not appear in any way alarming to an adult, calls for prompt separation of the child from the situation. That being excluded, neither immediate demonstrated affection nor punishment is particularly useful: to kiss and cuddle the child may be to yield to emotional blackmail and ensure repetition; to smack or scold him is unfair, since his emotions are temporarily out of his control, and it is

a cruel response to what may be an expression of desperate need. It is generally best to ensure that the child is so placed that he cannot seriously hurt himself, to show neither resentment nor concern but to leave him to howl for a few minutes, and then to seek to divert him with a new toy or a favourite game. Where tantrums are frequent psychological investigation may be needed.

In general, temper tantrums are a reaction to frustration, and most parents experience some such worry when their children disregard prohibitions and make a scene when they are not allowed to do as they wish. This sort of behaviour is very common in the toddler and is characteristic of his stage of development. It must be handled intelligently and not allowed to become an invariable pattern of reaction because this leads to the eventual emergence of the petulant, childish and resentful adult.

The child of 2 to 4 years taxes his parents' forbearance because he has become able to understand what is said to him and his offence is greater when he ignores it. His temper tantrums must be dealt with by insistence on a sensible regular routine maintained with firmness and patience. Restrictions should be as few as possible and must not reflect parental whim, impulse or inconsistency. They should also be explained by simple reason and logic capable of being appreciated by the child, and they must be adhered to and enforced. Children are also influenced by simple cause-and-effect punishments such as taking away their crayons if they refuse to stop scribbling on the wallpaper.

Conformity may be secured by compromise such as the imaginative substitution of some pleasurable alternative activity instead of adopting coercion which only aggravates anger and obstinacy. When a full-blown tantrum develops it is best dealt with by standing aside and letting the child expend his wrath without interference. To give in is fatal, but after the emotional outburst has subsided of its own accord the parents ought not to scold or show disapproval – comforting and pleasurable distraction are required instead. It is important to avoid making issues and having direct clashes. Imagination and ingenuity will suggest alternatives to divert a child from his immediate frustration. Many prohibitions result from fears for a child's safety. It is better to arrange the environment so that safety is inherent and the prohibitions unnecessary.

At a somewhat later age (3 to 7) tantrums sometimes result from what is known as the Oedipus (or Electra) complex: boys try to replace their father in their mother's affections and vice versa for girls.

Demonstrations of affection between the parents arouse envy and anxiety and may result in unexplained bouts of temper or nightmares. Usually these anxieties can be resolved if the child is treated particularly affectionately by the parent who is envied and whose removal is secretly desired.

Reactions of anger occur at other ages too. Even in the infant, too many caresses and too much emotional involvement may so condition it to being fondled that subsequent relationships seem cold and unsatisfactory by comparison. Thus the 1-year-old, suddenly deprived of intimate nursing contacts, feels neglected and strives for attention by inordinate demands which turn to sulkiness and temper when not fulfilled. Over-indulgence is particularly likely when a mother's own emotional life is unsatisfactory. Although adequate nursing intimacies are important for proper psychological development they should not be excessive and should be withdrawn gradually and replaced by other satisfactions if trouble is to be avoided.

Older childhood and adolescence are periods of growing independence. The school child increasingly makes to make his own decisions and do things for himself. Inevitably he is much slower and less accomplished than an adult, but if he is laughed at, or ignored, or prevented, or given no encouragement, he again becomes bewildered and angry. Nevertheless, to be allowed to decide for himself is the only way to develop beyond the stage of impulse. If he is prevented from carrying out his own ideas he reverts to the childish practice of temper tantrums or other aberrations of behaviour.

Similarly, adolescence is a period in which there is still further rebellion against established ways of life and this may be reflected in vandalism and delinquency unless constructive outlets are provided for the impatience and enthusiasms of youth.

tendinitis. Inflammation of a tendon, often caused by unusual and excessive use. The tendon becomes both painful and tender and may creak on movement. Rest is the main treatment, but severe cases may be helped by injections of hydrocortisone, and in some cases physiotherapy is needed after the inflammation has subsided.

tendon. A tough band of dense connective tissue which attaches a muscle to a bone. Typical tendons are the short, thick ones attaching the biceps muscle to the shoulder, and the long, thin ones that run from the forearm across the back of the wrist and hand to the fingers.

tenesmus. A constant sensation of weight and discomfort in the lower bowel, with desire to visit the lavatory, accompanied by straining in attempts – often unsuccessful – to empty the rectum. Tenesmus may be caused by the bowel being loaded with hard masses of faeces or by various diseases of the rectum, e.g., fissure or polypus; and it is also common in dysentery and other forms of diarrhoea. Warm hip baths or hot fomentations often

help, but if the symptom continues it requires investigation.

tennis elbow. See ELBOW.

tenosynovitis. Inflammation of the sheath surrounding a tendon and also of the tendon itself. Causes include a focus of sepsis (bacterial infection) elsewhere, damp, draughts and over-use of the muscle. The main symptom is pain, which is worse on movement, and in later stages worse in cold or damp weather and also worse on going to bed at night. Treatment involves looking for and removing the focus of sepsis, providing local heat and massage, supplying analgesics for the pain, and sometimes giving injections of hydrocortisone.

tension. Mental or emotional strain or strained personal relations. Tension arises mainly from the non-satisfaction of various needs (e.g., for affection, work success or social status). It sometimes expresses itself in outbursts of temper or in prolonged irritability, in which case the person is getting rid of his tension, however unpleasant the process may be for others. In other cases the tension is repressed into silent brooding or worrying, and in this eventuality it may lead to headaches, backache, cramps and various psychosomatic diseases.

Physical activity is often a good way of providing relief from a domestic or work situation that is creating tension. So is discussion of the particular problem with a trusted friend or relative.

terminal. At the end; when used describing an illness it indicates the approach of death.

tertian fever. See MALARIA.

testicle. One of a pair of glands in the male reproductive system, also known as the testis. The right and left testes are suspended in the scrotum by the spermatic cords which contain blood vessels and a secretory duct, the vas deferens. Each testis is an egg-shaped glandular body about 2.5 cm. by 3.8 cm. (1 in. by 1.5 in.) in size, made up of germinal tissue which produces spermatozoa or male germ cells and other tissue which supplies the male hormone testosterone.

Attached to the rear border of the testis is the epididymis which is a twisted tube receiving spermatozoa from the seminal tubules and continuing into the vas deferens.

Diseases. Inflammation of the testicle (orchitis) may occur in gonorrhoea, in almost any infection spreading from the urethra or prostate gland, or – quite often – in mumps. The main symptoms are swelling, pain and tenderness. Orchitis of bacterial origin responds well to antibiotics. Orchitis as a complication of mumps subsides in a few days without treatment other than rest and warm applications but may cause permanent sterility.

Cysts are of two types, dermoid cysts, which are essentially foetal remnants, and spermatoceles, which are swellings due to obstruction of the central tubes of the testis and are usually found in elderly men. Solid tumours occur rarely and are more often benign than malignant.

Variocele is essentially a varicose condition of the veins of the spermatic cord, and hydrocele is an accumulation of fluid in the capsule of the testis.

Treatment of cysts, tumours, variocele and hydrocele varies with the cause and the size of the swelling, but in some cases surgical treatment is needed.

testicle, undescended. Retarded or absent descent of the testicles. The testicles are formed in the abdomen of the developing male child and remain there in fish and birds. In man and other mammals they normally pass downwards into the scrotum before or soon after birth. In about 7 per cent of boys one testicle or both fail to descend by the age of one year. Causes of failure include anatomical abnormalities, endocrine deficiencies, and possibly abnormalities of the sex chromosome. In most of these cases the descent occurs spontaneously before the age of 8 years but in cases where descent does not occur by that age (about 1 boy in every 500) hormone treatment or surgical operation may be needed, because the internal temperature of the abdomen is too high to allow the testicles to function normally, so that the person with undescended testicles may be unable to manufacture live sperms.

test meal. A procedure for investigating the chemical function of the stomach by the analysis of small fractions of its contents at intervals during the process of digestion.

In the morning the patient swallows a thin rubber tube (Ryle's tube). The fasting gastric juice is withdrawn and measured, its content of bile and mucus is noted, its acidity is determined and it is also tested for starch (because presence of starch suggests some degree of obstruction at the ring of muscle that separates stomach from duodenum). A measured quantity of gruel is then given and further samples of gastric juice withdrawn at intervals for the next three hours. The acidity of each sample is measured and the sample is tested for starch, bile and blood. Consideration of the results is of help in diagnosis because characteristic findings are obtained in such conditions as gastritis, gastric ulcer, duodenal ulcer, cancer and pernicious anaemia.

For some purposes, however, the test meal is now replaced by a simpler procedure: a resin containing quinine is given by mouth, an injection of histamine stimulates release of quinine if the stomach contains hydrochloric acid, and the amount of quinine excreted in the urine is measured.

A test-feed for infants suspected of suffering from UNDERFEEDING involves assessing only the quantity of milk taken.

testosterone. Male hormone, an internal secretion produced by certain cells (cells of Leydig) in the testis and responsible for the development and function of male sexual characteristics. Originally extracted from bull's testes (by McGee in 1929) it can now be prepared synthetically from cholesterol. A range of similar substances (androgens) has been developed and of these the one mainly used therapeutically is either testosterone propionate or methyl testosterone. Androgens are employed as replacement therapy in castrated males and in those with similar symptoms from other causes. In the male climacteric they are of doubtful value. In the female they are used for the treatment of inoperable breast cancer, some cases of uterine bleeding, and dysmenorrhoea (pain during menstruation) because they counteract excess of the female hormone oestrogen, but they may cause signs and symptoms of masculinization. They are given by intramuscular injection, but more prolonged effects can be secured by using androgens in oily solution, or by implanting pellets below the skin.

tetanus. A serious disease caused by toxin of the tetanus bacillus (*Clostridium tetani*) which multiplies in infected wounds after contamination from soil and dust. Punctured or deep wounds are particularly suspect but tetanus can also develop after burns and may follow mere grazes or trivial disregarded injuries. A special type, tetanus neonatorum, occurs in infants through infection of the umbilical stump.

The incubation period is variable with an average of ten days and the initial symptoms are stiffness of the neck and jaw (lockjaw) followed by generalized rigidity and spasmodic contractions of the whole body with eventually death from respiratory and cardiac failure.

Treatment of the established disease is by anti-tetanic serum, penicillin and sedation, but cases should rarely arise if adequate attention is paid to prevention. Children should be actively immunized by tetanus toxoid from infancy and antitetanus injection should form an essential part of the routine treatment of injuries involving breaches of the skin.

tetany. A rare disease of the nervous system produced by a deficiency of calcium in the blood.

Infantile tetany occurs in young children usually as a complication of rickets or of diseases which lower the absorption of calcium, such as coeliac disease and severe diarrhoeal conditions. The condition may begin with a convulsion or series of convulsions. Spasm of the larynx may cause 'crowing' sounds (laryngismus stridulus) and result in breathing difficulty which may prove fatal. The hands and feet tend to adopt a characteristic posture (carpopedal spasm). Once recognized the symptoms yield readily to intravenous calcium and vitamin D.

Tetany in adults is usually due to injury or disease of the parathyroid glands or to gastro-intestinal disease interfering with calcium absorption. Long-term treatment with calcium and vitamin D is required. The apparently logical use of parathyroid hormone has not been very successful in practice.

tetracyclines. A class of antibiotics very useful in such diseases as whooping cough and influenzal meningitis. They sometimes have undesirable side effects and so need to be used with care.

thalamus. A part of the brain which acts as a relay station for sensory impressions, since it has extensive nerve connections with the cortex above and the spinal cord below, as well as with the cerebellum, optic tracts, and auditory nerves. Its functional level can be regarded as intermediate between the voluntary activity of the cortex and the reflex activity of the cord.

thalassaemia. A chronic progressive anaemia caused by a hereditary inability to use iron to manufacture haemoglobin. The disease is common in the Middle East, India and China, and is quite often found in immigrants from these parts.

There are two forms. In thalassaemia major there is very severe anaemia, enlarged abdomen through swelling of the spleen and liver, and often prominence of the forehead and sunken appearance of the bridge of the nose. This form of the condition is usually fatal during infancy, and there is no specific treatment although surgical removal of the spleen appears to help in some cases.

In thalassaemia minor the anaemia is only mild, the spleen and liver are only slightly enlarged, and the expectation of life is normal.

thalidomide. Extremely favourable reports about this drug (alpha-phthalimido-gluta-rimide) were first made public at a symposium in Germany in 1955. It was claimed to be an entirely new form of sedative and hypnotic free from the disadvantages of barbiturates, bromides and alkaloids. As a derivative of glutamic acid, a substance naturally involved in brain metabolism, it was regarded as particularly safe. In animal toxicity tests it had proved impossible to determine a lethal dose, and in clinical trials it was well tolerated even in severe liver insufficiency.

It was subsequently widely marketed under various trade-names for the treatment of anxiety, insomnia, migraine, asthma, and so on. It soon became well-established as a sedative producing calmness without confusion, and as a hypnotic restoring normal sleep-patterns.

Unfortunately, no one had done preliminary tests to determine if it was a drug affecting the foetus. The first note of alarm was sounded about 1960 when it was noticed that some mothers who had taken it during pregnancy were producing babies with serious deformities, particularly the absence or faulty development of limbs.

As soon as it was appreciated that this was due to thalidomide the drug was, of course, withdrawn (1961). Since then there have been prolonged legal battles to apportion blame and secure compensation for the victims (about four hundred in Great Britain alone).

It is easy to be wise after the event but perhaps it should have been foreseen that a drug which depressed adult nerve-cell activity so efficiently might also interfere with the function of embryonic nerve tissue on which other development depended.

therapeutics. The science and art of alleviating or curing disease. The term includes not only the giving of medicines and drugs but the use of other methods of treatment.

Therapeutics may therefore be (1) rational when the expected result of a remedy is based on accepted scientific knowledge of pathology and pharmacology; (2) empirical when a remedy is known to be effective although its action may not be fully understood; or (3) general when remedies are employed which are not medicines or drugs. This last includes measures like diet, climate, spa and bath treatment, massage, medical gymnastics and the use of physical agencies such as heat, light, electricity and radiation.

Therapy is the application of the principles of therapeutics. Usually a prefix indicates its precise nature, as for example physiotherapy, hydrotherapy, electrotherapy, deep x-ray therapy and so on.

thermometer. An instrument for measuring temperature. In principle, a simple conventional thermometer consists of a glass bulb containing a liquid (usually mercury or alcohol) which on heating expands along a very fine graduated and calibrated tube to give a reading indicative of the bulb's temperature.

Various thermometers are used in medical and nursing practice. Clinical thermometers measure body-temperature and are graduated from 35 °C. to 44 °C. or from 95 °F. to 110 °F. The ordinary oral type is used in mouth or armpit, and a stouter rectal type records temperature in the rectum. In clinical thermometers, the capillary-tube has a constriction so that the mercury-column separates when the bulb cools and remains in position until a reading can be taken. The column must then be shaken down before re-use. Low-reading clinical thermometers are graduated from 21 °C. and are required for the detection of hypothermia, usually in infants or the aged. Normal body TEMPERATURE is 36.9 °C. (98.4 °F.).

Conversion rules. To convert Fahrenheit to Centigrade first subtract thirty-two from the Fahrenheit reading, multiply the answer by five and then divide by nine; to convert Centigrade to Fahrenheit first multiply the Centigrade reading by nine, divide the answer by five and then add thirty-two.

thiamine. A complex organic compound

more familiarly known as vitamin B₁ or aneurin. Deficiency causes the disease beriberi.

Good sources of the vitamin are yeast, wheat and wheat-germ, brown rice (but not polished rice), egg-yolk, liver, chocolate, bacon and ham. Beriberi does not occur in Britain, but the intake of vitamin B₁ may be marginally insufficient under poor dietary conditions or in alcoholics. Signs of deficiency may include heart weakness and neuritis.

The daily requirements are 200 to 300 International Units for adults and proportionally less for children (1 IU = 3 micrograms). For prevention of deficiency one 3 mg. tablet daily is a usual prescription.

thigh. The upper part of the leg extending from the trunk to the knee. Its central support is a single bone, the largest in the body, known as the FEMUR.

thinking. Purposeful activity of the mind. It used to be common to divide conscious mental experience (i.e., ignoring the UNCONSCIOUS MIND) into feeling, willing and thinking, or in psychological jargon the affective, conative and cognitive aspects; but these tend to be very intermixed. Broadly, however, thinking presupposes two preliminary steps: first, perception, the stimulation of our sense organs by external sights, sounds and so on, the transmission of impulses from the sense organs to the brain, and their meaningful interpretation (e.g., as a distressed cry or as the appearance of a person); and second, the relation of perception to past experiences or to ideas (e.g., deciding that the distressed cry means that our child is hurt or in danger or that the person is the neighbour whom we desire to avoid). Real thinking begins when our perceptions and recollections of parallel experiences, ideas or imaginings alert us to a problem. The solution to the problem may be simple (e.g., that we should pick up and comfort the crying child or cross the street to avoid the neighbour) or it may be extremely complex and even beyond our abilities, but the attempt to solve it is the essence of thinking. The thinking may be misdirected if the perception is false (as in optical illusions) or if the relation to past experience is incorrect (as when we mistake the child's cry of joy for one of distress), but it is still thinking.

The purpose of thought is to solve problems by using and manipulating knowledge derived from immediate and stored perceptions. Many situations demand immediate action, and previous experience ensures that there is an answer ready. Thus a car-driver regulates his responses in accordance with traffic conditions and may appear to act almost reflexly, but actually these responses are being thought out on the basis of current stimuli and earlier perceptions. If no answer is immediately forthcoming the second stage of thought is to examine the

problem more closely – we 'stop and think'. The next stage is to attempt to resurrect from the mind the facts and principles necessary for a solution. This may take time – recognized by the traditional advice to 'sleep on it'. The recovery of latent ideas depends largely on association. If two ideas occurred together in the past, the calling up of one will tend also to recall the other, but what emerges may be affected unexpectedly by the immediate trend of thought.

Like other biological activities, thought can be influenced in many ways. It is for instance adversely affected by disease or by emotion which narrows the span of consciousness. When afraid or anxious we are unable to turn our thoughts from the object of our fear or anxiety. Mental disease in particular is essentially a disordered way of thought. On the other hand increased efficiency of thought can be developed with practice by building up our store of associations and by exercising our minds with problems so that we acquire an increased facility for the recovery of these associations from our subconscious.

thinness. Body-build is determined largely by constitutional and genetic factors. Many people in perfect health remain consistently thin despite an adequate or even generous dietary intake. This need cause no concern because the tall slender child and the 'skinny' adult with little or no subcutaneous fat are both within the limits of normality. Tabulated weights for height and age usually show only average values and a normal range can be 10 per cent above or below. There are some advantages in being thin; on the whole, thin people have fewer illnesses and live longer, because there is less strain on important systems, notably those of the heart, circulation, and joints.

Sudden or gradual loss of weight is, however, another matter. Thinness which develops as a result of this may be due to a variety of causes including disturbances of the endocrine glands, disorders of the digestive system, diabetes, tuberculosis, anaemia, malignant disease, alcoholism and depression. It calls for investigation.

Excessive thinness is known as emaciation when there is no suspected internal cause (e.g., the thinness that occurs in famine conditions), or cachexia when it is accompanied by signs of disease (e.g., the thinness found in cancer of the stomach). The emaciation which results from a neurotic refusal to eat is known as ANOREXIA nervosa.

thirst. The sensation of thirst arises from nerve-endings in the pharynx. It may be caused by drying of the mucous membrane in that area due to hot atmospheres, over-breathing, or drugs such as atropine which inhibit secretion; or it may indicate a real need of the body for water replacement. The latter is of course the plight of travellers stranded in the desert, but this kind of true thirst also arises in a variety of diseases and in various ways.

In feverish conditions there is generally excessive fluid loss because of high temperature and perspiration; and increased metabolic rate with sweating is also a feature of hyperthyroidism. Diarrhoea and vomiting occur in many diseases such as gastritis, enteritis, pyloric stenosis and cholera, and fluid loss in such cases is obvious.

Two specific diseases particularly characterized by thirst are diabetes mellitus and diabetes insipidus. In the former additional water is needed for urine which excretes some of the excess sugar, and in the latter a defect of the pituitary gland leads to massive passing of urine.

Infants suffer from thirst more often than is realized if kept too warm and given over-concentrated feeds. Crying and restlessness should not be interpreted indiscriminately as a demand for extra food if the requisite Calories for weight are already being provided. A bottle of sterilized water instead will often relieve the situation.

thoracic duct. The main channel by which lymph and chyle are conveyed to the blood-stream. Chyle is the milky fluid taken up by the lymphatic vessels of the intestine and is a mixture of lymph and emulsified fat. The thoracic duct drains the greater part of the body and discharges its contents into the veins in the root of the neck. A smaller right lymphatic duct drains the right upper half of the body and similarly joins the same veins on the right side.

thoracoplasty. An operation on the chest-wall to reduce the size of the underlying thoracic cavity.

Since lung-tissue is spongy, disease of various kinds may result in the formation of cavities. The sides of these cavities must be brought together so that they may heal over and this is achieved by compressing the affected lung tissue in a chest which has been made smaller by thoracoplasty. The scope of the operation required depends on the site and extent of the lung disease. In complete thoracoplasty the upper nine or ten ribs are removed so that the chest-wall can move inwards and compress the lung.

The procedure was formerly much used in the later stages of recovery from pulmonary tuberculosis but is now less necessary because of the introduction of effective drugs capable of arresting the disease before the occurrence of extensive tissue-destruction.

The operation is also employed in lung-abscess and bronchiectasis.

thorax. See CHEST.

threadworms. The threadworm *Enterobius vermicularis* is a very common intestinal parasite especially in children. The male is about 0.5 cm. and the female 1.0 cm. in length and they may often be seen in the faeces resembling short pieces of whitish thread. They inhabit the lower bowel and at night, with the patient warm in bed, may cause great discomfort and itching by emerging on to the skin around the anus where the female deposits her eggs. The skin becomes damaged and eczematous from scratching. Bladder irritability, frequency of passing urine, vaginitis and mucoid discharge from the anus may also occur. General health may be impaired by restlessness and sleeplessness. Persistent infection is maintained and spread to others by swallowing eggs transmitted on the hands contaminated during scratching. Diagnosis may be confirmed by microscopical identification of eggs in anal smears.

Effective treatment is available by appropriate drugs but complete eradication of the worms requires scrupulous attention to hand-washing, disinfection of night attire and bed-clothing, and simultaneous attention to other members of the household.

thrombocytes. See PLATELETS.

thrombosis. The clotting or coagulation of blood within living blood vessels. This may occur in the heart, arteries or veins, but it is commonest in veins where the blood is relatively slow-moving. If the clot remains attached it is a thrombus; if it floats away to lodge elsewhere it is called an embolus (see EMBOLISM). Thrombosis results from altered blood conditions as in anaemia or infection; from venous stagnation as in varicose veins or in prolonged bed-rest enforced by operation or illness; and from inflammation and degeneration of vessel walls.

Common sites of arterial clotting are the blood vessels of the heart (leading to CORONARY THROMBOSIS) and of the brain (leading to STROKE). Elderly persons with deteriorating blood vessels may also develop thrombosis of the retinal artery with loss of vision or of leg arteries leading to gangrene.

Venous thrombosis is most common in leg or pelvic veins and carries a risk of subsequent pulmonary embolism. It may occur after childbirth or abdominal operations and is one reason for the policy of encouraging early mobility in such patients.

The treatment of established thrombosis is by anticoagulant drugs and rest.

Thrombosis

thrush. Infection of mucous membrane by yeast-like fungi of the genus *Monilia*. The common species is *M. albicans*.

Thrush occurs mainly in young bottle-fed infants and appears as white patches of the fungus firmly attached to tongue or palate. In premature or debilitated infants the patches may spread to the pharynx, oesophagus or even the intestine. However, in most cases the extent of infection is limited to the mouth and its principal effect is to make the infant reluctant to feed and suck properly.

Treatment is relatively easy and effective. The traditional remedy was to paint the affected areas with a 1 per cent solution of gentian violet, but the fungicide nystatin as Nystatin Mixture applied locally by dropper is now generally preferred. Scrupulous attention must be paid to the cleaning and sterilization of equipment used in feeding infants.

thymus gland. A two-lobed ENDOCRINE GLAND, lying at the base of the neck, concerned with combating infection and possibly also with growth and development.

thyroid gland. An important ENDOCRINE GLAND lying in the neck and concerned with regulating the body's metabolic rate. Enlargement of the gland produces the condition known as GOITRE, and excessive secretion of thyroid hormone results in THYROTOXICOSIS.

thyrotoxicosis. The condition which results from hyperthyroidism or excessive secretion of thyroid hormone by the thyroid gland.

Primary thyrotoxicosis occurs in exophthalmic goitre (Graves' disease) which is characterized by enlargement of the glands, increased pulse-rate, prominent eyeballs, loss of weight, nervousness and tremors and an increased metabolic rate, which in turn causes sweating, thirst, increased appetite and sometimes other evidence of disordered metabolism – such as the excretion in the urine of sugar and the reduction of the level of cholesterol in the blood.

Secondary thyrotoxicosis is not essentially different. It results not from general over-functioning of the gland but from thyroid tumour. Signs of hyperthyroidism are less obvious and effects fall mainly on the cardio-vascular system. Auricular fibrillation (a type of disordered heart action) and signs of heart failure may develop before it is appreciated that these have a thyroid basis.

The treatment of thyrotoxicosis is now a very advanced speciality involving the use of drugs like thiouracil which stop or reduce the manufacture of thyroxine, and radio-active iodine which destroys over-active thyroid tissue; and sometimes surgery is necessary to excise part of the gland or to remove a tumour. Each case requires individual expert assessment.

tibia. The inner and larger of the two bones in the lower part of the leg. At its upper end it is enlarged to articulate with the thigh bone or femur at the knee-joint, and its lower end forms part of the ankle-joint.

Its front edge or crest lies just beneath the skin and is prominent at the shin and rather exposed to casual injury in such activities as football and cricket. It is also the bone most liable to show deformity as a result of rickets.

tic. Any sudden, rapid, twitching, involuntary movement that occurs repeatedly. Essentially tics are a group of nervous diseases in which there occur: (1) repetitions of sudden twitch-like movements, (2) sudden involuntary utterances, or (3) deliberate repetitive co-ordinated actions related to an imperative idea. Combinations of these types occur.

Simple tic usually shows in 'nervous' children by repeated blinking, grimacing, head-jerking, shoulder-shrugging and similar actions. Most cases recover spontaneously.

In convulsive tic spasmodic movements are more extensive and often accompanied by grotesque attitudes or apparent miming.

In psychic or verbal tic there is an uncontrollable impulse to repeat irrelevant words.

These two types affect older persons and often progress to mental deterioration.

The co-ordinated tic, sometimes seen in highly competent persons under stress, takes the form of purposeless repetition of complicated co-ordinated movements such as twiddling a pencil, jingling change in a trouser-pocket or fidgeting with a tie.

tic douloureux. See TRIGEMINAL NEURALGIA.

ticks. Arthropods of the class Arachnida which also includes scorpions, spiders and mites. Ticks and mites are similar and are grouped together as acarids. Most are very small, many are parasitic on a wide range of wild and domestic animals and some, in tropical and sub-tropical countries, are carriers of disease.

Ticks are usually oval or circular because their neck and abdomen are fused. Adult forms have eight legs and beak-like mouth parts adapted for sucking blood. Hard ticks (*Ixodidae*) have a shell while soft ticks (*Argasidae*) have no shell.

Hard ticks transmit tularemia and rickettsial infections and soft ticks spread African relapsing fever, and some animal diseases are also tick-borne. In countries where ticks are prevalent, preventive measures include the destruction of animals likely to infect sheep and cattle, and the dipping of flocks and herds. Workers in infested areas should wear a one-piece suit with tight fitting wristlets and anklets.

tinea. The scientific name for RINGWORM. Care should be taken to distinguish the term *Tinea* from *Taenia*, the latter being a generic name of TAPEWORMS.

tinnitus. See HEAD NOISES.

tobacco and health. See SMOKING.

toe. One of the five terminal members of the foot, corresponding to the fingers, and consisting essentially of two bones in the big toe and three in each of the other toes, with surrounding muscles, nerves and blood vessels. The toes play an important part in enabling us to maintain balance, e.g., when leaning forwards; and, where not stiffened by the habitual wearing of shoes, they can also bend considerably and so be of help in such activities as climbing trees. In communities habitually using footwear much of the mobility of the toes has been lost, but some people who have in early life lost the use of hands through illness or accident have learned to paint pictures and to operate typewriters with their toes.

Diseases. Congenital defects of the toes may take the form of extra toes (polydactylism), webbing or fusion of adjacent toes (syndactylism), contracted little toes, or enlargement of one or more toes. If any of these cause troublesome symptoms, they should be treated surgically.

Other conditions are related to the use of unsuitable footwear and symptoms are aggravated by the consequent development of corns, bursae, or arthritis. Gangrene of toes is quite frequently seen as a complication of diabetes and of diseases of small blood vessels. Acute arthritis, especially of the great toe, is common in gout, and ringworm may affect the nails and the skin between the toes (athlete's foot).

Onychogryphosis is a condition in which the toe-nails become enlarged and distorted, usually in elderly persons as a result of neglect.

Hallux valgus. Outward deflection of the great toe so that it may come to lie either above or below the second toe. The joint at the base of the toe is distorted and the head of the metacarpal bone projects on the inner side of the foot. Pressure on this causes arthritic changes, the overlying skin becomes thickened, and a BUNION may develop.

Hammer toe. A common deformity, usually affecting the second toe, in which the toe is bent in different directions at its various joints so that it takes the shape of an inverted 'v' with the apex projecting above the line of the other toes. The condition usually appears in adolescence and may be caused or aggravated by unsuitable footwear – too short, too pointed, or with excessively high heels. The subsequent development of corns, callosities or bursae over pressure-points will produce pain and disability.

In mild cases strapping down the toe or wearing a night-splint may secure improvement.

The surgical treatment of more severe cases is to remove the first joint (the apex of the 'v') and allow the bones to unite in a straight position. Amputation of the toe is not a good procedure since it allows the great toe to diverge sideways as in hallux valgus.

Ingrowing toe-nail. See NAIL, INGROWING.

toilet training. See INFANCY, PSYCHOLOGY OF.

The tongue

tongue. A muscular organ lying in the floor of the mouth. Its rear or pharyngeal part (the base) is relatively fixed while the front or oral part is freely mobile. It is covered by mucous membrane which is somewhat rough owing to the presence of projections called papillae. These are of various types, being small and velvety in front and much larger and more obvious behind. The tongue is concerned with SPEECH, SWALLOWING and TASTE.

Diseases. Superficial inflammation of the tongue is glossitis, usually associated with STOMATITIS, which is inflammation of the mucous membranes of the mouth. It may result from local sepsis as in dental caries and pyorrhoea; from gastric disorder and excessive smoking and drinking; or, in children, from infections by viruses and fungi (see THRUSH). A chronic variety is leukoplakia, where there are raised white hardened patches which may ulcerate and may become malignant.

Treatment varies with the cause, but usually the most important part of the treatment is the allaying of the fear of cancer, either by reassurance or, if necessary, by taking for laboratory examination a small scraping of the cells lining the tongue.

Deep inflammatory conditions of the tongue, which may lead to abscesses, occur when infection spreads to the substance of the tongue from superficial injuries or ulcers; they are also seen in mercurial poisoning, syphilis and actinomycosis.

Ulcers are usually the result of injury from teeth or of dyspepsia, but may be tuberculous, syphilitic or malignant.

Of tumours the commonest varieties are dermoid cysts and papillomata; cancer of the tongue is most often seen in men over 40 who are heavy smokers.

Black hairy tongue is a striking but unimportant condition due to overgrowth and staining of the papillae. An enlarged tongue is often seen in mongols and other mental defectives and is a congenital abnormality. TONGUE-TIE is described separately.

tongue-tie. On the under surface of the tongue the mucous membrane in the midline is raised up to form a crescentic fold known as the fraenum ('bridle'). If this is so formed as to restrict the movements of the tongue the condition is termed 'tongue-tie' and the front margin of the fold is sometimes snipped with scissors to free the tongue. However, a degree of tongue-tie sufficiently severe to interfere with sucking, or later with speech, is very rare. Usually the operation is carried out in ignorance of the normal appearance of the tongue and fraenum of the young infant. The operation is generally unnecessary.

tonsillitis. Inflammation of the tonsils from bacterial infection. Tonsillitis is a specific feature of diphtheria and measles but its occurrence in scarlet fever and rheumatic fever is due to infection by haemolytic streptococci, and the same organisms can nearly always be incriminated in less specific conditions such as outbreaks of pharyngitis and sporadic attacks of severe sore throat. Most cases occur in children of school age.

The symptoms are pain in the throat, especially on swallowing, general upset with malaise, fever and raised pulse-rate, and often enlarged neck glands. The tonsils appear swollen and red with spots of watery exudate. Pus may then develop producing an abscess or quinsy which will generally require surgical treatment.

Tonsillitis responds well to antibiotic drugs and should always be treated efficiently because of the risk of cardiac and rheumatic complications resulting from infection of the blood. Analgesics and antiseptic gargles also help to relieve the pain. Repeated attacks result in chronic tonsillitis and are usually an indication for removal of the tonsils and the associated adenoidal tissue in the pharynx.

tonsils and adenoids. The tonsils are two bean-shaped masses of lymphoid tissue lying on the side walls of the back of the soft palate on each side of the back of the tongue. They are easily visible when the mouth is widely opened. They are relatively large in children and usually shrink about the time of adolescence. Adenoids, possessed by all children, are pads of lymphoid tissue in the upper part of the throat behind the nasal passages. The pads tend to shrink about the age of 11 years. Tonsils and adenoids are part of the defence mechanism of the body. They help to waylay and destroy invading bacteria and also help to create immunity.

By a common misuse of words, 'tonsils and adenoids' is frequently employed to mean 'enlarged tonsils and adenoids'.

During pre-school and early school

The tonsils and adenoids

years both tonsils and adenoids often become enlarged as a result of repeated minor infections. Many children develop large smooth tonsils which cause no symptoms and later shrink. On the other hand, enlarged, rough-looking tonsils can be a focus of infection, causing enlargement of neck glands and general deterioration in health; over-growth of adenoids can cause nasal obstruction and mouth breathing, snoring, a stupid or vacant appearance, hoarse nasal speech, and sometimes deafness.

In the past enlarged tonsils and adenoids were removed almost routinely, but, while the operation is simple, removal of merely enlarged tonsils and adenoids deprives the body of organs that could perform useful functions. So the modern tendency is to remove them only if they are causing appreciable symptoms or if they are so chronically infected that they are harbouring germs instead of destroying them.

toothache. Sensations related to the teeth are transmitted by branches of the fifth cranial nerve, and dentists distinguish between odontalgia, or pain arising from effects on individual teeth, and neuralgia, in which pain may seem to arise in the teeth but is really from other conditions within the area of the face supplied by the same nerve, such as the nose and sinuses.

In odontalgia, disease of (or injury to) TEETH may expose the dental pulp, which is very sensitive to heat or cold and to the sweet, salt or acid constituents of food. Initially the pain is of a transitory twinge-like character, becoming more persistent and unbearable when the pulp becomes infected, inflamed, and begins to die. The usual cause is dental caries.

Gingivitis or inflammation of the gums leads to gum recession exposing the dentine below the necks of the teeth. This is particularly sensitive to stimulation by food substances which may produce severe

enamel — decay

pulp — dentine

Toothache

pain and prolonged aching thereafter. The onset of toothache in any form is an indication to seek early dental treatment.

torticollis. See WRY NECK.

touch. The skin can feel and differentiate touch, pressure, pain, heat, and cold. Of these, touch is the sensation elicited by, for example, brushing the skin with a wisp of cotton wool or applying a stiff hair, and as a further refinement, sensitivity is tested by using hairs of graded thickness and determining which one is just felt when applied with just sufficient force to bend it.

Touch is appreciated by special skin receptors and these 'touch spots' are not evenly distributed over the body. They are most numerous over the tips of the fingers, palms, soles and lips, and less so over areas such as the back and shoulders. On their closeness depends discrimination or the ability to recognize whether any contact is single or multiple. This is tested by a device like a pair of mathematical dividers or compasses in which the distance between two points can be adjusted. The finger-tips can feel two separate contacts when the points are 1 mm. apart; over the back a separation of 5 cm. may be required.

The very sensitive areas of the skin are characterized by hairlessness, but elsewhere the skin surface bears hairs which are either obvious or rudimentary. Hairs always slant in a definite direction and touch spots are found in the skin on their 'windward' side. Light contact with hair tips causes a sensation of touch since the hair acts like a tiny lever transmitting movement to its base and stimulating the touch receptor.

Sensations of touch travel from the receptors by nerves from the skin back to the spinal cord and thence upwards to the brain and its sensory centres.

Diseases. Alterations in skin sensitivity, of which touch is only one component, provides the neurologist with important diagnostic clues. Departures from normal may be (1) anaesthesia: loss of sensation, (2) hyperaesthesia: increased sensitivity or (3) paraesthesia: abnormal sensations such as burning, prickling or itching.

Each of these may be produced in many ways. Anaesthesia, for instance, may be caused by conditions as diverse as disease of the blood vessels of the brain or leprosy of cutaneous nerves; hyperaesthesia occurs in hysteria, the early stage of poliomyelitis, shingles, tabes, and often over inflamed underlying organs; paraesthesia is experienced in many skin diseases, in sciatica, and in degenerative conditions of the spinal cord. These are only given as examples; unexplained disorders of skin sensation require investigation.

tourniquet. Any appliance used to control haemorrhage from an injured limb by encircling it and applying pressure to its arterial blood-supply.

For first aid use a tourniquet can be improvised from a narrow-fold triangular bandage tied round the limb and tightened by passing a short rod through the knot and twisting.

Tourniquets are dangerous pieces of equipment in unskilled hands. Left on for more than half-an-hour they will cause gangrene of the limb. They must be loosened at least once every thirty minutes

handkerchief

penknife

hard object

An improvised tourniquet

to flush the limb with fresh blood, and only re-tightened if absolutely necessary. In most cases it will be found that clotting and retraction of injured vessels have either arrested the haemorrhage naturally, or have so reduced its force and volume that the slight pressure of a pad and bandage will be effective.

If a patient with a tourniquet is being transferred to the care of others (e.g., taken to hospital), the time of application of the tourniquet should be prominently indicated.

toxaemia. The presence or effects of poisonous substances in the blood-stream.

In bacterial toxaemia the multiplication of micro-organisms at some site of infection produces toxins which are then absorbed into the tissues and blood-stream with harmful results. These may be general, with fever, rigor, headache and vomiting, or related to individual tissues such as the heart or nervous system because of the special affinities of the particular toxin.

Non-bacterial toxaemia arises from deficiency or failure either in the body's breakdown of food substances or in its excretion of waste products. Toxic substances accumulate in the blood-stream and exercise harmful effects either by their abnormal presence or by their abnormally high concentration. Examples are uraemia in kidney disease; hyperglycaemia and acetonaemia in diabetes; thyrotoxicosis in toxic goitre; and cholaemia in obstructive jaundice.

toxic goitre. See GOITRE.

toxicology. The scientific study of POISONS.

toxin. Although the term is often used in a general way to include various harmful substances, toxins in the strict sense are poisons of complex protein nature produced by micro-organisms. Essentially they also act as antigens, i.e., they have the ability to induce the body to form specific antitoxins.

Toxins may be either exotoxins or endotoxins. The former are external products of bacterial growth which diffuse into the medium in which the organism is growing. When absorbed into the circulation they cause specific effects as in diphtheria, tetanus, and botulism. Endotoxins are poisonous constituents of the actual organism, liberated when it dies or disintegrates as the result of its destruction by body-defences. Their effects are less specific and shown by fever and tissue-degeneration.

The distinction is a fundamental one in treatment because exotoxins can be neutralized by appropriate antitoxin but endotoxins can be removed only by eradication of the germ itself.

toxoid. In addition to causing harmful effects, TOXINS also act as antigens. Their presence in the body brings about an immunity response and this normal defence mechanism results in the production of neutralizing antitoxin.

If toxins are mixed with formalin and incubated their toxicity is destroyed but their antigenic or immunizing properties are retained. Filtrates of bacterial cultures detoxicated in this way are known as toxoids, formol toxoids, or anatoxines and can be injected to induce active immunity against various diseases, particularly diphtheria, tetanus, and gas-gangrene.

toxoplasmosis. Infection by *Toxoplasma gondi*, a protozoon. It is a common parasite of many animals and birds. Human infection is perhaps mainly from cysts in meat but the parasite is easily destroyed by heating to 60 °C. (141 °F.) so cooking should protect. However, it has been shown that a large proportion of domestic cats harbour the organism in their intestinal tracts.

In the adult, severe symptoms are not common, as resistance develops rapidly, and diagnosis depends on laboratory tests. There have, however, been cases with fever and swelling of glands, and a few of these cases have been fatal.

Congenital cases are common and more important. Here an infected and often symptomless mother passes infection to her unborn child. In early pregnancy the parasite invades the developing nervous system and may cause brain damage or even death. Later in pregnancy it may cause enlargement of the liver and spleen. After birth the affected child may have swollen lymph glands for a few weeks, or in more severe cases may have permanent damage to brain and eyes.

Preventive measures are as yet uncertain. It is generally assumed that expectant mothers and very young children should avoid intimate contact with sick animals and birds and should probably also avoid close contact with cats and kittens.

trachea. The trachea or windpipe is a tube of cartilage and membrane which provides a channel for the passage of air to and from the lungs. It is about 2 cm. in diameter and 10 cm. long and extends from the larynx in the neck downwards into the upper part of the chest where it divides into the right and left bronchi. Its cartilaginous elements are a series of some twenty rings, incomplete behind. Their purpose is to stiffen the wall of the tube and prevent its collapse, especially while breathing in.

tracheotomy. A surgical operation to provide an alternative airway directly into the trachea or windpipe in the lower neck. Tracheotomy is required if there is dangerous difficulty in breathing due to obstruction of the upper air-passages. This may arise from foreign bodies, laryngeal oedema, diphtheria or tuberculous laryngitis, tumours of larynx or neck, and from some forms of laryngeal paralysis.

Surgical procedures on the mouth, tongue, pharynx or larynx sometimes require preliminary tracheotomy so that the airway may be packed off to prevent blood or septic matter from reaching the lungs.

In tracheotomy the skin and soft tissues are divided in the mid-line of the neck, the trachea incised and a special tube inserted (intubation). This has an inner sleeve that can be removed for cleaning.

A tracheotomy tube should be removed as soon as possible but some cases may require a permanent artificial opening. After a tube has been worn for some weeks the wound will heal with an established and well-defined track and patients soon learn to carry out routine management themselves and experience little inconvenience except from loss of voice, as air no longer traverses the larynx. Care must also be taken to avoid obstruction of the external opening by clothing.

trachoma. Severe, contagious inflammation of the membrane lining the eyelids, caused by a virus, and often resulting in blindness.

Trachoma is a disease of hot dry climates and therefore very rare in the U.K. The incubation period varies from four to seven days, and the inflammation, usually of both eyes, is generally mild at first and sometimes heals of its own accord without treatment. For some reason this spontaneous healing is commoner in children than in adults. More often the inflammation if untreated goes on to scarring of the eyelids, inability to close the eyes, and distortion of vision as a result of inflammatory tissue encroaching on the cornea.

Infection results from direct contact with eye discharges and is sometimes also spread by flies. High prevalence is associated with poor hygiene and crowded living conditions, and the disease is an immense problem in many under-developed countries. In other countries imported cases are occasionally seen, especially in sea-ports and amongst immigrants.

One attack confers no immunity to subsequent re-infection.

Unlike most virus diseases, trachoma responds well to treatment with either antibiotics or sulphonamides. The treatment most favoured nowadays is a combination of two antibiotics. With early treatment the outlook is good.

In warm developing countries where the disease is common it may be desirable to apply an antibiotic ointment to the eyes of contacts for five days a month for several months. Such preventive treatment is costly, however, and contacts can be very numerous.

traction. In fractures of the long bones of the limbs and of the fingers or toes, the muscles are put out of balance and often move the broken ends of the bone out of alignment. Healing in this faulty position will produce serious shortening or misalignment, and so in treatment the limb must be supported in a suitable splint or cradle and the muscle-pull overcome by extension in order to secure correct reposition.

Application of longitudinal counter-force to extend the limb and reduce the displacement is known as traction, generally provided by means of a cord, pulley and weights, or by elastic. The main problem is how to attach the extension force to the limb.

In skeletal traction this is done by the use of pointed callipers, wires, or pins of various design, which grasp or penetrate the actual bone of the lower fragment, and so provide a secure anchorage for the extension. This method is particularly required to oppose powerful muscle-groups as in thigh fractures. In skin traction the extension apparatus is attached to the skin of the limb by means of adhesive strapping.

The principle of traction also has other applications in the treatment of various bone and joint conditions when it is desired to rest the parts in a good position, to relieve pain, and to promote healing. Spinal fractures, 'slipped disc' and tuberculous hip-disease are examples.

traffic accidents. See ACCIDENTS.

trance. A state of profound or abnormal sleep, from which an affected individual cannot easily be roused, and not due to any organic disease or drugs. There is loss of voluntary movement, but consciousness and sensibility may be unaffected. Such a condition is particularly associated with hysteria, a psychoneurotic disease, in which symptoms of illness are assumed (albeit unconsciously) in order to secure some advantage. A trance represents therefore an extreme attempt to escape from some awkward real-life situation.

Stuporous conditions are common in mental disease and the problem in relation to diagnosis and treatment is to differentiate a trance which is a symptom of hysteria from similar manifestations in true psychosis like schizophrenia. This is a matter for expert assessment based on careful study of the patient's past and detailed observation. Hysterical and psychotic trance states have very different outlooks. Hysteria is likely to yield to effective psychotherapy, but in psychotic illness there are basic disorders much less easy to overcome.

tranquillizers. Ideally, a tranquillizer is a drug capable of allaying feelings of tension, worry, anxiety, restlessness and panic without impairing normal alertness and intellectual capacity.

There is now a wide choice of tranquillizers and the sedative range of such drugs has been classified by the World Health Organization as follows: (1) Hypno-sedatives: barbiturates; carbromol BP; glutethimide BP; methyprylone BP. (2) Tranquillo-sedatives: benzodiazepine type; propanediol type; diphenylmethane type. (3) Minor tranquillizers: phenothiazine derivatives such as promazine and promethazine. (4) Major tranquillizers:

phenothiazine derivatives such as chlorpromazine and chlorprothixene; reserpine; butyrophenones.

Barbiturates are widely used for mild symptoms but often an adequate dose causes sleepiness or incoordination. The benzodiazepines induce tranquillity without much sedation. Chlorpromazine is particularly used in the treatment of mental illness, especially schizophrenia and depressive states, but is probably not as effective as drugs of the benzodiazepine type in anxiety states.

The scientific names of all these drugs are very confusing. The following are some trade equivalents in the various groups now so widely prescribed and known that they have practically become household words: (1) Hypno-sedatives: Luminal, Gardenal, Medinal, Nembutal, Carbrital, Doriden, Noludar. (2) Tranquillo-sedatives: Librium, Valium, Mogadon, Miltown, Atarax. (3) Minor tranquillizers: Sparine, Phenergan. (4) Major tranquillizers: Largactil, Taractan, Serpasil, Harmomyl, Serenace.

transfusion, blood. See BLOOD TRANSFUSION.

transplant. Any tissue or organ transferred from one individual to another. The rectification of disabilities by the replacement of diseased parts is an attractive and logical idea. Transplant surgery has therefore developed considerably in recent years, but the difficulties are formidable and of three kinds: (1) limitations of surgical technique; the tendency of the body to reject tissue which its immune-system regards as 'foreign'; and (3) the supply of sufficient healthy tissue or organs to ensure that well-matched material, in fresh condition, can be provided promptly when required. Blood transfusion is a form of transplantation and its early success came about because these difficulties were minimal. It was easy to carry out; blood-types could be matched very exactly; and donors were readily available because they did not suffer and were able to regenerate what they donated.

Popular interest in transplantation has centred on more spectacular examples, such as heart and lung replacement, but some simpler procedures are becoming routine. The grafting of non-cellular tissues is relatively easy because they do not cause rejection reactions, and they are readily accepted by the living tissues of the recipient and become incorporated in their new position. Included in this category of transplant surgery (using healthy tissue from someone who has recently died) are the grafting of blood vessels, heart-valves and bone, and also corneal replacement.

The other large field with a considerable unsatisfied need is in kidney transplantation, still limited by problems of matching, rejection, and the supply of suitable organs. The matching problem is being tackled by a computer-system,

Eurotransplant, which retains a record of the tissue-characteristics of patients awaiting a transplant, and selects for operation the one who most closely matches an available kidney. The use of immuno-suppressive drugs and sera depress rejection responses, but an accurate match is of prime consideration because immuno-suppressive measures have the undesirable effect of simultaneously lessening body-defences against other infection. In the U.K. the problem of supply of kidneys has given rise to the Kidney Donor Scheme, which seeks to improve the supply of kidneys, usually taken from young healthy subjects who have died suddenly in accidents.

Heart transplantation gives rise to argument in respect of two of its aspects. Firstly, determination of the exact point of death: it is important that the heart be removed from the body of the donor immediately after death, and this being so, some people claim that, if a national celebrity is in urgent need of a transplant, there may be a temptation to expedite the death of the fatally injured victim of a traffic accident. Secondly, the expenditure of professional time: apart from follow-up, a heart transplant occupies a team of about seven doctors and nine nurses for the best part of a fortnight; some thinkers hold that, when most hospitals have long lists of patients awaiting less complicated treatment and in some cases dying for lack of such treatment, the heavy expenditure of staff time on one patient is unjustifiable.

The replacement of damaged parts of the body by structures made of metal, silicone or plastic is known as SPARE-PART SURGERY.

transvestism. A form of PERVERSION or sexual deviation characterized by the wearing of clothes appropriate to the opposite sex, and by the adoption of social and sexual behaviour conforming to the outward appearance so achieved. See HOMOSEXUALITY.

trauma. The effect on the body of any harmful external agency including violence, chemical substances, and physical phenomena such as heat, cold and radiation. By analogy the term has also become extended and qualified as 'emotional trauma', a term which embraces the ill-effects resulting from disturbing mental experiences which may be the root cause of psychoneurotic disorders.

travel sickness. Sensations of nausea, sometimes accompanied by actual vomiting, produced in susceptible persons by the irregular or rhythmical movements to which the body is subjected during travel in vehicles, ships or aircraft. It is due to the effect on the central nervous system of excessive stimuli received from the semi-circular canals (a balancing mechanism forming the labyrinth of the inner ear) especially if these conflict with impressions received from the eyes or other sense organs.

The well-known symptoms consist of a feeling of insecurity and visual disorientation, with dizziness, headache, loss of appetite, nausea, vomiting, double vision, and ultimately signs of shock, such as pallor, sweating, and prostration. The importance of visual stimulation is shown by the fact that very susceptible persons can become sea-sick on dry land merely from the sight of wave-movements. An attack closely resembles migraine, and migraine sufferers are generally bad travellers. Apprehension, anticipation, cold, travel smells and the sight of other victims all help to induce an attack.

Fresh air, or good ventilation, is very important, while for sea-sickness to lie down near the centre of the ship in a darkened cabin may help delay onset or minimize effects. Many effective sedatives are now available but travellers who have taken such drugs should be cautious about driving a car within four hours.

tremor. Involuntary muscular trembling or quivering, usually most obvious in the limbs, where alternate contractions of muscle-groups and their anatomical antagonists produce oscillations either general or limited in extent. Tremor may be physiological: shivering, for instance, is a normal reaction to cold or infection since muscular activity generates heat and warms the body; it also occurs when the body is tensed by nervous anticipation as in athletes and racehorses.

Otherwise, tremor is pathological; it may be caused by disease, such as multiple sclerosis, paralysis agitans, encephalitis, poliomyelitis, and certain brain diseases. Toxic effects on the nervous system cause tremor, as in alcoholism, metallic poisoning, hyperthyroidism, pernicious anaemia, vitamin B deficiency, and many infections.

The type of tremor may provide diagnostic help. It may be either 'fine' or 'coarse', the former more easily felt than seen. It may be induced by voluntary effort ('intention tremor'), as in multiple sclerosis, or inhibited when purposeful movements are made, as in chorea.

Treatment depends on the cause. Toxaemic tremors improve when toxaemia is removed or corrected but tremors caused by nervous disease present more difficulty. Advances have been made by the development of new drugs of which levodopa has achieved notable success in the management of PARKINSON'S DISEASE

trephine. A special type of bone-saw used for opening the skull by removal of a circular disc of bone. Basically it is a hollow steel cylinder one end of which is formed as a ring of saw-teeth extending upwards on the outside of the cylinder. At the other end is a cross-handle by which the cutting-edge can be rotated against the bone.

This rather old-fashioned instrument is laborious and difficult to use and has largely been superseded by electrically driven burrs and osteotomes (bone cutting tools). Larger areas of bone can be removed by drilling a succession of burr-holes and dividing the intervening bridges of bone by a flexible thread-saw.

trichinosis. A disease produced by the nematode worm *Trichinella spiralis,* a parasite of swine and many wild animals including rats. Human infection is mainly from undercooked pork or pork products containing living worm-cysts. In the intestine, encysted larvae mature to adult worms. These produce new larvae which migrate and encyst in muscles and organs of the human host.

Symptoms are mainly gastro-intestinal, but these are followed by oedema and nettle rash, and the affected muscles become painful, tender, and hard; swallowing, speech and respiration are also affected. In severe cases, fever, toxaemia and cardio-respiratory paralysis may lead to coma and death. Unless the disease is suspected, the diagnosis is easily missed, but it is confirmed by blood tests and laboratory investigation of muscle tissue.

Treatment is largely a matter of dealing with symptoms but vermicidal drugs should be given to destroy worms still in the intestine. Prevention is all important. Although natural distribution of the disease is world-wide it is now rare in most developed countries through control of pig raising (boiling swill; rat eradication, etc.), meat inspection and adequate cooking.

trigeminal neuralgia. The trigeminal (fifth cranial) nerve provides sensory fibres to the face and scalp, and motor fibres to the muscles of the jaw. Neuralgia is paroxysmal pain radiating in the area supplied by a sensory nerve and it frequently affects the trigeminal nerve to produce the condition sometimes known as tic douloureux.

This occurs mainly in older people and causes recurrent pain, which may be distressing and incapacitating, together with tenderness of face and scalp, often concentrated on eyebrow, nose and chin over the sites of the nerve branches. The condition is not fully explained, but it tends to be related to cold, damp, debility and overwork, and may be connected with the blood supply.

In treatment, potential causes such as decaying teeth or sinus infection should first be checked. If pain persists regular use of suitable analgesics is required. More radical surgical procedures are also available. These include injection of the nerve with alcohol or local anaesthetic, and severing the sensory nerve root.

tropical diseases. Conditions particularly prevalent in tropical countries or only found in such countries. A few of these diseases are wholly tropical infections, e.g., the tsetse fly that carries the organism of sleeping sickness does not breed in temperatures below 25 °C. (77 °F.). Many are infections which can occur anywhere but have been wholly or largely stamped out by preventive measures in temperate countries with adequate resources: malaria, cholera and leprosy are examples. Some are not infectious at all but diseases of malnutrition, e.g., pellagra, kwashiorkor and beriberi. In other words the diseases commonly termed 'tropical' are in part due to climatic conditions under which various organisms (and the mosquitoes, flies, ticks, mites, fleas and lice that carry them) can breed easily; in part due to ignorance, poor hygiene and absence of preventive measures; in part due to poverty; and in large measure due to a combination of these factors.

For the visitor to a tropical country, some precautions are obvious. Where the particular infections are still prevalent, vaccination is advisable against cholera, yellow fever, the typhoid group of fevers, poliomyelitis and tetanus. Appropriate antimalarial drugs should be taken when visiting malaria-infested areas (and for some weeks afterwards) and mosquito-nets should be used. Unless the water supply is known to be safe, as it now is in most large centres of population, water should be boiled or otherwise sterilized before being drunk or being used to wash food utensils. Care should be exercised in respect of all food that is not going to be thoroughly cooked. The danger of bites from snakes and poisonous spiders can be reduced by keeping feet and legs adequately protected. It is inadvisable to bathe in inland waters without assurance of their safety.

To prevent or treat tropical diseases occurring in the indigenous population is an enormous problem. Essentially it involves three things: (1) money, because schools, clinics, sewerage systems, agricultural machinery, etc. are all costly; (2) general education, e.g., with a view to improving agriculture and horticulture; and (3) health education to combat ignorance and harmful tradition.

Tropical diseases form a vast speciality and it is only possible to mention some illustrative examples, some of which are separately described elsewhere under their own headings.

1. Nutritional: beriberi; kwashiorkor; pellagra.

2. Bacterial and viral: cholera; plague (fleas); yellow fever (mosquitoes); leprosy; yaws; tularaemia (deer fly); relapsing fever (ticks); typhus (lice and ticks); typhoid fever; bacillary dysentery.

3. Protozoan: malaria (mosquitoes); kala-azar (flies); sleeping sickness (tsetse flies); amoebic dysentery.

4. Metazoan. Important metazoan parasites are mainly worms of three classes: (1) trematodes (with adhesive suckers): fluke infestation; schistosomiasis or bilharziasis (blood fluke disease); (2) cestodes (ribbon-like): many species of tapeworm; (3) nematodes (threadlike):

ankylostomiasis (hook-worm disease); filariasis (elephantiasis from mosquito-borne worms in lymph-channels); dracontiasis (guinea-worm under the skin – spread by cyclops, a small crustacean, in water supplies); Calabar swelling (subcutaneous infestation by mangrove flies); oncocerciasis (subcutaneous nodules caused by flies).

In the conquest of tropical diseases it has to be remembered that the introduction of methods and attitudes from advanced countries is not wholly a gain. There is some loss as well as much profit: for instance, as yaws declines syphilis increases, as leprosy becomes rare tuberculosis becomes commoner, and as malnutrition recedes the diseases of obesity begin to appear.

truss. A surgical appliance designed to give support to the site of a HERNIA (rupture), and to prevent its contents from protruding again after they have been replaced.

Design varies according to the site and size of the hernia, but the device is commonly used for the retention of inguinal, femoral, or umbilical hernias.

In adults, such treatment is merely for comfort, and an operation to cure the condition is generally preferable unless indicated inadvisable by age, ill-health, or the technical difficulties of securing a satisfactory result. In infants with inguinal or umbilical hernias the continuous use of truss for some time may eventually lead to a permanent cure.

trypanosome. A protozoan parasite causing trypanosomiasis or SLEEPING SICKNESS, and conveyed to man and animals by bites from infected tsetse flies.

tsetse fly. A biting and blood-sucking fly of Central Africa. The name includes various species of the genus *Glossina* which are of great importance because of their role in the spread of protozoan trypanosomes (which cause SLEEPING SICKNESS) to man and domestic animals from the many kinds of wild animals which harbour the parasites.

tuberculin. The fluid in which tubercle bacilli grow contains their toxins in solution, and this thick yellowish fluid is called tuberculin. This tuberculin is prepared as a sterilized liquid containing the standardized growth products of the tubercle bacillus, though some modifications have now been developed. Tuberculin is used in the diagnosis of tuberculosis both in man and in animals.

For a tuberculin test a standard quantity of tuberculin is injected into the skin. In non-tuberculous subjects no effect is produced (tuberculin-negative), but with pre-existing infection an inflammatory reaction results (tuberculin-positive).

tuberculosis. A communicable disease resulting from infection by the tubercle bacillus, *Mycobacterium tuberculosis*, of which there are four types – human, bovine, avian and piscine; only the first two usually affect man. As phthisis or

Reduction in tuberculosis before antibiotics in England and Wales
(deaths in thousands)

In pulmonary tuberculosis it is particularly likely to affect the lungs, but may affect any part of the body. Lymph glands (scrofula), bones and joints, skin (lupus vulgaris), nervous system (tuberculous meningitis) and larynx are all common sites, as are the intestinal, urinary and reproductive systems.

The disease is contracted by inhaling bacilli from an existing case, or by mouth from contaminated food, especially untreated milk.

As a first stage, a small inflammatory patch forms (the primary focus), usually in a lung but sometimes in the intestine or in a tonsil. The neighbouring lymph glands may become swollen but there are no other symptoms, and in course of time the primary focus becomes surrounded by fibrous tissue and shrinks to a small scar. When the disease was widespread (as it still is in many countries) most people developed the primary focus. The scar could be seen on x-ray examination and the TUBERCULIN test would indicate that the persons had been infected and had developed a defensive reaction. The person was not ill and was not infectious to others.

In a minority of cases the primary focus does not become walled off. Instead organisms spread through the lungs ('galloping consumption') or spread by the blood stream to various parts of the body (causing generalized or miliary tuberculosis, or tuberculosis of bones or joints, or occasionally tuberculous meningitis).

In yet other cases the walling off process starts but a sort of drawn battle ensues. The body develops sufficient resistance to prevent galloping consumption or miliary tuberculosis, but in the lung the pockets of infection (from the initial primary focus or from further infection) enlarge, forming cavities in the lung, with the development of such symptoms as fever, sweating at night, cough and loss of weight. In the absence of effective treatment the person, especially if young, may go downhill fairly quickly or, especially if elderly, may for years have practically no symptoms except a cough. In either case he is infectious to others.

Which of these three results will happen in a particular case depends on various factors. Some of these are: (1) the quantity of invading bacilli: most people have the bodily defence to ward off a few bacilli, but close and repeated contact with a highly infectious person may convert the invaders from a squad to an army, especially if the contact occurs in conditions of overcrowding and bad ventilation; (2) the body's health and capacity to resist: malnutrition greatly lowers this capacity, as do simultaneous illness and deep-seated grief; (3) age: in general susceptibility is greatest at 18 to 35 years and lowest in the middle-aged; (4) racial or family resistance or susceptibility: the disease was long deemed hereditary but it probably occurs in families mainly because one member infects another, and even the alleged susceptibility of some races may be explicable mainly on grounds of malnutrition.

In most infectious diseases invading bacteria either win rapidly or lose, but tuberculosis is different. Despite its activity in galloping consumption and tuberculous meningitis, the bacillus is usually fairly inactive, but it has a waxy coat which in part protects it from the body's defences. So it often causes little in the way of symptoms unless the patient's health declines from some other cause such as malnutrition or another respiratory disease; but though quiescent it nevertheless remains alive. Before the era of effective drug treatment it was rightly said that 'tuberculosis is never cured but only halted'.

Bones and glands. While the usual focus of infection is in the lung, so that 'tuberculosis' in ordinary speech generally means 'pulmonary tuberculosis', the disease can also affect bones, usually at or near joints: the spine (Pott's disease), hips, knees, ankles, shoulders and elbows are most commonly affected. Where joints are involved, the term used is tuberculous arthritis; bone disease alone is tuberculous osteomyelitis, and infection of lymph glands is tuberculous adenitis.

Either the human or the bovine organism can cause any form of tuberculosis, but it used to be held that the human type, mostly breathed in, usually selected the lungs, and that the bovine type, mostly drunk in infected milk or eaten in infected uncooked meat, affected bones and joints more often. Certainly, in countries with pasteurization and similar measures for sterilization of milk, and policies for eradication of tuberculosis from cattle, tuberculosis of bones and joints has become a rarity.

Prevalence. Tuberculosis in the nineteenth century caused one fifth of all deaths in developed countries like the U.K., and its dramatic reduction in such countries is due to a combination of social amelioration, health education and preventive measures, rather than to treatment. In less highly developed countries it is still common, and increasing, and is beginning to replace malaria as the biggest killing disease. It still infects at least fifty million people a year in the world, mostly in countries with a combination of poverty, overcrowding, malnutrition and rapidly growing population, and it causes about three million deaths annually.

Treatment. Formerly there was no specific treatment for pulmonary tuberculosis. Sanatorium treatment relied mainly on physical rest (complete bed rest at first, followed by carefully graded amounts of exercise), on absence of emotional and mental stress, on provision of a good and attractive diet, on ample fresh air (though its value was exaggerated) and, where appropriate, on artificial pneumothorax to collapse all or part of an affected lung and so facilitate its rest. However, in the middle of this century three effective drugs were discovered: streptomycin, para-amino-salicylic acid (PAS), and isoniazid.

In developed countries tuberculosis now seldom kills. For instance, as late as 1946, in England and Wales, 900 girls aged 15 to 25 years died from tuberculosis, as compared with 9 in 1961. Yet drugs, while reducing deaths, have not reduced cases. The reduction of tuberculosis is primarily due to prevention.

Prevention. Reduction of malnutrition has played the biggest part in combating tuberculosis. In the U.K., for instance, during the massive unemployment and consequent rise of poverty in the early 1930s, tuberculosis increased steadily; this was followed by a dramatic fall over the next twenty-five years as undernutrition decreased. Again, reduction of overcrowding has contributed enormously: in towns that vigorously replaced slums with corporation housing (like Barnsley in England and Aberdeen in Scotland) the disease dwindled. Not least, health education has made its contribution both by the primitive but accurate line of emphasizing that 'Spitting spreads disease' and through the advice of health visitors on budgeting and nutritional requirements and on matters like the importance of fresh air. In industry, attention to occupational hazards has helped. Pasteurization of milk and persuasion of the public to use it has greatly reduced tuberculosis of bones and joints. By 1951, when BCG was not yet available and when the new drugs for treatment were still in their infancy, the number of deaths from tuberculosis in England and Wales was 13,000, as compared with thrice that number even seventeen years earlier, and the number of notifications had fallen to 45,000 in the year.

As the prevalence of tuberculosis declined in developed countries two further measures became available: (1) mass radiography, i.e., efforts to persuade entire communities to accept x-ray examination in the hope of identifying the relatively few undetected carriers of the disease, with, in some areas, as much as three-quarters of the entire adult population being persuaded to accept the examination; and (2) the offer of BCG vaccination to children aged 13 years and also to such new-born infants as were deemed at special risk. By 1971 in England and Wales the number of deaths had fallen from the 13,000 mentioned above to just over 1300, and notifications in the year were down to 11,000. A problem, however, has arisen among immigrants in Britain and other developed countries: frequently undernourished in their strange new country, sometimes having a higher susceptibility to tuberculosis, and often living in overcrowded conditions, they suffer from about twelve times the proportion of tuberculosis found in indigenous citizens.

tularaemia. A specific infectious disease, primarily of wild animals, but also affecting man in North America, the U.S.S.R., parts of Europe, and Japan. It is transmitted by biting arthropods, particularly the deer-fly (*Chrysops discalis*), by ticks, and in Sweden by the mosquito *Aedes cinereus*. Infection may result also from handling infected carcases, and from eating imperfectly cooked rabbit-meat or contaminated water.

It is caused by a bacterium, *Pasteurella tularensis*. The incubation period is one to ten days and the onset is sudden, with chills, fever and prostration. Bites usually ulcerate and there may be enlargement or suppuration of lymph glands. Untreated cases run a long-continued fever with a 5 per cent death rate, but antibiotic treatment is effective and one attack protects. Vaccines are available.

Apart from direct infection during hunting and other open-air activities, cases occur in rabbit-handlers since infection persists even after refrigeration. Precautions should be taken against bites, and against casual infection from wild meat and water.

tumours. Growths of new tissue (neoplasms), whether benign or malignant.

Development of new cells is a normal occurrence, as when tissues grow to repair an injury, or a muscle enlarges to cope with repeated extra strain. Tumours, however, consist of cells that on microscopic examination often display abnormal or primitive characteristics (and are sometimes described as 'normal cells gone wrong'); in general they multiply much faster than do normal cells and are in no way an advantage to the body.

Benign or innocent tumours. These develop singly or, very rarely, in small groups; they displace adjacent tissues by size and pressure but do not infiltrate them, and they do not give rise to secondary growths (metastases). Examples are uterine fibroids and nasal polypi. Benign tumours usually have definite walls, so that their removal is relatively easy. Depending on their situation these neoplasms may cause no symptoms or cause symptoms only by pressure, e.g., a tumour situated on the root of a spinal nerve will gradually compress the soft spinal cord and so lead to paralysis.

As long as they do not produce symptoms through pressure and do not become unbearably unsightly, these tumours can be left in reasonable safety, although in a small proportion of cases an initially benign tumour later becomes malignant. If removal is desired, because of symptoms or appearance or fear of future malignancy, the surgical operation is straightforward, and there is no danger of secondaries and little chance of recurrence.

Malignant tumours. On the other hand this type of neoplasm infiltrates adjacent tissues, for example producing ulcers by breaking down subcutaneous tissues and skin, and the cells tend to travel by the lymphatic vessels or the blood vessels to create secondary tumours in other parts of the body. For fuller details, see CANCER.

twilight sleep. A popular name for a regime of sedation and analgesia once much used to allay anxiety and diminish pain during the first stage of labour. The drugs used were scopolamine and morphine given by injection under the skin and repeated at intervals according to the progress of labour and the condition of the patient. Although this form of treatment helped the mother it suffered from the great disadvantage that it also depressed the child's respiratory centre making it difficult to ensure resuscitation and natural breathing.

It has now largely been abandoned in favour of safer methods of analgesia.

twins. A pair of individuals whose birth results from the same pregnancy. The average frequency of twins in the general population is about once in ninety confinements but a tendency to bear twins is inherited and in some families the incidence is considerably greater.

Twins are of two types. Normally the ovaries release only one ovum during each menstrual cycle but when two or more are released each may be fertilized separately and a corresponding number of embryos will develop. Double or multiple ovulation may occur naturally but it is also particularly likely to happen if pituitary hormones or other 'fertility drugs' are being employed to stimulate ovarian activity for the treatment of infertility. If two separate ova are thus fertilized the result is fraternal, binovular or dizygotic twins. The ova are often released a month apart, so that one twin is really a month younger than the other, although they are born the same day. Whether really of the same age or not, fraternal twins are not necessarily of the same sex and are no more alike than are children of the same parents born at different times.

If, however, a single ovum is fertilized and during subsequent development it divides into two, this will produce identical, monovular, or monozygotic twins, with an identical genetic inheritance and resembling each other so closely in bodily and mental characteristics that they are difficult to distinguish. They do, however, have individual finger print patterns. The study of identical twins, especially where they have chanced to experience different environment in their early years, can do much to differentiate the influence of nature and nurture, since all differences in their personalities, careers and even diseases are clearly the result of factors affecting them after birth.

If this division into two separate embryos should not be complete, the result is undifferentiated or Siamese twins which are joined together to a variable extent. In many examples of this abnormality the degree to which organs are shared may mean that either one or both twins cannot survive, but many examples of surgical separation have been recorded.

Twins may present some problems of upbringing. Initially they may be small and difficult to rear because of their tendency to be born prematurely. If they are breast-fed a mother will seldom have sufficient milk for both and complementary feeds will generally be required. In most instances the exigencies of the situation with its large demands on maternal time and energy will make it desirable to resort entirely to artificial feeding with careful supervision of the intake of food, vitamins and iron.

There is also a great tendency to treat twins as a unit rather than as two individuals and to enhance their appeal and emphasize their similarity by dressing and treating them exactly alike. This is psychologically unwise. Each should be given a chance to acquire an individual personality with individual interests, accomplishments and friends. They should not be ostentatiously compared with each other to the disadvantage of one because this will inevitably engender feelings of inferiority.

tympanites. Distension of the abdomen from the presence of gas in the intestines. This may be either trivial or grave. Transient and insignificant cases are due to flatulence (commonly experienced with dyspepsia, gastritis and enteritis) and are also produced by over-consumption of fizzy drinks and fermentable foodstuffs, and by the nervous habit of air-swallowing. Appropriate dietary measures and carminative drugs usually bring relief.

More serious cases are the result of impaired intestinal function, resulting from obstruction, surgical shock after abdominal operations, local toxaemia as in typhoid fever, or general toxaemia caused by pneumonia or other infections. Cessation or reduction of intestinal movements from such causes is known as paralytic ileus and distension is aggravated by the proliferation of gas-forming organisms in the bowel. Treatment depends upon the exact cause. Obstruction requires operation but other measures available include enemas to encourage intestinal activity and the injection of muscle stimulants.

typhoid. The enteric fevers include both typhoid and PARATYPHOID fevers, which are specific infections caused by swallowing bacteria of the *Salmonella* group. Similar organisms are associated with certain types of food poisoning, and both *S. typhi* and *S. paratyphi* (A, B, and C) cause disease which has well-defined clinical characteristics. Paratyphoid fever differs from typhoid in being a less severe illness of different incubation period.

Infection is derived from patients or TYPHOID CARRIERS and is spread by contamination of water or food by their excreta, urine, or other discharges. Shellfish, raw vegetables and unwashed fruit, and milk and milk products are often involved. Flies may act as carriers between infected excreta and food awaiting consumption. Even tinned foods have been incriminated as a result of faulty processing. Carriers are a particular danger as food-handlers, and are also a risk to water supplies. Typhoid has a world-wide distribution and is common in undeveloped countries with primitive sanitary arrangements.

An incubation period of about two weeks (the range is from five days to over three weeks) is followed by an insidious onset with general discomfort, lassitude, abdominal uneasiness and increasing temperature with relatively slow pulse. Organisms within the bowel invade the lymphoid tissue of the intestine and soon spread to the blood stream as a bacteraemia. This widespread infection is shown in the second week by continued temperature, the occasional appearance of a few pink spots, enlargement of the spleen, increased intestinal disorder (pea-soup stools) and prostration, wasting, delirium, heart weakness, and other signs of severe blood poisoning. Intestinal haemorrhage or perforation may also occur and these contribute substantially to the death rate. In the third week temperature declines and symptoms abate, but convalescence is prolonged and relapses frequent. Bacteria may persist in faeces or urine for months and 2 to 5 per cent of cases may become permanent carriers.

Clinical diagnosis is often difficult: the disease can resemble various other conditions. However, if typhoid is suspected, the organism can be grown in a bacteriological laboratory and after the first few days blood tests become practicable.

Treatment in the past consisted mainly of skilled nursing and attention to symptoms, but in recent years the development of appropriate antibiotics has both reduced the number of deaths and shortened the course of the disease. The disease is notifiable in virtually all countries and patients are normally isolated in hospitals for infectious diseases.

Preventive measures include purification of water supplies; sanitation; fly-control; supervision of the processing, preparation and serving of food in public eating-places; control of shellfish; washing of food eaten raw; discovery and supervision of carriers; and health education of the public in general and food-handlers in particular. These measures between them have virtually eradicated typhoid in many of the developed countries, although a century ago it was the commonest of all fevers.

Specific vaccine protection is available by TAB vaccine. Travellers to countries in which the disease is still endemic should ensure that they observe this precaution with a primary course reinforced at not less than three-year intervals by subsequent injections.

typhoid carrier. A 'carrier' is a person who continues to harbour organisms of an infectious disease but displays no signs or symptoms of the disease.

The carrier state is particularly common after typhoid fever: between 2 and 5 per cent of cases after clinical recovery continue to discharge bacilli often for months or years. The organisms persist in the biliary or urinary system and are excreted in faeces or urine. Some 80 per cent of chronic carriers are women because of their greater liability to gall-bladder disease. The most famous carrier, 'Typhoid Mary', who was responsible for a large outbreak in New York (1903), finally had to be permanently isolated from 1915 until her death in 1938.

Prolonged courses of antibiotic therapy may ultimately cure the carrier state but for faecal carriers the most effective procedure is surgical removal of the gall-bladder.

Carriers need to be kept under regular supervision, precluded from acting as food-handlers, and specially instructed in personal hygiene. In Britain there are statutory powers for their control, and health departments maintain a register of former cases of typhoid to ensure supervision and suggest lines of enquiry in subsequent outbreaks.

typhus fever. The term now includes a variety of similar diseases caused by various species of *Rickettsia* and these are discussed under that heading. However, classical typhus fever, sometimes known as gaol fever, camp fever, or epidemic house-borne typhus fever, is caused by *R. prowazeki* and is one of the great epidemic diseases of history, always ready to appear under conditions of famine, war, and refugee movement, when deprivation, crowding and lack of hygiene, especially in cold or temperate climates, provide opportunities for lice to disseminate infection from man to man.

The onset is usually sudden with headache, shivering fever, general pain and a rash of discoloured spots on the fifth day. Toxaemia and prostration are pronounced. Untreated cases run a course of about two weeks and may recover spontaneously, but the death rate is high and may reach 40 per cent. Modern antibiotic treatment is very effective and there is a protective vaccine, but prevention by hygiene and louse-eradication is still essential.

Murine typhus or endemic flea-borne typhus has a world-wide distribution. It is less severe than classical typhus fever. It is caused by *R. mooseri*, and spreads from rats to man by fleas.

U

ulcer. An open sore on the surface of skin or mucous membrane where infection, inflammation and bacterial toxins cause gradual destruction of epithelium (surface cells) and underlying tissues, often with larger areas of dead tissue which fall away.

Ulcers are of many types. The common causes are: (1) superficial wound infections especially in tissues damaged by trauma, pressure, impaired circulation, disease or conditions affecting the spinal cord and nerves. Examples are slow-healing burns; mouth ulcers from jagged teeth or dental plates; bed-sores; varicose ulcers of the leg; and ulcers in various nervous diseases. (2) Specific infections such as tuberculosis or syphilis and, in the intestine, typhoid fever, cholera or amoebic dysentery. (3) Malignant disease. (4) DUODENAL ULCER, GASTRIC ULCER and ulcerative colitis in which psychosomatic factors may be involved.

Treatment necessarily depends on diagnosis but the principles of dealing with an accessible chronic pus-forming ulcer are to determine and remove the cause and secure rest, to improve circulation by posture, and to treat the accompanying disease. Locally mild antiseptics are usually followed by stimulating applications, and skin-grafting may be of help in the final stages of healing.

Ulcers of more specific causation require therapy appropriate to the exact diagnosis.

ulcerative colitis. Chronic ulceration of the colon and rectum, with diarrhoea, sometimes bleeding, and abdominal pain. Treatment involves rest and a high protein diet, and surgery may be necessary.

ulna. The larger of the two long bones in the forearm. It extends from elbow to wrist on the inner (or little finger) side of the limb. The relatively massive upper end articulates with the lower end of the humerus or upper arm bone and forms the greater part of the elbow-joint. This is a hinge-type joint and its stability is maintained by two bony projections of the ulna, the coronoid process in front and the olecranon process behind. The ulnar shaft runs parallel to the radius and diminishes in cross-section from above downwards to terminate at the wrist-joint. The prominent knob on the back of the wrist is the ulnar styloid process.

The olecranon process forms the 'point of the elbow', often fractured by direct violence in falls on the elbow. The shaft is subcutaneous and also liable to fracture by direct violence. Indirect violence, as from falls upon the outstretched hand, more commonly fractures the radius, but either the ulnar shaft or coronoid process may be involved if displacement is severe.

ultrasonics. Sound waves whose frequency exceeds about twelve thousand cycles per second are inaudible to the human ear but may still be heard by other animals. Such waves are utilized in the so-called 'silent dog-whistle' and are also employed by bats as a sort of 'radar' helping them to navigate in the dark. It is however possible to produce high-energy sound waves of much higher frequencies by means of the electrical excitation of a quartz-crystal (piezo-electric effect). These waves and their practical applications are called ultrasonics, and they have an important use in medicine.

Since depth of penetration and strength of return echo depends on the type of underlying tissue it is possible to scan parts of the body and by suitable recording equipment to map out underlying structures. By this method suspected tumours or abnormal situations of the placenta may be identified, and the technique is also proving useful for identification of conditions such as spina bifida in the early stages of pregnancy (with a view to termination of the pregnancy if necessary). The record produced is not unlike an x-ray plate, but the procedure is free from radiation hazard and is superior in soft-tissue examination.

Surgical applications of ultrasonics have also been developed. With suitable generating and localizing equipment waves are focused to a point, and small but accurately delineated portions of tissue can thus be destroyed without harming overlying structures. This technique has been employed for the treatment of Ménière's disease and is being developed in neuro-surgery, particularly in connection with Parkinson's disease.

ultra-violet radiation. A form of radiation occupying a position in the electro-magnetic spectrum just beyond the violet end of the visible light band and with shorter waves in the range of 3900 to 136 Angstrom units (one AU is one ten-millionth of a millimetre).

Ultra-violet rays are present in sunlight and are produced artificially by electric arc-lamps. Modern appliances have mercury-vapour arcs in quartz tubes.

The rays are absorbed by the skin, and as in sunburn, according to length of exposure, produce reddening or blistering followed by desquamation (the shedding of superficial layers of the skin) and tanning. They kill superficial germs, stimulate blood-supply to the skin, produce vitamin D by action on skin ergosterol, relieve pain by counter-irritation, and exercise some general tonic effect.

Therapeutically they are used locally or generally. Local applications are used for slow-healing ulcers, impetigo, acne, lupus and psoriasis and for the relief of fibrositic or neuritic pain. General irradiation is employed in rickets, malnutrition, anaemia, debility, recurrent respiratory infections and neurasthenia; but while it has its place both in prevention and treatment, the value of ultra-violet radiation was exaggerated in the past.

Proper supervision is required because of the risk of skin-burns and conjunctivitis (goggles are essential), and also because of potentially harmful effects in certain conditions such as pulmonary tuberculosis and eczema.

umbilical cord. The cord connecting the embryo to the placenta of the mother and containing the vessels – two arteries and one vein – through which nourishment reaches the child and waste products are removed from the child. The cord is normally tied with two ligatures immediately after birth and then cut between the ligatures.

Occasional abnormalities include knots, caused by the foetus slipping through loops in the cord and sometimes drawn so tight as to impede the circulation, thus damaging or even killing the unborn child; twisting may also occur, including twisting round the neck or round a limb.

umbilical hernia. The umbilicus or navel is a potentially weak area of the abdominal wall through which part of the intestine, enclosed in the peritoneum (the membrane lining the abdominal cavity), may protrude as an umbilical HERNIA.

Umbilical hernia is very common in infancy. The projecting umbilicus is well covered by skin and lined by peritoneum to form a small sac which quite often is not strictly a hernia since it may have no contents. The smallest sacs disappear spontaneously and the traditional treatment is to try to encourage this by the application of adhesive plaster strips either to retain a small pad or to invert the mid-line of the abdominal wall and so compress the sac between the opposed skin folds. These measures usually prove quite effective, but if the hernia persists, or is markedly unsightly, or poses a risk of damage to the protruding intestine, a repair operation will be required. This is best delayed until the age of 2 or 3, since abdominal operations in small infants are frequently followed by respiratory complications.

Occasionally infants are born with a large protruding sac of the peritoneum containing intestine or other organs. This congenital umbilical hernia is a developmental defect. It requires immediate surgery.

umbilicus. The navel or depressed scar in the centre of the abdomen which results after birth from the severance of the UMBILICAL CORD.

unconscious mind. The impulse producing a movement or action may originate consciously but the detailed execution is controlled unconsciously at a lower level. Similarly, incoming impressions are unconsciously monitored before they reach consciousness as perceptions. Both activities are influenced and modified by the stored-up results of earlier experience. To take a simple example, my eyes see seven people on the pavement; six do not really impinge on my consciousness, but the seventh is brought to my conscious mind as a friend whom I want to see, and I start walking without consciously telling my legs the order in which to move.

The existence of mental activity of which we are not conscious was only grudgingly admitted by the experimental physiologists of the nineteenth century, and even by the early schools of experimental psychology which followed them. These workers studied living systems from the outside and the operations of the conscious mind by introspection. In their views, physiology and psychology dealt with the same phenomena from different angles. The physiologists sought to explain how the brain and nervous system functioned, entirely in terms of reflex acts integrated and conditioned by experience, and the psychologists dealt only with what appeared in consciousness.

However, psychology soon altered out of all recognition and the concept that we take action only when our ideas are fully formed was turned round, so that it became accepted that we only have ideas when our unconscious mind has reached a state of readiness to act. Gradually it was realized that we are unaware of many of the factors which make us act in a particular way. Investigation, description, analysis, and measurement of consciousness had quite failed to explain important aspects of behaviour. It came to be recognized that since all experience was highly personal, subconscious abilities and attitudes were built up by the selection and classification of information continuously collected from the outside world. This background of experience is the basis of 'feeling' generated in the unconscious mind and the mainspring of its influence on action. The mental processes involved in desires and emotions are never conscious. It is only the end-products of motivational drives which become known directly, and the nature of underlying impulses can only be inferred from their conscious and behavioural consequences. That they do exist can be shown by their emergence in dreams and in states of consciousness modified by hypnosis or drugs.

Psychologists differ slightly about the levels of mental activity that occur without us being conscious of them, but the various terms – pre-conscious, fore-conscious, subconscious and unconscious mind – all mean nearly the same thing. They have been developed to fit explanations that are not widely different. Some see the unconscious as a seething cauldron of passion and desire; others regard it rather as a passive repository of instincts, habits and silent mental functions. At any rate, unconscious mental activity exists at various levels, some of which can be brought to consciousness. However, a distinction may profitably be made between the contents of the subconscious mind – symbols and feelings which can arise in consciousness but which at the moment are absent – and unconscious operations which are never appreciated consciously. Forgotten information, for example, may be dredged up by an effort of will; and names are recalled to consciousness with perhaps a transient feeling of strain, but with no exact awareness of how they are actually recovered.

From this it follows that behaviour is not simply conscious response to a stimulus or reasoning from that stimulus, but is in part based on feelings and ideas derived from past experience, with some of these never coming to consciousness.

Later workers were quick to realize that this provided a means of explaining the difference between logical thinking and the emotional thinking of complexes, so elucidating much that was mysterious in human behaviour. The fruition of this was psychoanalysis, dominated perhaps a little unfairly by Sigmund FREUD (1856-1939) since valuable but less sensational contributions were also made by many others.

Freud's theories were based on a distinction between the id, or unconscious mind, and the ego, or conscious mind. To this he later added the superego, which controlled the moral and judicious aspects of personality, and he also elaborated his definition of the id by recognizing two further principles. Emotional tensions resulting from sexual and other basic instincts he ascribed to an inner force which he called the libido. The conscious impact of this force was painful and unpleasant, and its relief gave pleasure. The second principle concerned destructive instincts which stimulated aggression and produced irrational hatreds and violence. Functionally he conceived that both the id and the superego operated by what he called cathexis or anti-cathexis to stimulate or restrain the ego. Anti-cathexis for example operates in connection with memory. If a person fails to recall something or makes a verbal slip it is because this unconscious censor is protecting the ego against some painful or disturbing association and so from the anxiety which recall would otherwise arouse. This is known as repression.

Anxiety is a crucial concept in the explanation of neurosis. Freud distinguished between objective, neurotic and moral anxiety. Objective anxiety is aroused by the recognition of a real danger, and moral anxiety results from shame induced by an active conscience, but neurotic anxiety is an expression of ill-formed fears resident in the id – so-called phobias. In the face of such stresses the ego develops various defence mechanisms designed to suppress or redirect the unpleasant, painful or anxiety-inducing cathexes – these impulses of sub-conscious origin. Such defence mechanisms include identification (adoption of discordant images as one's own), sublimation (the projection of an unworthy impulse on a more acceptable object), reaction formation (doing the exact opposite), fixation (persistence of a primitive mode of gratification) and regression (reversion to a more primitive personality).

However one now regards Freud, it was he who was largely responsible for first exploring the recesses of the unconscious mind. Others have built upon and adapted his fundamental ideas. Since man first emerged from his caves a cardinal tenet of human faith has been the belief that upward progress is inevitable through constant growth of knowledge and an increasingly rational approach to the problems of daily life. The developing theories of psychology do little to sustain this view. Rather they enforce the reflection that human conduct, to a great extent, still appears to be motivated by blind instinctual forces.

underfeeding. A common cause of failure to thrive in both breast-fed and bottle-fed infants. The underfed child fails to gain weight and is either fretful or apathetic; the skin is thin, inelastic, and wrinkled from loss of subcutaneous fat; the eyes appear sunken; muscular development and activity is poor; the abdomen appears relatively large; and the stools ('hunger stools') are often small and green.

In breast feeding, the mother's lactation may be insufficient, the nipples may be retracted or otherwise unsatisfactory, or there may be errors in nursing technique. The baby itself may be unable to suck properly because of a defective airway, congenital defects such as hare-lip or cleft palate, mouth infections, mental defect or intracranial injury. In artificial feeding, undernourishment results from giving insufficient or too dilute feeds, or from the infant failing to take in correct feeds through sucking difficulties, caused either by the disabilities already mentioned or by unsatisfactory equipment, particularly in relation to the design and openness of the teats.

A breast-fed baby should be weighed before and after a feed to determine how much milk it is actually getting; this is known as a test-feed. If underfeeding is confirmed a complementary artificial feed should be given after each breast feed. In artificially-fed infants the whole procedure should be carefully reviewed in detail and steps taken to ensure that the appropriate Calorie intake for the expected weight is both provided and taken.

Extreme degrees of underfeeding result in marasmus (extreme emaciation) and consideration should be given to the possibility of other diseases being present, such as congenital syphilis, chronic infection (especially tuberculosis or chronic enteritis), coeliac disease, parasitic infection or nervous and mental defect.

In primitive communities underfeeding may be particularly related to the protein component of the diet. This results, for example, in kwashiorkor, a condition characterized by malnutrition, anaemia, oedema and abnormalities of skin and pigmentation.

undulant fever. See BRUCELLOSIS.

uraemia. A condition of toxaemia due to retention in the blood stream of toxic waste-products normally eliminated by the kidneys. The symptoms generally include headache, nausea, vomiting, diarrhoea, diminished urinary output, itching, cramps, panting respiration with urinous smelling breath, restlessness, mental confusion, and eventually convulsions, coma and death.

Uraemia is not always due to kidney disease but may also be caused by metabolic disorders, poisons, or circulatory failure. In treatment the primary need is to identify the cause of the condition and give appropriate treatment, but the actual toxaemia may be relieved at least temporarily by the procedure of renal dialysis using an artificial KIDNEY MACHINE. Blood tests are employed to assess the gravity and progress of the condition.

urea. The breakdown of the protein in the diet produces urea, which enters the blood stream. Chemically, urea is carbamide $[CO(NH_2)_2]$, an organic compound of nitrogen; nitrogen is an essential constituent of protein. The normal level of urea in the blood is 20 to 40 mg. per 100 ml. and any in excess of this amount is excreted in the urine by the kidneys. This means that a diet rich in protein increases the urea in the urine, but a proportion of the daily output is also derived from the normal continuous disintegration of tissue-protein.

On an adequate diet, the healthy body maintains a nitrogen balance. Lost tissue-nitrogen is replaced from food and excess is excreted as urea. In starvation, nitrogen is lost by , tissue-wastage without replacement and the result is a negative nitrogen balance. Conversely, with an adequate diet, growth, pregnancy, physical training and convalescence all lead to a positive nitrogen balance.

In kidney disease urea excretion may be reduced. The estimation of blood-urea levels and the use of urea-clearance tests provide convenient methods of assessing renal efficiency, but urea retention alone is not wholly responsible for the toxic condition known as URAEMIA.

ureter. A tube which conveys urine from each kidney to the urinary bladder. Each ureter is about 25 to 30 cm. (10 to 12 in.) in length and is a relatively thick-walled narrow canal continuous with the lower end of the collecting funnel (or renal pelvis) of the kidney; it opens into the upper part of the bladder. See URINARY SYSTEM.

Calculi or 'gravel' produced by the precipitation of urinary salts may pass through the ureter or may become impacted or stuck at some point. The thick wall is composed of smooth muscle fibres and this muscular tissue makes spasmodic efforts to force the material downwards to the bladder or to overcome the impaction, so producing the painful symptoms usually called renal colic.

urethra. The passage through which urine from the urinary bladder is voided to the exterior.

In the female the urethra is short - only 4 cm. (1.5 in.) - and leads directly to an external opening situated immediately in front of the vagina. Its wall contains circular muscle fibres, particularly concentrated near the neck of the bladder to form the urethral sphincter.

The male urethra is much longer - 18 to 20 cm. (7 to 8 in.) - since it extends from the bladder to the end of the penis. Its first section, the prostatic urethra, is surrounded by the prostate gland and is there joined by ducts from that gland and from the seminal vesicles. The penile or cavernous part traverses the length of the penis. Between the prostatic and penile urethras is a short, narrow and compressible section, the membranous urethra, encircled by the muscle fibres of the urethral sphincter. In the male the urethra serves not only for the voiding of urine but also for the transmission of seminal fluid. In both sexes the outflow of urine is controlled by the sphincter muscle.

Urethritis. This is a condition in which there is inflammation of the urethra due to invasion of its mucous membrane by pus-forming organisms; there is a discharge with pain and difficulty in passing urine. In men, if the infection passes inwards to the posterior urethra, it may lead to further serious effects involving the prostate gland, seminal ducts, epididymis, and peri-urethral tissue, with possibilities of urethral stricture and deep abscess formation.

Most cases arise by infection from the exterior, and a common cause is gon-orrhoea transmitted by sexual contact. Infections due to intestinal organisms are not infrequent in women and also occur occasionally in elderly men. The condition may also follow use of a catheter or be a complication of cystitis.

In treatment the initial need is to

identify the infecting organism, to give appropriate antibiotics, and to maintain a copious urinary flow by a large fluid-intake and diuretics. Before the advent of effective antibiotics intensive antiseptic washes were used but these are now seldom required.

uric acid. A nitrogenous compound ($C_5H_4N_4O_3$) normally present in blood and urine. It is formed both by the wear and tear of body cells (endogenous or tissue-wastage production) and by the breaking-down of the nucleoprotein in certain foods (exogenous production). Fish, liver, kidney and sweetbreads are foods particularly rich in nucleoprotein, and tissue-wastage is increased in various acute fevers and in leukaemia.

In gout the excretion of uric acid in the urine is reduced and deposits of sodium urate occur in and around joints, causing the characteristically painful arthritis.

Pure uric acid is colourless, but in acid-urine deposits of it may sometimes be seen as small reddish crystals ('cayenne pepper' deposits). Larger aggregations occasionally form stones (calculi) in the urinary tract.

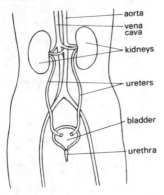

The urinary system

urinary system. Excess water and soluble waste products are eliminated from the body as urine, a pale yellow and usually slightly acid fluid. About 1200 to 1800 ml. (2 to 3 pts.) of urine are excreted per day. Urine is produced by the two kidneys and flows by the two ureters to the urinary bladder, where it is held until it is convenient to void it. Bladder emptying (technically termed micturition) is normally under voluntary control, urine being passed to the exterior through the urethra, which is short and direct in females but in males traverses the penis.

The complex part of this process is urine formation by the kidney, which consists of

The urinary system: structure of a nephron in the kidney

very many separate, microscopically small filtration units called uriniferous tubules or nephrons. Each nephron is associated with a tuft of blood vessels called a glomerulus (see diagram). Surrounding this tuft is the blind expanded upper end of the tubule, indented to enclose the glomerulus. The rest of the tubule is long and convoluted and finally opens into the interior of the kidney (known as the 'pelvis'). The glomerulus and surrounding tubule together act as a filter, removing from the blood stream water and all soluble constituents except protein. The upper end of the tubule thus contains, in effect, de-proteinized plasma. As this fluid passes along the convoluted part of the tubule, selective reabsorption takes place. Substances still required are recovered in accordance with body needs, while the excess water and unwanted waste products that remain pass on as urine, first to the hollow interior of the kidney, and thence to the bladder.

The main diseases of the urinary system are those involving the secretory organs, or KIDNEYS. Other structures have simpler functions related purely to collection, storage, and evacuation of urine. Congenital kidney defects are not uncommon and often prove rapidly fatal in infancy, but some may persist unsuspected to later life until symptoms make investigation necessary. Other kidney disease occurs as acute, sub-acute, or chronic NEPHRITIS (see KIDNEY) and may result from inflammatory, degenerative, or circulatory changes.

Bacterial infection can occur anywhere in the urinary tract. The resulting conditions are pyelo-nephritis (kidney and kidney-pelvis), cystitis (bladder), and urethritis (urethra), the last-named often of gonococcal origin.

Obstructions are common. They cause pain, frequency of passing urine, urinary retention, and local injury. They are usually due to stone (calculus), enlargement of the prostate, or stricture, and tend to lead to secondary infection. Chronic obstruction of urinary outflow from the bladder is practically confined to men with enlarged prostate or urethral stricture. Obstruction at any level eventually gives further trouble as back-pressure dilates ureters and kidney (hydronephrosis), thinning out and destroying kidney tissue.

Primary tumours affect mainly the kidney and bladder. Simple kidney tumours are rare, although occasionally cysts of congenital origin create symptoms in adult life. Hypernephroma is the commonest malignant tumour, usually occurring in older men, and often reaching a large size. Sarcoma and carcinoma are both rare.

The common bladder tumour is a papilloma, which has a strong tendency to become malignant. Bladder carcinoma also occurs as a sequel of hookworm disease (bilharziasis), and in industries which use carcinogenic solvents. Prostatic enlargement is frequent in older men. It is usually benign but may progress to malignancy.

urination. The act of passing urine. Urine, produced by the kidneys, flows to the bladder through the ureter. As the bladder distends the pressure rises and this invokes reflex contraction of its muscular wall, and the accumulated urine is voided through the urethra. In the normal person the reflex mechanism can be voluntarily restrained or initiated in accordance with circumstances.

Disorders of urination are obstruction, frequency (with or without pain) and incontinence. Obstruction may be due to urethral stricture, enlarged prostate or an impacted calculus (stone). Frequency is usually a symptom of cystitis. Incontinence occurs in the young child before control has been learned, in the aged because of failing control and lack of mental awareness, in spinal cord disease or injury, and often in women because of damage resulting from pregnancy.

urine. Normal urine is a fluid secreted by the kidneys and containing urea, uric acid, creatinine, phosphates, chlorides, and sulphates. It is straw-coloured (due to the presence of urochrome derived from the bile-pigment bilirubin), usually faintly acid, and possesses a characteristic odour; its specific gravity varies from 1.015 to 1.025.

The average daily adult output is 1200 to 1800 ml. (2 to 3 pts.).

Abnormal constituents indicate disease, and urine-testing should be a diagnostic routine. Alterations in colour may be due to blood or bile, but black urine occurs with certain tumours, and various drugs may colour it blue, yellow, green, or red. Bacterial infections split urea to give the smell of ammonia; and alcohol and some drugs also produce characteristic aromas. The specific gravity rises in diabetes mellitus and is reduced in diabetes insipidus and cirrhosis of the kidney. Urine of normal colour and smell may on examination be found to contain albumin, bile, sugars, or ketone bodies.

When normal urine is allowed to stand, a sediment collects; this is mainly phosphates, carbonates and urates, and occasionally uric acid. In diseased conditions the sediment may include blood-cells, pus-cells, bacteria, tumour-cells, fragments of tissue resulting from ulceration, and tube-casts, i.e., plugs formed in the kidney tubules as a result of inflammatory or degenerative kidney disease.

Incontinence. Loss of voluntary control over the passage of urine. This is common with the debility and muscular weakness of old age, but it can also occur in prostrating diseases and in surgical shock; in disease of the urinary tract; in pelvic injuries which damage bladder, urethra, or associated muscles; in mental stress from excitement or fear; in disease of the central nervous system; and in injuries to the spinal cord.

In true incontinence the bladder is empty and urine dribbles away as it is produced. In overflow incontinence the bladder is distended and small quantities of urine are passed involuntarily at intervals as pressure overcomes the obstruction. Overflow incontinence is often found in cases of enlargement of the prostate.

Stress incontinence usually occurs in women with pelvic muscles damaged by childbirth. Lifting weights or coughing tightens the abdominal muscles and raises the pressure within the abdomen, so compressing the bladder; and the extra strain overcomes the resistance of the spincter muscle of the urethra.

In stress incontinence a small operation to repair the damaged muscle may be needed. Nocturnal incontinence in old people can sometimes be helped by avoiding all drinks for three hours before bed-time (but taking care not to reduce the total daily intake of liquid). Where the condition persists incontinence pads are useful.

Suppression. Suppression of urine (anuria) is cessation of urinary secretion by the kidneys. It is a very serious condition, rapidly fatal if not relieved, since it leads quickly to uraemia. Anuria may occur in acute nephritis, whether caused by infection or by toxic substances; in the terminal stages of chronic nephritis; in severe fluid loss by other routes (e.g., with the diarrhoea of cholera or the vomiting of hyperemesis); in obstruction of both ureters (e.g., by stones); and occasionally after operations on the urinary tract, following severe surgical shock, or in association with circulatory failure in a disease of the heart. Treatment varies with the cause, but may include treatment with a KIDNEY MACHINE.

Retention. In urinary retention, urine cannot be passed although it continues to accumulate in the bladder. Lower abdominal pain results from distension of the bladder which can usually be seen and felt as a rounded swelling above the pubis, and there may be strangury, or painful attempts to pass urine.

Retention may be caused by the following: (1) mechanical factors such as calculus (stone), enlargement of the prostate, or stricture due to spasm, inflammation or such infections as gonorrhoea; (2) the effect of drugs, alcohol, shock, nervousness or hysteria on the centre of the brain controlling the bladder; (3) damage to the spinal cord which impairs the nerve supply to the bladder; (4) over-action of the sympathetic nervous system, especially after surgical operations; (5) pain inhibiting the passing of urine – this may be the result of such conditions as inflammation of the urethra; (6) muscular weakness in the aged and debilitated, or after childbirth, affecting the bladder itself or the muscles of the abdomen.

The condition may require relief by inserting a CATHETER, but if possible this should be a last resort because of the attendant risks of infection.

In cases due to temporary causes, difficulty can often be overcome by simple nursing measures to encourage relaxation (hot applications, a hot bath, or an enema).

urticaria. See NETTLE RASH.

uterus. The uterus or womb is a hollow, thick-walled muscular organ of the female pelvis, lying between the bladder in front and the rectum behind. During pregnancy it accommodates, protects, and nourishes the growing foetus. In the non-pregnant state it resembles a flattened pear (stalk end down), 7.5 cm. long, 5 cm. wide, and 2.5 cm. thick (3 in. by 2 in. by 1 in.). At its upper end on each side arise the uterine or Fallopian tubes through which ova, discharged from the ovaries, are conveyed to its hollow interior. Its lower third is named the cervix, a conical structure with a central canal, projecting into the upper end of the vagina.

The uterine cavity is lined by cellular tissue which is influenced by ovarian hormones and undergoes a regular cycle of changes, being shed each month during menstruation; however, if conception occurs it provides a lodging for the developing ovum. The lower part of the cervix has a different, more flattened type of cellular tissue, prone to degenerative or malignant change, and it is this which is

sampled in the preventive procedure of CERVICAL CYTOLOGY.

During pregnancy the uterus enlarges enormously. After childbirth it rapidly returns almost to its original size.

Diseases. Congenitally, the uterus may be duplicated, malformed developmentally, or undersized (hypoplasia). Sterility or difficulties with pregnancy or labour may result.

Normally the cervix and uterine body are directed upwards and forwards (anteversion), and the body is bent slightly forwards in relation to the cervical canal (anteflexion). Backward displacement (retroversion and retroflexion) is not uncommon after childbirth, following stretching of ligaments and weakening of muscles. It is in part preventable by good obstetric practice (avoiding injury), avoidance of over-long inactivity after the birth, prevention of bladder distension, and restoration of muscle-tone by appropriate exercises. Where the displacement occurs it may cause backache or menstrual pain and irregularity. Downward uterine displacement is partial or complete prolapse, usually following pelvic floor damage during childbirth. Pessaries or operative treatment may be advised.

Actual disease affects the cells of the wall of the cervix, the lining (endometrium) of the uterus, or its substance (myometrium). Erosion of the cervix is generally due to chronic inflammation (cervicitis) and produces vaginal discharge. Treatment may involve local applications, cauterization, or operation. Acute endometritis usually results from infection following childbirth, but may be gonorrhoeal or tuberculous in origin. Persistent chronic endometritis may be indicative of some other uterine condition. The appropriate treatment of endometritis varies with its cause.

Uterine tumours may be benign or malignant. Of the former, polyps grow from the cervical canal or from the endometrium, and fibroids, which may be multiple or of large size, develop from the myometrium. Cancer may arise either in the cervix or uterine body. Cervical cancer is commoner, most often seen after several pregnancies, and tends to spread rapidly to adjacent tissues. Conversely, cancer of the uterine body more often affects older women who have had no pregnancies and is slower to develop. The treatment of all these conditions is surgical and by radiotherapy.

The general symptoms of tumours are initially haemorrhage and discharge. Irregular bleeding or its post-menopausal recurrence indicates a need for full investigation.

Cervical cytology is a very simple procedure intended to detect pre-cancerous changes in the cervical epithelium so that treatment can be undertaken in good time. It should be a routine three-yearly precaution in all women over 35 years of age.

uvula. A flattened, conical projection, hanging downwards from the middle of the free border of the soft palate at the back of the mouth. It consists of muscle-fibres covered by mucous membrane. The function of the soft palate is to cut off the nasal passage from the mouth and throat, particularly during the act of swallowing; the uvula ensures that a more efficient seal is achieved.

V

vaccination. Although, strictly speaking, vaccination means anti-smallpox inoculation using smallpox vaccine administered intradermally (i.e., into the skin) by scratch or multiple-puncture technique, the term is now widely used to include any procedure for inducing active IMMUNITY which relies on preparations of killed or treated bacterial or viral cultures. These are usually given by injection under the skin, or even by mouth, as in active immunization against poliomyelitis. See IMMUNIZATION.

vaccine. A bacterium or virus so modified as to be no longer dangerous but capable of conferring IMMUNITY to the disease that it would normally cause. A dead or killed vaccine is one prepared by cultivating the organisms in an artificial medium and then killing them, e.g., by heat or by an appropriate chemical; there is no possibility of the vaccine producing the disease but it stimulates the defence mechanisms of the body to produce antibodies capable of dealing with invading organisms of the particular type. A live or attenuated vaccine is one prepared by cultivating the organism for many generations in an unnatural environment so that it completely loses its virulence but can still stimulate the defence mechanisms of the body. An autogenous vaccine is one prepared from organisms found in the patient's sputum, urine or other secretions; but as knowledge of the typing of organisms increases the need to prepare a vaccine specially for a particular patient clearly diminishes.

Vaccines are effective against a wide range of diseases, including smallpox, anthrax, rabies, cholera, plague, typhoid, paratyphoid, diphtheria, tetanus, whooping cough, poliomyelitis, tuberculosis, measles, rubella, mumps and influenza.

Some vaccines produce an almost perfect immunity: for instance it was virtually unknown for a person successfully vaccinated against smallpox to develop the disease during the next seven years, and the occurrence of diphtheria in a person immunized within the previous three years is an extreme rarity. Some, like rabies vaccine, are useful but by no means a hundred per cent effective. A few, like influenza vaccine, have to be altered frequently: there are many strains of influenza virus, and the vaccine prepared against a strain prevalent in one year may give only a partial protection against the strain prevalent a year later.

Vaccines have played an enormous part in the conquest of infectious diseases.

Examples are the eradication of smallpox from all countries in the world; the reduction of typhoid and paratyphoid in many countries by TAB; and the reduction of diphtheria in Britain from over fifty thousand cases and nearly five thousand deaths a year to around a dozen cases and no deaths. There are, however, some infections – from LASSA FEVER to the common cold – against which no vaccine is yet available.

vagina. The vagina, or female copulatory passage, is a musculo-membranous tube 10 to 12.5 cm. long (4 to 5 in.) extending upwards and backwards from its opening at the vulva to the uterus, the cervix of which projects into it at its upper end. It lies between the bladder and urethra in front and the rectum behind. In virgins the lower orifice is partially closed by the hymen. It forms part of the female REPRODUCTIVE SYSTEM, and during sexual intercourse it is penetrated by the male penis. It also serves as a channel for the menstrual discharge, and, much distended, as the birth-canal during childbirth.

Diseases. Inflammation of the vagina is known as vaginitis. The main symptom is vaginal discharge, but the vulva is usually involved as well (vulvo-vaginitis), giving rise to pain, irritation, itching, swelling, tenderness, and pain on intercourse. Long-standing cases sometimes develop mental depression. An abnormal discharge of white fluid from the vagina is known as leucorrhoea. The discharge of a little milky exudate a day or so before the beginning of the menstrual flow is not abnormal and simply indicates pelvic congestion, but persistent and copious discharge indicates infection or inflammation of the genital organs. Causes include chronic inflammation of the uterus or of its cervix, chronic infection of a cervical tear, gonorrhoea, and – if the discharge is purulent – either cancer of the cervix or presence of a sloughing fibroid. Since leucorrhoea is not a disease but a symptom, treatment clearly varies with the cause; but any persisting discharge demands medical investigation.

Smears should be examined bacteriologically to ensure a correct diagnosis. Treatment may require antiseptic douching, but many cases can be adequately dealt with by appropriate medicated pessaries and the use of systemic antibiotics and hormones. Tights, impermeable pants, and the imperfect rinsing of underwear washed in biological detergents have been blamed for a rising prevalence of vulvo-vaginitis.

vaginismus. A condition in which attempts

at sexual intercourse produce spasms of the muscles of vulva, vagina, and surrounding tissues, frustrating penetration or causing painful intercourse (dyspareunia).

Minor degrees of vaginismus may result from painful conditions such as lacerations of the hymen, caruncles (small fleshy excrescences), vulvitis, or vaginitis, and appropriate treatment should effect a cure. However, typical cases more often have a psychological basis due to a subconscious dread of inercourse. Psychotherapy may be required, combined with the use of vaginal dilators which the patient herself, after preliminary demonstration and instruction, can insert regularly, to implant in her mind a conviction that there is no physical basis for her difficulties.

vaginitis. Inflammation of the VAGINA.

vagotomy. Surgical severance of the VAGUS NERVE, certain fibres of which stimulate the stomach glands to produce gastric juice (pepsin and hydrocholoric acid). In ulceration of the stomach or duodenum a basic factor is excess acid secretion and the operation of vagotomy is designed to diminish this. It has to a large extent replaced partial gastrectomy, an operation to remove the part of the stomach in which secretory cells are most abundant.

vagus nerve. The vagus or tenth cranial nerve contains both afferent and efferent fibres, i.e., fibres bringing sensations to the brain and fibres conveying instructions to organs. It also contains fibres of the parasympathetic system. While other cranial nerves are concerned with the special senses and with the skin and muscles of the head and neck, the vagus – the name means 'wanderer' – travels downwards to the chest and abdomen, and supplies the pharynx, larynx, oesophagus, stomach, intestines, heart and lungs. Activity of the vagus slows the heart, narrows the bronchi and stimulates the process of digestion.

Valium. A TRANQUILLIZER.

valves flattened
by normal blood flow,
but filled out, thus
blocking the vein,
during back-flow

direction of blood flow

Valves in the veins of the leg

valve. Any flap-like fold of the lining of a blood vessel or duct acting as a one-way traffic director. When the pressure becomes higher on one side of the valve it forces the valve open so that fluid flows through to the other side. When the pressure rises on the other side it forces the valve shut, so that the fluid cannot flow backwards.

Perhaps the best-known valves are those of the HEART, but veins and lymphatic vessels also contain valves.

valvular heart disease. See HEART.

varicella. See CHICKENPOX.

varicocele. A varicose condition of some of the numerous, inter-communicating veins in the spermatic cord. They drain ultimately to the renal veins, and simple varicocele is almost invariably found on the left side because of anatomical differences between the venous junctions on the two sides.

There is usually no simple cause for varicocele but it can occur as a complication of renal tumour and the possibility of this should be investigated if varicocele appears suddenly.

Although the condition causes swelling of the scrotum and can be easily felt, giving an impression described as like a 'bag of worms', it generally gives little trouble and operation is rarely required. Any feeling of uncomfortable weight or strain can be relieved by wearing a net suspensory to support the scrotum. This is most often needed by young adults participating in athletic activities, or in older men, as ageing tissues provide diminishing support.

varicose veins. See VEINS, diseases of.

vascular. Containing or made up of blood vessels.

vasectomy See BIRTH CONTROL.

vector. Any insect or animal that transmits infection to human beings. Thus mosquitoes are vectors of malaria and yellow fever, lice are vectors of typhus, and flies can be vectors of typhoid and other food-borne infection. Some animals are themselves victims of the disease that they transmit, e.g., rabies reaches man through the bite of an infected dog, cat or wolf. In many cases the eradication of an infection transmitted by a vector depends more on control of the vector than on the much more difficult task of controlling the causal agent.

vegetables. Dietetically, a vegetable is a plant, or part of a plant, used for food, but excluding the parts surrounding its seeds, which are called fruits. This definition sometimes conflicts with ordinary usage. For instance, a marrow, although called a vegetable-marrow, is really a fruit; a tomato is also a fruit although some would regard it as a vegetable; and rhubarb, which is used as a fruit, is a leaf-stem and certainly a vegetable. Cereals are also a problem: they are usually described with the vegetables, but they are the fruits of grasses.

If cereals are included, vegetables may be classified as follows:

Cereals. The seed-grains of a variety of

cultivated grasses – wheat, rye, barley, oats, maize, and rice. They consist mainly of carbohydrate (in the form of starch), with variable amounts of protein, fat, minerals and vitamins. The protein is 'second class', in that it does not contain all the essential amino-acids. The minerals and vitamins are chiefly present in the husk and are largely lost in milling – hence the superiority of wholemeal bread, and also oatmeal, for which whole grains are ground or rolled. Cornflour is made from maize starch.

Pulses or legumes. Peas, beans, and lentils. These contain considerable amounts of carbohydrate and protein but are generally low in fat, with the exception of soya beans which have about 15 per cent fat. When fresh, the pulses are good sources of vitamin C.

Tubers and roots. Potatoes, carrots, parsnips and beetroot are all good sources of carbohydrate; carrots supply vitamin A; turnips provide little nutriment. The roots of certain tropical plants supply arrowroot and tapioca. Sago, also largely carbohydrate, is prepared from the pith of sago-palm stems.

Green vegetables. The commonest are cabbage, cauliflower and Brussels sprouts. They provide few Calories but are good sources of minerals and vitamin C. Lettuce and watercress are eaten without cooking and are particularly good since they do not suffer the losses caused in the others by over-boiling. Spinach contains about 3 per cent iron.

Vegetables thus form an important part of a normal DIET, and by their carbohydrate content contribute significantly to the total Calorie requirement. They have another important function in providing ROUGHAGE or residue – the plant material which is not digested and not absorbed from the human intestine. It is now recognized that roughage reduces constipation, prevents various colonic diseases, and plays a part in the burning up of fats.

vegetarian diet. A diet that excludes the flesh of animals, birds and fishes. There are two main types.

A lacto-vegetarian diet. This type rejects all forms of meat, fish, etc., but accepts milk, butter, cheese and eggs. Such a diet can easily provide a sufficiency of first class protein, vitamins and mineral salts. Although some people would find it a little monotonous to obtain all their first class protein from milk products and eggs, a lacto-vegetarian diet can be as adequate as any other diet. As an example, a day's ration containing 680 g. (24 oz.) bread, 170 g. (6 oz.) of cheese, 280 g. (10 oz.) of milk, 56 g. (2 oz.) of butter and 85 g. (3 oz.) of watercress would provide approximately 3000 Calories, about 100 g. of protein (half of it first class), adequate water-soluble and fat-soluble vitamins and reasonable amounts of most minerals.

A strictly vegetarian diet. Such a diet rejects all foods other than those of plant origin. Such a diet is subject to at least four main defects.

1. Since no vegetable food, however rich in second class protein, contains all the required amino-acids, the strict vegetarian cannot obtain all his protein from one or two sources (e.g., peas and beans or nuts and lentils) but requires to consume a judicious mixture of those vegetables that are rich in protein.

2. Most of the body's mineral requirements are normally supplied from animal sources, e.g., calcium and phosphorus from milk and cheese, iron from meat and eggs, and iodine from fish. The strict vegetarian requires rather a lot of green vegetables and nuts to supply his calcium, a quantity of peas or oatmeal to provide his iron, sufficient wheat germ to supply his phosphorus and water plants such as watercress to provide his iodine.

3. Much of the body's requirement of fat-soluble vitamins is normally obtained from animal fat. Hence the strict vegetarian may be in difficulties unless vitamins A and D are added to foods of vegetable origin, such as margarine.

4. A purely vegetarian diet tends to be very bulky: our nearest animal relations, monkeys, are essentially vegetarians but they devote their waking lives to finding food and eating it.

Nevertheless many people exist in good health on a carefully balanced vegetarian diet.

veins. The vessels which carry blood from the tissues of the body back to the heart. Veins have much thinner walls than arteries but the walls consist of the same three coats, i.e., an outer fibrous coat, a middle coat of muscular and elastic fibres, and an inner coat of elastic membrane. Most veins have VALVES which control the direction of the flow of blood.

normal vein   varicosed vein

Veins

Diseases. Veins are thin-walled and

often lie near the surface, so that they lack support and are exposed to injury.

Varicose veins are very common. Increased internal pressure produces dilation and lengthening. Lengthening causes twisting; and dilation, by further weakening the vein-wall and making internal valves incompetent, encourages further varicosity. Most frequently affected are the long veins of the legs, especially in persons whose occupation involves prolonged standing. Other common sites for varicose veins are around the anus (haemorrhoids or piles), the spermatic cord (varicocele) and at the junction between the oesophagus and the stomach, where they may rupture to cause gastric haemorrhage.

Severe varicose veins require surgical treatment either by removal or tying, or the injection of sclerosing (hardening) solutions. Elastic stockings help minor cases.

Inflammation of veins is called phlebitis; it may be either simple, from local injury or prolonged exhaustion, or infective. Infective phlebitis of leg-veins is common after childbirth, and is known as phlegmasia. Phlebitis causes clot-formation (thrombosis) within the vein, and detached clots may be carried elsewhere by the blood (embolism).

Phlebitis calls for rest and local symptomatic measures, with antibiotic cover for any infection.

venepuncture. Puncture of a vein in order to withdraw a sample of blood, or to release excessive blood, or to instil replacement blood, transfusion solutions or drugs.

venereal disease. Disease which is spread predominantly by sexual contact. The best-known conditions are syphilis, gonorrhoea, and soft chancre (chancroid), but some other diseases are spread in a similar manner. Lymphogranuloma venereum and granuloma inguinale (due to virus-like organisms) are diseases of sexual intercourse, and venereal clinics are also called on to treat non-specific urethritis and trichomonas infections.

Treatment has been effective since the introduction of antibiotic drugs in the 1940s. By the end of World War II it therefore seemed that venereal disease would be steadily reduced and perhaps ultimately eradicated, but this has not happened. Indeed, after a decline for a number of years, the tide seemed to turn. Syphilis remained fairly rare in the U.K. (around 1700 new cases in a typical year) but increased by about 300 per cent in the U.S.A., and in the 1970s experts estimated that there were about 50 million cases of infectious syphilis in the world (as compared with an estimate of about 20 million at the close of World War II). Gonorrhoea rose even more, to 70,000 cases in the U.K., about one and a half million cases in the U.S.A. and an estimated 150 million cases in the world,

making gonorrhoea the commonest infectious disease after the ordinary cold and influenza. Other venereal diseases also showed a rise. Most alarming of all is the increase - especially of gonorrhoea - in teenage youngsters.

Many medical and social factors are involved in attempts to control and reduce the venereal diseases, though clearly spread depends on the extent of promiscuity and on the size of the infector pool, i.e., the number of persons already infectious. Both moral and religious education and sex education should contribute to the reduction of promiscuity, but a trend operating in the reverse direction is prolonged separation of workers in our mobile society from their partners: venereal disease is notoriously common in merchant seamen, service-men, air pilots and air hostesses, persons working on oil rigs and long-distance lorry drivers. Again to some extent the professional prostitute, who could in many countries be legally subjected to periodical medical examination and who in any case would want to avoid infection or have it promptly treated, is being replaced by the 'good time' promiscuous girl, and this promiscuity is in large measure a part of the antisocial behaviour of adolescent rebellion. Although the increase in venereal disease started considerably before the contraceptive pill was in common use, removal of fear of pregnancy may contribute to the increase in promiscuity; however, experience in family planning clinics suggests that they are used by socially responsible people who are married or 'going steady' and virtually ignored by promiscuous girls.

As for reduction of the infector pool, clearly it is essential to provide adequate, accessible, confidential and free treatment centres; to ensure that these centres are open at hours suitable to the potential users; to spread information about the centres and about the dangers of untreated disease; and, in so far as is possible, to trace contacts and persuade them to undergo treatment.

In the U.K. the current stress is on contact tracing and contact persuasion. The former involves something of the interviewing skill of a detective and is difficult since the infected person may have met the contact casually, may not know the surname and may be poor at description; and contact persuasion involves much of the motivating skill of a health visitor and is even more difficult since the contact generally does not feel ill and in the majority of cases is found on examination to be uninfected. Perhaps it would be more useful to transfer the emphasis on the one hand to health education (with sex education as a component part) and on the other hand to ensuring that the positioning and hours of opening of treatment centres are satisfactory. Nevertheless the U.K. is dealing more successfully with the epidemic of venereal diseases than are various other countries.

venesection. An old-fashioned term for the cutting of a vein. Removal of blood was once a popular and often irrational form of treatment. One of the large veins at the bend of the elbow was simply exposed and deftly opened by a lancet-stroke, allowing the patient to bleed into a bowl. Bloodletting is perhaps still helpful in such conditions as polycythaemia, or in congestive cardiac failure with marked swelling of the veins, but nowadays it would be carried out by VENEPUNCTURE, using a wide-bore hollow needle and flexible tubing leading to a receiver.

venom. A general term for the poisonous substances produced by many different creatures, and injected into the body of a victim or adversary, by BITES AND STINGS. Venomous groups include many kinds of insects such as bees, wasps, hornets, and various tropical species, arachnids (spiders and scorpions), reptiles such as snakes and lizards (see SNAKE BITES), spiny fish and jellyfish.

The effects of venom injection may vary from local pain and swelling, as in bee and wasp stings, to rapid prostration and death, which may follow bites by vipers or cobras.

ventilation. The process of providing buildings, or individual rooms, with an adequate supply of fresh air.

When people are overcrowded, insufficient ventilation causes 'stuffiness', marked by feelings of oppression and bodily discomfort, with flushing of the cheeks, headache from swelling of the mucous membrane of the nose, nausea, and perhaps fainting and collapse. Such symptoms occur long before oxygen is seriously depleted or carbon dioxide concentration reaches dangerous levels, and are due entirely to the combined physical effects of increased temperature, increased humidity, and lack of air-movement.

Sufficient air-changes must be provided to avoid discomfort. About 28 to 56 cu. m. (1000 to 2000 cu. ft.) of fresh air are required per person per hour, and the appropriate number of air-changes per hour can be worked out from the cubic capacity of the room and the number of occupants. In ordinary dwellings, natural ventilation from windows, doors and chimney vents normally provides all the air-change that is needed, but in factories, offices and public buildings with systems of artificial ventilation, six changes per hour are generally recommended. Steps must be taken to prevent draughts by warming the incoming air and considering the position of inlets.

The katathermometer is used to assess the cooling-power of air in rooms. The dry katathermometer measures rate of heat-loss from radiation and convection. The wet katathermometer takes account of evaporation as well. Comfort for indoor sedentary work calls for a dry kata reading of about 6, representing a heat-loss from the previously-warmed thermometer of 6 millicalories per sq. cm. per second. If the readings are lower the room is too hot; if higher, it is too cold.

ventriculography. A procedure used in x-ray examination of the brain to visualize the lateral ventricles, which are cavities in the cerebral hemispheres of the brain filled with cerebrospinal fluid. Brain-tissue and cerebrospinal fluid are of uniform x-ray opacity and an ordinary plate is generally of little help in demonstrating suspected disease. In ventriculography the fluid is replaced by air or oxygen before x-ray examination, and since air is of different radiographic density it provides a contrast medium to outline the ventricles. Any displacement or alteration in their size and shape helps to determine the site or nature of the disorder.

The air is normally instilled through a hollow needle passed into the ventricles after a preliminary burr-hole has been made in the skull. An alternative method introduces air after lumbar puncture in the hope that it will rise and enter the ventricles.

vermifuge. Any drug used to expel parasitic worms. A similar word, vermicide, implies that the drug actually kills them.

A range of highly effective synthetic drugs (anthelmintics) is now available. Since worm-infestation causes much avoidable ill-health, this is an important advance. All these drugs require medical advice and supervision to regulate regimen and adjust dosage to body-weight, since some are mildly toxic.

verruca. A medical term for a WART.

vertebra. The thirty-three vertebrae, united to each other by intervertebral fibro-cartilaginous discs and by ligaments, are the bones which together form the SPINAL COLUMN.

vertigo. A term used to describe any sense of unsteadiness or movement experienced by an individual either when he seems to be spinning himself (subjective vertigo), or when the things around him seem to spin (objective vertigo).

Vertigo is always the result of direct or indirect disturbances of the balancing mechanism of the inner ear (labyrinth), of the vestibular nerve connecting the labyrinth to the brain, or of the cerebellum.

The possible causes are thus very numerous. They include diseases of the ear and its central connections; toxaemia from fevers, alcohol or drugs; cardio-vascular abnormalities causing high or low blood-pressure; anaemia; motion sickness; migraine and epilepsy; and organic brain disease, particularly if accompanied by raised intracranial tension.

Treatment depends on detailed investigation to determine an exact

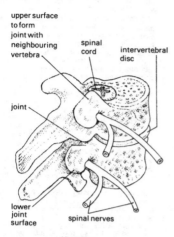

upper surface
to form
joint with
neighbouring
vertebra

spinal
cord

intervertebral
disc

joint

lower
joint
surface

spinal nerves

Vertebrae

diagnosis. See also DIZZINESS and HEAD NOISES (Ménière's disease).

vesicles. Small blisters occurring as an eruption on skin or mucous membrane, and conventionally not larger than a pea. If bigger, they are usually called bullae, or just blisters.

The horny layer of the skin is raised by exudation of clear or turbid fluid to form a roughly hemispherical protrusion, sometimes surrounded by a red, inflamed zone.

Vesicles occur in a variety of conditions: (1) specific infections: chickenpox; herpes; impetigo; (2) skin diseases: eczema; nonspecific pyogenic (pus-forming) infections; (3) parasitism: insect bites; scabies; lice infestation; (4) external irritants; and (5) drugs: iodides; mercury.

Careful study of the type, distribution, and development of vesicles may be of diagnostic help. Vesicle contents may also be sampled for microscopic examination and culture to determine any specific bacterial or viral cause.

Vincent's angina. A particular form of severe ulcerative inflammation of the mucous membrane of the mouth. In definitive cases two micro-organisms are constantly present: *Bacillus fusiformis* and *Spirillum vincenti*. These appear to act in association, but other factors are involved because the disease tends to be found in people suffering from debilitating general conditions such as continued fevers, blood diseases, metallic poisoning, and vitamin deficiencies. There is always pre-existing dental neglect and inflammation of the gums.

The condition is only mildly infectious with occasional outbreaks in residential institutions.

General symptoms are usually trivial. The gums are red, swollen and ulcerated, and shallow ulcers may form elsewhere in the mouth and pharynx, and on the tonsils, often with an adherent exudate resembling diphtheria. The neck glands are enlarged and the breath has a characteristic smell.

The occurrence of Vincent's angina should prompt a search for some general disease. Otherwise treatment is by antibiotics combined with suitable antiseptic mouth-washes or local applications. Oxidizing agents such as hydrogen peroxide or potassium chlorate are particularly effective. Thorough dental treatment is also required.

virilism. The development of male characteristics in a woman, with masculine distribution and growth of body and facial hair, deepening of the voice, and cessation of menstruation. Adiposity (excess of fat-containing tissue) is often an additional feature.

As a disease (adrenogenital syndrome), virilism is due to over-secretion of androgenic hormone and this results from changes in the adrenal gland, the endocrine gland which produces this hormone. These changes may be either benign growths (adenoma) or malignant (carcinoma). Surgical treatment is indicated.

Virilism also occurs as a side-effect of corticosteroid drugs, and of testosterone (male hormone) and other anabolic agents with similar properties. This usually calls for adjustment of dosage or change of drug, but androgens based on testosterone are used for some serious conditions such as advanced and inoperable breast cancer, and masculinization may have to be accepted as a lesser evil.

viruses. Extremely minute infective agents which are only visible by use of the electron microscope. It is helpful to think of their magnitude, by volume, as being roughly one-thousandth that of the bacteria.

Most larger infective agents (such as bacteria) can be cultivated in artificial media which do not require cells of living tissue, but no accepted virus has so far been grown in anything simpler than a tissue culture. Inability to multiply independently is thus part of the definition of a virus. This correlation between small size and dependence on living tissues probably means that viruses cannot provide internal enzyme systems for themselves and therefore are forced to rely on those of some convenient host. It is also possible that the virus misdirects in some way the host enzyme systems in its own interests, and that it is this alteration which causes disease in the host.

Research has now identified many specific types and varieties of viruses which are known to be responsible for a wide range of diseases in animals and plants. Conditions of human importance include smallpox, chickenpox, herpes, hepatitis, poliomyelitis, measles, German measles (rubella), mumps, yellow fever, lassa fever and rabies, as well as influenza, the common cold, and other less well-defined affections of the respiratory, gastro-intestinal, nervous and glandular systems. It is also quite likely that viruses play a part in the causation of CANCER.

In general, drugs and antibiotics have little effect on viral diseases, although there are prospects of future progress. Three products now available are: methisazone (for smallpox and the complications of smallpox vaccination), idoxuridine (for herpes, especially when the cornea is affected), and INTERFERON.

Control of important viral diseases depends largely on vaccination. Smallpox vaccination has eliminated the disease. Other vaccines in common use include those against poliomyelitis, measles, rubella, yellow fever, rabies, and influenza. With some viruses, vaccination or an attack produces solid and lasting immunity, but with others, such as influenza and the common cold, results are often brief and uncertain. This is probably due to the existence of several similar viruses only slightly different, and this variation means that a particular vaccine may not be exactly matched to a prevalent infection.

viscera. A collective term for the organs contained within the chest, abdomen, and pelvis.

visceroptosis. A condition in which the abdominal viscera tend to sag downwards.

It is most often seen in women, and is due to loss of tone in the abdominal muscles and to the stretching of suspensory ligaments, and is often caused by the effects of repeated pregnancies. Displacement may be general or limited to individual organs, particularly the stomach, liver, spleen, kidney, or colon. The lower part of the abdomen appears unduly prominent and the patient may suffer dragging pains, indigestion, and constipation, with more indefinite neurasthenic symptoms such as a sense of weight, lassitude, and depression.

The most satisfactory course is to provide a well-fitted abdominal support and to correct any prominent symptoms – physical or mental – by appropriate medical treatment.

vision. See EYE.

vitamin content of foods. Traditionally the amounts of vitamins A and D are stated in international units, and those of the B and C vitamins in milligrams, although the differentiation is no longer necessary: 333 units of vitamin A and 40,000 units of vitamin D each represent a milligram.

Many tables exist purporting to show the exact vitamin content of various foods. Such tables are useful to persons dealing with large quantities of food but are perhaps of less value for the ordinary householder.

To illustrate let us take the position of a householder who proposes to eat an apple, part of a cabbage and a helping of beef. A table will tell him that 100 g. of apples contain 3 mg. of vitamin C, that 100 g. of spring cabbage contain 60 mg. of that vitamin and that 100 g. of beef contain 35 units of vitamin A. However, before doing arithmetical calculations related to the particular weights of the foods that he is preparing to eat, the householder has various things to remember. Firstly, his concern is with the portion that he intends to eat: there is no point in his weighing the apple before removing the skin and a small bruised portion or weighing the cabbage before removing the outer leaves. Secondly, even when he has weighed only the part that he intends to eat, the table gives him only an average assessment. The amount of vitamin A in his piece of beef will vary appreciably according to how lean or how fat it is, and the vitamin C content of the apple or cabbage will vary with the exact type of the fruit or vegetable, with the climatic conditions under which it was grown, with the degree of ripeness when it was picked, with how long and under what conditions it was stored, and not least – if it is to be cooked – with the method of cooking.

The exact requirement of most vitamins for an adult of average size is known, although more may be required during pregnancy, lactation, strenuous work and illness, and growing children need more than in proportion to body weight. Inadequacy of any vitamin is serious. On the other hand, no quantity of the B and C vitamins has been known to do any harm, harmful excess of A would involve eating very large daily amounts of liver, carrots and spinach, and harmful excess of D would imply a quite inordinate fondness for sardines, herring and salmon. Excess of the fat-soluble vitamins can certainly be produced by over-dosage of vitamin tablets or of cod-liver oil or halibut-liver oil, but with any ordinary diet it is unlikely.

So, to save over-frequent studying of complicated tables, it is perhaps useful to set down the average content of foods rich in the various vitamins, so that, for example, a man who normally eats a helping of liver or a good portion of carrots or spinach can see at a casual glance that he is likely to have enough vitamin A.

Vitamin A. Daily requirement – 2,500 to 5,000 international units. (333 IU equal 1 mg.).

Average number of IU per 100 g.: halibut-liver oil – 1,950,000; cod-liver oil – 105,000; liver – 10,500; carrots – 6,000; spinach – 4,300; butter – 4,000; margarine (reinforced) – 3,000; dried apricots – 1,600; watercress – 1,600; cheese – 1,300; lettuce – 1,280; tomatoes – 980; kidney – 980; eggs – 980; dried prunes – 840; cabbage – 300;

vitamins

sardines – 270; peas and beans – 165; herring – 145; milk – 105.

Vitamin B₁. Daily requirement – 1.5 to 2.3 mg.

Average mg. per 100 g.: yeast – 4.3; nuts – 0.9; chicken – 0.7; duck – 0.7; ham – 0.7; boiled rice – 0.7; bacon – 0.6; pork – 0.5; liver – 0.4; wholemeal bread – 0.32; peas – 0.3; egg – 0.14; mutton – 0.14; potatoes – 0.11; spinach – 0.10; beef – 0.07.

Vitamin B₂. Daily requirement – 2.2 to 3.3 mg.

Average mg. per 100 g.: yeast – 4.4; liver – 3.0; cheese – 0.5; egg – 0.4; nuts – 0.3; herring – 0.25; bacon – 0.20; beef – 0.20; chicken – 0.20; pork – 0.20; salmon – 0.20; spinach – 0.20; cream – 0.20; wholemeal bread – 0.18.

Nicotinic acid. Daily requirement – 15 to 25 mg.

Average mg. per 100 g.: yeast – 72; liver and kidney – 13; nuts – 9; ham – 6; duck – 6; chicken – 6; pork – 5; mutton – 4; oily fish – 3; beef – 2.5; white fish – 2; wholemeal bread – 2; boiled rice – 1.

Vitamin c. Daily requirement – 70 mg.

Average mg. per 100 g.: blackcurrants – 200; cherries – 200; brussels sprouts – 80; cauliflower – 70; cabbage – 60; strawberry – 60; spinach – 60; orange – 56; lemon – 40; tomato – 24; new potato – 14.

Vitamin D. Daily requirement – 400 to 800 international units. (40,000 IU equal 1 mg.)

Average number of IU per 100 g.: halibut-liver oil – 210,000; cod-liver oil – 10,500; salmon – 870; oily fish – 800; tinned salmon – 600; margarine (reinforced) – 350; butter – 60; eggs – 60; cheese – 35; milk – 1.

Shortage of vitamin A is uncommon in adults in developed countries except for people with many dietary pecularities, but can fairly easily occur in children and in particular in babies. Shortage of the B vitamins is fairly frequent among the poorer sections of the community and the elderly, and is also common among heavy consumers of alcohol. Shortage of vitamin c is common in areas in which people eat insufficient fruits and green vegetables, whether from tradition or from the cost of these commodities. Shortage of vitamin D is rare in southern countries (because to a considerable extent it can be manu-factured under the skin in the presence of sunlight) but is quite common in northern countries, especially in immigrants from countries of greater sunshine. Exact bodily requirements of vitamin E are not yet known.

In many developed countries multiple vitamin tablets are on sale commercially. A typical one might contain about 2,500 IU of vitamin A (or most of the day's supply), about 0.5 mg. of vitamin B₁ (or about a quarter of the day's supply), possibly a little vitamin B₂ and nicotinic acid (but most tablets lack these either entirely or partially), about 13 mg. of vitamin c (or roughly a quarter of the day's supply) and about 250 IU of vitamin D (or about half of the day's supply). With adequate diet such supplements should theoretically be unnecessary but they can be useful in northern climates during winter months, when in particular little vitamin D is manufactured in the body, vegetables and fruits are scarcer and may have lost some vitamin c by cooking, storage with exposure to light, etc., and intake of the B vitamins may be restricted by cost.

vitamins. A group of complex organic compounds essential in small amounts to normal body metabolism. Insufficient intake of vitamins causes various DEFICIENCY DISEASES.

Vitamin A. Carotene; 'anti-infective' vitamin which is fat-soluble. Sources: fish-liver oils, egg-yolk, liver, dairy products, carrots and green vegetables. Deficiency causes xerophthalmia (corneal degenera-tion), night-blindness, and susceptibility to infection. Excess may cause severe symptoms, with loss of appetite, periostitis (inflammation of the fibrous membrane covering bones), bone-pains, spontaneous fractures, and enlargement of liver and spleen.

Vitamin B-*complex.* A group of water-soluble vitamins essential to many ENZYME systems concerned in the utilization of carbohydrate, protein, and fat. Although each factor has specific importance there is also overlap and interdependence.

Vitamin B₁. Aneurin or thiamine. Sources: wheat-germ, cereal husks, yeast, egg-yolk, liver, pork, and legumes. Deficiency causes beriberi or in lesser degrees of deprivation neuritis, mental dullness, cardiac and general weakness.

Vitamin B₂. Riboflavin. Sources: milk, egg-white, liver, offal, beef, tomatoes, and green vegetables. Deficiency causes angular stomatitis (cheilosis, i.e., inflammation of the mucous membrane of the lips and angles of the mouth) and seborrhoea (excess secretion of oil from sebaceous glands) of nose and lips, not infrequently seen in elderly people on a poor diet.

P-P Factor. Pellagra-preventive factor or nicotinic acid (niacin). Sources: yeast, milk, pork, beef and offal. Deficiency causes pellagra.

Vitamin B₆. Pyridoxine or 'anti-dermatitis' factor. Sources: yeast, wheat-germ, milk and vegetables. Deficiency is probably related to pellagra syndrome.

Folic acid (formerly vitamin M). Sources: yeast, spinach, liver. Deficiency causes large-celled anaemia as seen in sprue, steatorrhoea, coeliac disease, and pregnancy. In pernicious anaemia it represents the 'extrinsic factor'. It relieves the anaemia but not the associated nerve-degeneration. 'Intrinsic factor' (B₁₂) is also required. Interaction takes place in the liver to produce restoration of satisfactory red-cell formation.

Vitamin B₁₂. Cyanocobalmin: 'intrinsic factor'. Derived from enzyme activity in the stomach. Deficiency causes pernicious anaemia. Interaction with folic acid controls red-cell formation.

Other vitamin B factors are of lesser human importance but their absence causes disease in laboratory animals, or retards bacterial growth. Pantothenic acid (B₃) has effects similar to those of riboflavin and is claimed to be of value in arthritis; biotin neutralizes avidin, a constituent of egg-albumen, which causes dermatitis, emaciation and death in rats fed exclusively on egg-white. Choline, inositol, and para-amino benzoic acid affect bacterial growth.

Vitamin C. Ascorbic acid or cevitamic acid. This is water-soluble and not produced or stored in the body; daily needs are increased by fever. Sources: blackcurrants, citrus fruits, other fruits, green vegetables. Deficiency increases capillary permeability and causes scurvy, and there is much speculation about its role in infections and other conditions. Large doses (1 g. or more per day) have been advocated for prevention and cure of common colds, and this theory has gained some popular experimental support.

Vitamin D. Calciferol or 'anti-rachitic' vitamin. This is fat-soluble or can be derived from a precursor, ergosterol, by ultra-violet irradiation, and this change can occur in exposed skin. Sources: fish-liver oils, animal fats, egg-yolk, summer milk. Vitamin D controls calcium absorption, and deficiency causes rickets. Children and pregnant and nursing mothers require supplies. It is stored by the body and excess can produce hypercalcaemia and kidney damage from calcium deposition.

Vitamin E. Alpha-tocopherol or 'anti-sterility' vitamin, which is fat-soluble. Sources: wheat-germ oil, cereals, egg-yolk, milk and green vegetables. Deficiency effects are not definite in man, but in animals its absence causes testicular degeneration, abortion, muscular and myocardial degeneration, thrombosis, and defects in bones, teeth and pelts. Because of this experimental evidence it is used clinically for treating habitual abortion, menopausal disorders, senile vulvo-vaginitis, male infertility, and peripheral vascular disease. Despite scepticism there is probably much still to learn about vitamin E function in man, and particularly about its role in fat digestion, which has implications related to cardio-vascular disease and ageing.

Vitamin K. Phytomenadione, which is water-soluble. Sources: green vegetables mainly, but it can be manufactured in the gut. It is concerned in blood-clotting and deficiency delays clotting and arrest of haemorrhage. Bile-salts are necessary for its absorption, and deficiency states are associated with obstructive jaundice, some types of haemorrhagic disease of the new-born, ulcerative colitis, and feverish wasting diseases, which increase demand and interfere with its manufacture in the gut. Although vitamin K is valuable in selected cases, its use in premature infants needs care to avoid destruction of red blood corpuscles. It is also used as an antidote for anticoagulant drugs and in the treatment of dental haemorrhage.

General. Most people on a normal diet get adequate quantities of vitamins although it may be necessary to supplement the diet at critical periods such as pregnancy, lactation, growth, and acute illness. Exceptions occur chiefly amongst alcoholics, food-faddists, psychotics, mental defectives, impoverished old persons living alone, and sometimes in institutions with bulk-cooking and poor menus. Deficiencies are usually of the B group and if one symptom is recognized it can be assumed that other B factors are minimal too. Those living alone are also prone to scurvy because they do not bother much about fruit and vegetables (see VITAMIN CONTENT OF FOOD).

During illness, deficiencies arise from defective absorption (see DIGESTION) particularly in chronic intestinal disease, after operations on the stomach, and in obstructive jaundice. Indefinite ill-health is often ascribed to vitamin deficiency but not often proven. Even rickets needs care in diagnosis and x-ray confirmation.

Complaints of mental origin may mimic vitamin deficiency, but a feature of deficiency diseases is that they are very rapidly relieved by doses of the appropriate vitamin. If this therapeutic test fails, it can be safely assumed that there is some other cause.

vocal cords. See VOICE.

voice. The larynx or voice box is a part of the respiratory system, situated at the front of the neck. It is a chamber made of cartilage containing the vocal cords, which are two bands of elastic tissue capable of being separated, drawn together, or tensed by muscular action. When the vocal cords vibrate in a current of air expelled from the chest, the result is the sound called voice, or phonation. Modification of this sound by changes in the size and shape of pharynx and mouth, and by positional alterations of tongue, teeth, and lips, is called articulation and produces vowels and consonants, linking to form words, or SPEECH.

Voice has loudness, pitch and timbre. Loudness is dependent on the force with which air is expelled, i.e., it varies with amplitude of vibration. Pitch is related to length and tension of the vocal cords, which is to say that it is determined by frequency of vibration. Length can be altered only slightly. Men normally have longer cords than women and children, and their voices are naturally deeper in the same way as the longer strings of a cello produce deeper notes than the short strings of a violin. Basically length determines range, but within individual range pitch is changed by altering tension, as with a violin string. Timbre depends on the presence and intensity of overtones, which are influenced by the shape and capacity of resonating chambers and these are provided by chest, trachea, pharynx, nose and mouth.

Individual voices are unique since no two persons have identical resonating chambers and articulators. Devices have therefore been made to record 'voice prints' and can be used to study emotional factors influencing speech.

In whispering, a current of air is articulated by the tongue, teeth and lips but the vocal cords are not brought into play.

epiglottis

trachea, below vocal cords

vocal cords

larynx wall

Vocal cords viewed from above

volvulus. Intestinal obstruction resulting from a twisting of the bowel. This is usually precipitated by some abnormality of the mesentery, the pleated membrane which supports the bowel; it may be congenitally lax, stretched by over-loaded bowel, or deformed and contracted by disease. Bands or adhesions from previous intra-abdominal disease can also lead to entanglement of the intestinal coils. The pelvic colon, caecum, and small intestine are most commonly involved. Large bowel volvuli tend to occur in older patients with chronic constipation. Those of the small bowel are commoner in children.

The condition is serious because twisting both obstructs the bowel and cuts off blood-supply, so that gangrene rapidly occurs. Volvulus is an emergency requiring immediate operation.

vomiting. Regurgitation of stomach contents, usually preceded by nausea and salivation. After a deep intake of breath, followed by closure of the glottis (the entrance of the main airway), the stomach is compressed by contraction of the abdominal muscles and descent of the diaphragm so that its contents are squeezed upwards through the oesophagus, pharynx, and mouth. In the projectile vomiting of pyloric stenosis the stomach plays a more active part, contracting forcibly while the pyloric sphincter at the lower opening of the stomach is closed. A similar mechanism produces the regurgitant vomiting of intestinal obstruction.

Vomiting is most usually a reflex act resulting from irritation in the gastro-intestinal tract, but is also produced by the effects of toxaemia on the vomiting centre in the brain, as in poisoning, kidney disease, uraemia, and other metabolic disturbances. Other causes are the psychic effects of anxiety, fear, or disgust, and the over-stimulation of receptors in the inner ear, producing sea-sickness.

Drugs producing vomiting are called emetics. Some, like tartar emetic and salt-solution, act by irritating the stomach. Others, such as apomorphine, act on the brain like toxins.

Cyclical vomiting, or repeated attacks in children occurring without obvious cause, are often ascribed to acidosis. Although ketone bodies may be demonstrable in the urine, acidosis is not a completely satisfactory diagnosis, and possibilities to be considered include migraine, faulty diet (particularly related to fat-intake), respiratory infection, and psychological causes such as school-phobia and other factors which have given rise to anxiety.

voyeurism. A condition in which a person becomes sexually excited or satisfied by looking at sexual acts or even simply at the genitals of the opposite sex. To a minor extent this is quite a normal phenomenon in part created by the conventional secrecy in which the naked body is held; and it is the main psychological source of the fairly common interest in pornographic pictures. In more extreme varieties it is classed as a PERVERSION and shows itself in the 'Peeping Tom' behaviour, in which the person with this particular sexual deviation attempts to gain satisfaction by looking through bedroom windows or key-holes.

vulva. Those parts of the female REPRODUCTIVE SYSTEM which lie on the body surface.

W

warts. Localized small growths formed on the skin. They vary in size and shape and are in most cases caused by a virus.

The commonest warts or verrucas occur in children and young adults, especially on the hands. In many cases they ultimately disappear without treatment. Unless they are very unsightly they are best left untreated.

Plantar warts, on the sole of the foot, quite common in persons frequenting swimming baths, are caused by a fungus and are infectious.

Large, soft, moist warts sometimes occur in the genital area and may cause itching. Treatment, where necessary, varies with the type of wart and its situation.

wasp sting. See BITES AND STINGS.

Wassermann test. The most widely used test for the diagnosis of syphilis. The test ascertains whether blood from the person examined forms antibodies which react with a substance that exists in normal blood. A negative reaction means the patient does not have syphilis, but there are two possible exceptions: (1) a patient who has received considerable antisyphilitic treatment may appear as negative, and (2) during the first two months after infection a patient may still be negative. A positive reaction is normally taken as proof of syphilis, but temporary false positives occur in glandular fever, yaws, leprosy and one or two other conditions.

Most workers nowadays prefer to use the Wassermann and another test simultaneously.

wasting. Shrinkage of muscles and loss of weight occur after prolonged inactivity, as in any disease necessitating bed-rest for a lengthy period. Nowadays, however, a policy of getting patients out of bed much earlier than in the past, together with physiotherapy treatment for persons still confined to bed, make wasting as a consequence of treatment rather uncommon.

More common is wasting as a symptom of advanced disease, e.g., as an indication of cancer or tuberculosis. In particular wasting in children may occur as a result of many conditions, from intestinal worms to worry over homework. In general any appreciable loss of weight or in a child failure to gain weight over a sizeable period warrants medical investigation.

water. At one time or another, water – inwardly or outwardly – has been declared a remedy for almost all human ills; and certainly it ranks next to air as the second most urgent of the body's needs. Water accounts for between 50 and 65 per cent of the weight of the body, being nearer the lower figure in the average middle-aged woman (with more fat) and nearer the higher figure in the average young man. Even under conditions when water intake is limited, the daily loss of water seldom falls below 1.7 litres (3 pints): a minimum of 600 ml. (1 pint) in urine without which the body cannot get rid of poisonous waste products; at least 300 ml. (0.5 pint) in evaporation from the lungs; a little in faeces; and anything from 600 ml. (1 pint) upwards in perspiration, with the quantity increasing rapidly if the external temperature is high or if the body is freely exercised. Without water intake we die in three or four days. The minimum intake for continued survival in a temperate climate is about 3 pints (1800 ml.) of which about 1 pint is provided in an average diet (e.g., potatoes are more than half water) and the rest has to be drunk as water, tea, milk, coffee or other liquid. For health an intake of 2 to 2.5 litres (4 to 5 pints) is desirable for the average adult; roughly one-quarter of this is included in food.

Dehydration, or water deficiency exhaustion, occurs in persons deprived of fresh-water intake (e.g., adrift at sea or lost in a desert) or in cases of extreme diarrhoea and vomiting (where the accompanying nausea may prevent drinking). The symptoms include thirst, dryness of mouth and tongue, fatigue and giddiness, and later delirium, coma and death. Minor deficiency through not drinking quite enough manifests itself in dry skin, pasty appearance and constipation.

Treatment includes rest in a cool room, a high fluid intake if the patient can take it, and intravenous injection of saline solution if the person is unconscious or unable to swallow. Salt depletion often occurs simultaneously with water depletion, and if this is suspected the drink given should contain roughly half a teaspoonful of salt for each tumbler of water.

Since children have smaller reserves of water than have adults, dehydration in children – especially young children – is not uncommon. It should be remembered that any disease involving perspiration or rise of temperature increases the loss of water and that the intake should rise correspondingly.

Insufficiency of water renders it difficult for the kidneys to excrete poisonous products in the urine; and an adequate supply of water helps to prevent constipation and its attendant evils. Whether water is consumed hot or cold and whether it is drunk as water, tea or some other liquid matter little, but it is useful to drink at least a tumblerful each morning and each evening, although elderly people often find that excessive night rising is avoided by taking the evening drink some hours before retiring to bed.

It is difficult to take too much water. In general excess is simply excreted, causing no symptoms except increased urination. Water intoxication – with restlessness, muscle twitching and confusion – is a rarity which occurs when the kidneys are defective and cannot cope with the excretory problem. Oedema (dropsy) is not caused by too much water but by retention of salt, with water retained in the tissues to keep the salt in dilute solution.

While water is necessary and is in general beneficial to health, dangers arise from water that is too hard, too soft, lacking in certain MINERAL SALTS and, worst of all, polluted.

Water which is too hard causes indigestion as well as causing 'furring' of kettles and other domestic utensils. Temporary hardness, created by the water containing a large amount of soluble bicarbonates, can be removed by boiling, but permanent hardness (mainly from chlorides and sulphates) is removable only by fairly elaborate processes. Until recent years it was thought that hard water was completely disadvantageous – necessitating the use of more soap and the frequent replacement of kettles and boilers as well as creating dyspepsia, especially in persons previously accustomed to softer water. Recently, however, it has been shown that soft water is associated with a higher incidence of degenerative heart diseases, and it would appear that one of the minerals in hard water has some protective effect against these conditions.

Soft water can absorb lead from pipes of that metal, and lead gradually accumulates in the body to a level that is poisonous. For many years the use of lead for cold water pipes has been discontinued, but some old lead pipes are still in use. Apart from the lead danger soft water is very pleasant for washing and quite pleasant for drinking. It is sometimes alleged to cause constipation, and it is more likely than hard water to be deficient in some of the mineral salts.

The presence or absence of such mineral salts as calcium, magnesium and iron does not really matter: we get our supplies from other sources and the amounts in even the hardest waters are minute. Deficiency of iodine, however, as in parts of Derbyshire and in the Calders area of Scotland, causes simple goitre which can be prevented by adding a small amount of iodine to table salt; and deficiency of fluorine in water is associated with greatly increased incidence of dental caries. See FLUORIDATION.

Where water is polluted it can cause a large number of diseases. See WATER-BORNE DISEASES. A water-borne outbreak is characterized by an explosive outburst, with many cases occurring almost simultaneously. When such an outbreak occurs the public should be warned to boil all water – including water to be used for washing their persons or their dishes – until such time as the source has been identified and the whole water supply adequately sterilized by chlorination.

For external use of water see HYDROTHERAPY.

water-borne diseases. The term is normally restricted to diseases caused by infective agents transferred by water. In such cases the water has been polluted or contaminated by faecal matter or urine – as in the use for drinking purposes of water that has already received the sewage of houses or factories, or water that has been contaminated by floods or heavy rains which carried transport or farm excreta to the drinking water, or water that has been polluted from labour camps or by holiday makers. Water-borne outbreaks in this sense tend to have an abrupt onset, rise very rapidly to a peak of cases, and decline rapidly. Cholera (mainly spread by water), typhoid (sometimes spread by water) and less frequently bacillary dysentery, poliomyelitis, infective hepatitis, Weil's disease (infectious leptospirosis), amoebic dysentery, hookworm infestation and filariasis are examples.

The halogen deficiency diseases (e.g., goitre from lack of iodine in the water and dental caries from deficiency of fluorine) and metallic poisonings (e.g., plumbism from absorption of lead by soft water) are not usually included under the heading of water-borne diseases; and somewhere on the borderline are gastro-intestinal upsets from consumption of bacteriologically satisfactory water containing excessive amounts of vegetable matter.

water brash. A regurgitation of clear acid fluid from the stomach to the mouth, sometimes accompanying HEART-BURN. The cause is excessive secretion of hydrochloric acid by the stomach and temporary loss of control over the sphincter muscle that normally closes the entrance to the stomach. Immediate treatment consists of a short rest and the swallowing of a mild alkali, such as milk of magnesia. If the condition recurs frequently medical investigation may be required.

watering eyes. Tears are normally secreted by the lacrymal duct on the outer side of the eye, then pass across the eye with cleansing effect and are discharged by a duct on the inner side of the eye to the nose. Watering of the eye may be the result of pressure on the nasal duct (as in some diseases of bone), blockage of the duct (which if left untreated may cause a painful abscess), laxity of the tissues of the lower eyelid (quite common in elderly women) or exposure to wind and cold. Treatment varies with the cause, but in general medical advice is necessary if the condition continues for more than two or three days.

wax. A normal secretion of the glands in the skin of the ear canal. In most people the amount of secretion of wax is balanced by extrusion of dried particles, but where secretion is extensive the wax may accumulate and obstruct the passage, causing temporary deafness. Such deafness is particularly liable to occur if water enters the ear during washing and causes the wax to swell.

The instillation of a few drops of hydrogen peroxide into the ears about once a week tends to prevent accumulation of wax. Where it has accumulated to the extent of impairing hearing the wax should be softened by introducing a few drops of sweet oil of almonds (or olive oil), leaving it in place for twenty-four hours with a plug of cotton wool to prevent its exit, and then the ear should be gently syringed to remove the softened wax. Gentleness is essential to prevent damage to the ear drum.

weal. See WHEAL.

weight. A solitary measurement of weight gives little or no information. If, after allowance has been made for height, bone structure and (in the case of a child) age, the weight of the child or adult is very appreciably above or below the average, the information merely confirms what the doctor or health visitor initiating the weighing already knew; and if the weight, after taking into account the factors already mentioned, is a little above or below the average, there are too many imponderables for the measurement to point to undernutrition or the beginning of a disease associated with loss of weight, or to suggest the start of obesity from hereditary, endocrine, dietetic or other causes. On the other hand, change of weight, as shown by measurements at intervals of two or three months, can provide important information.

The optimum weight for children is a very complex calculation, dependent not only on height but also on age. See DEVELOPMENT.

Tables of HEIGHT AND WEIGHT of adults are subject to the limitations that average is not 'optimum' and that a person of large frame will clearly have a higher optimum weight than a small-framed person of the same height. While allowance has to be made for the type of frame, insurance companies claim that expectation of life is greatest in persons a few pounds below the average for their height. Being under-weight is alleged to increase the chance of death slightly below the age of about 40 years but thereafter to carry no penalty unless it is so marked as to constitute actual malnutrition or to indicate existing disease. Being 10 per cent overweight substantially increases the chance of early death from about 35 years onwards, and to be 20 per cent overweight increases the

mortality risk by about one-third.

For estimation of weight change it is important that there should be little variation in the amount of clothing. In particular the weight of shoes varies considerably, and people carry variable weights in their pockets. Where circumstances necessitate a person being weighed fully dressed an appropriate allowance has to be made for the weight of the clothes.

weight, excessive. See OBESITY.

weight, loss of. An adult's loss of weight or a child's failure to gain weight as a result of starvation, privation, under-feeding or deliberate dieting (as in the treatment of obesity) is generally easily recognized. Other causes of weight loss include cancer, various diseases of the digestive tract, diabetes mellitus, some diseases of the kidneys, syphilis, tuberculosis, some diseases of the pancreas, a few nervous diseases (e.g., anorexia nervosa) and prolonged errors of diet.

Unless the cause is obvious, medical investigation is desirable; and in general the physician – looking first for common causes – should initially think of the possibility of cancer in the second half of life, of diabetes in persons aged 20 to 50, of tuberculosis in adolescents and young adults, and of gastro-enteritis or defective feeding in infants. Treatment varies with the cause but clearly includes the provision of adequate, appetizing, attractively served meals in circumstances conducive to their enjoyment.

Weil's disease. A serious infectious disease caused by a spirochaete (a corkscrew-like micro-organism) which frequently infects rats and mice and less often cats and dogs. The organism passes from the urine of infected animals to ponds, canals, rivers and swamps; man contracts the disease sometimes by eating food contaminated from such water but more often by the organism passing through the damaged skin of a person bathing or working in infected water. Weil's disease is also called leptospirosis, spirochaetal jaundice and swamp fever.

The incubation period varies from three to twenty-one days but is usually about ten days. The onset of the disease is characterized by high temperatures, rigors, severe headaches, muscle pains and gastro-intestinal disturbances with nausea and vomiting. Jaundice appears about the fifth day. Between 10 and 40 per cent of victims die, the proportion varying largely with the quality of nursing services available, and in the remainder convalescence begins after the second week.

Antibiotics – especially benzylpenicillin and streptomycin – are of some value, but recovery depends in large measure on good nursing and prevention of dehydration.

Weil's disease is in the main preventable. Preventive measures include the use of rubber boots and gloves by workers in water, swamps or mines liable to contamination by the urine of rodents; avoidance of bathing in dubious waters; protection of food from contamination from such water; drainage of swamps; and measures for rodent control.

wet dream. See NOCTURNAL EMISSION.

wheal. A small, swollen, burning or itching area of the skin. Weals or wheals (the spelling is variable) may result from sharp blows or from the stings of insects, nettles or jelly fish. See NETTLE RASH.

wheezing. Breathing with difficulty and with a whistling or grating sound. The symptom is found in bronchitis, asthma, some other diseases of the respiratory tract, and congestive heart failure. The cause is either a narrowing of the smaller bronchial tubes (as occurs in asthma) or their partial clogging with mucus (as happens in bronchitis). Treatment is that of the causal condition.

whiplash injury. An injury, not uncommon in car collisions, in which the head and neck are jerked violently backwards and then flick forward like a whiplash. In most cases there is considerable pain and stiffness of the neck. Painkillers will generally relieve the pain but a special supporting collar may be required for several weeks. Occasionally, however, a whiplash injury is so severe as to dislocate a vertebra. Car headrests reduce the frequency of the injury.

white leg. A term used for two different complications of childbirth.

1. Femoral thrombosis, the formation of a clot in any part of the femoral vein, usually appears about nine or ten days after delivery, and is characterized by high temperature, stiffness followed by pain in the leg and some swelling of the affected limb. The vein is tender to the touch and can be felt as a hard line running down the leg. Treatment consists of rest in bed, immobilization of the limb by sandbags on each side, hot boracic fomentations with some lead and opium added, and mild sedatives. The pain usually subsides in a few days and the swelling disappears in two or three weeks.

2. Phlegmasia alba dolens, now rare, is essentially a blockage of the lymphatic vessels at the root of the thigh, with the affected leg becoming greatly swollen, and the skin white and glossy. Treatment is as for femoral thrombosis but the condition may last for several months and in some cases the leg remains permanently swollen.

Both conditions are said to be more common in anaemic women, but the exact causes are still disputed.

whitlow. See HAND.

whooping cough. An acute infection (medically known as pertussis), found mostly in children under the age of 6 years but liable to occur at any age, involving the trachea and bronchi, and characterized by a paroxysmal cough which ends with a crowing, inspiratory 'whoop'. It is caused by *Haemophilus pertussis*, which is transmitted by droplet infection, and the infectivity is greatest during the early catarrhal stage before the typical cough has appeared. The incubation period is seven to ten days.

The initial manifestations, raised temperature and short dry cough, are those of almost any respiratory infection; but in a few days the characteristic paroxysmal cough and whoop appear, and a paroxysm is often followed by vomiting. There is no specific treatment. For the first few days the patient is best kept in bed and given a largely fluid diet; and after he is allowed up he should be isolated from unimmunized children who have not had the disease. Infectivity ends – and the patient may be allowed to associate with susceptible persons – in about three weeks, even though the cough and whoop continue for another fortnight or so.

Occasional serious complications include broncho-pneumonia, infection of the middle ear, convulsions, and hernia.

The disease was formerly very common. For instance, in 1950 there were 157,000 notifications of whooping cough in England and Wales, and of these roughly 1 in every 400 died, most of the deaths being in children under 2 years of age. Antibiotics, increasingly employed in the 1950s and 1960s, do not cure the disease but reduce some of the complications, and so reduce the number of deaths, but not the number of cases.

The big advances in the control of whooping cough were the production of a vaccine (extensively used since the middle 1950s), the improvement of that vaccine and the persuasion of the public to accept vaccination. By 1971 notifications in England and Wales numbered 15,933, and of these, 23 – or roughly 1 in every 700 – died. In extremely rare cases (e.g., a child suffering from convulsions or with a family history of epilepsy) the vaccine is not advisable because of a very remote chance of brain damage, but to omit vaccination in a child not suffering from such conditions is simply needlessly to run the risk of a serious and occasionally fatal disease.

A vaccine which confers a high degree of immunity is normally combined with the vaccines employed for protection against diphtheria and tetanus. For a normally healthy baby such triple vaccination should be started by the age of 6 months.

Widal test. A blood test for diagnosing typhoid fever. The test is useful but has two limitations: firstly, that a positive reaction does not usually appear until about the seventh day of the illness, so that a provisional decision to treat a case as typhoid (or to exclude typhoid from the diagnosis) has to be made in advance of the test; and secondly, that a person who is not suffering from typhoid but has had TAB vaccination within recent months may give a slightly positive reaction.

windpipe. See TRACHEA.

womb. The common name for the UTERUS.

women, diseases of. With obvious exceptions, such as diseases of the prostate in men and of the uterus in women, men and women are subject to the same ailments and disabilities, and greater frequency of a condition in one or other sex sometimes provides a clue to causation.

The term 'diseases of women' is, however, normally restricted to illnesses peculiar to women. An alternative term is gynaecological diseases. Examples of such diseases are: cancer, fibroid, displacement or inflammation of the uterus; inflammation, tumour or cyst of the ovaries; salpingitis and other diseases of the uterine tubes; inflammation of the vagina; and disorders of menstruation. While the symptoms vary with the particular disease, common symptoms of gynaecological conditions include – pain below the level of the umbilicus, pain associated with menstruation, pain associated with performance of the sexual act, absence of menstruation, excessive blood loss during menstruation, haemorrhage between menstrual periods, and vaginal discharge. Accurate diagnosis is, of course, a necessary preliminary to treatment.

The branch of medicine specializing in the study of diseases of women is known as gynaecology.

word blindness. A rather vague term for a condition in which, as a result of disease or injury of the speech area of the cerebral cortex or more frequently as a result of disease or injury of the nerve tracts communicating with that area, a person becomes unable to associate meanings with words. According to the nature of the damage he may on the one hand be able to speak coherently but be unable to appreciate the meaning of written words even though he can spell out the letters composing the words, or he may on the other hand also lose all appreciation of words even as spoken by himself, so that his speech becomes totally unintelligible.

Where word blindness occurs in a previously normal adult the diagnosis is obvious. Where it is suspected in a young child the condition of DYSLEXIA should not be regarded as confirmed until defects of sight, hearing and general intelligence have been eliminated. The treatment of genuine word blindness is not easy but most cases ultimately recover.

World Health Organization. An international organization, of which virtually all countries are members. Its aims are (1) to transmit epidemiological information rapidly from country to country, (2) to provide medical and nursing help at the request of a government, and (3) through expert committees, to provide the best advice on improvement of health and reduction of disease. Its biggest successes to date have been the elimination of smallpox and the reduction of malaria.

worms. A rather ill-defined division of the animal kingdom containing creatures that do not possess appendages. Many species are parasites in the bodies of man and animals, and some of these species cause diseases.

Parasitic ROUND WORMS include the large *Ascaris lumbricoides*, sometimes as long as 40 cm. (16 in.), the whip worm (about 5 cm., or 2 in., long) and the tiny but common THREADWORM (*Oxyuris vermicularis*) which is a frequent source of anal irritation in children. Parasitic flat worms include the pork and beef TAPEWORMS (*Taenia solium* and *T. saginata*) and the FLUKES responsible for schistosomiasis.

Many worms are transmitted through the eating or drinking of material that contains their eggs, but some diseases, such as FILARIASIS, are passed to man through the bites of blood-sucking insects. Effective treatments for most worm infestations are now available. See VERMIFUGE.

wound. Any breach of the skin with damage to underlying tissues. Wounds are normally classified thus:

1. Clean-cut or incised wounds, caused by a sharp-edged instrument. The edges are definite, and bleeding is generally abundant.

2. Bruised or contused wounds, caused by a blunt instrument. Bleeding is usually scanty or even absent.

3. Punctured wounds or stabs, caused by a pointed instrument. Bleeding may be abundant. If the stab is deep there is danger of involvement of internal organs and also danger of sepsis from the introduction of germs.

4. Torn or lacerated wounds caused by animal bites or contact with moving machinery. The edges are ragged and bleeding is usually scanty.

The classification is not completely satisfactory. For instance, a bullet wound may well be both punctured and lacerated. More important than the type of wound is whether it is clean or potentially septic through introduction of germs.

The main points in the treatment of a wound are: (1) Stop the bleeding if serious: see HAEMORRHAGE. (2) With thoroughly cleaned hands (preferably washed in water containing an antiseptic) cleanse the wound with a mild antiseptic solution or (failing that) water that has been boiled, and apply a sterile dressing, and cover the dressing with a bandage. (3) Keep the part at rest – with a sling or splint if necessary. (4) Treat symptoms of SHOCK. (5) If the wound may have been contaminated by garden or field soil or stable refuse, contact a doctor swiftly so that the patient may receive anti-tetanic serum. See also First Aid section at the end of the book.

wrinkles. Ridges or folds, especially of the skin of the face, produced through decrease of the natural elasticity of the skin as age advances. The natural process of development of wrinkles is accelerated by prolonged worry, by malnutrition, by excessive use of tea, coffee, alcohol or tobacco, and by lack of fresh air and exercise. There is no reliable cure. Operations to remove wrinkles tend to produce small scars instead of folds, and injection of material under the skin is liable to create deformity. Suitable lotions can often render wrinkles less visible.

wrist. The region between the forearm and the hand. The wrist joint is formed by the lower ends of the radius and ulna and the eight carpal bones. The joint has only fairly moderate sideways movement but very extensive upwards and downwards movement. Both because of the wide range of movement and because a person who falls forward tends to put out his arm and take the strain on his outstretched hand, dislocations and sprains of the wrist are very common. Fracture is also not uncommon (COLLES' FRACTURE). Stiffness of the wrist is sometimes caused by arthritis.

Wrist-drop. In this condition the hand droops at the wrist and there is difficulty in extending the wrist. Probably the commonest type is crutch palsy, where pressure of an inadequately padded crutch in the elbow damages the large nerve of the arm. A similar but more temporary effect is sometimes observed when a person sleeps with the head resting on the upper arm. Other causes include chill and the neuritis created by lead, arsenic or, rarely, alcohol. Forms due to pressure on the nerve or to chill respond to rest, with, if they appear to be lasting too long, the addition of massage or electrical treatment. Where wrist-drop is a result of neuritis induced by poisoning, the source of the poison must, of course, be identified and removed.

writer's cramp. A disease of gradual onset produced by habitual repetitive use of one set of muscles and characterized by pain, weakness and spasm of the muscles concerned. The condition occurs most commonly in manual writers – hence the name – but is also found in typists, seamstresses, musicians and indeed in any occupation demanding precise, finely co-ordinated movements of a set of small muscles, a fact which gives rise to its alternative name of occupational palsy. In a typical case the movements of the pen become more difficult and the writing irregular, the pen is grasped harder and harder, the writing becomes heavier, the hand feels heavy and tired, and ultimately cramp develops almost as soon as writing is started.

Preventive measures include teaching less constricted methods of manipulation, encouragement of the use of either hand, avoidance of excessive hours at the particular work and adoption of a policy of gradualness after any appreciable absence. Treatment includes a period of rest, removal of adverse environmental factors, attention to general health and attempts to remove tensions and anxieties. While treatment is completely successful in some cases, in many cases change of occupation is essential, and in a minority occupational palsy occurs also in the new occupation.

wry neck. A condition, technically called torticollis, in which the head is permanently twisted to one side.

1. Wry-neck in infants or young children is often called congenital torticollis but it is seldom truly congenital in the sense of being inherited or resulting from intra-uterine influences. Most commonly it follows injury to one of the sterno-mastoid muscles (which run from base of neck to base of skull) caused during childbirth, especially in breech births. The muscle-fibres are accidentally torn; a swelling filled with blood forms and fibrous tissue grows into it; the relatively inert fibrous tissue restricts muscle growth; and so the muscle becomes shorter than the one on the opposite side of the neck and produces the typical deformity.

2. The condition of ocular torticollis is not usually as marked as the congenital variety and is caused by a weakness or paralysis of one of the muscles controlling the position of the eyes. The head is twisted into the abnormal position in an attempt to keep the eyes parallel and prevent a squint. In this case the sterno-mastoid muscle is not defective and treatment usually involves eye surgery.

3. Spasmodic torticollis, occurring mostly in the middle-aged and more in women than in men, is a condition of doubtful cause. Some cases appear to be of rheumatic origin while others may be due to psychological factors. There is fairly general agreement that no form of surgery is useful and that treatment should start with a period of rest in bed, but there is considerable argument about the value of other forms of treatment – a plain indication that no one form of therapy benefits the majority of patients.

XYZ

xerophthalmia. Dryness and ultimately thickening and opacity of the front of the eye with consequent effect on vision. The condition, rare in highly developed countries, is produced by prolonged deficiency of vitamin A.

x-rays. Electromagnetic radiation consisting of radiated energy of very short wavelength (appreciably shorter than even that of ultra-violet rays) which can penetrate soft tissues · and can register on photographic film. X-rays discovered in 1895.

Radiological diagnosis. Dense, heavy substances (e.g., bone and various metals) are opaque to x-rays and therefore cast dark shadows, while air and soft tissues are transparent to these rays and so cast no shadows or very light shadows. Because dense substances cast heavy shadows x-rays have obvious value for the detection and exact localization of fractures and of such foreign bodies as bullets and needles. Since the lungs, mainly filled with air, cast very little shadow x-rays can be used to identify abnormalities such as the consolidation of pneumonia or the presence of tuberculosis or cancer in the lung.

Soft tissues which would normally cast little shadow can be rendered temporarily opaque by instillation of a suitable heavy substance: for instance, to confirm the presence or absence of an ulcer the stomach and duodenum can be photographed after the patient has taken a meal containing an adequate amount of barium or bismuth, and the kidney and urinary system can be studied after the injection or swallowing of a compound containing iodine. Conversely, the brain can be studied by injecting air into the ventricles which then show up as white shadows.

In recent decades radiography has become a supremely important diagnostic tool in many branches of medicine and surgery.

Preventive applications. Where an infectious disease is spread largely by mild cases almost without symptoms (e.g., the mild tuberculosis formerly common in the elderly) the development of a system of rapid and inexpensive x-ray photography – mass miniature radiography – provides a useful method of identifying and bringing under treatment persons who may be transmitting the disease. Similarly, where a person's occupation would render him a danger to others if infectious (as in the case of a health visitor, school teacher, midwife or nurse) radiological examination can identify such conditions as early tuberculosis. Again, when tuberculosis has become rare in a country, radiological investigation may be useful in the case of immigrants arriving from a country in which the disease is still widespread.

Therapy with x-rays. See RADIOTHERAPY.

Dangers of x-rays. Sufficiently large doses of radiation destroy all forms of life; and even fairly moderate doses can damage the blood-forming tissues and the sex glands. For patients receiving treatment not only is the dosage carefully regulated but also the rays are directed only to the particular tissues for which they are required. In other words, the patient's blood-forming tissues and sex glands are not at risk. Much care, however, is needed on the part of the operator, who is in constant danger of exposure to radiation. Modern forms of apparatus minimize that risk, but in addition the working hours of radiologists and radiographers are restricted, and they are periodically examined for early indications – such as anaemia – of excessive exposure to x-rays.

yawning. An involuntary reflex action in which the mouth is opened and the breath slowly exhaled. The typical morning yawn is essentially Nature's attempt to stimulate blood circulation and respiration. Yawning during a conversation or while listening to a formal address may imply sleepiness or boredom but more frequently occurs in persons whose blood pressures are low and who normally rely on movement to help the circulation of the blood.

Frequent yawning is usually a sign of insufficient sleep or inadequate exercise.

yaws. An infectious disease – common in South America, the West Indies and parts of Asia and Africa – characterized by lesions in the skin and bones. It is caused by a spirochaete (*Treponema pertenuae*) which closely resembles that of syphilis, but infection is usually transmitted not venereally but by direct contact or on the feet of flies, the contact being generally through abrasions in the skin. The incubation period is three to six weeks.

The primary lesion is a nodule, most often found on the legs or buttocks. Crops of secondary lesions occur, months or even years apart, on any portion of the skin, each batch of nodules tending in the main to subside painlessly but with a nodule occasionally giving rise to an ulcer. Secondary lesions also occur in bones where they cause pain, tenderness and deformity. Sometimes tertiary lesions occur in the form of indolent ulcers and nodules on the skull and breast-bone.

The disease responds quickly to

treatment with penicillin and is now becoming rare.

yeast. A fungus which ferments sugar and is used in the brewing of beer, the distilling of spirits, the making of wine and the raising of bread. Yeast contains large amounts of the various B vitamins and so tablets of dried yeast are sometimes used in disorders due to deficiency of one or more of these vitamins.

yellow fever. An acute and often fatal infectious disease, caused by a virus and transmitted by the bite of a female mosquito (*Aedes egypti*) which breeds in small quantities of water. The incubation period is three to ten days and the disease occurs in two distinct forms. The mild form, found mostly in persons normally resident in areas in which the disease is endemic, is an influenza-like illness characterized by fever, severe headache, nausea and vomiting, with recovery usual in about four days. The severe form has an acute onset with high fever, fast pulse, chills and rigors, severe headache, backache and limb pains, followed by nausea and vomiting, with the vomit sometimes black as a result of the presence of altered blood; there is often an apparent remission about the fourth day with the pulse rate decreasing more than in proportion to the fall of temperature, and then a second phase of high fever, severe vomiting, jaundice, and bleeding from mucous membranes. The fatality rate in the severe form is about 80 per cent, with death usually occurring on the seventh or eighth day. If the patient survives, convalescence begins about the twelfth day.

There is no specific treatment. Sulphonamides and antibiotics are not helpful. Skilled nursing is probably the most important factor in improving the chance of recovery. Small, frequent glucose drinks are useful, and foods of high protein content are said to help if the patient can swallow them; intravenous saline is required if the patient is dehydrated and vitamin K is sometimes helpful.

Three major measures of prevention are as follows: (1) In areas where the disease is endemic, destruction of mosquitoes and especially of their breeding grounds, e.g., drainage of swamps. (2) Strict anti-mosquito control of all aircraft travelling from an infected area to an area in which the mosquitoes could breed, and vaccination of all travellers on such aircraft. (3) Vaccination of persons travelling to infected areas; such vaccination gives a powerful immunity which develops in ten days and lasts for at least six years, but in Britain vaccination is not advocated for children under the age of 9 months.

zinc protamine insulin. A suspension of insulin hydrochloride combined with protamine and zinc. It is slowly liberated and absorbed from the site of injection. A diabetic patient who is unsuitable for modern oral preparations might require three injections of ordinary soluble insulin daily, whereas with a mixture of ordinary soluble insulin and zinc protamine insulin a single daily injection will usually suffice – the soluble insulin beginning to act almost at once and its effect starting to fade after four or five hours, and the protamine zinc insulin beginning to act in about four hours and continuing to do so for at least a further twelve hours, so that the patient has at worst only a few hours each day of excess blood sugar.

zoonosis. A collective term for infections transmitted to human beings from infected animals. Examples are anthrax, plague, rabies, psittacosis, typhus, undulant fever (brucellosis), the bovine type of tuberculosis and many varieties of worm infestation. Measures of prevention vary with the disease but clearly involve the collaboration of medical and veterinary experts. The virtual eradication of the bovine variety of tuberculosis and the progress towards eradication of undulant fever in several developed countries are instances of the success of that collaboration.

zygoma. The arch of bone which forms the prominence of the cheek, to which is attached the masseter muscle of mastication. One of the minor variations in mankind is that the arch is higher in some races than in others.

zygote. The fertilized ovum. See REPRODUCTION.

FIRST AID

People do not usually have heart-attacks or accidents involving serious bleeding or poisoning, gassing or apparent drowning immediately outside a hospital gate or in close proximity to a doctor or nurse. Again and again in accidents and sudden illnesses the victims endure very considerable needless pain and suffering, and some of them needlessly die, simply because the persons present do not have the knowledge to undertake emergency resuscitation, to control bleeding, to cope with poisoning or to treat shock.

It is therefore important that every intelligent adult should acquire a reasonable working knowledge of first aid – the efficient rendering of immediate assistance to a person who has suddenly become ill as a result of disease or accident – because that intelligent adult may well be the only person available to offer prompt help in an emergency. Thirty hours of theoretical and practical instruction (three hours a week for as short a period as ten weeks) may easily make the difference between the death and the life of a relative or a friend in a subsequent emergency.

Yet it is almost equally important to emphasise that a person who has gained a working knowledge of first aid should not attempt to do too much. Where the illness or accident has occurred far from available skilled help the efforts of the first-aider may easily be life-saving; but where such skilled help is available within minutes the first-aider should content himself with doing what is immediately necessary and should appreciate that, while he has spent thirty or forty hours in learning to cope, the doctor or nurse has had years of full-time professional preparation.

Commonsense judgment is always required. To get the airways clear, to attempt mouth-to-mouth resuscitation if breathing has stopped, to control serious bleeding, to begin heart massage if the heart has stopped, and to treat poisoning if the source is known are always useful and sometimes life-saving; but to try to act as a professional by using treatment that goes beyond the limits of first aid and to delay the summoning of skilled help means that the first-aider is accepting a responsibility that he is wholly untrained to bear. In other words, there is a considerable difference between the type and extent of first aid usefully attempted in accident or illness on a lonely mountain and the type and extent in a situation where an ambulance or a doctor may be expected to arrive within a few minutes.

There are many excellent small books on first aid, such as those published by the British Red Cross and the St. John's and St. Andrew's Ambulance Associations, but neither these books nor the even briefer guide below are a substitute for practical training. Information about courses can be obtained from any local branch of an ambulance association or from the nearest ambulance station.

The short outline that follows begins with a few general principles and then discusses individual matters, such as the stopping of bleeding and the restoration of breathing. Clearly the seven general points and their order of priority have to be considered in the light of the particular situation.

Some general principles

1. Keep cool. A quiet, calm demeanour allays excitement and inspires the patient with confidence if he is conscious.

2. Protect the patient from obvious physical dangers. In some cases, e.g., fire or serious gas leak, this may involve moving him.

3.   Clear a space, both to give the victim air and to give yourself room for action.

4.   Unless the injury appears trivial send for a doctor with such information as is immediately available, not forgetting the exact place at which the patient is. Information such as 'Probable fracture of femur following bicycle accident' or 'unconscious and said to be diabetic' may help a doctor to assess priorities between two urgent calls and may also help him to decide what apparatus and instruments to bring.

5.   Quickly observe both the surroundings and the patient. A weapon or a bottle that contained poison or alcohol can disappear easily but its existence may be important both for early diagnosis and for criminal proceedings. Also note the victim's posture, position, expression and position of injuries.

6.   Give immediate first aid.
There are several things which you should check and act on straight away.
   Airways. Check that the air-passage is open so that the patient can breathe. Clear the mouth and nostrils of any blood or vomited material, and if vomiting or bleeding in mouth or nose is continuing turn the patient's head to the side so that the material can leak out without obstructing breathing. Loosen tight collar, belt or corset.
   Bleeding. Keep the patient's head low and if practicable raise the bleeding part. If there is appreciable bleeding stop it by direct pressure of the fingers on the wound. Types of bleeding are considered later, but essentially in a case of a smooth trickle of purplish blood there may be time to get a sterile dressing if available or even a clean handkerchief, or to wash dirty fingers; but where bright red blood is spurting out there is not time for such measures.
   Breathing. If the patient is not breathing attempt mouth-to-mouth or mouth-to-nose resuscitation; but in a case of apparent drowning another form of artificial respiration may be better.
   Circulation. If the pulse cannot be felt (at the wrist or just in front of the ear) start massage of the heart.
   Fainting. Keep the head low and make sure that the air-passages are clear.
   Fractures. Run your hand gently along the limbs to detect a possible fracture. If there is one, avoid all rough movement and if possible immobilise the fracture before moving the patient at all. An immediate commonsense decision must be made between avoiding worsening of the fracture and protecting the patient: for instance in a burning building or a car likely to go on fire the person must be moved at all costs.
   Shock. Virtually every serious injury produces a considerable amount of shock. Unless there is some reason for moving the patient or altering his position, leave him lying recumbent but protect him from cold by covering him with a blanket or coat. If he is unconscious or has an abdominal injury, give nothing by mouth. If he is conscious and collapsed and has no apparent injury of the digestive tract, let him sip a cup of hot tea or coffee. Do not give alcohol, because while it is helpful in some emergencies it is definitely harmful in others. Keep the patient comfortably warm. Sudden serious illness or injury is terrifying to the victim, so, if he is conscious, remember the importance of reassurance: the patient may well think he is about to die and may be vastly helped by such remarks as 'I think you have had a mild heart attack but are already beginning to recover. Just try to rest easy until the doctor arrives'.

7.   Examine the patient and give less immediate first aid. If he is conscious he may be able to supply useful information, and in some cases of serious disease or injury he may lapse into unconsciousness before skilled help arrives. If a limb is injured, remove the clothing from the uninjured side first and then if necessary rip down the seam on the injured

side; and in re-applying the clothing for warmth replace it first on the injured side. If he is unconscious, look for wounds, swellings or depressions of the skull; and notice whether the pupils are contracted or dilated, whether they are equal in size and whether they contract on the admission of light. If the doctor has not yet arrived, examine the jaw, ribs and spine, looking for irregularities, grating sound on touch, and tender spots; and look generally for wounds of the body.

Bright red spurting blood means bleeding from an artery and its prompt arrest is essential. Darker, smoothly flowing blood means haemorrhage from a vein and is usually much easier to stop. Pallor, rapidity of pulse, gasping or sighing respirations, cold and clammy skin and other signs of severe collapse and shock suggest haemorrhage – internal bleeding if no blood is visible. Fracture is suggested by loss of function, tenderness, unnatural mobility of the part, swelling and deformity. Unconsciousness with flushed, congested face, may be due to cerebral haemorrhage (stroke), a specific fever, or drunkenness. Powerlessness of the arm and leg on the same side, in the absence of fractures, suggests cerebral haemorrhage or cerebral thrombosis. Unconsciousness with dilated pupils may mean belladonna (nightshade) poisoning or pressure on the brain or – if the pupils react to light – severe shock. Contracted pupils may be due to morphia poisoning but have some other possible causes. Bleeding from the ear or nose after a head injury generally means a fractured skull. The coughing up of bright red frothy blood suggests lung injury or lung disease, while the vomiting of dark blood suggests damage to the stomach.

Sudden vomiting may be the result of dietetic indiscretion, food poisoning, excess alcohol, gastric ulcer, abdominal obstruction, some diseases of the kidneys and some diseases of the brain. Also it may follow a blow on the abdomen; it may be a symptom of pregnancy; and in a child it may herald the onset of a fever, e.g., scarlet fever or measles.

Fainting may be caused by terror, emotional shock of any nature, severe pain, external bleeding, internal bleeding, extreme heat, physical or mental exhaustion, or various diseases that interfere with the blood supply to the brain.

Severe pain in the region of the heart and stomach is likely to be related to the stomach in persons under 40 years and likely to be related to the heart in persons above the age of 50. Severe pain on the right side of the lower abdomen may well be appendicitis.

Procedures

The first-aider should remember that detailed diagnosis is not his function. His function is to give such immediate aid as will be helpful (and sometimes life-saving) and to supply such information as will facilitate diagnosis and treatment.

Bleeding. The three types of external bleeding are described under HAEMORRHAGE but are here summarized. Capillary bleeding is a steady reddish ooze from cut tissues; venous bleeding is a steady purple stream; and arterial bleeding is bright red and spurting. Although bleeding is a very common emergency and one which calls for prompt and effective treatment, it is really only arterial haemorrhage which presents the first-aider with much difficulty.

For any appreciable bleeding it is useful to keep the head low (to allow adequate flow of blood to the brain) and to raise the affected part. For capillary or venous haemorrhage a dressing and a cotton-wool pad secured by a firm bandage will generally achieve all that is required. Ruptured varicose veins of the leg, however, will bleed heavily as long as the patient is upright: in that case it is essential to get the patient to lie down and to raise the leg, so as to reverse the pressure of blood.

When a large artery is severed a great deal of blood escapes in a short time, and even a small artery can soon pump out the litre or so of blood whose loss can endanger life. The obvious immediate method of controlling arterial bleeding is by direct firm pressure on the wound (or on the wound and on the side of it nearer to the heart). Fingers are available for this pressure, and there is no time to wash them or to secure a sterile dressing to place between the fingers and the wound. Certainly dirty fingers can cause infection, but infections can be treated; whereas if the bleeding is not stopped quickly the patient will die.

As soon as is reasonably practicable the fingers can be replaced by a sterile dressing and pad above the dressing, secured by a firm bandage. If the bleeding does not stop, the dressing and pad should be reinforced by towels or other soft material, again secured by a firm bandage.

An alternative method for wounds in the region of the groin, armpit, knee or elbow is forced flexion. A pad is placed in the bend of the joint and the joint is then fully bent and secured in the bent position by a firm bandage.

Many manuals on first aid stress the importance of pressure points at which (nearer the heart than the wound) an artery can be compressed against an underlying bone. Some of these pressure points are described and illustrated below:

Scalp area. The temporal artery can be compressed just in front of the ear opening and the occipital artery about 2 cm behind the ear.

Face. The facial artery can be compressed where it crosses the border of the lower jaw about 2 to 3 cm in front of the angle of the jaw.

Head and neck. The common carotid artery can be reached in the neck alongside the windpipe and about 3 cm above the shoulder blade, but its compression requires considerable expertise.

Arm. The brachial artery can be compressed against the shaft of the humerus about half way down the upper arm, and the axillary artery can (less easily) be pressed against the head of the humerus at the top of the armpit.

Leg. With great pressure usually involving two hands the femoral artery can be pressed against the brim of the pelvis near the middle of the groin.

These pressure points have been mentioned because they are emphasised in most books on first aid. They can be useful to a person who has received considerable training in first aid; but a person with little knowledge of first aid is more likely to stop arterial bleeding by firm pressure on the wound, followed by a firm pad and bandage, than by groping for a pressure point.

A TOURNIQUET is suitable only for use on the arms and legs and then only if other methods fail. It may be improvised from a narrow folded triangular bandage or any similar strip of material, tied round the limb and twisted by any form of short rod. It has to be placed between the wound and the heart, tightened only enough to control the bleeding and not left on continuously for more than 25 to 30 minutes at a time.

In arterial bleeding to stop or reduce the bleeding is a matter of life and death. It is also important to send for medical help as quickly as possible, and to be alert for – and ready to treat – stopping of the heart (see p. 434) and signs of severe shock (see p. 431).
See also BANDAGES AND BANDAGING.

Burns and scalds. Irrespective of whether these are caused by fire, electricity, boiling liquids or chemicals, the essentials of treatment are to separate the casualty from the danger, to bathe the damaged part freely in cold water in order to reduce pain and heat, and thereafter to apply a sterile non-adherent dressing and to cover the dressing with available soft materials, such as cotton-wool and a bandage. (See BANDAGES AND BANDAGING.)

The application of greasy substances (such as butter) was at one time recommended, but these substances probably do more harm than good. Similarly cold tea, because of its tannic acid content, was much advocated but it is doubtful whether it is more useful than plentiful cold water.

In severe burns and scalds dangers to be watched for – and treated if they arise – include stopping of breathing, stopping of the heart and serious shock (see p. 433, 434, 431).
See also BURNS AND SCALDS for more information.

Choking. The various causes of choking are indicated in the article on that subject. Where choking is due to a foreign body (e.g., a lump of food) in the throat it is often possible to remove the object with the fingers.

Failing this, the object may be dislodged by a couple of hard slaps on the upper part of the back between the shoulders. Clearly the dislodging will be easier if the object can simply fall out. So a young child before the slaps can be held up by the legs with the head downwards, and an older child can be placed over an adult's knee with, again, the head downwards.

After the object is removed it is essential to ensure that the airway is clear, so that the person can breathe. If breathing has actually stopped, artificial respiration will be required (see p. 433).

Drowning accidents. It is useful to remember as a preliminary that every child should be taught not only to swim but also to float: a person who is able to float and to tread water is seldom in immediate danger. (See also DROWNING.)

Rescuing the person. Anything that floats (e.g., a branch of a tree) can be thrown to the victim to make it easier for him to float, and similarly anything that floats (e.g., a pair of trousers knotted at the ankles and filling with air as the rescuer enters the water) will give the rescuer additional buoyancy.

To make a life-line from the shore or bank a rope or belt or large towel is useful, and it can be thrown more accurately if the end is weighted with a shoe or a small piece of wood (but not with something so heavy that it may cause injury to the person in difficulty). The 'human chain' method of rescue, useful in strong currents, involves several rescuers facing opposite directions, clasping hands wrist to wrist and stretching from shore to victim. It is important that the rescuer on the shore is a strong person and is firmly stationed on solid ground.

A swimmer proposing to effect a rescue should use his strength reasonably. There is little point in reaching the drowning person a couple of seconds earlier than would have normally been anticipated if, as a result of his burst of speed, the swimmer lacks the strength to tow the victim to land.

Treatment of the apparently drowned. If the person has stopped breathing the first essential is to make an attempt to expel water from the lungs by placing the patient face downwards, raising the lower part of his body and allowing water to run out through the mouth and nose. Thereafter artificial respiration has to be started. The rhythmical compression of the chest according to Schafer's method is perhaps the most desirable here: it also helps to expel water and leaves the drowned person in the best position for getting rid of the water; see p. 434.

The mouth-to-mouth (kiss of life) method is very effective once the air passages are reasonably clear but cannot be expected to succeed with a seriously waterlogged patient.

If the ordinary respiration does not restart, artificial respiration should be continued for half an hour before hope of recovery is abandoned.

When the patient is breathing, either never having stopped or having restarted in response to artificial respiration, it has to be realised that he may well be in a condition of shock, and shock has to be treated (see p. 431).

Electric shock. If the victim is still in contact with a high tension wire it is unwise to attempt to rescue him. However callous it may seem the best action is to notify an expert and await his arrival.

If the victim is still in contact with ordinary domestic electric current, disconnect it by turning off the appropriate switch or jerking the plug from its socket, or, if both of these are impossible, try to push the victim away from the wire using insulating material, e.g., a dry walking stick. Do not attempt to cut live wires.

After the victim is no longer in contact with the wire, treat as for burns, and if breathing has stopped apply artificial respiration (see p. 431).

Fractures. Often the victim, if conscious, will be able to tell you that he heard or felt the bone snap and that he now has pain and tenderness at the site of the break and cannot move the limb. In any case the limb looks deformed in shape and often appears shorter than the opposite limb, and in the case of fracture of a flat bone (e.g., in the skull) there may be either a depression or an elevation. While abnormal mobility and a grating sensation when the broken ends are moved against each other are commonly stated as additional evidence of fracture, the first aid worker is strongly advised not to look for these signs: excessive examination can easily convert a simple break into a compound fracture.

Where a fracture is suspected the immediate aims should be (1) to prevent further damage by rough handling or needless movement, (2) to treat shock (see p. 431) which is often considerable, and (3) to secure prompt medical attention. In general the patient should not be moved unless he is in a position of danger; and if it is necessary to move him the injured limb should first be fixed in as good a position as the circumstances allow. For this purpose a splint should be improvised out of any available suitable material, e.g., walking sticks, umbrellas or boards. A splint should be rigid enough to immobilize the broken bone, long enough to reach from beyond the joint above the break to beyond the joint below it, and preferably wider than the limb. If practicable the splint should be padded with cotton-wool or similar material. It should be firmly fastened by bandages or strips of clothing (e.g., neckties or braces) and should prevent movement without obstructing the circulation or causing pain.

In measuring the length and breadth of the required splint there is no need to use the injured limb and possibly cause pain. Any measurement can be done on the opposite limb. It is very difficult for one person to apply a splint. Ideally three are needed: one to hold the upper part of the broken limb, one to pull very gently on the lower part, and one to apply and fix the splint. The knots of bandages, straps or tapes – preferably reef-knots – should be over the splint, not over the bone.

When the splinted patient is being moved to a stretcher or to a vehicle one person should have the sole duty of supporting the injured limb with both hands.

Much that has been said above also applies to a fractured spine or pelvis, but the danger of moving the patient is greater, so that if possible he should be left lying until a doctor arrives. As mentioned at the beginning of this note, there is likely to be a considerable degree of shock and it is important to treat it.

Frostbite. The condition is diagnosed by the affected part (usually toes, fingers, tips of ears or tip of nose) becoming very white and hard. The best treatment is to bathe the part gently with cold water, delaying the use of warm water until the part has thawed.

The old treatment of rubbing the frozen part with snow is no longer advocated. The rubbing can damage the tissues.

Poisoning. Many substances, harmless or even beneficial when taken in appropriate quantities, are poisonous when consumed in considerable excess. Aspirin tablets and iron tablets are examples. So three commonsense measures are: (1) to keep all medicines, tablets, cleansing fluids, disinfectants and so on completely out of reach of young children and to explain their dangers to older children; (2) to ensure every potentially poisonous substance in the house is clearly labelled – both to lessen the chance of anybody consuming it by mistake and to ensure that if some is swallowed the nature of the substance is immediately known; and

(3) in no circumstances to extract something from the medicine cupboard and swallow it in the dark – since two containers of similar shape can easily become interchanged in position.

On the other hand it is worth remembering that, apart from cases of deliberate suicide, death from poisoning is an extreme rarity. Apart from strong acids and strong alkalis the overwhelming majority of substances found in an ordinary house or garden are less serious in their effects than is sometimes imagined.

Where the poisonous substance is unknown. If it has been swallowed an immediate drink of milk will dilute it and so make it less harmful. If it has been inhaled fresh air will probably help and artificial respiration may be needed if the breathing shows signs of stopping. If it has got into the eyes the lids should be held well apart and the eyes bathed with a gentle stream of warm – but not hot – water. If it is on the skin, thorough washing with soap and water is likely to remove it. Clearly decision about whether to seek immediate medical aid is difficult if the poison is not known. One has to be guided largely by the condition of the patient.

Where the poisonous substance is known. It is manifestly not possible to list every possible poison in a single article, but acids, alkalis and petroleum products would be generally recognized as such, and, for these, vomiting would be positively harmful as it would bring the substance back into the throat. For any other substance deemed to be poisonous or probably poisonous, a fairly sound procedure is to give a drink of milk and then try to induce vomiting.

Poisons may be divided into five groups. The following three groups are the main ones for which vomiting is definitely harmful: (1) If the poison is a corrosive acid (e.g., sulphuric or nitric) do not on any account induce vomiting; give milk or milk of magnesia or very soft white of egg in large quantities and seek immediate medical aid. (2) If the poison is a strong alkali (including some floor strippers and oven cleaners) again do not on any account induce vomiting: give large amounts of milk or water, followed by diluted vinegar or lemon juice, and seek immediate medical help. (3) For petrol products (including lighter fluid and turpentine) again do not try to induce vomiting: give large quantities of milk, attend to the breathing and seek immediate medical aid.

In the remaining two groups an attempt to induce vomiting should be made: (4) For many moderate, non-corrosive poisons (e.g., alcohol, antifreeze, hair dyes, household antiseptics and methylated spirits) try to induce vomiting with syrup of ipecac if available or by pushing a finger to the back of the throat. After vomiting has occurred, check with hospital or doctor as to whether any further treatment is necessary. (5) For the vast majority of non-corrosive poisons (e.g., arsenic, boracic acid, camphor, carbon tetrachloride, iron tablets, marking ink, moth balls, naphthalene, most of the poisonous plants, most sleeping tablets and strychnine) try to induce vomiting and – without even awaiting its occurrence – bring the doctor to the patient or the patient to the doctor.

If the patient has to be taken to a doctor or to a hospital, it is important that the substance (if known) and the approximate amount consumed are notified to the person dealing with the patient; or, failing fuller information, the partially empty container can be taken along with the patient. The doctor is placed under a very severe handicap if he is merely told that the person has swallowed some unspecified poisonous material.

Shock. To a greater or lesser degree shock occurs in all serious injuries and in many cases of sudden, severe illness. The face becomes pale, the skin cold and clammy, the pulse weak, the breathing shallow, the eyes sunken and the pupils dilated.

Immediate treatment is to keep the patient lying down, if practicable indoors and in bed, and with the head preferably a shade lower than the feet so as to allow easy flow of blood to the brain; keep the patient comfortably warm, e.g., by placing warm – but not overwarm – water bottles at the feet, armpits and groin. If the person is lying on a bed or sofa it is fairly easy to raise the foot slightly by using bricks or other solid materials. If there is a possibility of a water-bottle being too hot a blanket can usefully be placed between the bottle and the patient's skin.

If the patient is conscious he will require reassurance and he should be encouraged to sip hot sweetened tea or coffee unless the shock is due to abdominal injury.

Occasionally in severe shock breathing becomes difficult and artificial respiration may be needed.

Wounds. Where the skin is broken there are three essentials of first aid treatment – to stop the bleeding, to cleanse the wound and to combat shock. Bleeding is discussed on page 425 and shock in the preceding paragraph. For cleansing a wound it is best to start by bathing it with warm, boiled water, then to swab with any available disinfectant in appropriate dilution (using boiled water as the diluting agent), and finally to cover the wound with any available sterile dressing or with a piece of wet linen that has been boiled.

While the stopping of serious bleeding (see page 425) is an essential first priority, the vast majority of wounds and cuts do not involve arteries or large veins. Where blood is merely oozing out or slowly trickling out the person proposing to apply first aid should, where practicable, thoroughly wash his hands before starting treatment.

If the implement that made the cut is liable to have been contaminated by garden or field soil or by street dust or stable refuse, a doctor should be consulted because the patient may require anti-tetanus serum. In other cases there is no need for a doctor unless the wound is large enough to require stitching or unless the wound becomes inflamed and throbbing, indicating that it has become infected.

Unconsciousness. Irrespective of the cause five essential measures in dealing with an unconscious patient are: (1) to stop serious bleeding if there is any (see p. 425); (2) to maintain a clear airway, involving turning the head to the side so that saliva or blood can trickle out, removing dentures and loosening clothing at neck and waist; (3) to ensure that breathing continues, using mouth-to-mouth respiration if breathing stops (see p. 433); (4) to keep the patient lying down with no unnecessary movement; and (5) to keep him warm (e.g., by covering with blankets) except in unconsciousness due to heat-stroke. A sixth general point is a negative one: no attempt should be made to give an unconscious person anything by mouth.

Beyond these points treatment varies with the cause and a competent first aid worker should attempt to make a provisional diagnosis, both because of possible additions to the immediate treatment and because of possible aid to the doctor when he arrives.

The main causes are: (1) injury: concussion, shock, bleeding, electrocution, and heat-stroke; (2) diseases of the nervous system: apoplexy (stroke), epilepsy, and hysteria; (3) poisoning: alcohol, opiates, hypnotics, other drugs and chemicals; (4) toxaemia: diabetes and uraemia; (5) lack of oxygen to the brain: fainting and heart disease; and (6) asphyxia: gas poisoning, drowning, choking and strangulation.

Information from a friend of the unconscious person may be helpful: for instance the friend may be able to state that the person is subject to epileptic fits or suffers from diabetes or from kidney disease. Information about the mode of onset is useful: in apoplexy the unconsciousness is usually sudden whereas in diabetic coma it is usually gradual. Inspection of the patient provides many clues: a head injury is often obvious; a flushed face and noisy breathing suggest apoplexy; foaming at the mouth suggests epilepsy. To smell the breath is often helpful: in uraemic coma (kidney disease) the breath smells like urine, in diabetic coma it smells like apples, and in unconsciousness due to alcohol the smell is characteristic (but if the first-aider is not the person first on the scene he should check that an odour of alcohol is not a result of a misguided attempt to help the patient by pouring whisky into his mouth). In opium or morphine poisoning the pupils are contracted, whereas in most forms of unconsciousness they are not. In heat-stroke the skin may feel hot (and the patient should not be kept warm).

In all cases of unconsciousness except a faint with recovery of consciousness within three minutes medical aid should be sought immediately.

General

The eleven occurrences so far discussed – bleeding, burns and scalds, choking, drowning, electric shock, fractures, frostbite, poisoning, shock, wounds and unconsciousness – are the emergencies most likely to be encountered; but five important matters have still to be considered – what to do if breathing stops, what to do if the heart stops, how to move the patient if movement is necessary, how to reduce some hazards, and what sort of medicine chest can reasonably be provided in an ordinary house.

Artificial respiration. If breathing stops the patient will die or suffer irreparable damage within minutes unless oxygen is pumped into his lungs until such time as natural breathing returns. Even where some breathing continues but is clearly difficult – with the face becoming blue and the veins of the neck enlarged – artificial respiration is needed.

Kiss of life. Except for drowning cases the mouth-to-mouth method is generally best as well as easiest. After separating the patient from the cause and ensuring that the airway is clear (including removing dentures and loosening tight clothing), lay the patient on his back, kneel beside his head, use one hand to press the lower jaw upwards and forwards (so that the head is tilted back thus providing a straighter airway) and the other to close his nostrils, pinching them between thumb and forefinger. Take a deep breath, place your lips firmly round the patient's mouth and breathe out into the patient's mouth. If you are doing it correctly you should see the patient's chest beginning to rise as the lungs fill. If the chest fails to rise, check that you have closed the nostrils and check that your mouth is firmly round the patient's mouth. If the chest is duly rising, remove your mouth and take another deep breath while the chest is falling. Then reapply the mouth and breathe into the patient. Aim at about ten to twelve breaths a minute, and every three minutes desist for a single breath in and out, to see whether natural breathing has been resumed. If it is not resumed, continue for half an hour before abandoning the attempt.

Schafer's method. In drowning accidents this is better because it facilitates the escape of water and mucus from the air passages. Clear the airway, place the patient on his stomach with the head turned to one side, kneel across his buttocks or on one side of his back facing the head, place your hands over the lowest ribs on the back one on each side, quite slowly throw the weight of your body on the hands (thus pressing the back of the chest downwards), then slowly raise your body to remove the pressure but leaving the hands in position, and repeat this double movement about twelve times a minute. If there is no evidence of resumption of natural breathing, continue for a full hour before abandoning hope.

After breathing has been restored, whether by mouth-to-mouth or by Schafer's method, remember to treat the patient for shock (p. 431).

Stimulation of the heart. Even if the patient is breathing his brain will be damaged unless oxygen reaches it.

The pulse is more easily felt in front of the ear than at the wrist.

If the circulation stops and the pulse cannot be felt, start by separating the patient from the cause, clearing the airway and trying half a dozen breaths of mouth-to-mouth respiration (see p. 433). In most cases this re-establishes the heart beat.

If no heart beat can be detected, begin massage of the heart. Place the patient on his back, kneel beside his chest, place the palm of one hand on the lower end of the sternum (breastbone), cover the one hand with the other, with arms straight rock forwards over the patient until your shoulders are vertically above your hands (thus pressing downwards), rock backwards releasing the pressure, and repeat the double movement about sixty times a minute for an adult. For a child less pressure is needed: place one hand on the lower part of the sternum and the other on the ground; and aim at between eighty and ninety double movements per minute. In both cases pause occasionally to see if the natural heart beat has been restored, but in the absence of restoration continue the massage for at least half an hour.

A highly skilled person can sometimes manage to combine heart stimulation and mouth-to-mouth respiration. If both breathing and circulation have stopped and if the only person available cannot manage both techniques, he is probably wiser to concentrate on respiration: as indicated above, a few breaths will often restart the heart, but a restarting of the heart will not re-establish breathing.

Moving the patient. The broad general rule is 'don't'. Needless movement may increase bleeding, may make a fracture worse and may do other damage; but clearly there are circumstances in which a patient has to be moved for his own safety.

Where removal for a few yards is necessary (e.g., from the road to the pavement) the sound procedure is to attend to serious bleeding, to clear airways, to hold any fractured limb to minimize its movement and to move the patient as gently as is possible.

In an extreme emergency (e.g., an adult overcome by smoke in a burning house) the easiest way to move a heavy person quickly is to pull his hands over your shoulders and crawl out, dragging him behind you. An alternative which leaves your hands free is to tie his wrists with a belt and loop his arms over your neck.

Reduction of hazards. Excepting the degenerative conditions of old age most diseases and injuries are in large measure preventable. Much of this entire book is devoted to prevention, and it is manifestly impossible in a single short section to deal with matters like the prevention of infections or the prevention of coronary thrombosis, even though these have their first aid aspects. All that will be attempted here is to pick out five sets of common hazards and to offer a few hints about their reduction.

Home accidents. Check the safety of gas and electrical appliances. Attend to the safety of the kitchen, the most dangerous room in the house. Keep sharp implements, matches, medicines and cleansing liquids out of reach of the toddler. Avoid placing articles where you could trip over them if you have occasion to rise during the night. Beware of polished floors and of inadequately lit stairs. Don't smoke in bed. Remember that all these points apply to your holiday cottage or temporary residence just as much as to your permanent home. See also ACCIDENTS.

Motor accidents. Check the efficiency of brakes, etc., from time to time. Concentrate when driving. Keep a reasonable distance behind the next vehicle in case it stops suddenly. Take special care at cross-roads, crossings and bends and on roads made slippery by ice or sudden rain after a drought: change down when in doubt. Make a habit of using your driving mirror and of giving your signals in plenty of time. See also ACCIDENTS.

Hiking accidents. Learn in advance about anticipated weather conditions and about your intended route. Leave information about your route and your expected time of return. Learn the rudiments of first aid. Dress sensibly and remember the importance of carrying matches, a knife and a whistle. If hill-walking always take a map, compass and emergency rations as well. Remember that weather conditions can rapidly turn fierce in mountains even in summer, so take spare clothing and waterproofs. Preferably hike with a companion, not alone. When forced to walk on the road keep to the side facing oncoming traffic.

Sunbathing hazards. In warm climates use a sunburn preventive cream; sunbathe sparingly for the first few days until you are used to the climate, trying as a start ten minutes a day if you are more than four hundred miles nearer the equator than in your home and five minutes a day if you are more than seven hundred miles nearer the equator; and until used to the climate do not sunbathe between the hours of 10.30 a.m. and 3.30 p.m. Remember that when the sun is partially obscured by light cloud the danger of sunburn is increased, not decreased.

Bathing accidents. Don't swim in an unfamiliar place and don't let your child swim in such a place without learning about currents. To swim alone is always dangerous. If you get into difficulties, try to float and don't panic. When swimming or bathing in a warm sea, beware of stings by a Portugese man-of-war or a jellyfish: if bitten, place dry sand over the part, gently scrape it off, avoid rubbing, apply methylated spirits as soon as practicable, and if badly stung seek medical aid.

Medicine chest for the family. Sudden illnesses and injuries occur in every household, and a medicine chest – containing first aid materials and household remedies – is an obvious necessity. A chest with a lock is in general undesirable, because if the key is left in position the chest can be opened by a child, and if the key is removed it tends to be momentarily lost at the very time access is urgent.

Ideally it should be a small wall cabinet, well out of reach of young children but easily opened by any adult. Such a cabinet should be used for storing any medicines currently prescribed for a member of the family, simple home remedies such as aspirin and antiseptics, dressings and other basic first aid requirements. It should not be used to store other items. Any medicine remaining at the end of a prescribed course of treatment should be removed and destroyed, as should any medicine which has been kept for a long period. The medicine chest should be kept closed except when an item is being removed or replaced.

The following articles might be regarded as a useful list of contents of the medicine chest:

adhesive plaster dressings for minor cuts and wounds; absorbent gauze dressings for minor burns; cleansing tissues; cotton wool; narrow bandages (2 cm.); wide bandages (5 cm.); safety pins; dressing scissors; soluble aspirin; junior aspirin; calamine lotion; antihistamine cream; a mild laxative; sal volatile or brandy; tincture of iodine.

Probably no two doctors would agree on the exact contents of a medicine chest and much depends on available space, but the above is a reasonable list.